Essentials of Practice Management in Dermatology and Plastic Surgery

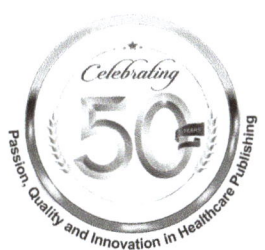

Essentials of Practice Management in Dermatology and Plastic Surgery

Editor-in-Chief

Venkataram Mysore
MD DNB DipRCPath (Lond) FRCP (Glasgow) FISHRS
Director
Consultant Dermatologist
Hair Transplant Surgeon—Dermatopathologist
Venkat Center for Skin and Plastic Surgery
Bengaluru, Karnataka, India

Editors

Manish Gautam
MBBS DVD DNB (Dermatology)
Chief Dermatologist
Skin Solutions—Skin, Hair and Laser Centre
Navi Mumbai, Maharashtra, India

BS Chandrashekar
MBBS MD DNB
Chief Dermatologist
Medical Director and Founder
CUTIS Academy of Cutaneous Sciences
Bengaluru, Karnataka, India

Sanjay Parashar
MBBS MS DNB (Plastic) MCh (Plastic Surgery) FICS
Consultant Plastic and Aesthetic Surgeon
Craniofacial Fellow
Royal Australasian College of Surgeons
Chairman Scientific, Emirates Plastic Surgery Society
Chairman, Cocoona Centre for Aesthetic Transformation (UAE and India)

Associate Editor

Aniketh Venkataram
MBBS MS MCh (Plastic Surgery) FDAFPRAS (Belgium) FASAPS (USA)
Consultant Plastic Surgeon
Venkat Center for Skin and Plastic Surgery
Bengaluru, Karnataka, India

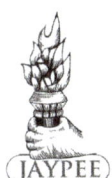

JAYPEE BROTHERS MEDICAL PUBLISHERS
The Health Sciences Publisher
New Delhi | London

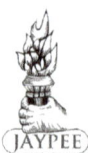 **Jaypee Brothers Medical Publishers (P) Ltd.**

Headquarters
Jaypee Brothers Medical Publishers (P) Ltd
4838/24, Ansari Road, Daryaganj
New Delhi 110 002, India
Phone: +91-11-43574357
Fax: +91-11-43574314
Email: jaypee@jaypeebrothers.com

Overseas Office
J.P. Medical Ltd
83 Victoria Street, London
SW1H 0HW (UK)
Phone: +44 20 3170 8910
Fax: +44 (0)20 3008 6180
Email: info@jpmedpub.com

Website: www.jaypeebrothers.com
Website: www.jaypeedigital.com

© 2021, Jaypee Brothers Medical Publishers

The views and opinions expressed in this book are solely those of the original contributor(s)/author(s) and do not necessarily represent those of editor(s) of the book.

All rights reserved. No part of this publication may be reproduced, stored or transmitted in any form or by any means, electronic, mechanical, photocopying, recording or otherwise, without the prior permission in writing of the publishers.

All brand names and product names used in this book are trade names, service marks, trademarks or registered trademarks of their respective owners. The publisher is not associated with any product or vendor mentioned in this book.

Medical knowledge and practice change constantly. This book is designed to provide accurate, authoritative information about the subject matter in question. However, readers are advised to check the most current information available on procedures included and check information from the manufacturer of each product to be administered, to verify the recommended dose, formula, method and duration of administration, adverse effects and contraindications. It is the responsibility of the practitioner to take all appropriate safety precautions. Neither the publisher nor the author(s)/editor(s) assume any liability for any injury and/or damage to persons or property arising from or related to use of material in this book.

This book is sold on the understanding that the publisher is not engaged in providing professional medical services. If such advice or services are required, the services of a competent medical professional should be sought.

Every effort has been made where necessary to contact holders of copyright to obtain permission to reproduce copyright material. If any have been inadvertently overlooked, the publisher will be pleased to make the necessary arrangements at the first opportunity. The **CD/DVD-ROM** (if any) provided in the sealed envelope with this book is complimentary and free of cost. **Not meant for sale.**

Inquiries for bulk sales may be solicited at: jaypee@jaypeebrothers.com

Essentials of Practice Management in Dermatology and Plastic Surgery

First Edition: 2021

ISBN: 978-93-89776-02-7

Contributors

Aditi Jaiswal MBBS
Resident
Department of Dermatology
DY Patil University School of Medicine
Navi Mumbai, Maharashtra, India

Aditya N Patil MS MRCS MCh (Plast) DNB (Plast)
Consultant
Department of Plastic and Reconstructive Surgery
HCG Hospital
Bengaluru, Karnataka, India

Amit Gupta MS DNB (Plastic Surgery)
Plastic Surgeon
Founder and Director
Divine Cosmetic Surgery
New Delhi, India

Amiti Shah DNB (Plastic Surgery)
Consultant Plastic and Cosmetic Surgeon
Shah Superspecialty Clinic
Mumbai, Maharashtra, India

Aniketh Venkataram
MBBS MS MCh (Plastic Surgery) FDAFPRAS (Belgium) FASPAS (USA)
Consultant Plastic Surgeon
Venkat Center for Skin and Plastic Surgery
Bengaluru, Karnataka, India

Anil Dashore MBBS DVD
Director
Dashore's DHL Center
Indore, Madhya Pradesh, India

Anil Ganjoo MBBS MD
Consultant Dermatologist and Director
Skinnovation Clinics
New Delhi, India

Anil Kumar Garg MS MCh ABHRS Fellow ISHRS
Plastic Surgeon and Director
Rejuvenate Hair Transplant Center
Indore, Madhya Pradesh, India

Ankur Talwar MD (Dermatology)
Consultant Dermatologist
Talwar Skin Center
Lucknow, Uttar Pradesh
Associate Professor
Department of Dermatology
Hind Institute of Medical Sciences
Lucknow, Uttar Pradesh, India

Anuradha Jindal
MBBS (Gold Medalist) MD FRGUHS (Dermatology)
Fellowship Trainee
Venkat Center for Skin and Plastic Surgery
Bengaluru, Karnataka, India

Apratim Goel MD DNB FAGE
Managing Director
CUTIS Skin Solution
Mumbai, Maharashtra, India

Aseem Sharma MD
Assistant Professor
Department of Dermatology
LTMMC & LTMGH
Sion, Mumbai, Maharashtra, India

Ashish Davalbhakta
MBBS MS MCh (Plastic) FRCS (Glasg)
Professor
Department of Esthetic Plastic Surgery
An MUHS Accredited Esthetic Surgery
Fellowship Centre
Aesthetics Medispa
Pune, Maharashtra, India

Ashwini L Hirevenkangoudar MBBS MD (DVL)
Fellowship Trainee
Venkat Center for Skin and Plastic Surgery
Bengaluru, Karnataka, India

Atulkumar K Shah LLM (Gold Medal)
MCh (Plastic and Reconstructive Surgery) MPhil
(Cosmetology) MPhil (Health and Hospital Systems
Management) PG Diploma (Medical Law and Ethics)
Consultant
Cosmetic, Plastic, Reconstructive and
Burns Surgery
Vadodara, Gujarat, India

Avitus John Raakesh Prasad DDVL
Managing Director
SP Derma Center
Madurai, Tamil Nadu, India

Bhanu Prakash MD DHM PGDMLE
Professor
Department of Dermatology
Vydehi Institute of Medical Sciences
Bengaluru, Karnataka, India

BS Chandrashekar MBBS MD DNB
Chief Dermatologist
Medical Director and Founder
CUTIS Academy of Cutaneous Sciences
Bengaluru, Karnataka, India

CP Thajudheen MD
Dermatologist
Dr Thaj Laser Skin and Hair Clinic
Thalassery, Kerala, India

Deepak Vedamurthy MBBS MD FHM
Associate
Division of Hospital Medicine
Christiana Care Health System
Newark, Delaware, USA

Dinesh Kumar D
MBBS MD FIAMS MRCPS (Glasgow)
Consultant Dermatologist
Dr Dinesh's Skin and Hair Clinic
Chennai, Tamil Nadu, India

Dipak Kulkarni MD (Skin and VD)
Chief Dermatologist and Proprietor
Alok Clinic
Center for Dermatology
Panvel, Maharashtra, India

Ganesh S Pai MD
Senior Consultant Dermatologist
Derma-Care
Skin and Cosmetology Center
Mangaluru, Karnataka, India

Harsha Siddappa
MD DVL FRGUHS (Dermatosurgery)
Junior Consultant
Department of Dermatology
CUTIS Academy of Cutaneous Sciences
Bengaluru, Karnataka, India

Jaishree Sharad MBBS DVD FAAD
Cosmetic Dermatologist
Department of Dermatology
Medical Director
Skinfiniti Aesthetic and Laser Clinic
Mumbai, Maharashtra, India

James Roy Kanjoor MS MCh FRCS
Consultant Cosmetic Surgeon
Department of Cosmetic Surgery
Roy's Cosmetic Surgery Center
Coimbatore, Tamil Nadu, India

Jyothi Kannangath MD
Dermatologist
Dr Thaj Laser Skin and Hair Clinic
Coimbatore, Tamil Nadu, India

Contributors vii

Jyotsna Vinayak Deo MD (Skin) DDV DNB
Consultant Dermatologist
CUTIS Skin and Laser Center
Navi Mumbai, Maharashtra, India

K Feroz MBBS DDVL PG Dip (Med Cosmetol)
Consultant Dermatologist
Dr Feroz's Skin Care Clinic
Kannur, Kerala, India

Kapil S Agrawal MS MCh (Plastic Surgery)
Professor (Addl.) Plastic Surgery
Department of Plastic Surgery
Seth Gordhandas Sunderdas Medical
College (GSMC) and
The King Edward Memorial (KEM) Hospital
Mumbai, Maharashtra, India

Karishma Kagodu
MS MCh (Plastic Surgery) FDAFPRS (Italy)
Managing Director
Dr Karishma Aesthetics Clinic
Bengaluru, Karnataka, India

Karthik Ram DNB (Plastic Surgery)
Chief Cosmetic Surgeon
Chennai Plastic Surgery
Chennai, Tamil Nadu, India

KHS Rao
MD PGDMLE PGDHHM Dip STD/AIDS (Bangkok)
Principal Consultant
Department of Dermatology
Central Health Service
Bengaluru, Karnataka, India

Kiran Godse MD PhD FRCP (Glasgow)
Professor
Department of Dermatology
DY Patil University School of Medicine
Navi Mumbai, Maharashtra, India

Koushik Lahiri
MBBS DVD (CAL) FAAD FFAADV FRCP (Glasgow) FRCP
(Edin) FRCP (London)
Professor and Senior Consultant
Department of Dermatology
Apollo Gleneagles Hospital
Kolkata, West Bengal, India

Krupa Shankar DS MD DVD FRCP
Consultant Dermatologist
Department of Dermatology
Mallige Hospital
Bengaluru, Karnataka, India

Kshama Talwar MD (Dermatology)
Consultant Dermatologist
Talwar Skin Center
Lucknow, Uttar Pradesh
Assistant Professor
Department of Dermatology
Hind Institute of Medical Sciences
Lucknow, Uttar Pradesh, India

Lakshyajit D Dhami MS MCh (Plastic Surgery)
Cosmetic, Laser and Plastic Surgeon
Vasudhan Cosmetic and Laser Surgery
Mumbai, Maharashtra, India

Lokesh Kumar MS MCh FICS
Director and Head
Department of Plastic and Cosmetic Surgery
BLK Superspecialty Hospital
New Delhi, India

Lawrence M Field
Inaugural International Traveling Chair of
Dermatologic Surgery (International Society
for Dermatologic Surgery), University of
California, San Francisco (Dermatologic
Surgery) (Emeritus 2006), and Stanford
University Medical Center, Stanford, California
(Emeritus 2006), USA

Madhulika Mhatre MD FRGUHS
Consultant Dermatologist
Wockhardt Hospital
Mumbai, Maharashtra, India

Madhuri Agarwal MD (Skin and VD) DDV
Founder and Medical Director
Department of Dermatology
Yavana Aesthetics Clinic
Mumbai, Maharashtra, India

Madura C MBBS MD DVL FRGUHS (Dermatosurgery)
Consultant Dermatologist
Dermatosurgeon and Hair Transplant Surgeon
Department of Dermatology
CUTIS Academy of Cutaneous Sciences
Bengaluru, Karnataka, India

Malcom Noronha MBBS MD FRGUHS (Dermatology)
Fellowship Trainee
Venkat Center for Skin and Plastic Surgery
Bengaluru, Karnataka, India

Manjot Marwah MD (Dermatology)
Consultant Dermatologist
Dr Manjot's Clinic
Jalandhar, Punjab, India

Manjunath R MD (Skin and VD) PGDMLE (NLSIU)
Consultant Dermatologist
Spoorthi Skin and Hair Care Clinic
Kollegal, Karnataka, India

Manoj Khanna MBBS MS MCh DNB FICS
Consultant Cosmetic and Plastic Surgeon
CMD, Enhance Clinics, India
National Secretary of India of ISAPS-2005 to 2023
Ex-President IAAPS 2016
Ex-President AHRS-I 2012

Maya Vedamurthy MD MAMS FRCP (Edin)
Consultant Dermatologist
RSV Skin and Laser Research Center
Apollo Hospitals
Chennai, Tamil Nadu, India

Medha Bhave MS DNB MCh DNB (Plastic Surgery)
Consultant Plastic Surgeon
Department of Plastic and Cosmetic Surgery
Lasercosmesis
Thane, Maharashtra, India

Milan Doshi
MS MCh (Plastic and Reconstructive Surgery)
Medical Director
Allure MedSpa
Vardan Hospital
Mumbai, Maharashtra, India

Milind S Wagh
MS (Gen Surg) MCh (Plastic Surgery)
Consultant Plastic and Cosmetic Surgeon
Make A Change
A Center for Cosmetic Surgery
Mumbai, Maharashtra, India

Namitha Chathra MD FRGUHS
Assistant Professor
Department of Dermatology
BR Ambedkar Medical College
Bengaluru, Karnataka, India

Nayeem Sadath Haneef MBBS MD
Professor and Head
Department of DVL
Deccan College of Medical Sciences
Hyderabad, Telangana, India

Neeta Patel MS MCh
Consultant Plastic and Reconstructive Surgeon
Founder Member
ISPRES
Past President
Indian Association of Aesthetic Plastic Surgery

Neha Chauhan
MS (General Surgery) MCh (Plastic Surgery)
Consultant Plastic Surgeon
Chinmaya Mission Hospital
Bengaluru, Karnataka, India

Omprakash HM MBBS DVD
Consulting Dermatologist
Department of Dermatology
Samastha Skin Clinic
Mysuru, Karnataka, India

P Prasanna MD
Senior Consultant Dermatologist
Samprithi Skin Clinic
Mysuru, Karnataka, India

Prashant Palwade MBBS MD (Skin)
Consultant Dermatologist
Satej Skin Hair Laser Center
Aurangabad, Maharashtra, India

Praveen Kumar SP BPT MHA
Chief Operating Officer (COO)
CUTIS Academy of Cutaneous Sciences
Bengaluru, Karnataka, India

Preethi B Nayak
MBBS MD DNB FRGUHS (Dermatosurgery)
Junior Consultant Dermatologist
CUTIS Academy of Cutaneous Sciences
Bengaluru, Karnataka, India

Priyanka Agarwal MD
Consultant Dermatologist
Department of Dermatology
Gurugram, Haryana, India

Putta Srinivas
MD (Dermatology) DD (Diploma in Dermatology)
Director
Government Medical College
Mahabubnagar, Telangana, India

Rabinder Kant Sikri BTech MBA
Principal Consultant and CEO
Energy and Energy Consultants
New Delhi, India

Rajat Gupta MBBS MS DNB DNB (Plastic Surgery)
Consultant Plastic and Cosmetic Surgeon
Director
Skinnovation Clinics and Excel Medical Centers
New Delhi, India

Rajat Kandhari MBBS MD Msc
Consultant Dermatologist
Dr Kandhari's Skin and Dental Clinic
New Delhi, India

Rajesh Buddhadev MD (Dermatology)
Chief Dermatologist
Nu Skin World
Surat, Gujarat, India

Rakesh Bharti MD
Consultant
Bharti Derma Care and Research Center
Amritsar, Punjab, India

Rakesh Kalra MBBS MS MCh
Consultant Esthetic and Plastic Surgeon
Ashirwad Hospital
Dehradun, Uttarakhand, India

Rasya Dixit MD (Dermatology)
Medical Director
Dr Dixit Cosmetic Dermatology Clinic
Bengaluru, Karnataka, India

Ravi Hiremagalore
MD Fellowship Pediatric Dermatology
Consultant
Dermatology and Pediatrics
Manipal Hospital, Center for Human Genetics
Bengaluru, Karnataka, India

RG Torsekar MD FCPS DDV
Founder Member and Medical Director
Disha Skin and Laser Institute, Thane
Consulting Dermatologist
Fortis Hospital, Mulund, Mumbai
Thane, Maharashtra, India

Rohit Batra MD
Consultant Dermatologist
Department of Dermatology
Sir Ganga Ram Hospital
New Delhi, India

Sajin Alexander MBBS MD (DVL)
Fellowship Trainee
Department of Dermatology
Venkat Center for Skin and Plastic Surgery
Bengaluru, Karnataka, India

Saloni Katoch MD
Consultant Dermatologist
Department of Dermatology
Dr KN Barua Institute of Dermatological Sciences
Guwahati, Assam, India

Sandeep Sattur MCh (Plastic Surgery)
Founder Member and Past President
AHRS, India
Member, ISHRS
Member, Hair Research Society of India
Consultant Hair Restorative Surgeon
Hairrevive—Center for Hair Restoration Mumbai
Wockhardt Hospital
Mumbai, Maharashtra, India

Sanjay Labh
Chartered Accountant
Ghaziabad, Delhi NCR, India

Sanjay Parashar
MBBS MS DNB (Plastic) MCh (Plas) FICS
Consultant Plastic and Aesthetic Surgeon
Craniofacial Fellow
Royal Australasian College of Surgeons
Chairman Scientific, Emirates Plastic Surgery Society
Chairman, Cocoona Centre for Aesthetic Transformation (UAE and India)

Sanjeev Aurangabadkar MD (Dermatology)
Consultant
Skin and Laser Clinic
Hyderabad, Telangana, India

Satish Bhat
MS DNB (Surg) MCh DNB (Plastic Surgery)
MRCS (Edin, UK)
Consultant Plastic and Cosmetic Surgeon
Linea Cosmetic Clinic
Mangaluru, Karnataka, India

Savitha AS MBBS MD (DVL) DNB FRGUHS
Associate Professor
Department of Dermatology
Sapthagiri Institute of Medical Sciences and Research Center
Bengaluru, Karnataka, India

Seema Garg MBBS MSc ABHRS
(Diplomate of the American Board of Hair Restoration Surgery)
Hair Transplant Surgeon
Member, ISHRS, AHRS, India
Rejuvenate Hair Transplant Center
Indore, Madhya Pradesh, India

Shashi Kumar BM MBBS MD (DVL) FIADVL
Associate Professor
Department of Dermatology
Mandya Institute of Medical Sciences
Mandya, Karnataka, India

Shehnaz Z Arsiwala MD DDV
Founder and Director
Renewderm Center
Consultant Dermatologist
Saifee Hospital
Rince Aly Khan Hospital
Mumbai, Maharashtra, India

Shuken Dashore MBBS MD DNB
Director
Dashore's DHL Centre
Indore, Madhya Pradesh, India

Sonali Langar
MD Postgraduate Diploma (Aesthetics American Academy of Aesthetic Medicine)
Consultant Dermatologist
Department of Dermatology
Apollo Hospital, Skin Remedies Clinic and Laser Center
Noida, Uttar Pradesh, India

Subodh P Sirur
MBBS DVD DNB (Dermatology) LL.M; FIII
Consulting Dermatologist
Specializing in Medical Law
Wockhardt Hospital, Mumbai
Apollo Spectra
Mumbai, Maharashtra, India

Contributors

Sumit Gupta MBBS MD (Dermatology)
Consultant Dermatologist
Department of Dermatology
Skinnovation Clinics
GNH Excel Medical Center
Sir Ganga Ram Hospital
Northern Central Railway Hospital
New Delhi, India

Surajit Gorai
MBBS (Hons) MD (Gold Medal) DNB MNAMS (Dermatology)
Consultant Dermatologist
Department of Dermatology
Apollo Gleneagles Hospital
Kolkata, West Bengal, India

Suresh Talwar MD (Dermatology)
Consultant Dermatologist
Talwar Skin Center
Lucknow, Uttar Pradesh, India

Sushil Tahiliani MD DV&D
Consultant Dermatologist, Mumbai
Honorary Dermatologist
Department of Dermatology
Hinduja Hospital and Research Center
Mumbai, Maharashtra, India

Tanay Tulsaney MBA
Co-Founder, CEO and Director
DigiLantern
New Delhi, India

Tejaswani Diwakar
MBBS MS DNB DNB (Plastic Surgery)
Consultant Plastic Surgeon
Max Hospital
Saket, New Delhi, India

Trupti Agarwal MBBS MD
Senior Consultant
Department of Dermatology
Cloudnine Hospital
Mumbai, Maharashtra, India

Umashankar Nagaraju MD
Consultant Dermatologist and Honorary
Secretary General
Department of Dermatology
Indian Association of Dermatologists,
Venereologists and Leprologist (IADVL)
Rajarajeswari Medical College and Hospital
Bengaluru, Karnataka, India

Vani Yepuri MBBS DDVL FRGUHS
Consultant Dermatologist
Venkat Center for Skin and Plastic Surgery
Bengaluru, Karnataka, India

Venkataram Mysore
MD DNB DipRCPath (Lond) FRCP (Glasgow) FISHRS
Director
Consultant Dermatologist
Hair Transplant Surgeon—
Dermatopathologist
Venkat Center for Skin and Plastic Surgery
Bengaluru, Karnataka, India

Viral Desai MCh DNB MS
Cosmetic and Plastic Surgeon
Hair Transplant Surgeon
Co-Founder and CMD-CPLSS
Sarla Hospital, DHPL, DHV, DHI India
Mumbai, Maharashtra, India

Vishalakshi Viswanath MD DNB DDV
Founder Member and Medical Director
Disha Skin and Laser Institute, Thane
Professor and Head
Department of Dermatology
RGMC & CSMH
Thane, Maharashtra, India

Zeba Chhapra MBBS DDVL
Dermatologist
CUTIS Skin Solution
Mumbai, Maharashtra, India

Assistant Editors

Anuradha Jindal
MBBS (Gold Medalist) MD FRGUHS (Dermatology)
Fellowship Trainee
Venkat Center for Skin and Plastic Surgery
Bengaluru, Karnataka, India

Ashwini L Hirevenkangoudar MBBS MD (DVL)
Fellowship Trainee
Venkat Center for Skin and Plastic Surgery
Bengaluru, Karnataka, India

Deepthi Malayanur MD FRGUHS
Consultant Dermatologist
Venkat Center for Skin and Plastic Surgery
Bengaluru, Karnataka, India

Harsh Tahiliani MD
Consultant Dermatologist
Tahiliani's Clinic
Mumbai, Maharashtra, India

Madhulika Mhatre MD FRGUHS
Consultant Dermatologist
Wockhardt Hospital
Mumbai, Maharashtra, India

Malcom Noronha MBBS MD FRGUHS (Dermatology)
Fellowship Trainee
Venkat Center for Skin and Plastic Surgery
Bengaluru, Karnataka, India

Namitha Chathra MD FRGUHS
Assistant Professor
Department of Dermatology
BR Ambedkar Medical College
Bengaluru, Karnataka, India

Nitya Malladi MD DNB MNAMS
Assistant Professor
Department of Dermatology
HBTMC and RN Cooper Hospital
Mumbai, Maharashtra, India

Priyadarshini P Gaddagimath
MBBS DDVL FRGUHS
Consultant Dermatologist and Pediatric Dermatologist
Venkat Center for Skin and Plastic Surgery
Bengaluru, Karnataka, India

Rasya Dixit MD (Dermatology)
Medical Director
Dr Dixit Cosmetic Dermatology Clinic
Bengaluru, Karnataka, India

Sajin Alexander MBBS MD (DVL)
Fellowship Trainee
Department of Dermatology
Venkat Center for Skin and Plastic Surgery
Bengaluru, Karnataka, India

Vani Yepuri MBBS DDVL FRGUHS
Consultant Dermatologist
Venkat Center for Skin and Plastic Surgery
Bengaluru, Karnataka, India

Preface

A book about practice management for doctors (dermatologists and plastic surgeons) would have appeared strange and irrelevant until a few years ago. Earlier doctors would have just started their practice, often in their garage and gradually learnt the art, on the job through trial and error, acquired patients by word-of-mouth, but success took its own time, some times up to five decades. Saying used to be that doctors took time to settle which they did by gradually working their way up from cycle to scooter to car to a house. Life and practice were simple, many hard years spent in gaining knowledge of the science of medicine in a medical college was the only investment needed. A few tips from friends and well-meaning seniors was the only guidance to start off medical practice.

Alas, the milieu is not the same anymore! The changing trends over the last decade have ensured that medical practice is a far more complex art and involves mastering myriad skills. Possession of excellent soft skills, utilization of web and social media for advertisement, maintaining electronic medical records, managing human resources, investments and loans, operating devices and machines, well structured clinic with pleasing interiors, awareness about local acts and laws such as clinic regulations and pollution control, taxes including GST, insurance, medicolegal law and Consumer Protection Act are necessary tools. Advent of cosmetic dermatology and cosmetic surgery have transformed a patient into a client. Practice does not just cater to diseases but to desires and demands as well.

And as the young doctor sets in to this bewilderingly complex world of medical practice, he is expected not just to handle complex medical cases and problems, but these weighty practice management issues as well. The problem is rendered even more difficult as the rigorous medical education engages and engulfs the student totally but leaves him entirely ill-prepared and ill-equipped to handle these pragmatic issues. This lack of preparation can be a huge hindrance and deficiency, especially in these days of deteriorating doctor-patient relationship and declining trust in the medical profession prevalent in the society.

Our book seeks to fill this void and hopes to prepare doctors in dermatology and plastic surgery for the life ahead—be it a budding doctor starting the practice, a doctor seeking to expand his/her practice into multiple clinics or start a larger center, in small towns or large cities. The book is covered in two separate sections—Dermatology and Plastic Surgery. All aspects listed above are covered extensively by experienced practitioners with expertise in the specific area. There is a separate section on "How I did it" by senior doctors who recount and reminiscence about the journey of their career. The chapters are written in an easy readable style with personal anecdotes and tips. Where needed, contribution of non-medical experts such as chartered accountants have been included. Since there can be many approaches in practice, there is some overlap in different chapters—this is deliberately left unedited. We hope that readers will choose the approach that suits them. While this book is primarily meant for these two specialists, most chapters are relevant to all specialities and hence all doctors across all specialities will find it useful.

The book is and has been a unique experiment, an experience enjoyed by the editors who have learnt and unlearnt along the way. Medical practice is changing and evolving and will continue to do so. Our ability to adapt to this evolving situation determines the success of our profession.

"The only way that we can live, is if we grow. The only way that we can grow is if we change. The only way that we can change is if we learn. The only way we can learn is if we are exposed. And the only way that we can become exposed is if we throw ourselves out into the open. Do it. Throw yourself."

—C JoyBell C

The Editor-in-Chief wishes to extend special thanks to the editors, Drs Manish Gautam, BS Chandrashekar, Sanjay Parashar and all the authors. In particular, special thanks to our corresponding editor Dr Manish Gautam and Dr Aniketh Venkataram, our energetic associate editor for plastic surgery who put in long hours of toil, without which this book would not have been completed. Our thanks to the entire publishing team at Jaypee publications for their diligent work.

Venkataram Mysore

Acknowledgments

I would like to thank the authors of all the chapters, who have taken the time and effort off from their busy work and family. I am grateful to Shri Jitendar P Vij (Group Chairman), Mr Ankit Vij (Managing Director), and Ms Chetna Malhotra Vohra (Associate Director-Content Strategy) of M/s Jaypee Brothers Medical Publishers (P) Ltd, New Delhi, India, for bringing out this edition.

Contents

PART 1: DERMATOLOGY

Section 1: Dermatology

1.1 **Introduction to Dermatology Practice** — 3
Venkataram Mysore, Namitha Chathra

1.2 **The Road Ahead After Residency!** — 6
Madhulika Mhatre, Aseem Sharma, Trupti Agarwal

1.3 **Choosing your Subspecialty** — 16
Madura C, Harsha Siddappa

Section 2: Setting-up a Clinic

2.1 **Understanding Needs and Demands in Practice** — 21
Sumit Gupta

2.2 **How to Choose the Location for Your Clinic?** — 26
Rasya Dixit

2.3 **Architecture of a Basic Skin Clinic** — 28
Dinesh Kumar D, Namitha Chathra

2.4 **Designing an Esthetic Clinic** — 33
Madhuri Agarwal

2.5 **Ideal Practice (Clinic) Management Software** — 38
Prashant Palwade

2.6 **Accreditation** — 43
Venkataram Mysore, Bhanu Prakash

2.7 **Biomedical Waste Management** — 48
Bhanu Prakash, Malcom Noronha, Venkataram Mysore

Section 3: Spreading your Wings

3.1 **Group Practice** — 55
RG Torsekar, Vishalakshi Viswanath

3.2 **Involving Other Dermatologists in Building Your Team** — 59
Dipak Kulkarni

3.3	Managing 120 Plus OPD with Cosmetic Practice *Anil Dashore, Shuken Dashore*	64
3.4	All in the Family: Practicing Dermatology with Family Members *Ankur Talwar, Suresh Talwar, Kshama Talwar*	68
3.5	Lasers to Invest in Practice: Which, When, and How *Sanjeev Aurangabadkar*	74
3.6	Expansion Dilemma: Partnership Firm, Limited Liability Partnership or Private Limited? *Dipak Kulkarni*	79
3.7	Building Bridges: Interspecialty Interaction in Practice *Sushil Tahiliani*	83
3.8	Role of Doctors as Assistants, Fellowship Training and Academic Work in Dermatological Practice *Venkataram Mysore*	86
3.9	Interaction with Industry *BS Chandrashekar*	88

Section 4: Hiring and Managing Staff

4.1	Staffing Needs of a Dermatology Center *BS Chandrashekar, Praveen Kumar SP*	94
4.2	Role of Counselors and Technicians *Venkataram Mysore, Vani Yepuri*	99
4.3	Time Management *Venkataram Mysore, Anuradha Jindal*	104

Section 5: Finance and Planning

5.1	Investments for a Medical Practitioner (Esthetic Dermatologist) *Ganesh S Pai*	109
5.2	Professional Indemnity for Dermatologist *Omprakash HM, P Prasanna*	112
5.3	Tax Planning for Dermatologists *Shashi Kumar BM, Sanjay Labh, Savitha AS*	117
5.4	Creating a Business Plan in Practice *Krupa Shankar DS*	122

Section 6: Marketing: Ethics and Means

6.1	Ethical Marketing: Best within Limits *Rohit Batra*	127

6.2	**Traditional Marketing in Practice** *Rajat Kandhari, Tanay Tulsaney*	130
6.3	**Digital Marketing: Website as a Marketing Tool** *K Feroz*	138

Section 7: Medicolegal Aspects in Practice

7.1	**Informed Consent** *KHS Rao*	143
7.2	**An Overview of Laws and Acts Applicable to Medical Professionals in India** *Manjunath R*	147
7.3	**Malpractice and Related Issues** *Subodh P Sirur*	158
7.4	**Quackery** *Putta Srinivas, Rajesh Buddhadev*	161
7.5	**Medicolegal Cases in Dermatology** *Venkataram Mysore, Saloni Katoch*	173
7.6	**Esthetic Procedures: Whose Domain it is?** *Putta Srinivas*	182
7.7	**Safe Medical Practice** *Venkataram Mysore, Ashwini L Hirevenkangoudar*	185
7.8	**Code of Medical Ethics** *Putta Srinivas, Nayeem Sadath Haneef*	188
7.9	**Out-of-Court Settlement: Why, When, and How** *Venkataram Mysore, Subodh P Sirur, Satish Bhat, KHS Rao*	202
7.10	**Healthcare Professionals and Consumer Protection Act, 2019** *Atulkumar K Shah*	208

Section 8: Doctor–Patient Interface

8.1	**Hand-holding (Mentoring) in Healthcare Practice** *Rakesh Bharti, Rabinder Kant Sikri*	213
8.2	**Handling Celebrity Patients** *Jaishree Sharad*	218
8.3	**Managing an Angry/Difficult Patient** *Apratim Goel, Zeba Chhapra*	219

8.4	**Handling Negative Reviews Online and Offline** *Anil Ganjoo*	225
8.5	**Means to Retain Esthetic Patients in Practice** *Jyotsna Vinayak Deo*	229
8.6	**Ensuring an Unforgettable Esthetic Experience for a Patient** *Sonali Langar*	232
8.7	**Empathy and Ethos of Clinical Practice** *Koushik Lahiri, Surajit Gorai*	238

Section 9: Managing Special Clinics

9.1	**Setting Up and Managing Esthetic Dermatology Clinic** *Shehnaz Z Arsiwala*	247
9.2	**Trichology Practice** *BS Chandrashekar, Preethi B Nayak*	252
9.3	**Setting Up and Managing Allergy Clinic** *Kiran Godse, Aditi Jaiswal*	258
9.4	**Setting Up and Managing Laser Clinic** *Avitus John Raakesh Prasad*	260
9.5	**Setting Up and Managing a Pediatric Dermatology Clinic** *Ravi Hiremagalore*	266
9.6	**Establishing Hair Restoration Surgery Practice** *Venkataram Mysore, Sajin Alexander*	269

Section 10: How I did it?

10.1	**Journey from Lotions to Lasers** *Ganesh S Pai*	273
10.2	**Single Clinic to Multiple Clinics** *CP Thajuddin, Jyothi Kannangath*	275
10.3	**Dermatology to Dermatopathology to Hair Transplantation, the Journey** *Venkataram Mysore*	280
10.4	**Small Town, Big Success: How I did it?** *Manjot Marwah*	282
10.5	**How I did: Establish a Large Dermatology Center** *BS Chandrashekar*	286

10.6	**Adopting/Incorporating New Techniques in Practice** *Maya Vedamurthy, Deepak Vedamurthy*	291
10.7	**Managing Association Work with Practice: Striking a Balance** *Umashankar Nagaraju, Priyanka Agarwal*	295

Epilogue

	(Great) Grandfatherly Advice for Young(er) Dermatologists and Dermatologic Surgeons *Lawrence M Field*	298

PART 2: PLASTIC SURGERY

Section 11: Starting Off

11.1	**An Introduction to Plastic Surgery Practice** *Sanjay Parashar, Aniketh Venkataram*	303
11.2	**Acquiring Skills and Mastering the Art of Plastic Surgery** *Karishma Kagodu*	304
11.3	**Golden Rule of Success: Mastering Personality Development** *Sanjay Parashar*	308
11.4	**Setting-up Documentations in your Practice** *Milind S Wagh*	312
11.5	**Patient versus Client** *Lokesh Kumar*	326
11.6	**Three Pillars to Success: Quality, Service and Safety** *Medha Bhave, Amiti Shah, Neha Chauhan*	328
11.7	**Setting-up a Day Care Esthetic Surgery Clinic** *Rajat Gupta, Tejaswani Diwakar*	337
11.8	**Setting-up Inpatient Clinic with Operation Theater** *Lakshyajit D Dhami*	343

Section 12: Marketing

12.1	**Developing your Brand** *Karthik Ram*	347
12.2	**Websites and Search Engine Optimization** *Aniketh Venkataram*	350
12.3	**Traditional Marketing (Offline)** *Sandeep Sattur*	353

12.4	Online and Social Media Marketing Amit Gupta	361
12.5	In the Box Thinking, Salesmanship Sanjay Parashar	367

Section 13: Growth

13.1	Setting-up Goals James Roy Kanjoor	372
13.2	Expanding your Practice Manoj Khanna	375
13.3	Facial Esthetic Plastic Surgery: A Business Perspective Ashish Davalbhakta	378
13.4	Building a Rhinoplasty Practice Kapil S Agrawal	383
13.5	Body Contouring Practice Milan Doshi, Aditya N Patil	386
13.6	Building a Breast Surgery Practice: "Reconstructing" the Doctor-Patient Relationship Neeta Patel	393

Section 14: Essentials

14.1	Financial Management Viral Desai	398
14.2	Legal Issues in Clinical Practice Satish Bhat	407
14.3	Practice Management in Skin and Plastic Surgery: Challenges and Roadblocks Commonly Faced—How to Overcome them? Rakesh Kalra	419
14.4	Incorporating Research into your Practice Anil Kumar Garg, Seema Garg	422

Index   *427*

Part 1
Dermatology

- Section 1 Dermatology
- Section 2 Setting-up a Clinic
- Section 3 Spreading your Wings
- Section 4 Hiring and Managing Staff
- Section 5 Finance and Planning
- Section 6 Marketing: Ethics and Means
- Section 7 Medicolegal Aspects in Practice
- Section 8 Doctor-Patient Interface
- Section 9 Managing Special Clinics
- Section 10 How I did It?

SECTION 1

Dermatology

1.1 Introduction to Dermatology Practice

Venkataram Mysore, Namitha Chathra

RISE OF DERMATOLOGY IN INDIA

The roots of dermatology, as we know, in India can be traced back to 1876 when Dr Henry Vandyke Carter, appointed by the British Government to assess skin diseases in the country, published his epidemiological study. The first chair of dermatology was established at Grant Medical College, Bombay, India, in 1895 as a result of the pioneering efforts of Major C Fernandes. For most of the 20th century, the field witnessed a steady growth with assimilation of dermatology, venereology, and leprosy.[1] Although the practice of dermatology in India has largely been a reflection of the Western medicine, unlike the west, dermatology in India had limited itself to being a medical specialty and had not explored the surgical dimensions until recently. Also, dermatology has minimal share in the curriculum and almost negligible stake in the qualifying examination of medical graduates in India.[2] Thus, for several decades dermatology was at the bottom of the list of postgraduation aspirants in India.

In the last few decades, the winds have changed for dermatology. The addition of esthetic practice, explosive growth of dermatosurgery, and recent advances in clinical dermatology have been a shot in the arm for the field. Now, it is one of the few branches of modern medicine that can boast of having both medical and surgical aspects. In addition to the stupendous and rapid growth of the field, the fact that dermatology practice can be contained to suit the practitioner's schedule has made it one of the most sought-after branches among young doctors. However, there is a yawning gap between what is learnt by postgraduate students in a medical college and what is needed to establish in dermatology practice. This book intends to fill up this chasm and serve as a guide to dermatologists keen on venturing into private practice.

EVOLUTION OF DERMATOLOGY PRACTICE

From being a triple specialty branch in the days of yore, the field of dermatology has flourished vigorously to include several subspecialties such as cosmetic dermatology, dermatosurgery, pediatric dermatology, dermatopathology, and teledermatology, to name a few. Among these, undoubtedly cosmetic dermatology is the fastest growing specialty.[3] Cosmetic dermatology and dermatosurgery, together known as interventional dermatology, have caused a paradigm shift in a specialty which limited to armchair practice for several decades.

The rise in demand, predictability and safety of therapy, and better monetary benefits have led to a constantly increasing number of dermatologists opting to practice cosmetic dermatology, sometimes exclusively. In several countries, patients seeking a cosmetic botulinum toxin injection have more swift access to dermatologists than those needing urgent dermatology appointments.[4]

It is feared that the fall out of this scenario is an increasing dependence on nondermatologists and quacks for treatment of diseases of skin.

However, as the old adage goes, "change is the only constant." Many other specialties such as otolaryngology, cardiology, and radiology have diversified into newer subspecialties. Similarly, in dermatology, rather than being confined to just writing prescriptions, technical advances in cosmetic dermatology such as better molecules, laser, and light devices can be utilized to treat dermatological problems that have not responded well to medical management.

Therefore, a holistic practice that combines medical, cosmetic, and surgical dermatology is ideal.

VARIOUS MODELS OF DERMATOLOGY PRACTICE

After completion of postgraduation, a dermatologist has the privilege of choosing among various practice settings. Joining a medical college as faculty will ensure continuation of academic pursuits, research activities, interaction with students, and standardized patient care. Association with an already established practice or a corporate hospital has the advantages of an increased monetary benefit and flexibility with regard to the working hours. Setting up a private clinic, although a challenging endeavor, gives the reward of absolute autonomy and the scope for unlimited expansion. However, starting a private practice also implies that the dermatologist should be familiar with a gamut of issues including investments, software, communications, human resource management, medicolegal matters, etc.

A dermatologist opting to start a private practice can choose from the following models:

- *Solo practice:* Individual practice at a self-owned or rented place (most common)
- *Group practice*: Single specialty or multispecialty
- *Corporate-owned*: Corporate organization ownership wherein the dermatologist works full time or part time
- *Integrated health care delivery system*: Multispecialty hospitals wherein the dermatologist works full time or part time
- *Others:* As part of digital/mobile health technology services[5]

Solo practice entails single-doctor ownership, managing the practice with the benefits of individual freedom, and the ability to set his/her own growth pattern. However, the drawbacks of working in this way include longer working hours and more financial risks. In contrast, working in large clinics as an employee or as a partner ensures shorter working hours and fixed income, albeit with lesser freedom and a predictable but slow growth curve. Currently, there are several commercial chains operating successfully in India. These chains offer training in interventional dermatology, a regular income, and medicolegal protection. Naturally, this model has found many takers among the young dermatologists. However, it must be borne in mind that these clinics have their presence in multiple areas and thus undermine the individual dermatologist's practice.

Clarity on the nature of practice one intends to begin with is of utmost importance. Depending on the affinity, affordability, and training received, a dermatologist can choose to start:
- Traditional disease-based clinical dermatology practice
- A combination of diseased-based and esthetic dermatology practice (a common and preferred scenario, where a dermatologist begins with general practice and minor cosmetology procedures, and once the foundation is built, the practice is escalated to include lasers, injectables, and dermatosurgery)
- Specialized cosmetic dermatology practice, which offers services of a plastic surgeon, Medispa, etc.

TRANSITION FROM A PATIENT TO A CLIENT

Currently, India has more than 10,000 qualified dermatologists and an equal or more number of nonqualified or underqualified medical personnel treating skin diseases and practicing esthetic medicine. The quasiskin specialists have resorted to atrocious promotional tactics relying heavily on misleading promises. Patients who are exposed to these marketing strategies expect a similar result when they visit a dermatologist.

Unlike patients undergoing medical treatment, most patients undergoing esthetic procedures tend to behave like consumers. They seek a physician after researching about the treatment options. They regard esthetic practitioners as service providers and expect to be provided with a high-quality service. Increased paying capacity of the patients seeking cosmetic dermatology services has contributed to this. Meeting these elevated expectations consistently is a difficult task. To maneuver this, the dermatologist must understand the opinions and the preferences of the patient and should build the patient's trust on his/her expertise. The dermatologist must also ensure that consultation charge and the cost of the procedures should be more or less on par with the community standard.

Possession of excellent communication skills by the staff of the clinic will also serve as a great asset in developing rapport with patients.

Building the clinic as a brand, ensuring a healthy presence online, and hiring and retaining dedicated and efficient staff are perquisites for patient satisfaction in today's era.

THE ROAD AHEAD FOR A BEGINNER

The challenges faced by a beginner are different from those faced by an established practitioner. There is very little documented guidance that can be availed by a beginner; the training is on the job and hence the learning curve becomes longer. Nevertheless, the successful dermatology practice can be achieved with perseverance, hard work, entrepreneurship, and by taking the first step. To quote an ancient Chinese philosopher Lao Tzu, "A journey of thousand miles begins with one step."

REFERENCES

1. Mukhopadhyay AK. Dermatology in India and Indian dermatology: a medico-historical perspective. Indian Dermatol Online J. 2016;7(4):235-43.
2. Thappa DM, Kumari R. Emergence of dermatology in India. Indian J Dermatol Venereol Leprol. 2009;75:86-92.
3. Sandhu JK. Cosmetic dermatology: an integral part of current dermatology curriculum. Indian J Dermatol Venereol Leprol. 2019;85:1-2.

4. Resneck JS Jr, Lipton S, Pletcher MJ. Short wait times for patients seeking cosmetic botulinum toxin appointments with dermatologists. J Am Acad Dermatol. 2007;57:985-9.

5. Vishalakshi V. Group Practice in Cosmetic Dermatology. Dermapractice: The Dermatology Practitioner's Guide. IADVL Practice Management Cell. Volume 1; 2016.

1.2 The Road Ahead After Residency!

Madhulika Mhatre, Aseem Sharma, Trupti Agarwal

INTRODUCTION

The journey from graduation to postgraduation is definitely full of hard work and turmoil and hours and hours of preparation and dedication, not to mention the sleepless nights spent pouring over books and articles trying to assimilate the quantum of knowledge out there in order to educate ourselves and treat our patients better. However, receiving that much-coveted degree at the end of it that qualifies one to practice in their chosen field of dermatology is truly worth all the efforts. Though many may think that the quest ends here, this is not entirely true. Residency programs are, in fact, merely the beginning of learning—the time when a young doctor gets exposed to the vast glory of dermatology, in all its faces and facets. And the proverbial iceberg is revealed when residency ends and the search begins—the search for academic or nonacademic pursuits, mentors, trainers, courses, fellowships, observerships, preceptorships, and so on. However, these opportunities as well as facilities for learning are not uniform and vary greatly from center to center across India.[1]

The field of dermatology has expanded beyond the conventional clinical and histopathological realms, with new and newer specialized arenas such as lasers, esthetics, injectables, dermatosurgery, trichology, onychology, dermoscopy, and so on, requiring an entirely distinct skill set and dedicated training, which postgraduate courses often fail to impart. Thus, young postgraduates, even after 3 years of dermatology training, feel the need to expand their armamentarium and acquire either specialized training opportunities in these fields, exposure to private practice or a sense of autonomy, and dealing with patients on their own before stepping into an active patient care setup.

A checklist for a fresh postgraduate would read as follows:
1. Joining a medical institute
2. Training under the preceptorship of an established dermatologist
3. Corporate practice (hospital/clinic chain)
4. Starting one's own private practice
5. National fellowships
6. International training opportunities

JOIN A MEDICAL INSTITUTE

One can opt to join a medical institute (central/state government, semigovernment, municipal or private) as a senior resident or a lecturer. The process involves scouring newspapers and social media buttons for the advertisement (especially government institutions, as those can easily be missed!), applying for the post, and going through a round of interviews. It is imperative to state here that central government institutes, including armed forces institutions, have a slightly more complicated procedure involved, and it would be prudent to contact someone from those organizations for further information. The option for joining a medical institute is usually fruitful due to the various pros and cons:

Pros:
- Enormous clinical variety and acumen development
- Improves clinical diagnostic and procedural skills
- Guidance of seniors and professors in case of difficulty—teamwork
- Helps to tackle difficult, complicated, and chronic cases
- Limited working hours, and hence a good professional–personal life balance
- Continuous process of learning and academics
- Open doors for clinical or laboratory-based research
- Platform to publish papers and research and attain fame
- Opportunities for professional development and teaching
- Time to attend various clinical meets and conferences to upgrade your skills
- Interaction with other specialties
- A stable income (maybe even a pension!)

Cons:
- Monotonous lifestyle
- High inter institute variability (Choose your institutes wisely!)
- Expectations may not culminate into reality
- Low or no exposure to certain subspecialty—esthetics, dermatosurgery, trichology, lasers
- Slow, time-bound, and vacancy-dependent growth

TRAINING UNDER THE GUIDANCE OF SENIOR DERMATOLOGISTS

For young dermatologists and their basic understanding of the know-how of a private or clinic-based practice, there is no better way than to shadow a well-established dermatologist and learn the intricacies of what goes on behind a successful dermatology clinic. This mentorship opportunity is totally at the behest and discretion of the senior dermatologist. The junior dermatologist or junior consultant will get an opportunity to examine patients, maybe get hands-on on procedures, as well as get exposure about various technologies that the clinic has to offer—lasers, esthetics, dermatopathology, vitiligo surgery, etc. This is a one-on-one learning opportunity.

Pros:
- Better learning
- Guidance
- Job security
- Comfortable environment to work in
- Opportunity to learn various new techniques
- Good patient exposure
- Less stress
- Learn to manage staff
- Management of resources and pharmacy

Cons:
- Restricted responsibility
- No freedom to make your decisions
- Set pattern of practice
- Less creative options
- No flexibility in working hours
- Poor income

CORPORATE PRACTICE

A corporate practice essentially takes forward the learning that one acquires from a private practice—a hospital or a healthcare chain.

It is also the perfect exposure for someone transitioning from a government setup to private practice. Corporate hospitals usually employ young postgraduates on a fixed-hour scenario, laden with incentives. It also exposes a young doctor to the functioning of a department or a clinic, including the nits and grits—human resource management, utilities—electricity, water and so on, machine management, and the basic functioning of a scaled setup.

Pros:
- Can negotiate on working hours and salary
- Salary not affected by the ups and down of the market
- Transfer options to a different state
- Contracting and terminating, debt claims accumulation endeavors, patient and staff booking, preparing, and all the rest are normally dealt with by the corporate office
- Discounted rates
- Good exposure for new graduates

Cons:
- Stress on sales
- Leaves have to be planned in advance
- Growth and skills limited to technology available
- Your treatment plans might be investigated by corporate administration
- You will probably not be able to evaluate new, cutting-edge methods or procedures
- Limited decision-making ability
- Lengthy approval process

STARTING YOUR OWN PRIVATE PRACTICE

This is another option that senior practitioners always tell youngsters at meets and conferences. Starting as a fresher gives you the obvious edge in terms of a patient base, a head start in terms of visibility, and a continuation of a family practice, if applicable. It also gives one an autonomous, "learn-as-you-go" approach. The downsides to an immediate practice are the numerous glitches and the hows and whys of it all, which have been delineated under the previous heading—"Training under a senior dermatologist." Another noteworthy option here would be the establishment of a group practice between three or more dermatologists. The benefits and difficulties in starting your own practice are as follows.

Pros:
- Independence and autonomy—freedom to make your decisions
- You control who you work with
- Limited working hours or working hours of your choice
- More creative options
- Sense of accomplishment
- Learning marketing skills
- Learn through your mistakes

Cons:
- No guidance, unless family is in the same profession
- Costs are high rent, equipment, staff salary, etc.
- Building patients from scratch
- Hiring staff and training
- Flexible and unpredictable income
- Increased responsibility and stress

INDIAN SCHOLARSHIPS AND FELLOWSHIPS[2]

Indian Association of Dermatologists, Venereologists and Leprologists (IADVL) as well as other associations have recognized these unmet needs of residents and young dermatologists during residency training and instituted some programs to facilitate the learning process and bridge the glaring gap. Scholarships, fellowships, observerships, mentorships, workshops, online education, and research grants are some of the varied tools available, to provide necessary exposure and training in these new arenas of dermatology.

Scholarships

- Residents are encouraged to become provisional members of dermatology associations, such as our national body IADVL (www.iadvl.org), Association of Cutaneous Surgeons of India (ACSI; http://www.acsinet.net/), and Cosmetic Dermatology Society of India (CDSI; http://www.cosdermindia.in/). These associations encourage residents to participate in their conferences by offering scholarships to those presenting posters and oral or award paper presentations.
- The IADVL provides scholarships to both national (MIDDERMACON and DERMACON) and international conferences (World Congress of Dermatology, International Congress of Dermatology, Asian Dermatology Congress, and South Asian Regional Conference of Dermatology) to their provisional life members (residents). Members can avail one national and one international scholarship during their lifetime. The announcements for the scholarship are available at www.iadvl.org and the respective conference website.
- The American Academy of Dermatology (AAD) offers two reciprocal scholarships and two Strauss and Katz World Congress scholarships to IADVL members to attend the AAD annual conference every year. Candidates are selected through application by a three-member jury appointed by the IADVL. Similarly, several other associations offer assistance for attending their international meetings, e.g., Asian Society for Pigment Cell Research (ASPCR), European Academy of Dermatology and Venereology (EADV), Dermatology and Aesthetic Surgery International League (DASIL), World Congress of Dermatology (WCD), World Congress of Hair Research (WCHR), and New Zealand Dermatological Society Inc (NZDSI). Details of the same can be obtained from their respective websites.

Fellowships or Observerships

- These are offered by the IADVL, ACSI, universities, and individual centers in India. The IADVL, by means of the IADVL Academy, and ACSI, through their Central Council, offer observerships for a period of 2–4 weeks, depending on the age of the candidate. As of 2018, the IADVL offers observerships in clinical dermatology, dermatopathology, dermatoscopy, dermatosurgery, hair transplantation, HIV medicine, immunofluorescence, lasers and esthetic dermatology, pediatric dermatology, photodermatology, trichology, and urticaria in 22 centers across India. A nominal stipend of ₹15,000 is also given to life members (LMs) aged <35 years on completion.
- The IADVL also offers an international dermatopathology observership, with a stipend of ₹1 lakh, to each candidate, in a liaison partnership with three centers in USA and one center in Taiwan, to six LMs, annually.

These observerships/fellowships are through invited applications and the selection is by the respective associations and universities or institutes based on the requisite criteria, by independent juries.

Table 1.2.1: Prominent fellowships offered by Indian universities and institutes.

University	Institute	Fellowship	Duration
Rajiv Gandhi University of Health Sciences (www.rguhs.ac.in/)	Bangalore Medical College and Research Institute (BMCRI), Bengaluru (www.bmcri.org)	Dermatosurgery, esthetic dermatology, pediatric dermatology	1 year
	Venkat Center for Skin and Plastic Surgery, Bengaluru (www.venkatcenter.com)	Esthetic dermatology	1 year
	St. John's Medical College, Bengaluru (www.stjohns.in)	Dermatosurgery	1 year
	CUTIS Academy of Cutaneous Sciences, Bengaluru (www.cutis.org.in)	Dermatosurgery, esthetic dermatology, pediatric dermatology	1 year
	Kempegowda Institute of Medical Sciences (KIMS), Bengaluru (www.kimsbangalore.edu.in)	Esthetic dermatology	1 year
Maharashtra University of Health Sciences (www.muhs.ac.in)	KEM Medical College, Mumbai (https://www.kem.edu/)	Diagnostic dermatology	1 year
	Lokmanya Tilak Municipal (LTM) Medical College, Mumbai (http://www.ltmgh.com/frontview/index.aspx)	Trichology	1 year
All India Institute of Medical Sciences (AIIMS) (www.aiims.edu/en.html)	AIIMS, New Delhi	Contact dermatitis, sexually transmitted infections, dermatosurgery, dermatopathology, lasers and pulse therapy	Contact AIIMS

Apart from the short fellowships, there are intensive, long courses offered by universities or institutes, directly. The detailed procedure can be looked up at their websites. The prominent fellowships are appended in **Table 1.2.1**.

INTERNATIONAL TRAINING OPPORTUNITIES[3]

There are various institutes in USA, UK, Europe, Bangkok, and Singapore that provide opportunities for fellowships and preceptorships. These can be either application-based travel grants, preceptorship opportunities, or paid-training programs.

International Observership Program in Dermatology, New York

- The Ronald O Perelman Department of Dermatology at the New York University (NYU) School of Medicine offers an International Observership Program in Dermatology for select physicians in other countries around the world. This Program is designed to enhance knowledge in general dermatology and dermatological subspecialties, increase familiarity with technological advances in dermatology, and provide exposure to dermatological care as practiced in one of the foremost training centers in the United States.

The program is of 1 month's duration and begins on the 1st day of the month between September and June.
- Tuition is 3000 USD which is the responsibility of the applicant.

For more information: http://www.med.nyu.edu/dermatology/education/international-observership-program-dermatology.

International Traveling Mentorship Program

The International Traveling Mentorship Program (ITMP) was established in 2010 through the Lawrence Field, MD, International Dermatologic Surgery Education Exchange Fund. The ITMP enhances the exchange of information and body of knowledge of dermatologic surgery between the US and international community of dermatologic surgeons. The American Society of Dermatologic Surgery (ASDS) allows dermatologic surgeons to visit a host institution in another country, or host a dermatologic surgeon from another country, for a defined period of teaching, surgical demonstration and table-side exchange.

Requirements
- Be a member of American Society of Dermatologic Surgery (ASDS) or other member (ASDS acceptance of "Other" membership contingent on applicant providing evidence of international equivalence in dermatology certification/training).
- Have completed a residency/fellowship in dermatology and have a minimum of 7 years of practice experience.
- Be in possession of special skills needed in the dermatologic surgery community.

For more information: https://www.asds.net/itmp/.

ASDS International Preceptorship

The ASDS International Preceptorship Program sends an international dermatologic surgeon to the US to shadow a Preceptor, observing a variety of treatments and advanced techniques, consulting with patients and more. This helps foster an exchange of dermatologic surgery knowledge between international colleagues and helps to improve patient care. Limited funding is available. One international dermatologist is selected annually.

For more information: https://www.asds.net/international-preceptorship/.

St John's Institute of Dermatology Visiting Professional Programme, Dermatological Surgery and Laser Unit, UK

The Dermatological Surgery and Laser Unit Programme has been designed by leading surgical consultants within St John's Institute of Dermatology, which is part of Guy's and St Thomas' NHS Foundation Trust. The program offers international visiting professionals with the opportunity to experience cutting-edge skin cancer services (including Mohs) and laser devices.

For more information: www.guysandstthomasevents.co.uk

Post-residency Fellowships, Canada
- The University of Toronto program for Mohs Surgery is an official 1-year fellowship accredited by the American College of Mohs Surgeons (ACMS; http://www.mohscollege.org/acms/). It is open to Canadian dermatologists as well as international dermatologists. USMLE is not required.
- The Dermatologic Laser Surgery and Aesthetic Medicine Fellowship is a 1-year

clinical fellowship designed to help improve the fellow's knowledge and skill in the area of noninvasive dermatologic laser surgery and esthetic medicine. It is open to Canadian dermatologists as well as international dermatologists—self-funded. For additional information, email: shelley.racicot@Sunnybrook.ca.

ISD Mentorship Programme

The International Society of Dermatology (ISD) provides opportunities to ISD members to enhance dermatological knowledge and skills through a fellowship program for 3 months. This fellowship is open to dermatologists from developing countries as well. Applications are invited once a year and candidates can give their choice of mentor from a list of international mentors approved by the ISD. Resident applicants who are 35 years old and below are given priority. Only two awards per country are given each year.
For more information: www.intsocderm.org

Ramathibodi Hospital, Mahidol University, Thailand

The Ramathibodi Skin Laser Center provides short-term training fellowships in dermatology, dermatosurgery, and laser medicine. The fees are 2,000 USD per month/1,200 USD for 2 weeks.
For more information: http://med.mahidol.ac.th/ramalaser/.

Siriraj Hospital, Mahidol University, Thailand

A short-course training fellowship in dermatosurgery is also offered at Siriraj Hospital, Thailand. It is a 1-month fellowship with a fee of 50,000 Thai baht. Interested applicants can apply through the website.
For more information: http://www.sirirajlaser.com/academic/#short-court-en.

Seoul National University Hospital, Seoul

The Department of Dermatology of the Seoul National University Hospital offers short-term fellowships of 2 weeks, and 4 weeks, duration, which include training in basic dermatology, dermatosurgery, Mohs, lasers as well as hair transplantation. Fellows are also encouraged to participate in research trials.
For more information: http://www.snuh.org/english/snuh/snuh03/sub01/index1.jsp.

The International Master Course on Aging Sciences Academy

The International Master Course on Aging Sciences (IMCAS) Academy offers an online platform for training in various esthetic procedures. Through its various online courses and webinars, one can get the required know-how regarding a wide range of esthetic procedures.
For more information: http://www.imcas.com/en/academy/webinar.

Fellowships and Training in Hair Transplantation

- The International Society of Hair Restoration Surgery (ISHRS) Fellowship Training Committee has formalized the Policies, Procedures, and Guidelines for ISHRS-recognized Fellowship Training Programs.
For more information: http://www.ishrs.org/member-fellowship-training.php
- The International Academy of Hair Transplant Surgery provides a comprehensive education in the hair transplant industry for a total duration of 12 months, providing top education concerning theoretical issues, practical skill development, and hair restoration business management.

For more information: http://www.iahts.org/doctor/fellowship-program.aspx.

In addition to the aforementioned centers, individual countries have their own fellowship criteria for their board-certified dermatologists and due to the limited scope of this chapter and vastness of the available content, we have not included them. Additionally, for Indian trained dermatologists looking for short-term training and fellowships abroad, in addition to the above-mentioned centers which have international repute, there are various other individual practitioners and private centers that offer training and exposure.

Fellowships and Training in Dermatopathology[4]

Of the multitude of options, the US has the highest number and the best-structured programs **(Table 1.2.2)** for international medical graduates, who aim to return to their own countries after completion of training.

Other dermatopathology fellowship options are:
- Mackay Memorial Hospital, Taipei, Taiwan
  - *Program Director*: Dr. Yu-Hung Wu
  - *Duration of observership (for those not holding a Taiwan medical license)*: 3, 6, 12 months
  - *Prequalification*: Board certified in dermatology or pathology
  - *Fee*: 10,000 New Taiwan dollars per month; scholarships available
  - Living expenses in Taipei are roughly 12,000–15,000 NT dollars per month
  - *For more information*: mmhedu@ms2.mmh.org.tw
- National Skin Centre, Singapore
  - *Program Director*: Dr Joyce Lee
  - *Duration of fellowship*: 1 year
  - ICDP-UEMS (see below) accredited training center
  - Accepts both dermatologists and pathologists
  - No tuition fee charged, but administration fee charged by the National Skin Centre (contact Mr Naim at naim@nsc.com.sg for details)

For more information: joycelee@nsc.com.sg

The pros and cons of post-doctoral/fellowship courses can be summarized as follows.

Pros:
- Invaluable experience
- You are pushing yourself, and the envelope
- Interaction with international students
- More learning opportunities
- Experience of new and latest technologies
- Building of an international network
- Educational diversity

Cons:
- Expensive
- You are out of your comfort zone
- Difficulty in communication
- Racism
- People have too many expectations
- Recognition of your degree by other countries
- Loneliness may creep in, especially in the longer courses

No matter what the chosen path, this chapter would be rendered incomplete without a mention of marketing, finances, communication skills, and medicolegal aspects. These are, undoubtedly, the cornerstones of any new practice or setup. Unfortunately, we do not undergo hands-on or formal training when it comes to these aspects, and most of us end up learning this the hard way.

Table 1.2.2: American fellowships and training programs in dermatopathology.

Institute	Director	Duration	Fee ($)	Specimen accessions/year
Ackerman Academy, New York	Dr Geoffrey Gottlieb, Dr Ying Guo	4–12 months	1,000/month	100,000
Boston University School of Medicine	Dr Jag Bhawan	1 or 2 years	15,000/year	30,000
Wake Forest School of Medicine, Winston-Salem, North Carolina	Dr Omar Sangueza	1-year observership	22,000/year	17,000
University of California, San Francisco	Dr Philip LeBoit Contact: Mary-kate.fitzsimon@ucsf.edu	1 year	10,000/year	92,000
Medical College of Wisconsin, Milwaukee, Wisconsin	Dr Saul Suster Contact: Ssuster@mcw.edu	1 year (meant for pathologists only)		
Medical University of South Carolina	Dr John S Metcalf Dr Dirk Elston elstond@musc.edu	–	–	12,000
University of Vermont Medical Center	Dr Deborah L Cook	Educational Commission for Foreign Medical Graduates (ECFMG) certificate required		
MD Anderson Cancer Center, Houston, Texas	Dr Victor G Prieto	1 year American Board eligible dermatologists or pathologists may apply; is one of the four centers for the IADVL International Dermatopathology Observership program	–	–

(IADVL: Indian Association of Dermatologists, Venereologists and Leprologists, ECFMG: Educational Commission for Foreign Medical Graduates)

FINANCES

This significant factor ought to be considered as the foundation stone of one's business. One has to appropriately recognize the sources through which one will acquire this. Private practice is akin to a business and cannot be sustained without inflow of resources, especially financial. The financing example is one of the most significant components to consider before beginning a business. This by and large incorporates the capital that you start up with. In corporate hospitals, things get a bit more complex with the board of directors having a major role to play in the scheme of things.

Assets can be obtained for business, through either present moment or long haul credits. A clear financial approach needs to be in place, the correct approach to banks, private loan specialists, and other means.

Tangible and intangible assets need to be assessed and acquired, to make the most of the capital and resources. In due course of time, and with smart cost accounting and management, these assets can start repaying a setup.

MARKETING

Medicinal practices are not perceived as pure business models, and in some ways, they should not be. But once clear goals have been established, an ideal plan should be formulated, which would blend various types of promotion, such as website, internal, print, and special events. Attention is to be given to each and everything, opportunities should not be missed, the opposition must be investigated thoroughly, and multimedia promotion techniques should be employed.

A paper by Sachdev et al. makes for further reading into the other, lesser touched-upon aspects of practice management, and in general. An interesting concept is the 14 Ps of Practice— Place, Person(s), Purpose, Patients, Procedures, Photography, Professional skills, Products, Publicity, Promote, Protection to name a few.[5]

COMMUNICATION

Communication or "soft skill training" is another aspect which is never taught during formal medical education programs. This is an extremely-important-yet-often ignored aspect, even though it is a dictum in the corporate world. This is pertinent especially to young doctors from understaffed, overworked government hospitals, wherein a cyclical process of unlearning, learning, and relearning must take place. Individuals or young dermatologists should acquaint themselves in this fine art of communication, as this will help them in creating a good rapport with patients, dealing with irate patients, convincing their patients for treatments and compliance, dealing with colleagues and coworkers, and also helping train their staff in these aspects. Such training can be acquired through various institutes or agencies offering a soft-skills training program, which are aplenty. A bit of this can also be imbibed whilst under a mentor in the setting of a senior dermatologist's clinic. Limited knowledge can also be obtained by reading books on the pertinent subject, but like everything else, a hands-on or on-job training is unparalleled.

MEDICOLEGAL ASPECTS

Conventional medical education has a single-point focus—to prepare experts who will preserve mankind; eliminate, control, and prevent disease; and spread health awareness. Unfortunately, medical schools, even postgraduate schools, do not prepare these experts to deal with the nitty-gritties of ethos, ethics, torts, and other legal implications of medicine. Despite the fact that medicine and law have gone hand in hand for a considerable amount of time, there exists a significant knowledge gap between this marriage. Albeit there are emerging concepts that attempt to bridge this gap, such as "medicolegal rounds," dedicated legal case discussions, and intensive medicolegal workshops, there is a pressing need for concentrated medicolegal education.

As a young dermatologist, in today's era of increased public awareness and litigation, it is mandatory to learn the legalities involved and practice safe and sound dermatology. Various books are available on the subject and we recommend that dermatologists should make it a part of their reference/reading material as soon as they step into the world of clinical practice. Alternatively, IADVL does have a medicolegal cell that can help, in times of need.

PRACTICE TIPS TO AVOID MEDICOLEGAL HASSLES

- Get professional indemnity insurance
- Counseling
- Communication
- Meticulous documentation
- Legal coverage

TIPS FROM EXPERIENCE

- Do not rush.
- Decide your area of focus.
- Choose the option that gives you maximum exposure to concerned subspecialty.
- Talk to seniors/colleagues—learn from their mistakes and experiences.
- Most scholarships/international training opportunities are merit based—work on strengthening your CV.
- Attend CMEs and conferences—keep learning and networking.
- Read journals—stay updated.

CONCLUSION

The road after residency is a complex one, with multiple roads and inroads available at every juncture. This complexity acts a double-edged sword. On the one hand, it provides for further learning, new avenues, and expanding horizons—both physical and mental, and makes us strive to push our envelopes whereas on the other hand, with more and more people embarking on these journeys, the value of our core postgraduate degree (or diploma) is diminishing. The authors' perspective on this dilemma can be summed up, best, as an improvisation on Robert Frost's poem—the road less travelled is still better than the road not taken.

REFERENCES

1. Mysore V. Scholarships, grants, and training opportunities for dermatology residents in India by Indian Association of Dermatologists, Venereologists and Leprologists. Indian Dermatol Online J. 2016;7:3-5.
2. Kolalapudi SA, Valia AR, Pandhi D. Clinical training and research opportunities for dermatology residents in India. Indian Dermatol Online J. 2018;9:231-3.
3. Mhatre M, Mysore V. International Training for Aesthetic Dermatology. In: Mysore V (Ed). ACSI Textbook of Cutaneous and Aesthetic Surgery, 2nd edition; New Delhi: Jaypee Brothers Medical Publishers; 2017.
4. Laskar S. Training avenues in dermatopathology for an Indian dermatologist or pathologist. Indian J Dermatol Venereol Leprol. 2018;84: 506-9.
5. Sachdev M, Britto GR. Essential requirements to setting up an aesthetic practice. J Cutan Aesthet Surg. 2014;7:167-9.

1.3 Choosing your Subspecialty

Madura C, Harsha Siddappa

INTRODUCTION

Dermatology has grown enormously from being one small department next to department of psychiatry to the current enviable huge department with various subspecialty wings. It is now one of the most commonly sought-after postgraduate degree courses because of the rapid growth in the field of esthetic dermatology and dermatosurgery. The current budding dermatologist has a wide range of subspecialties to choose from. However, most of the postgraduates have very little insight regarding the various subspecialties available to them. This is because of the lack of information and exposure to these various subspecialties during their postgraduation training. This chapter aims at guiding the young dermatologists and/or postgraduates in choosing the subspecialty practice in dermatology.

HOW TO CHOOSE THE SUBSPECIALTY?

Though most of the youngsters have an inclination toward esthetic practice, it is worth knowing about other growing subspecialties enlisted in **Box 1.3.1**.

Esthetic Dermatology/Medical Cosmetology

This has major attraction for most of the youngsters. It includes procedures such as chemical peels, microdermabrasion, lasers for hair removal, pigmentation, etc., body and facial contouring with energy-based devices, injectables (botulinum toxin, fillers, injection lipolysis), and thread lifts. Good esthetic practice needs good location with target population, good ambience, and initial investment for lasers. Also, one needs keen eye appreciation of beauty, patience, and finally greater communication, counseling, and artistic skills to excel with good rewards.

Dermatosurgery

It is one of the subspecialties for postgraduates or residents who have surgical inclination. Apart from having surgical orientation, one should have delicate hands (good skills), lion's heart (ability to handle complications), and stamina for long hours of surgery. It includes procedures such as basic surgeries (lipoma, cyst, corn, and mole excisions), vitiligo surgeries, nail surgeries, acne scar revision, and advanced surgeries such as scar revision, tumor excision followed by reconstruction surgery with flaps and grafts, blepharoplasty, breast augmentation, hair transplantation, liposuction, and fat transfer. The major advantages are that dermatosurgery can be practiced in any area. Based on the target population, it gives immediate results with higher patient and doctor satisfaction rates, but it has a long learning curve. One needs to invest at least 1 year in specific training. Though basic surgeries can be learnt faster, advanced surgeries always need long training through fellowship programs. If one needs to do only dermatosurgery, then his/her option is restricted to institutional practice. Therefore, one can choose focus practice on either liposuction and fat transfer, or hair transplantation to make it advantageous. The main investment in dermatosurgery is to install a well-equipped operation theater and appointing, retaining, and maintaining technical staff.

Box 1.3.1: Various subspecialties in dermatology.

- Esthetic dermatology/Medical cosmetology
- Dermatosurgery
- Pediatric dermatology
- Trichology
- Laser medicine
- Diagnostic dermatology (dermatopathology, immunofluorescence, dermoscopy)
- HIV medicine and AIDS
- Sexual medicine
- Geriatric dermatology
- Dermatological research

(AIDS: acquired immunodeficieny syndrome; HIV: human immunodeficiency virus)

Laser Medicine

Nowadays, lasers are part of both clinical and esthetic practice. There are lasers for hair removal, pigmentation, tattoo, body and facial contouring, scars, and hyperhidrosis. One needs the ability to understand laser physics and its applications. It needs you to hire good technical staff and train them. The major disadvantage is the heavy cost involved in the initial investment to buy the laser machines, but it adds to the esthetic practice.

Trichology

It is an upcoming subspecialty, rapidly growing due to special interest in hair transplantation. Trichology practice includes not only hair transplantation but also all hair-related disorders, excision surgeries of scalp, and procedural interventions involving hair growth. The advantage is that it is a focus practice with good financial rewards. The only investment is a well-equipped operation theater and hiring, retaining, and maintaining the technical staff.

Pediatric Dermatology

It is a focused and specialized branch of dermatology focusing on childhood skin disorders from birth through adolescence including procedural interventions. Special training is required for this field as the challenges faced in pediatric population are different ranging from the inability of patients to correctly specify their problems to handling them in a hospital setup. One choses this subspecialty, more for the joy and self-satisfaction, and not for the financial reward.

Dermatopathology

Dermatologists are the best dermatopathologists worldwide. They see the dermatology clinical cases and if they have the knowledge of dermatopathology, their clinical acumen and diagnostic skills improve. This aspect bears an upper hand in comparison to a pathologist who does not get to see clinical cases. So a fellowship in dermatopathology following postgraduation helps them to get trained in identifying different structures and patterns in the biopsy specimen. They can also be trained in immunofluorescence and immunohistochemistry. Dermatopathology is for respect and academic satisfaction and not for the financial reward.

PRESELECTION WORKUP/WHAT YOU NEED TO DO BEFORE CHOOSING A SUBSPECIALTY?

There are many factors that influence or help in choosing the specialty. This chapter gives residents a few pointers which can help them choose a subspecialty suited for them.

- *Research the availability of specialty*: First, the residents have to research regarding the availability of the fellowships and observerships and make a list of the courses they will be eligible for.
- *Field of interest:* This is the most important factor. It is always good to first go through the curriculum of the courses, to see what interests you, and if you have the passion for it. It could be motivation by mentors or seniors during postgraduation, who create special interest for you in the subject. You can also seek the guidance of seniors who have passed out or current fellowship/observership students for further information regarding the courses, the experience and challenges they had, and what made them choose the particular field.
- *Self-assessment*: Residents must assess themselves and consider if they have the

- skills required for the particular specialty they are choosing. This is especially important for dermatosurgery and trichology where fine surgical skills are required.
- *Choose a backup specialty*: It is always safe to have a secondary option.
- *Area of practice*: Rural/urban/semiurban, and the interest of target population in the practice area
- *Duration of fellowship*: Residents must consider the duration of fellowship/observership. Subspecialties such as esthetic dermatology, dermatosurgery, trichology, and pediatric dermatology have a course of 1-year duration, whereas subspecialties such as dermatopathology, dermatoscopy, and HIV medicine have courses ranging from 1 to 3 months.
- *Financial rewards*: Subspecialties such as trichology, esthetic dermatology with lasers, and dermatosurgery have good financial rewards. Diagnostic dermatology, pediatric dermatology, and HIV medicine and AIDS are more for joy and keen interest toward the subject and adds to their practice, not for financial rewards.
- *Number of specialties*: It depends on multiple interests in subjects. Either choose a single subspecialty or opt for multiple subspecialties. There are many renowned dermatologists who practice multiple subspecialties together.
- *Preparing a good CV:* It is very important to prepare a detailed and authentic curriculum vitae (CV) before sending them for interviews. It should highlight your skills which can help in the particular subspecialty, your interest to improve in the field, and any research work correlating with it.
- *None of the above (NOTA):* Residents can choose not to pursue further subspecialty training and instead focus on just clinical dermatology. In time if they develop any interest in any of the fields, they can pursue it further

WHAT ARE THE TRAINING OPTIONS?

The Indian Association of Dermatologists, Venereologists and Leprologists (IADVL) and many individual institutions offer observerships and fellowships in various subspecialties (after completing postgraduation) to help them fine-tune in their field of interest. As there are limited seats available in these courses, there is high competition to enroll in them. The IADVL and Academy and Association of Cutaneous Surgeons of India (ACSI) offer observerships for a duration of 4 weeks across 22 centers and 5 centers, respectively, in India. This is available annually and only to members of their respective organizations. Information regarding application for these observerships will be available in their respective websites (www.iadvl.org, www.acsinet.net). The subspecialties offered here are clinical dermatology, dermatopathology, immunofluorescence, dermatoscopy, esthetic dermatology, dermatosurgery, hair transplantation, lasers and esthetic dermatology, HIV medicine, pediatric dermatology, photodermatology, trichology, and urticaria.

Many government and private institutions offer fellowships in various specialties such as esthetic dermatology, dermatosurgery, trichology, pediatric dermatology, diagnostic dermatology, and dermatopathology. These fellowships run for a duration of 1 year and help in complete training and fine-tuning the residents in the respective specialty.

Table 1.3.1: University/Institutes offering fellowships.[1]

University	Institute	Fellowship	Duration
Rajiv Gandhi University of Health Sciences (http://www.rguhs.ac.in/)	Bangalore Medical College and Research Institute (BMCRI), Bengaluru (www.bmcri.org)	Esthetic dermatology Dermatosurgery Trichology Pediatric dermatology	1 year
	St John's Medical College, Bengaluru (http://www.stjohns.in/)	Dermatosurgery	1 year
	Venkat Charmalaya, Bengaluru (http://www.bangalorehairtransplant.com/)	Esthetic dermatology	1 year
	CUTIS Academy of Cutaneous Sciences, Bengaluru (http://cutis.org.in/)	Esthetic dermatology Dermatosurgery	1 year
	Indira Gandhi Institute of Child Health, Bengaluru (http://www.igich.in)	Pediatric dermatology	1 year
Maharashtra University of Health Sciences (http://www.muhs.ac.in/)	KEM Medical College, Mumbai	Diagnostic dermatology	1 year
	Institute of Skin Cosmetology and Lasers, Solapur	Basic phototherapy and lasers in clinical dermatology	1 year
AIIMS (http://www.aiims.edu/en.html)	AIIMS, New Delhi	Contact dermatitis, dermatopathology, dermatosurgery, lasers, pulse therapy, sexually transmitted infections	–

Information regarding application to these fellowships will be available in their respective websites **(Table 1.3.1)**.[1]

CONCLUSION

With the availability of these many subspecialties, it can be a daunting question to the resident when frequently asked about his/her plans after postgraduation as they would have had minimal or sometimes no exposure to any of these specialties. Whatever the subspecialties one chooses, the basic denominator always remains clinical dermatology. If one wants to excel in the chosen subspecialty, their knowledge in clinical dermatology must be strong.

ACKNOWLEDGMENTS

We acknowledge Dr Nitin Barde, Consultant Dermatologist and Hair-transplant Surgeon, Nagpur, and Dr Eshwari L, Associate Professor, Bangalore Medical College, Bengaluru, for their valuable inputs.

REFERENCE

1. Kolalapudi SA, Valia AR, Pandhi D. Clinical training and research opportunities for dermatology residents in India. Indian Dermatol Online J. 2018;9:231-3.

SECTION 2: Setting-up a Clinic

2.1 Understanding Needs and Demands in Practice

Sumit Gupta

INTRODUCTION

Understanding "need and demands" in medical practice is akin to learning about the epidemiology and burden of a disease before reading further about it. It is not a static, one-time exercise that we as medical practitioners should indulge in before setting up practice. It is a constant and dynamic process that helps us not only to keep up with the times, but also to develop into more worthy and effective medical professionals.

CONCEPT

Understanding needs and demands is essentially a marketing concept and forms the core of all marketing decisions and strategy. "Marketing" is often considered a derogatory process or word, especially by us, Medical Professionals. We have been trained as technocrats who are supposed to know and excel only in our sphere of expertise. Also, most people believe that marketing is synonymous with advertising and as per the medical ethics, medical professionals/institutes should not indulge in it. However, advertising is a small component of the comprehensive marketing management process. Let us have a look at what "marketing" is defined as.

- The American Marketing Association defines marketing as "the activity, set of institutions, and processes for creating, communicating, delivering, and exchanging offerings that have value for customers, clients, partners, and society at large."
- The Chartered Institute of Marketing defines marketing as "the management process responsible for identifying, anticipating and satisfying customer/client/partner/society's requirements profitably."
- The famous Marketing Guru and Author Philip Kotler defines marketing as "satisfying needs and wants through an exchange process."

So, whatever be the field of endeavor, if it has to do with people and society at large and related to fulfilling any requirements of perceived or nonperceived value, it is inconceivable to perform it without marketing. Formally and informally, people and organizations engage in a vast number of activities which we call marketing. For corporate organizations, finance, operations, accounting, and other business functions will not really matter without sufficient demand for products and services so the firm can make a profit or create value. In the healthcare industry, medical skills, diagnostic capability, treatment algorithms, technology and infrastructure will have no meaning until there are either patients who can benefit from them or they are atleast aware that they can benefit from them. So, marketing is essentially about identifying and meeting human and social needs.

Needs are the fundamental human requirements such as for food, clothing, shelter, and health. Humans also have potent needs for education, comfort, social interaction, recreation, and entertainment. These needs become *wants* when directed to specific objects that might satisfy the need.

A person in Mumbai needs food but may want to eat *vada pav* at a food stall. Similarly, a person in Kochi needs food but may want to eat curd rice and fish curry. Our needs are essentially the same, but wants are shaped by our cultural behavior and society.

Demands are wants for specific products or services, supported by an *ability to afford*. Many people want to buy the latest I-Phone, but only few can afford one. Companies must measure not only the aspirational value of their products or services (wants), but also the willingness and ability to buy them (demands).

Now, many people can argue that healthcare is an essential need and medical services have no potential of being categorized as wants and demands. However, there are many examples in the healthcare field of wants and demands. Access to healthcare is a *need*, but access to healthcare with minimum and comfortable waiting time is a *want*. For providing this facility, a medical practice will have to invest in appointment management software, queue management system, trained receptionist, etc. The practice may also have to invest in a comfortable, air-conditioned waiting room with ample furniture for patients and their chaperones. The medical practice may have to monetize these facilities by charging a little high for its medical services. Now, some people may find it worthwhile to pay the extra amount (*demand*) while some may not. Investing in this type of infrastructure and mentioning "consultation by appointment" or "for appointment contact: XYZ" on prescription/hoarding/clinic board, etc., is an act of marketing which is catering to this very demand.

Many practices also have a provision of ancillary professionals who help in achieving healthcare requirements comprehensively. For instance, an orthopedic practice may have a provision of a physiotherapist and physiotherapy-related equipment. It results in convenience to the patient so that his/her particular healthcare need is being comprehensively catered to at one location. Similarly, a provision or availability of a dietician, counselor, lab technician/equipment, pharmacy, etc., in a medical practice, adds to the convenience of the patient. These conveniences may result in better compliance, proper monitoring, holistic care, and more positive outcomes. But the availability of these conveniences will require investment by the medical establishment which will increase the cost of service to the patient. The medical establishment has to assess which want has become an overwhelming demand in its space of operation and has to add services or equipment accordingly.

In a medical establishment, investment is also related to the level and scope of medical establishments. A medical establishment or practice that positions itself as a referral center will have to invest in more sophisticated equipment and more trained specialists, as its purpose is to cater to rarer conditions than a more general level establishment.

In addition to healthcare needs, most dermatology practices also cater to desires. With the rise of cosmetic and procedural dermatology, the field of dermatology has evolved over the years to extend its scope beyond treating skin diseases. Cosmetic dermatology helps in fulfilling the *desire* of people to look good. As distinguished to needs, *desires* are associated with passionate, emotional dimensions. Marketing pundits have used psychological research on how desires can be stimulated to find more effective ways to induce consumers into buying a given product or service. Desire for a product or service can be stimulated by advertising or awareness campaigns, which attempt to give buyers a *sense of lack or wanting*. For example, a line like: "grow your hair and confidence back!" would appeal to a bald person's low self-esteem due to baldness and urge him to do something about it.

So, understanding the marketing principles of needs, wants, demands, and desires specific to the field of practice is paramount in its successful functioning.

PROCESS

The process of understanding needs, desires, and demands starts at the conception of an establishment and should be constantly and indefinitely carried out since its functioning. Businesses and establishments that continuously fail to perform need/demand analysis are at the risk of becoming outdated and losing relevance.

In recent years, the descent of companies such as mobile phone giant Nokia and the photography behemoth Kodak are hidden from none. People's needs and demands evolve over time as competition, society, and cultural practices evolve. Failure to keep up with them, is failure to survive.

Particularly, for a dermatology practice, the information of needs or demands, etc., of a certain population can be obtained by the following sources:

- *Epidemiological data of diseases*: Epidemiology of diseases or conditions defines the scope of practice in different geographical areas. One of the examples is melanoma. Since the incidence of melanoma in South Asian skin is very low, dermatology practices in India are very unlikely to develop mole mapping protocols or invest in mole mapping technologies. Likewise, within India, different zones have different disorders which are more prevalent. It is important for a dermatologist to have in-depth knowledge of the prevalent diseases and conditions in the zone he/she plans to practice.
- *Demographic data*: Population characteristics such as age, gender, education, marital status, occupation, income level, family structure, etc., influence health-seeking behavior of people. A predominant population of well-educated young adults living either alone or in nuclear families, employed in multinational IT companies with enough disposable income, are more likely to be influenced by global trends in cosmetic dermatology and surgery. Similarly, they are more likely to search online for treatment guidelines, recommended dermatologists, drug side effects, etc. We need to modify our practice, communication, and services offered accordingly. For example, a considerably young, cosmetically conscious population in a city like Bengaluru or Gurugram are more likely to be bothered about problems such as hair loss and facial melanosis. Hence, the demand, suitability, and hence; market for a procedure such as hair transplant or a technology such as Q-Switched Laser are likely to be more in these areas. Cultural influences play an important

role in determining people's needs and demands. In places like Punjab and Haryana, where facial hair in women is a big taboo, laser hair reduction is probably a more prudent first laser technology to invest in.

- *Established practices*: An analysis of services offered by already established dermatology practices in a certain area, will tell the current consumption pattern of the populace. It is important to evaluate this type of information meticulously. There might be a service which is offered by almost all well-established practices. This may mean that either there is an overwhelming and still unfulfilled demand (supply < demand) for that service or it has already reached a level of saturation (supply > demand). Generally speaking, pricing of services drops if saturation occurs. Dropping of prices may increase demand, as now the service is in reach of a wider population. Soon, a new level of saturation will occur, causing the cost of services to drop further if feasible. Different geographical areas are often on different levels of this demand and supply curve. An understanding of the prevalent services and pricing can help set standards for any ensuing endeavors. This analysis can also present some unexplored avenues and *unmet needs* that might exist in a particular area.
- *In-clinic queries*: Patients may enquire about some treatments or services either during consultation or at clinic reception. With time, there might be an increase in the number of queries about a particular treatment. It is important to keep track of the pulse of clientele's needs and demands to catch any new trends. Both the medical and the nonmedical staff (especially front-desk, telephone call responder), should be sensitized enough to record these queries for analyses.
- *Google search analytics:* Analysis of Google searches made in a particular geographical area can be studied for certain keywords featuring diseases, treatments, and procedures. This can give an insight into the search and interest patterns of a population. It is important to look out for the correct keywords in this exercise. For example, a patient in a Tier II city in India is more likely to search for words "pimple treatment" instead of "acne treatment."
- *Continuing Medical Exams (CMEs)/ Workshops*: If there are increased and sustained conversations, discussions, or sessions on a certain type of procedure in conferences, it indicates a rising trend. For example, until 2015, most dermatologists in India were probably not even aware of "eyebrow microblading" meant. Now, many national or regional conferences have sessions or workshops on this procedure.
- *Social media feedback*: Many clinics, nowadays have social media presence in form of online profiles/pages where they upload educational videos, blogs and posts. Increased feedback or engagement on post related to a particular condition or treatment can indicate interest patterns. Nowadays, many practices also store databases of patient contact details. Practices could also conduct online surveys through emails in order to assess awareness levels regarding specific services.
- *Peer opinions/analyses*: Well-intentioned experienced practitioners are a wealth of wisdom about patterns and trends in needs and demands. It is always

beneficial to interact with them and gain their insights.
- *Evidence-based medicine/guidelines*: In this era of internet, even patients have access to medical literature published in major journals. There are websites, internet fora, and online support groups which educate patients about medical literature and management guidelines. If there is an overwhelming recommendation of a specific medical service for a particular disorder in published medical literature, especially association guidelines, aware patients sooner or later are going to enquire about that medical service. For example, patients of nonsegmental vitiligo involving a large body surface area, are very likely to enquire about whole-body narrow-band Ultraviolet B (NBUVB) Phototherapy Treatment.

RESPONSE

Sometimes, the above-metioned process can result in a clear-cut trend, pointing toward an overwhelming demand. For an establishment, it is important to respond appropriately on the basis of its understanding of the needs and demands of its clientele. As a strategy, medical establishments need to calibrate their responses as per the following:
- *Defining factors*: The scope and positioning of the medical establishment or the mission statement of the organization can affect its response to a rising demand. A clinical dermatology practice of a tertiary level which takes pride in its core competence is unlikely to respond to increasing queries for facial rejuvenation procedures whereas a focused esthetic dermatology practice may even consider commencing wellness or spa services and evolving into a medical spa-like establishment. An establishment should know its strengths and disposition well.
- *Qualitative factors:* Before responding to an identified trend, its robustness should be properly analyzed. Often, there are some passing "fads of the season" that do not stand the test of time and scientific scrutiny. Practices should look for an established "Proof of Concept" (the medical service has been successfully introduced and is giving positive outcomes in a similar practice and similar population for a prolonged duration) and then work toward adopting the concept.
- *Outcome analysis:* The expected outcomes of introducing a service at a medical practice should be properly analyzed. Both types of outcomes—tangible and non-tangible—should be taken into consideration. Tangible outcomes may include financial profit, increased electricity consumption, increased maintenance or consumable costs, marketing costs, modification of clinic room plans, better patient retention, more new patient enrolment, etc. Non-tangible outcomes include improved positioning of the establishment, better disease management, better patient and physician satisfaction, more word-of-mouth publicity, etc. This type of analyses will also help in deciding the cost of the service (if any), charting a return on investment plan, and judging the short-term and long-term viability of the service. Outcome analyses will also help in monitoring the effect of introduction of the service in the practice.

CONCLUSION

Understanding needs, wants, desires, and demands in practice is not an option but a necessity. Before setting up a dermatology practice, thorough investigation of the prevalent needs and demands will help in laying out the plan, scope, and extent of the establishment. While running a practice, such pursuits will enable us to stay relevant and be more effective care-providers. We may do it informally by keeping ourselves receptive to "sources of information" or adopt a more systematic approach where the information is actively gathered, documented, and periodically scrutinized. Keeping our clientele's interests and requirements at priority can help us introduce scores of positive changes—be it improving patient experience by introducing efficient appointment management systems, imparting patient information materials, etc., or expanding the clinical services available by introducing new medical technologies—and eventually guide our evolution into a more valuable organization.

2.2 How to Choose the Location for Your Clinic?

Rasya Dixit

One of the most important decisions that you make in your career as a private practitioner, is to choose the location of your clinic. This space is where you will spend the maximum time during waking hours, and it will also be a physical representation of you. Also, the location of the clinic will have big impact on the costs and therefore the revenues of the clinic. So, you will need to spend some time to go through some important factors before making your decision.

HOW MUCH SPACE DO YOU NEED?

Before you even start looking for a space, make a list of your present requirements depending on your chosen specialty. For example, if you choose to invest in lasers, you need to have one or two additional rooms as treatment rooms or if you plan on doing hair transplants and dermatosurgical procedures, you may need an operation theater (OT) set up. If you are a fresher, you can consult your seniors to understand the requirements based on your specialty or area of interest.

You will also have to consider any rules and regulations pertaining to minimum space recommendations which may be specific to the state that you are planning the clinic in. For example, starting a pharmacy in the clinic means you need to set aside a minimum of 120 sq ft, below which the license will not be issued. Similarly, the Tamil Nadu Medical Council set a rule that a consultation room should be a minimum of 100 sq ft.[1]

Once you understand the space requirement, it is always advisable to add 20% extra to allow for expansion and growth over the next few years, inorder to avoid moving to a new, bigger set up, every few years.

WHERE SHOULD THE CLINIC BE LOCATED?[2]

The location of the clinic will depend on the patient demographics. Centrally located clinics may be more accessible to patients all over the city, but the cost of real estate rentals may be significantly higher. Looking for a neighborhood which has a good mix of residential and commercial activities, may help in estimating footfalls throughout the day and week. Also, knowledge of demographics such as a patients' age and where they are distributed help junior doctors set up practices in new areas of development, which offer an opportunity to begin with no or minimal competition. It is also important to consider the age demographic of the patients in a particular area. For example, a pediatric clinic is better located in a residential area and a sports orthopedician may do better next to a training area for sport athletes.

Visibility of the clinic is another important factor to consider. A clinic located on the main road which is well visible and easily spotted by moving traffic, helps recall for patients and helps to increase walk-ins. Look for a well-built building with nice exteriors, as this forms part of the first impression for the patient. Nearby landmarks such as financial institutions or important city landmarks help to guide patients to the location easily.

The disadvantage of being on a main road can often be the lack of parking space. Look for a space which offers parking for a few two-wheelers and a couple of cars or at least make sure that safe and easy parking is available nearby. This makes a large impact on the positive experience of the patient as he/she accesses the clinic.

DOES THE NEIGHBORHOOD HAVE RESTRICTIONS ON COMMERCIAL SPACE UTILIZATION?

Knowledge of the city sanction policies, including zoning restrictions as residential, commercial, and semi-commercial areas, is invaluable to the doctor looking for a new clinic space. In every city, there are many restrictions as well as rules to be followed that are laid down by the neighborhood welfare associations. It is prudent to look for a complete commercial space and make sure that all the taxes and occupancy certificates are approved for commercial use before going ahead with the location.

Some doctors prefer the use of their homes for clinics. Though in most cities, this is permitted, it blurs the line between personal and professional space and time and the doctor may always have to be available to the patients. Also, completely commercial spaces offer a professional outlook to the practice and are the preferred choice of most physicians today.

However, make sure that the clinic is close to your residence so you do not have to waste precious time on the commute. An ideal situation is where you can walk to work so that you can enjoy both the work and the home environments.

WHO ARE YOUR NEIGHBORS?

The immediate neighbors play an important role in forming part of the first impression of the clinic. A clinic is expected to be in a clean and hygienic place, and hence, make sure that the clinic surroundings are clean and noise free. See if there are offices or workspaces nearby, so that you can benefit from their employees being your patients.

Having hospitals and doctors of different specialties can be beneficial as cross-referrals are easily possible, increasing footfalls into the practice. Also, nearby hospitals become a good place to refer emergency patients or patients who need more intensive care and cannot be managed at the clinic.

Accessibility of the clinic makes it easy for patients to reach the clinic. Make sure that there are various means of transport to reach the clinic. Locations near bus stops, metro stations, or auto stands make for good landmarks. In a study of insured children and their dental visits, it was noted that closer proximity to the clinics contributed to higher utilization of services.[2,3] However, the increased use of app-based transport solutions has made most locations easily accessible to most of the internet-savvy patients.

Competition analysis is required when starting a clinic is important to know the location of the doctors practicing similar specialties in the nearby vicinity. The increase in the number of doctors increases the options for the patients. Setting up a practice near that of established doctors means that you will have to put in a lot of efforts in carving a space and making a name for yourself.

OTHER FACTORS TO CONSIDER

Having the ground floor space is probably the best for any practice. However, if the space is on the higher floors, there must be provision for a lift. Wheelchair access to a clinic is a very important consideration which not only helps differently abled patients to access services, but also proves very beneficial in case of an emergency to shift out a patient.

HOW MUCH ARE YOU WILLING TO SPEND?

Rent comprises the major portion of your ongoing facilities expense, but consider extras such as utilities—they are included in some leases but not in others. If they are not included, you need to factor them in. Make sure you find out what kind of security deposits will be required, so that you can develop an accurate move-in budget along with the budget that you will require for doing up the interiors of the clinic. As rent is the most important recurring cost, make sure that you have a final budget in mind before you set out to discover your dream location.

REFERENCES

1. Health and Family Welfare Department Tamil Nadu Clinical Establishments (Regulations) Rules, 2018. [G.O. Ms. No. 206, Health and Family Welfare (Z2), 1st June 2018, Vaikasi 18, Vilambi, Thiruvalluvar Aandu - 2049.] No. SRO A-30(b)/2018. In exercise of the powers conferred by sub-section (1) of section 14 of the Tamil Nadu Clinical Establishments (Regulation) Act, 1997 (Tamil Nadu Act 4 of 1997).
2. Griffin PM, Scherrer CR, Swann JL. Optimization of community health center locations and service offerings with statistical need estimation. IIE Transactions. 2008;40(9):880-92.
3. McKernan SC, Pooley MJ, Momany ET, Kuthy RA. Travel burden and dentist bypass among dentally insured children. J Public Health Dent. 2016;76(3):220-7.

2.3 Architecture of a Basic Skin Clinic

Dinesh Kumar D, Namitha Chathra

A well-designed clinic is an amalgamation of form and function. While planning a clinic, it is vital to keep the operational aspect of the clinic in the foreground along with maintaining adequate attention to the esthetics of the clinic. A clinic with a pleasant atmosphere can help in creating a positive first impression in a patient. Ambience of the waiting room, cleanliness of the clinic, and temperament of the staff can tremendously influence patient satisfaction.[1,2] The layout of the clinic should be able to respond to the future demands of services and patient load while meeting the frequent constraint of restricted space and budget. For a dermatologist, the specifications of a clinic vary depending on the services offered. This chapter focusses on the requirements for a standard dermatology clinic.

STANDARD DERMATOLOGY CLINIC

A basic dermatology clinic is adequate for a dermatologist who seeks to establish predominantly prescription-based practice of dermatology (skin, hair, and nail) with the inclusion of a few minor diagnostic and therapeutic procedures. The objective is to treat patients of skin, hair and nail disorders with medical line of management and to do minimal intervention procedures such as punch biopsy, comedone extraction, electro/radiocautery in an office or clinic setting without inpatient services or day care facilities.

SERVICES PROVIDED IN A BASIC DERMATOLOGY CLINIC

- Consultation for skin, hair, and nail disorders and treatment of the same through medical line of management (prescription) and follow-up
- Facilities for diagnostic procedures such as punch biopsy, Wood's lamp examination, dermoscopy, and trichoscopy
- Provision to perform a few minor therapeutic procedures such as comedone extraction and electro/radiocautery
- Optional facilities such as pharmacy, blood collection for laboratory investigations.

CLINIC SPACE

The clinic should be spread over an area of 200–500 sq ft and should comprise of a reception cum waiting area, a consultation room, and a procedure room. If there is adequate space, there could an area earmarked for dispensing medicines.

Reception cum Waiting Area

The Clinical Establishments Act specifies that a clinic should have a reception cum waiting area. The front desk, which is the first zone of interaction between the patient and the clinic staff, should be uncluttered at all times. The seating arrangement for the receptionists should be compact yet comfortable. The chairs for the patients have to be arranged in a way that the space is utilized adequately without imparting a claustrophobic feeling to the patients. Neatly arranged latest magazines or newspapers in English and regional languages, playing light music in the background and a television playing neutral content are a few ways to ensure that the patient stays pleasantly occupied during the waiting period. The consultant's name and credentials should be displayed prominently in the reception area and also his/her consultation timings **(Fig. 2.3.1)**.

The patient should be able to easily locate the restroom without any prompting from the clinic staff. Since most people naturally attempt to exit the same way they entered, the entry and exit path should be the same.[3] This will reduce frequent and repetitive questions which may hinder clinic flow.

In the reception area, if possible, a provision has to be made to dispense medicines.

Consultation Room

The Clinical Establishments Act mandates that a consultation room should not

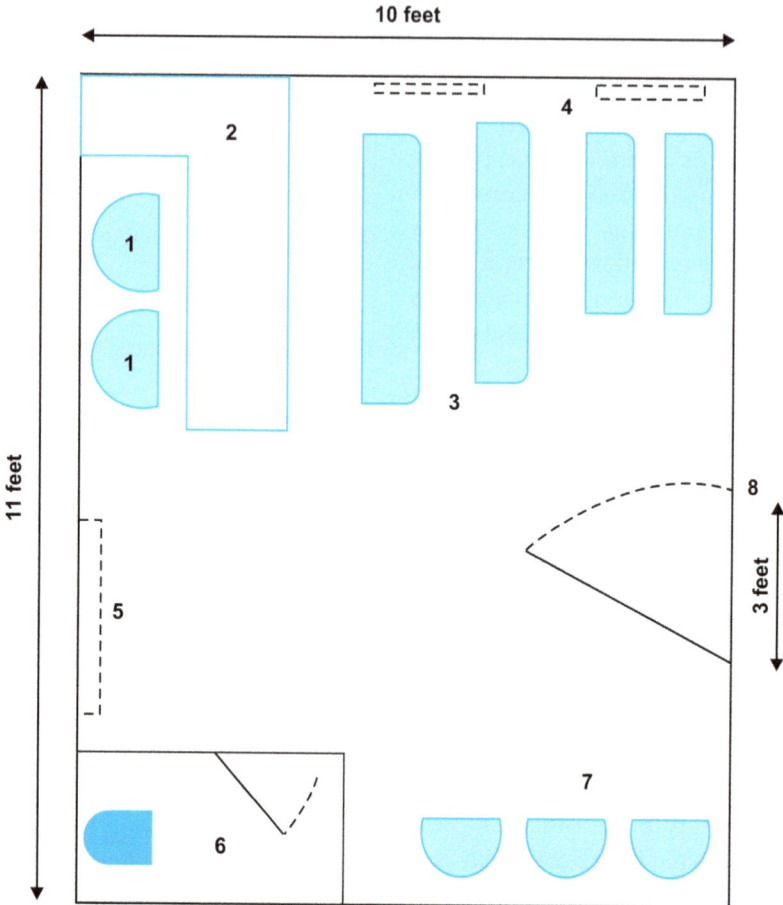

Fig. 2.3.1: Example of a reception area layout: (1) Compact yet comfortable chairs for the front desk staff. The wall behind serves as a display area; (2) Front desk with attached storage—5 feet (W) × 3 feet (D); (3) Patient seating area; (4) Wall-mounted magazine rack; (5) Entry to the consultation room; (6) Toilet—4 feet (D) × 3 feet (W); (7) Additional seating area; (8) Common entry and exit.

be <100 sq ft in size and should harbor sufficient light and ventilation.[4] The room should have a comfortable desk and chair for the doctor, a revolving stool for the patient, and chairs for the patient's attendants. There should be an examination bed, accompanied by floor-length curtains which can be drawn when in need of privacy. It is recommended to install a wash basin and a tap in the consultation room. An examination lamp is another necessary fixture in the consultation room. Readers can refer to the sample layout plan **(Fig. 2.3.2)** and modify according to the configuration of the available space.

Procedure Room

In a procedure room, a bed with an adjustable headrest is of great convenience. The emergency medicines should be stored in an accessible manner, preferably on a mobile trolley. The trolley can also be used to station equipment. The equipment and materials needed for simple procedures are

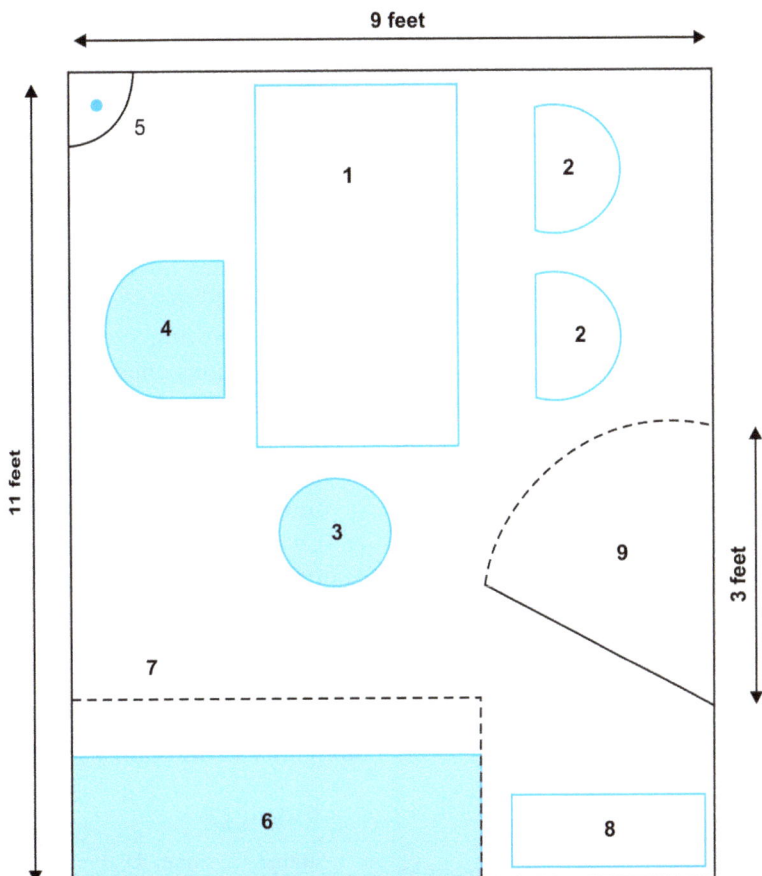

Fig. 2.3.2: Layout of a consultation room meeting the minimum space requirement criteria: (1) Table cum storage area—5 feet × 2.5 feet; (2) Chairs for patient and the attenders; (3) Revolving stool for the patient; (4) Revolving chair for the doctor; (5) Wash basin with a wall-mounted mirror; (6) Examination bed/adjustable chair—6 feet × 3 feet; (7) Drawable curtains; (8) Storage area; (9) Door with an automatic closer—3 feet wide to accommodate wheelchairs.

mentioned below and these can be stored safely in a sterile manner in a cupboard in the room. The storage area should be away from areas of high patient traffic and should have stringent safety measures to prevent access to unauthorized individuals.

If there is no provision for a separate procedure room, these can be incorporated within the consultation room.

Essential equipment for a standard dermatology clinic includes:

- *Diagnostic*: Magnifying lens, Wood's lamp, dermascope, stethoscope, blood pressure apparatus, punch biopsy probes, handheld torch, thermometer
- *Therapeutic*: Electro/radiocautery, minor surgical equipment such as forceps, comedone extractors and scissors
- *Emergency drug kit*: Consisting of adrenaline, atropine, betamethasone/dexamethasone, hydrocortisone, deriphyllin, ranitidine, pheniramine maleate, IV set, syringes, artificial tears, eye drops
- *Miscellaneous*: Digital camera, dark-colored wall to serve a background for

photographs, examination bed, examination or spot light, trolley, consumables (such as slides, gloves, local anesthetic injections, topical anesthetic creams and antibiotic creams), autoclave, formalin chamber, weighing apparatus, mirror

- *Computer/laptop:* Preferably two, one in the reception and one in the consultant's room. Computers are essential in the modern clinic to manage the appointment schedules, store the electronic medical records, send mailers and lab reports to patients, maintain accounts, etc. If possible, the consultant can have a CCTV camera in the reception and monitor the activities of the reception in his computer.
- *Stationery:* Visiting cards, patient education or awareness material, receipt books, etc.
- *Housekeeping materials:* Toiletries, tissue papers, room fresheners, etc.

MISCELLANEOUS TIPS

- An exclusive phone number for the clinic is a must.
- There should be an intercom connection between the consultation room and the reception area so that the doctor need not hunt for staff to give verbal orders. Alternatively, a light signaling system or electronic health record may be used to transmit the information.
- The secretary must be trained to instruct the patients on nearby parking options and the availability of the restroom facilities in the building.
- The clinic must be accessible by a wheelchair and there should be enough space for its mobility.[3]
- The Medical Council of India (MCI) code of ethics regulations considers it improper for a physician to use an "unusually large" signboard and write on it anything other than his name, qualifications obtained from a university or a statutory body, titles and name of his specialty, and registration number including the name of the State Medical Council under which it is registered.

A well thought-out plan that reckons the available finances and the intended nature of practice is instrumental for successful and smooth functioning of the clinic. Remember that those who plan well do better than those who do not, even if they rarely stick to the plan.

REFERENCES

1. Renzi C, Abeni D, Picardi A, Agostini E, Melchi CF, Pasquini P, et al. Factors associated with patient satisfaction with care among dermatological outpatients. Br J Dermatol. 2001;145(4):617-23.
2. Smith RJ, Lipoff JB. Evaluation of dermatology practice online reviews: Lessons from qualitative analysis. JAMA Dermatol. 2016; 152(2):153-7.
3. Wang JV. Layout and flow of dermatology clinics: principles from operations management. Dermatol Online J. 2018;24(4).
4. The Clinical Establishments (Registrations and Regulations) Act, 2010.

2.4 Designing an Esthetic Clinic

Madhuri Agarwal

INTRODUCTION

Esthetic medicine is an amalgamation of the science of clinical, corrective, and surgical dermatology. With recent advances and dynamicity in medical esthetics industry, starting a new esthetic practice can be exciting and challenging at the same time for a dermatologist.

There is no universally accepted definition for esthetic medicine as of today. The American Board of Cosmetic Surgery has characterized corrective surgery as "a subspecialty of medicine and surgery that exceptionally limits itself to the upgrading of visual appearance through surgical and nonsurgical techniques. It is particularly concerned with keeping up one's physical appearance, enhancing it, progressing toward an artistic level."[1,2]

The aim of designing an esthetic clinic should be to create an exclusive and personalized place for your esthetic patients. Interior and architecture of a clinic is the focus point of an esthetic clinic. All the elements of a clinic, from the layout, color scheme, décor to lighting, should be designed to put the patients at ease in the clinic environment.

FOUNDATION/EARLY STAGES, PLANNING/CONCEPTION

Before proceeding with any structural work, spend time in understanding and researching the kind of clinic space and functionality you want to create in your esthetic clinic. Esthetic clinic presentation is a little different from the regular outpatient clinics. It has to look more appealing and artistic with touch of warmth and comfort to the patient. It has to be spacious and well lit with suitable bright colors.

The vibe of the clinic should be such that it makes the patient look forward to visit again. Use of newer themes and materials will help in planning such a clinic.

Some tips that help to start the process of clinic planning are as follows:
- Choose a template and trailor according to your needs by visiting various websites on line.
- All the ideas that crops in the mind should be jot down, about the color and appearance. This would help in conceptualizing the final look while finalizing the project with the architect.
- While planning, it is also important to assess how the space will function, where each room should be positioned, and which equipment will be placed in each room. I had multiple meetings with my architect and design consultant. We drew each room plan on paper, put down furniture of every room, the machines that will be placed in every room, how the waiting room and consulting rooms movement will flow seamlessly, the free space, the door clearance, the position of reception and back office, product display, pharmacy, etc. Since esthetic treatments require privacy, a glass door partition was planned to separate the waiting and consultation area from the treatment rooms. If you have adequate space, plan a separate exit for the high-profile patients

who seek confidentiality with regard to their visits and treatment. An essential point to remember is that males are increasingly seeking esthetic treatments. Therefore, the interiors of an esthetic clinic must be designed to have a unisex appeal and not too feminine.

Location

Location is one of the prime requisites while setting up an esthetic clinic. The clinic can be located on a plush street or on a byway, but the most important aspect is its visibility and whether it is well connected.

Logo and Concept

Logo is the face and recall value of an esthetic clinic. Tailor-made professional logo and clinic concept catches the attention of patients. It also gains the trust and confidence of patients and imbibes a feeling of familiarity in patients. A theme or concept-based architecture of the clinic looks professional and attractive.

THE CLINIC PLAN

The key elements that are to be kept in mind while planning the design of a clinic are given in the following text.

Reception or Waiting Room

This is the area that can create a positive first impression in your patients and it also provides the best opportunity to put them at ease. The seating has to be in a manner such that there is proper balance of making the best use of available space, providing adequate personal space, and comfort of seating (**Fig. 2.4.1**). The choice of marketing material is very crucial as you will have a diverse crowd of patients coming to your clinic. At times, the person accompanying

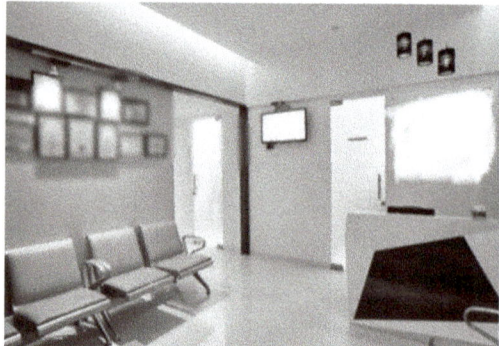

Fig. 2.4.1: A well-planned waiting room is essential.

the patient can also be your potential patient. Hence, the information displayed in the waiting area must be versatile enough to take care of all concerns. You can have a smart television that showcases your procedure videos and products seamlessly. It can also be compiled from different online and media sources. A regular floor unit or a floating wall unit can be fixed in the waiting room that is at an eye level to exhibit your brochures, pictures, products, etc. This assists to increase the clinic portfolio awareness in patients and adds to your product sales.

Office

An important part of the clinic, this space is required for patient records, daily clinic operation materials, billing documents, relevant official documents, and marketing materials.

Storage

There is a need for a secure space where you can keep your treatment stock such as peels, fillers, and botulinum toxin locked and out of easy access. You will require space to store your fumigator, incubators, and autoclave. There has to be provision for a laundry unit where the dirty towels, uniforms, and gowns can be stored for washing.

Staff and Pantry Room

A room where your staff can change their uniforms, groom, take a break, and eat their meals is a desirable. In an esthetic clinic, patients opting for procedures such as laser hair removal and hair transplant will have to stay in the clinic for a long period of time. Having a provision for a small pantry will help in serving refreshments such as tea and coffee which will put them at ease.

Closure Room

Esthetic patients are usually uncomfortable in discussing their treatment, financials, and payments in a waiting or reception room with people around them. Hence, a place where the billing can be done discreetly makes a huge difference. This is a place where your clinic staff can use to address any patient queries and share package details, and at times certain elite patients can wait for their appointments in privacy.

Photography Space

As before and after photos are essential in esthetics, a space with adequate lighting and a dark, nonreflective background can be planned. It can be a treatment room that doubles up as a photography room if there is space constraint.

Pharmacy

A pharmacy that stocks the products of your choice is a great add-on and convenient for your patients. Try to position the pharmacy near the exit of the clinic or at the reception. This makes it easy for patients to access the pharmacy and boosts your retail sales. In the planning stage, check the regulatory mandatory rules for setting up the pharmacy.

Restrooms

This is essential again for patients who are in your clinic for long periods of time. An esthetically made restroom with good hygiene is a necessity.

Hair Transplant Room and Hair Wash Space

In case your practice offers hair transplant, you will require to plan a hair wash station. The restroom can be modified to include a hair wash area if there is space constraint. You can design the hair transplant room in a manner that it is not intimidating and offers a sense of comfort and well-being to the patient.

Treatment Rooms

This is the heart of your clinic where your patients spend their maximum time after consultation. The rooms should be designed to have a positive vibe with fresh, relaxing colors and comfortable beds. If you have sufficient space, you can allocate rooms for different technologies (**Fig. 2.4.2**). Hair removal lasers have to be set up in a separate room as they require specific cooling controls, electricity set up, and varying hygiene levels. A room can be allocated for minimally invasive procedures such as botulinum toxin, dermal fillers, and threads. Procedures performed with energy-based devices and other lasers can be given the third room, and a fourth room can be allocated for medifacials and relaxing treatments. Ideally, a minimum of five to six rooms are recommended to divide and house different treatments. In case there is paucity of space, the same room can be used for multiple treatments. The different technologies can be stored in an adjacent small room and brought to the treatment room when required.

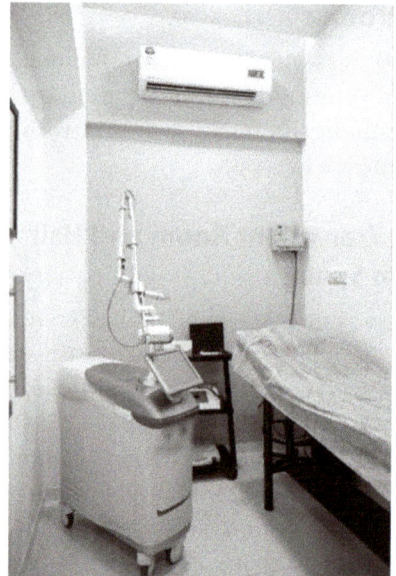

Fig. 2.4.2: Separate rooms for individual technologies and machines.

Furniture

The layout of the clinic should be planned to respond to the future demands of expansion of services and patient load. This helped us to keep newer laser machines along with the existing equipment in a room at the same time. Decorative items and artwork can be placed strategically to add to the ambience. Potted plants and greenery also add a soothing touch. The reception counter must be at a comfortable height and allow patients to easily approach and talk to the receptionist. The counter should provide sufficient cover to the clinic front desk so that confidential work can be carried out discreetly. Appropriate arrangements have to made to help patients fill the clinic forms comfortably.

Flooring

As the clinic will have a regular inflow of a variety of people, the flooring should be durable to withstand it and not look worn out with time. Since the clinic has to adhere to strict hygiene practices, the floors have to be disinfected and cleaned frequently throughout the day. It is advisable to have a hardwood or nonslippery flooring that is esthetically pleasing and sturdy.

Lighting

Appropriate lighting is crucial to enhance the ambience and to maintain the patient`s comfort in the clinic. A poorly lit room will appear unwelcoming to patients. Lighting serves two purposes in an esthetic clinic— to produce a visual impact and the regular utilitarian purpose. The lighting in the waiting room should be warm and less bright to evoke a sense of calm in the waiting patients. I have added a mix of lower power white LEDs with shadow lights in my waiting room to dispel the clinical image. Identify sources of natural light and maximize their use in clinic spaces such as reception, staff room, and certain treatment rooms. Natural light adds to the alertness and feel good vibes in the clinic. Consultation and treatment rooms require bright, strong lights. Avoid strong ceiling lights in treatment rooms where the patient has to be lying flat and looking up at the ceiling for long periods of time. You can have provision for soft lights in the room where you plan to conduct medifacials or make the patients sit with numbing cream for procedures. Mobile focus lights can be added in rooms for injectable and minor dermatosurgery procedures.

Client Record Management

Cloud-based software is ideal for the management of patient records and storing clinic data such as details of the stock, utilized billings, and employee details. It is prudent to have a hard copy as backup. The system should also have the option of recording and retaining patient treatment photographs in a systematic manner. It should also have easy accessibility for future use.

Technology and Treatments

The clinic should display expertise in all aspects of dermatology and esthetics by keeping up with all the recent advances. Make sure that you are offering the best treatment to the patient by investing in the right technology and equipment.

Medical esthetic practice diverges into medical practice and the cosmetic boutique. The medical practice caters to dermatology complaints, surgical procedures, and treatments for skin disorders. The cosmetic boutique focuses on providing cosmetic skin and hair care consultations and treatments to those patients who desire more youthful, wrinkle free, and healthy skin and hair. You can plan to offer a bouquet of treatments ranging from medifacials and microdermabrasion to advanced options such as injectables and transplant.

Start with basic esthetic procedures; steadily gain new skills and once confident, gradually upgrade to advanced procedures. It is often sensible to rent technologies till the clinic has a steady flow of patients before investing in them.

PEARLS

- Invest time in understanding and researching the kind of clinic space and functionality you want to create before embarking on actual work.
- Ensure adequate privacy in the clinic with the use of glass door partitions.
- Consider gender neutral themes while designing the interiors of the clinic.
- Create dynamic spaces with modular furniture to facilitate future expansion plans.
- Color and lighting should be customized according to the space and to put the patients at ease and optimize the functionality.

CONCLUSION

Steve Jobs rightly said "You got to start with the customer experience and work back towards technology-not the other way round." The design of an esthetic clinic is pivotal for its success. It defines and differentiates the clinic experience of patients. The focus of design should be to conceptualize a place with a unique esthetic individuality, reflection of your values and ideology, and a vision of future clinic evolution. A unique and special patient experience is what marks the long-term success of an esthetic clinic.

REFERENCES

1. Chang D. 6Rs of aesthetic medicine. Cosmetol Oro Facial Surg. 2018;4:e108.
2. Sachdev M, Britto GR. Essential requirements to setting up an aesthetic practice. J Cutan Aesthet Surg. 2014;7:167.

2.5 Ideal Practice (Clinic) Management Software

Prashant Palwade

INTRODUCTION

As a medical graduate we are well versed with medical textbooks, medical terminologies, and diseases, their treatments, and procedures. We are trained for that and we keep upgrading ourselves on it. As medical professionals, we are utilizing our knowledge as per our potential. But that is not sufficient enough to run a clinic, hospital, or an institute. One needs a system which takes care of patient appointments, patient records, billing, hospital purchases and expenses, financial reports, patient photographs, laboratory reports, staff records, and many more. We are not trained for all this and everyone goes though a learning curve and comes out with his or her own unique method to handle it. With increasing workload, it becomes cumbersome to handle all this. With advances in computer science, which have touched every aspect of our lives, health sector has been witnessing a "sea of changes" in its working pattern. Many multispecialty hospitals have installed customized software to manage appointments, prescription generation, and record keeping. With rapidly evolving technology, there is emerging need to shift from manual methods of administration of clinics to a full-fledged software handling your clinic.

WHY IS CLINIC MANAGEMENT SOFTWARE REQUIRED?

A clinic management software for a medical practitioner is required for following reasons:

- Registering patients with unique registration numbers
- Storing all the medical information related to patient
- Generating prescription with instructions in local language
- Billing for the services offered including all relevant taxes
- Storing images in relation to the respective patient
- Retrieving all the patient-related information whenever required
- Analysis of data financially and disease wise

The records in software stays for a longer period of time compared to the hand written records and can be retrieved at a click of button. This helps in patient management to a great extent.

WHAT SHOULD CLINIC MANAGEMENT SOFTWARE IDEALLY DO?

Clinic management software should be tailored to suit every individual person's working pattern. It should be able to handle all the work related to clinic functioning.

A clinic management software should have the following features:

Registering Patients

Registering patients in the software with respect to name, age, sex, mobile number, city, birth date, and type of visit (new case/follow-up/procedure). A specific registration number should be assigned to every patient. Also one should be able to enroll multiple patients using same mobile number. This page should be visible at both the reception and doctor end. This is helpful in some situations where a physician has to enroll patients, e.g., when a person accompanying the patient wants to take an additional consultation or in the absence of a receptionist. The patient registration data should be modifiable at both reception and physician end. This helps to correct spelling or any other mistakes in the data filled. Enrollment of patient using birth date helps to calculate age of patient automatically and also with every passing year the age keeps changing in the software, so that one need not change it manually. If one desires, a birth day message can be sent to the patient on that particular date. Once a patient is registered in the system, patient details are reflected on doctor screen. Time of enrollment should also be visible so that one knows at what time a particular patient has arrived and this way we can calculate average waiting time for patients in our OPD. In addition, the software should be able to tell, depending on prefilled time per consultation, likely time when patient would be taken for consultation. This feature helps patient plan his other works and then come for consultation at approximate time calculated by the software.

Searching Data

The software should have a search field where patients can be searched by their name, mobile number, or by specific registration number generated by the software. This feature should be available at both the ends. This feature helps to enroll follow-up patients in a fraction of second and all previous records of the enrolled patient should be visible to the physician when clicked. During enrollment of follow-up cases coming directly for procedures, there should be a system wherein the procedure enlisted in the software is selected and a bill is generated as per procedure bill already filled in the software. This feature helps save time and speeds up the system. One should be able to search patients by diagnosis as well. This helps to list, identify, or contact all patients suffering from a particular disorder.

Writing Prescription

Once a patient is enrolled, there should be a single window to enter all findings related to health condition of that person. It should include general health parameters such as pulse rate, blood pressure, respiratory rate, weight, height, general examination, and systemic examination. Then it should have skin-specific parameters to detail the history such as complaints, history, skin examination, investigations, and diagnosis. There should also be a column to write a special comment if one wants to add and does not want it to be printed in the prescription. The drug list specific to the specialty should be readily available in the software database. The drug list should have a generic name and a trade name in the bracket or vice versa as per physician's choice. If a drug name is not in the software database, one should be able to add it right there and should be saved for future use. Once a drug name is entered in the field, the specific instruction stored as per choice of physician for that drug should appear in the instruction field. The instruction should come on the screen in English and should be modifiable at physician's wish. If there is no instruction assigned to the drug, then one can add instruction right there without going back to the software database. After instruction, there should be a field for number of days of treatment and quantity of medications to be dispensed. There should be field for general instructions wherein instructions related to a particular disorder, dietary habits, and specific precautions related to a particular disorder are written and appear on prescription paper in a language the patient understands. There should be field for follow-up visit wherein a date appears by default as fixed earlier in the software as per physician's choice. This date should be modifiable. Once everything is filled, prescription should be saved and previewed for confirmation before one orders printing.

Adding Procedures

While writing prescription, there should be a separate field in the same window for procedures. It should have two parameters—suggested procedure and procedure done and its details. In suggested procedure, one should be able to write whatever procedure has been suggested and costing for the same if required. In the procedure done, prefilled procedure details should come such as name of procedure, area treated, parameters of the procedure, charges, discount in rupees or percentage, goods and services tax (GST) or any other taxes, and a field for comment like number of sessions for the same procedure. The procedure details and its charges should be prefilled in the system so that adding procedure should be an easy job. One should be able to add multiple procedures in the same field. Also there should be a field to add packages if one is doing procedures as package. Once all the necessary fields are filled, the page should be saved and one should be able to print all clinical details related to this in the area below routine prescription fields.

Image Capturing, Linking, and Retrieving

Ideally, the software should be able handle this in the simplest possible way. An image should be clicked with a camera and once submitted should automatically be attached to patient's records with patient name, diagnosis, and date. On follow-up, all the images should be available for comparison. This is possible with a mobile app and an internet connection which transfers images to the software. One should be able to download or share images from the software as well for communication with others. One should be able to retrieve images for a particular disorder or for a particular patient at any point in time.

Follow-up

Once a follow-up case is entered in the software, one should be able to see all previous follow-up visits as per date and could see all past prescriptions as well, if required. The prescription field should show last prescribed drugs with instructions, days, and quantity prescribed along with general instructions and procedures done. If one wants to keep the same prescription, one should just click print, if not then, one should make whatever modifications required and print with a follow-up date. This way, adding follow-up data would be an easy job.

Billing

At the end of printing prescription, one should bill the patient as per consultation and/or procedure. The billing should be done at physician end and/or at the reception end. The billing window should show all chargeable heads along with discounts given and taxes applicable and a final figure in numbers and letters should be visible. The entire bill to be printed should be available for preview before printing.

Appointments and Managing Waiting Patients

There should be a system in the software to enroll patients as per timing and it should show all appointments in different color codes or as per appointment time. The prefixed appointments can be limited to a certain number as per physician's choice. There is another system wherein patient registers with the software through an app and can take appointment as per available slot shown by the software. One should be able to restrict such appointments to a certain number to avoid more time committed working and give preference to walk-ins depending upon type of practice. There is another system wherein a virtual queue is created and patients can download the app and check real-time changing consultation time. If a physician is late or in a procedure, he/she can pause the queue and the notification regarding the same goes on patient's app and he/she can schedule his arrival to the clinic accordingly. Alternatively, the software should be able to give approximate waiting time to the patient depending on time per consultation fixed in the software.

Analysis

The software should be able to give financial analysis for chosen dates. It should show clinic-wise collection for the date, collection from procedures, GST collected, and a total amount collected for the day. It should also show expenses added to it for the day and a final amount, if deposited in bank, and its details. At the end of the month, one should be able to take out a report of amount collected per day, expenses, taxes collected, and amount deposited in bank, so that auditing accounts becomes an easy affair.

OFFLINE SOFTWARE

The offline software runs within the clinic setup with one server and other computers in LAN (Local Area Network) with it. As the name suggests, it works without internet connection. So it is independent of internet speed. The software has to be installed in the computer physically before it starts functioning. It is usually onetime investment with or without maintenance chances. For any trouble shooting, the service person has to get connected to the system through specific software or physically solve the problem. It cannot be used on all operating systems. Based on its program language, it can be used in specific versions of operating system. It is important to use the version of operating system compatible with the software. Data backup is important as any malfunctioning of the system may lead to loss of all the data. As the data increases, there are chances of software showing decreased speed.

ONLINE SOFTWARE

It is a web-based application, which runs on internet only. It works on any internet-connected device, be it desktop, laptop, tablet, or a mobile phone. It works on all operating systems. The speed of software depends on internet speed. If there is no internet connection the software can not function. All the data is stored in cloud system located at remote destinations within the same country or any other country. Data can be accessed from any place anywhere. One has to check the security parameters of data storage. High levels of data security assure safety of data. Even if the local operating system gets corrupt, the data is safe at remote locations.

DATA SAFETY

The concerns of data safety are more often talked about online software as in these software data is stored at remote locations. There are data safety norms and if the service provider adheres to it, it should not be a major issue. One should read the data safety part of service agreement carefully.

Offline versions are seemingly well protected against data theft, but the service provider can have access to all the data during repairs and upgradation of the software. Hence, it is matter of ethics that a service provider follows, be it an online or offline software. One whom you can trust is the one whom you should go ahead with and use the services from.

DISADVANTAGES OF A SOFTWARE

There is a slight learning curve for practitioners who are not well versed with computers. So the time required for typing, filling details, and finally taking out a prescription may take a little longer in the initial phase. But with time, as the clinician gets used to the system, the time required is much lesser than usual.

While one is typing on computer system eye-to-eye contact with the patient may be lost. But that usually happens in the initial phase. But with time, as prescription is ready in a short while, there is more time to interact with patient.

If data is not protected and saved, there is possibility of data loss or data theft.

As data increases the server may get slower unless upgradations are done periodically.

CHOOSING A SOFTWARE (TIPS AND PEARLS)

While choosing a Practice Management Software, it is important to go through the positives and negatives of both offline as well as online softwares. Unless one reads and understands both the types, one will never be able to understand the benefits of the software for enhancing practice and making it more organized. One has to invest some time understanding it and then trying it in practice.

Those with internet issues should go for offline software. Understanding the utility of it, using it regularly, regular data back up, and upgrading it with time are important aspects of it to get the maximum out of the software. All technical issues have to be solved manually by the service provider at the site, either personally or through internet access to the server.

Those who are comfortable using internet, an online software will be of great use. Space constraint in hard disk is not an issue with it. As it can be accessed from any corner of the world, virtually all the data is with you and is available at the click of a button from any device. The data is password protected and you can change the password as you wish. Communicating with patients and organizing images becomes much easier. All software upgrades happen from the server at remote place and all users get the upgrades at one go, as against in the offline software, where one has to upgrade it manually at every user's server.

WHAT IS THE FUTURE?

With advances in computer science and information technology and with the advent of artificial intelligence (AI), it is a high time we gear up ourselves and start using software for managing our practice. Using web-based software, a patient app, and a physician app to coordinate working of your practice will go a long way in organizing your practice in times to come. The AI may help us getting close to the diagnosis depending on patients signs and symptoms, it may help us monitor patient who are on drugs which require regular monitoring by regularly sending reminders of the laboratory tests to be done, and it can help us give an alarm about the likely side effects of a drug, a patient is on by popping up a window of its side effects. The AI may help us and patients by reminding of the dosage schedule of the drugs. The list is unending and it will keep increasing. It will definitely add to our clinical expertise and help manage our patients better.

2.6 Accreditation

Venkataram Mysore, Bhanu Prakash

INTRODUCTION

The demand for quality in healthcare services is rising constantly due to factors such as insurance, corporate hospitals, and competition. Social media highlighting numerous instances of poor patient care, medical negligence, inadequate resources and facilities, lack of information, and suspicion about unwanted medical interventions have led to increased friction, mistrust, and plethora of medicolegal cases (MLCs) thus creating a huge gap between the service provider and the receiver. In India, the problem is further worsened by the fact that different types of healthcare organizations and institutions deliver different levels of patient care—government hospitals, private clinics, NGO hospitals, medical colleges and hospitals, corporate hospitals, AYUSH (Ayurveda, Yoga & Naturopathy, Unani, Siddha, Sowa Rigpa and Homoeopathy) clinics and hospitals, etc. Several acts and regulations were created to check the allegations and assure patient safety. Chief among them were: *The Consumer Protection Act; The Clinical Establishment Act; The Insurance Companies Regulation; empanelment policies adapted by agencies such as Directorate General of Health Services (DGHS), Ex-servicemen Contributory Health Scheme (ECHS), corporates, and MNCs; Medical Tourism; and import of patients from outside countries for treatment in India.*

There are no exceptions for Dermatologists. The lack of awareness or concern for the developments will harm us in a great way. We are dealing with cosmetology where people come with great and unrealistic expectations and deal with drugs which can cause many adverse effects sometimes leading to a lot of morbidity and sometimes even to mortality. Unless we learn to accept this reality and turn into an evidence-based and ethical practice, it is a matter of time before we head into a plethora of medicolegal cases.

To overcome these problems, to improve effectiveness, to reduce errors and cost of the care, and finally to increase patient safety, a quality assurance mechanism has been created through various accreditation systems. The systems in the accreditation process help improve access, affordability, efficiency, quality of health care, and cost-effective care. Healthcare services can acquire accreditation through various national and international bodies such as NABH, JCI, ISO, ISQua, and CRISIL Rating. Among the various accreditation systems, the NABH accreditation evolved by the Quality Council of India is the most popular and standard form. It is the principal accreditation system for hospitals in India.

The National Accreditation Board for Hospitals and Healthcare Providers (NABH) is defined as "A self-assessment and external peer assessment process used by healthcare organizations to accurately assess their level of performance in relation to established standard and then to implement ways to continuously improve it."

Table 2.6.1: NABH standards.

Patient-centered standards	Organization-centered standards
Access, Assessment and Continuity of Care (AAC)	Continuous Quality Improvement (CQI)
Care of Patient (COP)	Responsibility of Management (ROM)
Management of Medication (MOM)	Facility Management and Safety (FMS)
Patient Right and Education (PRE)	Human Resource Management (HRM)
Hospital Infection Control (HIC)	Information Management System (IMS)

HISTORY

The idea of standardization is more than a century old when in 1917, the American College of Surgeons established a set of minimum standards for hospitals. In 1951, the American College of Surgeons joined several other professional associations to form the Joint Commission on Accreditation of Hospitals. Accreditation has assumed importance only in the last two decades since the establishment of NABH in 2006.

The first edition of standards was released in 2006 and after that the standards have been revised every 3 years. Currently, the 4th edition of NABH standards, released in December 2015, is in use.

NABH guidelines are composed of 10 chapters. These chapters project all departments of a hospital for delivering standard care. Among these 10 chapters, 5 are patient centered and 5 organization centered **(Table 2.6.1)**. Each chapter has got specific standards (105 in whole). Each standard has certain "Objective elements," 683 as a whole.

NABH conducts various accreditation and certification programs to nearly 21 types of HCOs. Since we dermatologists practice more in clinics or in polyclinics, this chapter focuses on the accreditation program in this category, called Allopathic Clinic.

STANDARDS FOR ACCREDITATION OF CLINICS PRACTICING MODERN SYSTEM OF MEDICINE (ALLOPATHIC)

Section 1—Standards for Accreditation of Clinics Practicing Modern System of Medicine (ALLOPATHIC):
01. Access, Assessment and Continuity of Care (AAC)
02. Care of Patients (COP)
03. Patient Rights and Education (PRE)
04. Infection Control (IC)
05. Continuous Quality Improvement (CQI)
06. Responsibilities of Management (ROM)
07. Facility Management and Safety (FMS)
08. Community Participation and Integration (CPI)

Section 2—Guidebook to Standard for Accreditation of Clinics: Modern System of Medicine (Allopathy) Practicing:
01. Access, Assessment and Continuity of Care (AAC)
02. Care of Patients (COP)
03. Patient Rights and Education (PRE)
04. Infection Control (IC)

05. Continuous Quality Improvement (CQI)
06. Responsibilities of Management (ROM)
07. Facility Management and Safety (FMS)
08. Community Participation and Integration (CPI)

For convenience, the standards are grouped into eight chapters with the same headings as described above.

Section 1 comprises chapters having a description which explains its purpose. Each chapter contains a number of standards and objective elements which indicate the structures and processes necessary to deliver the standard.

Section 2 gives a brief detail of the objective elements providing interpretation and remarks. It explains the objective element and methods to achieve the same wherever possible.

Definition of clinic: A standalone healthcare facility that provides allopathic services.

Healthcare facility	Definition
Clinic	A standalone healthcare facility for services (other than OPD of a hospital)
Polyclinic	A clinic which provides services in two or more areas working in cooperation and sharing the same facilities and specialties
Dispensary	A clinic, which in addition to patient care, provides for dispensing medicines

In addition, a "clinic" may have add-on services such as laboratory, imaging, and other support services like: pharmacy, physiotherapy, nutrition, and counseling.

A clinic shall exclude the following: Daycare centers that have admitting beds; services such as ambulatory surgical procedures, dialysis, and chemotherapy; and includes nonallopathic systems of medicine such as ayurvedic, AYUSH, homeopathic, and wellness centers.

The entire list of licenses and statutory obligations might not be applicable to all the clinics. The clinic operator or owner has the responsibility to identify and update applicable state-level licenses or statutory obligations and maintain them.

1. AERB Act and Rules of Safety Code Building Permit (From the Municipality)
2. No objection certificate from the Chief Fire Officer
3. License/regulations under Biomedical Management and Handling Rules, 1998
4. No objection certificate under Pollution Control Act
5. Radiation Protection Certificate in for all X-ray and CT scanners from Bhabha Atomic Research Center (BARC)
6. Excise permit to store Spirit
7. Income tax PAN
8. Permit to operate lifts under the Lifts and Escalators Act
9. Narcotics and Psychotropic Substances Act and License
10. Sales tax registration certificate
11. Vehicle registration certificates for Ambulances
12. Retail drug license (Pharmacy)
13. Wireless operation certificate from Indian post and telegraphs (if applicable)
14. Air (Prevention and Control of Pollution) Act, 1981, and License
15. Arms Act, 1950 (if guards have weapons)
16. Atomic energy regulatory body approvals
17. Biomedical Waste Management Handling Rules, 1998
18. Boilers Act, 1923
19. Cable Television Networks Act, 1995
20. Central Sales Tax Act, 1956
21. Consumer Protection Act, 1986
22. Contract Act, 1982
23. Copyright Act, 1982

24. Customs Act, 1962
25. Dentist Regulations, 1976
26. Drugs and Cosmetics Act, 1940
27. Electricity Act, 1998
28. Electricity Rules, 1956
29. Employees Provident Fund Act, 1952
30. ESI Act, 1948
31. Employment Exchange Act, 1969
32. Environment Protection Act, 1986
33. Equal Remuneration Act, 1976
34. Explosives Act, 1884
35. Fatal Accidents Act, 1855

Most of these above mentioned documents are required if not all. The responsible person should co-ordinate all activities related to accreditation by becoming familiar with the existing standards. A copy of standards can be downloaded from the website www.qcin.org.

PROCEDURE FOR NABH ACCREDITATION

1. Obtain a copy of NABH Standards (From NABH office).
2. Understand the standards and objective elements and implement them.
3. Obtain a copy of application form (From NABH website).
4. Fill and submit the application along with other required documents and application fees (to NABH Secretariat).
5. Acknowledgment and Scrutiny of application by NABH.
6. Assessment of clinic.
7. Review of assessment report.
8. Recommendation for accreditation by AC.
9. Approval for accreditation by NABH Board.
10. Issue of accreditation certificate by NABH Secretariat.

After step 5, feedback to the clinic will be given and necessary corrective action will be taken by the clinic.

QUALIFYING CRITERIA FOR ACCREDITATION

- All the regulatory legal requirements should be fully met.
- No individual standard should have more than one zero to qualify.
- The average score for individual standards must not be less than 5.
- The average score for individual chapter must not be less than 7.
- The overall average score for all standards must exceed 7.

Accreditation to a clinic shall be valid for a period of 3 years. NABH conducts one surveillance of the accredited clinics in one accreditation cycle of 3 years. The surveillance visit will be planned during the 2nd year, i.e., after 18 months of accreditation. As part of surveillance, some reports may be asked by NABH from the accredited clinic from time to time. The clinics should apply for renewal of accreditation at least 6 months before the expiry of validity of accreditation for which reassessment shall be conducted. NABH may call for an unannounced visit, based on any concern or any serious incident reported by an individual or organization or media.

ACCREDITATION TIMELINE (TABLE 2.6.2)

The recommended prior steps are: (1) obtain a copy of NABH standards and guidebook and (2) attend NABH awareness programs conducted by continuous quality improvement (CQI).

BENEFITS OF ACCREDITATION

- To the organization
  - Becomes easier to get empaneled with insurance companies.
  - High-quality patient care and better outcomes enhance word-of-mouth

Table 2.6.2: Accreditation timeline.

Accreditation steps	Approximate timeline
Submission of application (along with fee amount) + self-assessment tool kit + documents + signed copy of terms and conditions	
(a) Registration and acknowledgement to healthcare organization along with unique reference no (b) Reflect same on website	Within 10 days of receiving application form and fees
Preassessment	Within 3 months of fee deposition
Take corrective action and send report to NABH secretariat	Within 3 months of date of assessment
Final assessment	Within 6 months of preassessment
Take corrective action on nonconformities raised during final assessment and send report to NABH secretariat	Within 3 months of final assessment
Review by accreditation committee	
Verification assessment (as and if decided by AC)	
Surveillance assessment	Within 15–17 months of accreditation
Take corrective action on nonconformities raised during surveillance assessment and send report to NABH secretariat	Within 1.5 months of surveillance visit
Reassessment	Before 6 months of expiry of accreditation

publicity, and increases patient numbers, thus leading to increased business generation.
- Provides staff an increased satisfaction with continuous learning, good working environment, leadership, and ownership.
- Focuses on continuous quality improvement.
- All equipment, of regularly maintained and calibrated, reduce operational costs in the long run and ensure patient safety.
- Reliable and certified information on facilities, infrastructure, and level of care.
- Reduces medicolegal issues or cases.
■ To the patients
- High standards of patient care and safety.
- Patient satisfaction is evaluated regularly which results in more courteous staff, less confrontations and better services.
- Rights are respected and protected with better communication.
- Access to organization and staff which have good credentials.

CHALLENGES FOR ACCREDITATION

About 1% of hospitals and nursing home put together have taken up accreditation. The remaining are not able to face the challenges involved. The recent Insurance Regulator and Development Authority of India (IRDAI) move mandating 33,000 hospitals empaneled with it to meet the preaccreditation entry-level standards laid down by the NABH within 2 years should make the HCOs to take up the accreditation program.

NABH has developed *Pre Accreditation Entry Level Certification* standards, in consultation with various stakeholders in the country, as a stepping stone for enhancing the quality of patient care and safety. The aim is to introduce quality and accreditation to the HCOs as their first step toward awareness and capacity building. Once Pre Accreditation Entry Level Certification is achieved, the HCO can then prepare and move to the next stage—*Progressive* level and finally to *Full Accreditation* status. This methodology provides a step-by-step and staged approach, which is practical for the HCOs. The applicant hospital must have conducted self-assessment against NABH Pre Accreditation Entry Level standards after implementing it for at least 3 months before submission of application and must ensure that it complies with the standards.

Organization Challenges

The commitment of the management in implementation is very important in setting up of high standards and following them. Lack of commitment by the top management is a sure recipe for failure of the program. A committed management helps in creating and sustaining motivation among the staff by continuous education to increase the knowledge and skills such as documentation, interaction with patients, problem-solving methods, etc.

Financial and facility resources: The financial cost of accreditation, as the program involves an ongoing continuous program and sustaining, is very important. Importance of infrastructure such as space, machineries, medications, computerization, financial, and other resources can be a threat to the success of this program.

CONCLUSION

The accreditation standard for hospitals helps to focus on patient safety and improve quality of healthcare services and processes. It is the most frequently used external quality assessment of healthcare organizations to prove its effectiveness and performance. As of today, NABH standards serve as the highest benchmark standard for hospital quality care in India. Patients are the biggest beneficiaries of this program.

2.7 Biomedical Waste Management

Bhanu Prakash, Malcom Noronha, Venkataram Mysore

INTRODUCTION

Healthcare waste, also termed biomedical waste (BMW), contains infectious, contaminated, and hazardous waste such as discarded sharps, blood, body parts, toxic chemicals, pharmaceuticals, medical devices, and radioactive substances.

Biomedical waste is defined as "any solid, fluid and liquid or liquid waste, including its container and any intermediate product, which is generated during the diagnosis, treatment or immunization of human being or animals, in research pertaining thereto, or in the production or testing of biologicals and the animal waste from slaughter houses or any other similar establishment." If not managed properly, it carries a substantial risk to the hospital staff, the patients, and the community, public, and environment.

BACKGROUND

According to the World Health Organization (WHO) nearly 85% of all waste generated by hospital is general waste (non-hazardous waste); only about 15% waste is BMW (hazardous waste). Of these, infectious waste accounts for 10% and noninfectious waste such as radioactive and chemical wastes accounts for 5%. But when hazardous waste is not segregated at the source of generation and is mixed with nonhazardous waste, then the entire waste becomes hazardous.

PROBLEM SITUATION

The WHO has estimated that in the year 2000, injections with contaminated syringes caused 21 million hepatitis B virus (HBV) infections, 2 million hepatitis C virus (HCV), and 260,000 HIV infections. In a large tertiary care hospital in India, the waste generated is about 1-2 kg/bed/day as against 2.8 kg/bed/day from a similar sized hospital in USA. There are 198 common biomedical waste treatment facilities (CBMWF) in operation and 28 are under construction. 21,870 health-care facilities (HCFs) use their own treatment facilities. 1,31,837 HCFs use probably shared or common CBMWFs. In India, the BMW problem is compounded by health workers handling healthcare waste with no gloves, masks, or shoes etc. There is also the problem of reuse of syringes and other instruments without appropriate sterilization.

NEED OF BIOMEDICAL WASTE MANAGEMENT

- Injuries from sharps may lead to infection (AIDS, hepatitis, etc.) to hospital personnel, waste handlers, and at times to general public, causing serious threats to human health.
- Poor waste management can lead to nosocomial infections.
- Risk associated due to hazardous chemicals, drugs, and spurious drugs
- Risk of recycling of "Disposables"
- Risk of environmental pollution—air, water, and soil pollution

Thus, hazardous waste can result in infections, genotoxicity, chemical toxicity, radioactivity hazards, and physical injuries etc. This leads to depletion of resources in terms of money, manpower, and materials. Scientific disposal of BMW minimizes the loss of the resources and limits damage to humans.

EVOLUTION OF THE BIOMEDICAL WASTE MANAGEMENT SYSTEM

In a WHO meeting in Geneva, in June 2007, the core principles for achieving safe and sustainable management of health care waste were developed. There are three international agreements and conventions which are particularly pertinent in BMW management. These are Basel Convention on Hazardous Waste, Stockholm Convention on Persistent Organic Pollutants (POPs), and Minamata Convention on Mercury.

BIOMEDICAL WASTE (MANAGEMENT AND HANDLING) RULES, 1998

In India, "Biomedical Waste Management and Handling Rules" were framed and came into force on July 20, 1998. Since then, the onus lies on the health care institutions to ensure proper health care waste management (HCWM). These rules apply to all persons who generate, collect, receive, store, transport, treat, dispose, or handle biomedical waste in any form.

The rules have been modified in 2000, 2003, 2011, 2016 and recently in 2018.

SALIENT FEATURES OF BIOMEDICAL WASTE MANAGEMENT RULES, 2016

Rules have been amended to improve compliance and strengthen the implementation of environmentally sound management of biomedical waste in India.

- The ambit of the rules has been expanded to include vaccination camps, blood donation camps, surgical camps, or any other healthcare activity.
- Phase out the use of chlorinated plastic bags, gloves, and blood bags within 2 years.
- Pretreatment of the laboratory waste, microbiological waste, blood samples, and blood bags through disinfection or sterilization on-site in the manner as prescribed by WHO or National AIDS Control Organization (NACO).
- Provide training to all its healthcare workers and immunize all health workers regularly.
- Establish a Bar-Code System for bags or containers containing biomedical waste for disposal.
- Biomedical waste has been classified into 4 categories instead of 10 to improve the segregation of waste at source.
- Procedure to get authorization simplified. Automatic authorizations for bedded hospitals. The validity of authorization synchronized with the validity of consent orders for bedded HCFs. One-time authorization for nonbedded HCFs.
- The new rules prescribe more stringent standards for the incinerator to reduce the emission of pollutants in the environment.
- Inclusion of emission limits for dioxin and furans.
- State government to provide land for setting up a common biomedical waste treatment and disposal facility.
- No occupier shall establish an on-site treatment and disposal facility, if the service of a common biomedical waste treatment facility is available at a distance of 75 km.
- Operator of a common biomedical waste treatment and disposal facility to ensure the timely collection of biomedical waste from the HCFs and assist the HCFs in conduct of training.

The steps in the management of biomedical waste are as follows **(Flowchart 2.7.1)**:

- Generation
- Segregation
- Collection
- Storage
- Treatment

Flowchart 2.7.1: Management of biomedical waste.

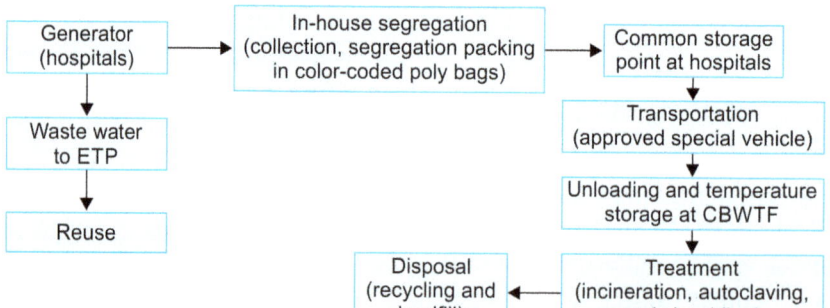

(CBWTF: common biomedical waste treatment facility; ETP: effluent treatment plant)

- Transport
- Disposal

Segregation, pretreatment, collection, storage, and transportation are exclusive responsibilities of an HCF. The CBWTF operator is primarily responsible for treatment and disposal barring laboratory and highly infectious waste which is pretreated by the HCF.

Duties of Occupier (Hospital/Healthcare Facility)

- To provide a safe, ventilated, and secured location for storage of segregated BMW within premises
- As per the Biomedical Waste Management (Amendment) Rules, 2018, use of chlorinated plastic bags (excluding blood bags and gloves) has to be phased out by March 27, 2019.
- Provide training to all its healthcare workers and others involved in handling of biomedical waste at the time of induction and once a year thereafter and maintain records for the same.
- Immunization against hepatitis B and tetanus for workers.
- Establish a Bar-Code System for bags or containers containing biomedical waste to be sent out of the premises by March 27, 2019 as per the Biomedical Waste Management (Amendment) Rules, 2018.
- Maintain and update the biomedical waste management register daily and display the monthly and annual record on website.
- Report major accidents such as needle stick injuries, broken mercury thermometer, accidents caused by fire, and blasts during handling of biomedical waste and the remedial action taken and record the same in Form 1.

Segregation, Packing, Storage, and Transport

- *Biomedical waste is classified into four categories based on treatment options.* BMW should not be mixed with other wastes. It should be segregated into containers or bags at the point of generation and labeled prior to its storage, transportation, treatment, and disposal.
- No untreated BMW shall be mixed with other wastes. Untreated BMW has to be transported only in a vehicle which is authorized by competent authority as specified by the government.
- Untreated human anatomical waste, animal anatomical waste, soiled waste, and biotechnology waste shall not be stored beyond a period of 48 hours.
- If required to store beyond 48 hours, the authorized person must take permission of the prescribed authority and the occupier shall ensure that it does not affect human health and the environment.

Annual Report

- Every occupier or operator of CBWTF shall submit an annual report to the prescribed authority by June 30 every year.
- The prescribed authority shall compile, review, analyze, and report to the CPCB on or before July 31 every year.
- The CPCB shall submit a report on the same to the Ministry of Environment, Forest and Climate Change by August 31 every year.
- The annual reports shall be available on the websites of the occupier.

Maintenance of Records

Records in relation to generation, collection, reception, storage, transportation, treatment, and disposal shall be maintained for 5 years as per rules.

Accident Reporting

In case of a major accident, the authorized person shall intimate immediately and submit a report within 24 hours regarding the remedial steps taken.

SALIENT FEATURES OF BIOMEDICAL WASTE MANAGEMENT (AMENDMENT) RULES, 2018

Biomedical waste generators including hospitals, nursing homes, clinics, dispensaries, veterinary institutions, animal houses, pathological laboratories, blood banks, healthcare facilities, and clinical establishments will have to phase out chlorinated plastic bags (excluding blood bags) and gloves by March 27, 2019.

- All healthcare facilities shall make available the annual report on its website within a period of 2 years from the date of publication of the Biomedical Waste Management (Amendment) Rules, 2018.
- Operators of common biomedical waste treatment and disposal facilities shall establish bar coding and global positioning system for handling of BMW in accordance with guidelines issued by the Central Pollution Control Board (CPCB) by March 27, 2019.
- The State Pollution Control Boards (SPCB)/State Pollution Control Committees (SPCCs) have to compile, review, and analyze the information received and send this information to the Central Pollution Control Board in a new Form (Form IV A), which seeks detailed information regarding district-wise BMW generation, information on healthcare facilities having captive treatment facilities, and information on common biomedical waste treatment and disposal facilities.
- Every occupier, i.e., a person having administrative control over the institution and the premises generating BMW, shall pretreat the laboratory waste, microbiological waste, blood samples, and blood bags through disinfection or sterilization on-site in the manner as prescribed by the WHO or guidelines on safe management of wastes from healthcare activities and WHO Blue Book 2014 and then sent to the common biomedical waste treatment facility for final disposal.

BMW management is guided by rule of Central Pollution Control Board, Ministry of Environment, Government of India, which calls for mandatory registration with appropriate authorities for pollution control and waste disposal. This set of rules might vary from state to state, and dermatologists should consult the concerned authority in their respective states. It is mandatory that all clinics should register with the concerned authorities and engage agencies for waste disposal.

Steps of Biomedical Waste Management

- *Step 1*: Segregation and pretreatment of waste at the site of generation
- *Step 2:* Collection of segregated waste from all areas of the hospital
- *Step 3:* Transportation of waste from various areas of the hospital to storage site
- *Step 4:* Weighing of bags at storage site
- *Step 5:* Transportation for final disposal

Step 1: Segregation and Pretreatment of Waste

Staff should segregate the waste at source in the clinic/hospital into leak proof and puncture proof high density plastic container with proper color-coded polythene bag inside for proper disposal of the generated waste. The biohazard logo should be displayed bold and clear on the containers and bags.

Highly infectious and laboratory waste such a needles and syringes, scalpels, blades and vials are pretreated with 1% sodium hypochlorite and then disposed off in color-coded bags or bins at the site of generation.

Posters detailing a segregation list of items are displayed in each area of the hospital. BMW generated from patients positive for hepatitis or HIV is collected in a separate bag and is labeled as positive along with the area and date of generation.

Categories of biomedical waste:
- *Category 1—Human anatomical waste*: Human tissues, organs, body parts
- *Category 2—Animal waste:* Animal tissues, organs, body parts, carcasses, bleeding parts, fluid, blood and experimental animals used in research, waste generated by veterinary hospitals, colleges, discharge from hospitals and animal houses
- *Category 3—Microbiology and biotechnology waste:* Wastes from laboratory cultures, stocks or specimens of microorganisms, live or attenuated vaccines, human and animal cell culture used in research and infectious agents from research and industrial laboratories, wastes from production of biologicals, toxins, dishes, and devices used for transfer of cultures
- *Category 4—Waste sharps:* Needles, syringes, scalpels, blades, glass, etc., that may cause puncture and cuts. This includes both used and unused sharps
- *Category 5—Discarded medicines and cytotoxic drugs:* Wastes comprising outdated, contaminated, and discarded medicines
- *Category 6:* Solid waste (items contaminated with blood and body fluids including cotton, dressings, soiled plaster casts, line beddings, other material contaminated with blood)
- *Category 7:* Solid waste (waste generated from disposable items other than the waste sharps such as tubing, catheters, intravenous sets, etc.)
- *Category 8—Liquid waste:* Waste generated from laboratory and washing, cleaning, house disinfection by chemical, and disinfecting activities
- *Category 9—Incineration waste:* Ash from incineration of any biomedical waste
- *Category 10—Chemical waste:* Chemicals used in production of biological and in chemical treatment, etc.

A segregation list of common items in hospital as per Biomedical Waste Management Rules 2016 is given in **Table 2.7.1**. This should be noted in English and Hindi.

Containers should be noncorrosive disposable plastic bags or containers of a specific color code. They should be tied with only three-fourth filled. They should not be allowed to overfill. They should be labeled with date of packaging, waste category number, waste class and description, destination, biohazard/cytotoxic symbol, weight of the pack, and emergency contact number. Labels should be nonwashable and prominent **(Fig. 2.7.1)**. Containers should be transported in the hospital by a handcart wheeled trolley. They should be stored in separate rooms.

Step 2: Collection of Segregated Waste

Segregated waste is then collected from all over the hospital in waste trolleys. The frequency of waste collection varies depending on various sections of the hospital—OT/lab/OPD/offices, etc.

Step 3: Transportation of Collected Waste

Waste collected from all over the hospital is transported to the collection site in color-coded, handcart wheeled waste trolleys. The

Table 2.7.1: Color coding and disposal of waste after categorization.

Yellow	Red	White	Blue
• Human anatomical waste • Animal anatomical waste • Soiled waste • Expired or discarded medicines and cytotoxic drugs along with glass or plastic ampoules, vials, etc. • Chemical waste • Micro, biotechnology and other clinical laboratory waste • Chemical liquid waste • Discarded linen, mattresses, beddings contaminated with blood or body fluids	*Contaminated waste (recyclable):* Vacutainers, tubing, bottles, intravenous tubes and sets, catheters, urine bags, syringes (without needles), and gloves	*Waste sharps including metal sharps:* Needles, syringes with fixed needles, needles from needle tip cutter/burner, scalpels, blades	*Broken/discarded glass:* Medicine vials and ampoules except those contaminated with cytotoxic wastes. *Metallic body implants*

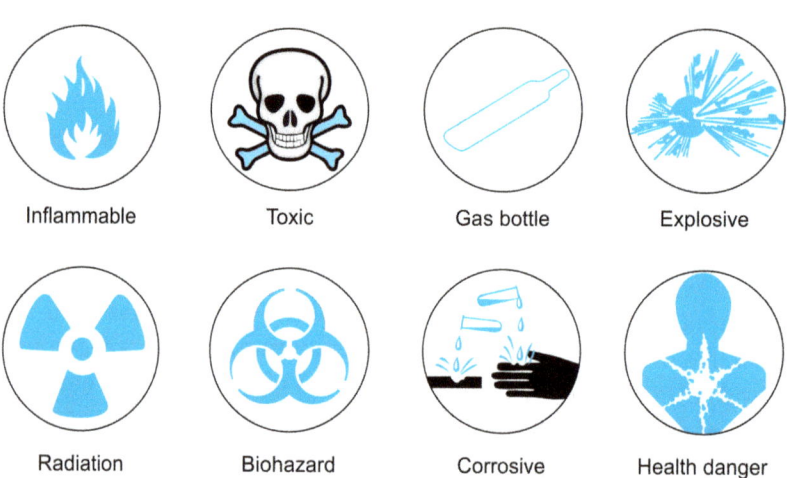

Fig. 2.7.1: Labels of hazard warnings.

workers transporting the waste must use personal protective equipment (PPE) such as boots, gloves, masks, and aprons. The collected waste is not stored for >48 hours.

Step 4: Weighing of Waste Bags

At the collection or storage site, bags are weighed before transportation for final disposal.

Step 5: Transportation for Final Disposal

This is usually done by the external agency.

CONCLUSION

Dermatologists do not contribute much of BMW. Waste generated from lasers, peels, and radiofrequency are minimal but some surgical procedures such as liposuction might lead to generation of significant BMW. Nevertheless, all clinics are supposed to register for BMW disposal under regulations set by the Central Pollution Control Board, Ministry of Environment, Government of India. So, it is important for a dermatologist to be familiar with rules and regulations and procedure of BMW disposal.

SECTION 3
Spreading your Wings

3.1 Group Practice

RG Torsekar, Vishalakshi Viswanath

INTRODUCTION

The changing scenario in the Indian healthcare system has witnessed entry of corporates in a large scale in private practice, which was the domain of individual doctors' clinics, polyclinics, nursing homes, and few large multispecialty hospitals in the past. Technology has played a pivotal role in the evolution of dermatology practice as evidenced by use of newer equipment and information technology, and this has been coupled with higher patient expectations. The subject of dermatology is a blend of disease dermatology (clinical dermatology) and desire dermatology (cosmetic dermatology), and integrating these aspects helps to provide comprehensive dermatological or esthetic solutions to the patients or clients. However, in a private set up, the clinical, entrepreneurial, and managerial skills to address the varied domains professionally and sustain them successfully by a single individual though not impossible, may be daunting. A group practice may be a solution for achieving a successful, sustainable integrated practice.

TRENDS IN DERMATOLOGY PRACTICE

The American Academy of Dermatology (AAD) practice profile survey has shown an increase in female dermatologists and a decrease in the percentage of dermatologists in solo practice (44% in 2005 to 35% in 2014). Solo practice dermatologists are 50 years or older, whereas dermatologists aged 49 years and younger are in group practice. Use of electronic health records and teledermatology is also on the rise.[1]

The business models of dermatology practice are outlined in **Table 3.1.1**. In an office-based private set up, a dermatologist can address the traditional consultation-based practice, cosmetic and surgical components at different levels[2] **(Table 3.1.2)**. Level 3 or integrated dermatology practice is most conducive to a dermatologist-owned group practice. The current trend in Western countries is consolidation of dermatology practices.

Table 3.1.1: Models of dermatology practice.

Models	Practice characteristics
Solo practice	Individual practice at a self-owned or rented place (most common)
Group practice	Single specialty or multispecialty
Corporate-owned	Corporate organization ownership wherein the dermatologist works full time or part time
Integrated healthcare delivery system	Multispecialty hospitals wherein the dermatologist works full time or part time
Others	As part of digital or mobile health technology services

Table 3.1.2: Levels of dermatology practice.

Levels	Practice characteristics
Level 1	A traditional disease-based clinical dermatology practice along with equipment such as hyfrecator, chemical cauterizing agents and other minor equipment
Level 2	A minor focus on cosmetic procedures with use of chemical peels, intense pulsed light (IPL) systems or microdermabrasion
Level 3	A good combination of 'disease and desire' based practice coexists with use of lasers, lights, radiofrequency equipment and injectables along with dermatosurgery
Level 4	Specialization in procedures comprising total cosmetic dermatology practice may be integrated with a plastic surgery or medispa setting

GROUP PRACTICE

A group practice involves:
- Teaming of a diverse group of people
- With complementary abilities
- Who collaborate to accomplish common goals
- For which they are accountable together

A dermatology group practice involves a team of two or more dermatologists. It may be a single-specialty group (only dermatologists) or a multispecialty group (dermatologists with plastic surgeons, dieticians, etc.) practice. Though group dermatology practice in the Western countries has been present since the last century, it has started gaining popularity in India recently. For doctors, forming and running a group practice is however not an easy venture since "organizing doctors is like herding cats because of their fiercely independent spirit and lack of unity."[3] Dermatologists-owned group practice with an equity-based partnership can help in achieving a good integration between clinical and cosmetic dermatology. Based on the our experience, it is possible to provide comprehensive dermatological healthcare services with focus on affordable, ethical, and quality care to all strata of the society under one roof with such a practice model. In contrast to a corporate group owning the practice or being the equity investor, a dermatologist-owned group has direct control on policy decisions.

The most important aspect for long-term sustenance and success of a group practice is the nature of the constituent members. The group should be composed of like-minded individuals committed to quality patient care and development of the organization rather than self; they should have a long-term vision and be committed to achieve the goals together. The group can consist of both young and senior dermatologists; this helps to have a good mix of enthusiasm and experience. At the start of group practice, it is important to delineate the functional and financial terms, strategies, and policies. Dilemmas and differences in opinion with respect to practice management and growth strategies can occur in founders, and this needs to be addressed by brain-storming sessions within the group and by networking with experts in respective fields.

GROUP PRACTICE MANAGEMENT: KEY COMPONENTS

A successful medical practice needs a mixture of science, arts, and commerce. Identifying the 7 Ps are important for setting up a practice.[4,5] For managing a group practice, various aspects need to be addressed—clinical, administrative, human resources, financial, legal, information technology, and marketing. With multiple heads, the management aspects are dynamic and complicated and need continuous monitoring and standardization. The key components to address these complexities in a group are outlined in **Box 3.1.1** and **Figure 3.1.1**.

Financial Aspects[6]

A group practice can adopt various types of business organization models—partnership firm, limited liability partnership, private limited company, or a public limited company. Registration of business needs to be done as per legal norms. Budgeting, risk analysis, return on investment, and good financial practices need to be adopted. In general, a cosmetic dermatology set up

> **Box 3.1.1 : 7 Ps of a group practice.**
>
> 1. *Plan*: Following initiation and development of a like-minded group, planning of policy decisions pertaining to all aspects of practice management is vital.
> 2. *Place*: Location is a key factor for a successful practice and the place needs to be accessible to the clinicians, employees, and most importantly the patients/clients. A larger space may be needed for a group practice compared to other models. Scope for expansion and specialization should be considered, especially in view of the high investment costs and long-term sustenance.
> 3. *Personnel*: Development of a patient or client base is most vital for a successful practice, and this can develop faster when the group consists of a mix of young and senior, experienced dermatologists. Trained medical and administrative staff is essential in a group practice.
>
>   *Medical staff*: The core group can employ qualified dermatologists and physician assistants (nurses/counselors) and establish networks with experts in dermatosurgery, hair restoration surgery, plastic surgeons, dermatopathology, laboratory services, statisticians, and research personnel. By implementing this model, the authors' group practice has been able to provide the patients or clients with ethical, quality care at a one-stop place for their dermatological or esthetic problems.
>
>   *Administrative staff*: The front desk staff and ancillary support staff should be well trained, well groomed, polite and of a pleasant personality. The core group of doctors is responsible for the various practice management aspects (human resources, financial, legal, marketing, information technology, and marketing) in the initial phase. However, with growth, it becomes difficult to manage both the clinical and the nonclinical managerial aspects efficiently. Hence, it is beneficial to employ reliable full-time or part-time staff to address the management aspects.
> 4. *Protocols and processes*: Development of processes and implementation of standard operating protocols (SOPs) with periodic revision based on the changing needs are mandatory. A group practice is inherently dynamic (multiple heads) and as the practice grows, there is an increase in the number of human resources to manage the practice and this may be ever-changing. Hence, SOPs are extremely important.
> 5. *Procedures and products*: Investment in standard high-quality equipment and retailing of products can be done. The pricing of various procedures and products should be monitored and revised based on the change in the trends of the services offered. Increased and better utilization of the machines can be done in a group practice due to the increased physician pool, networks, and referrals.
> 6. *Promotion*:[8] Continual marketing strategies should be formulated, and each member of the group should strive to keep up with the latest advances in technology to promote the practice. The traditional marketing strategy is "word of mouth." In a group practice, all forms of external, internal, and internet marketing should be utilized wisely based on practice needs. External marketing (print media, radio/television, networking, conducting workshops, educational programs) and internal marketing (cross-referrals, creating awareness about newer therapies amongst existing clients, loyalty appreciation) strategies should be implemented. Internet marketing (website, search engine optimization, e-mails and social media, YouTube, blogs, teledermatology) is a promising avenue in recent times.
> 7. *Progress*: A vigilant and active approach to setting strategies and policies, brainstorming to address key administrative and clinical issues, adoption of newer research or technology and sustenance of quality control measures is vital for progress in group practice. SWOT (Strengths, Weaknesses, Opportunities and Threat) analysis should be done by the founder directors at regular intervals at the individual level and collectively to address all practice management aspects. Accreditation need for expansion and development of franchisees or chains can be thought of as one progresses in the practice. Specialization in particular segments can be individually taken up at various locations based on the locality needs and group members' interests. Staff retention, staff or owner burn out issues should be identified and tackled immediately.

is a high-investment- and high-income-generating practice model. Due to inherent financial burden, recovering investment may be a priority rather than providing cost-effective care. However, the goal to achieve a balance between cost-effective quality care and sustainable financial returns can be better achieved with an integrated group practice.

The most complex issue in a group practice is the compensation formula or income distribution for stake holders; hence, policy decisions should be taken at the outset and the compensation plan should be kept simple. A split in income based on equal pay (all partners work equally and get an equal pay) or productivity-based compensation (added incentives given to more productive people) may be adopted. Various practices on income distribution have been detailed in an article at the American College of Physician website.[7] As the practice progresses, retention of key employees becomes important and profit-based sharing or equity-based sharing amongst employees can be considered.

Advantages and Disadvantages

A group practice setup benefits the patients or clients by providing a one-stop place for their healthcare. However, there are advantages and disadvantages for the physicians involved in group practice (**Table 3.1.3**).

CONCLUSION

Group practice is a relatively new concept in the Indian dermatology healthcare scenario. It typically passes through entrepreneurship cycle phases (stimulatory, support, and sustenance) wherein the group as a whole

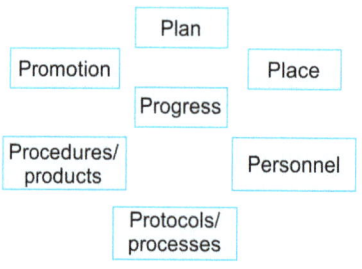

Fig. 3.1.1: 7Ps of a group practice.

Table 3.1.3: Advantages and disadvantages.	
Advantages	Disadvantages
• Shared clinical experience, patient responsibilities, and valued second opinions in difficult-to-manage cases • Shared investment (finances contributed by individual physician minimum) and better management of financial risks • Shared administrative responsibilities • Sharing of machines, newer technology, and research ideas • Good networking and referral systems • Talent pool creation • Direct control on policy decisions (dermatologists-owned group practice) • Better professional advancement and new skills development for group members • Flexible scheduling and better time management • Better work–life balance • Employee benefits better • New avenue for freshly passed dermatologists	• More administrative staff • Higher overhead costs—administrative, utilities purchase and maintenance, rentals, larger space • Delays in decision-making since policy decisions to be approved by all • Multiplicity of management issues with growth of organization • Conflicts in new-entry segments, clinical and administrative aspects • More bureaucracy • Different days, different physicians • Disparity in knowledge, skills, and therapeutic aspects • Less autonomy and control for individual physician in the group

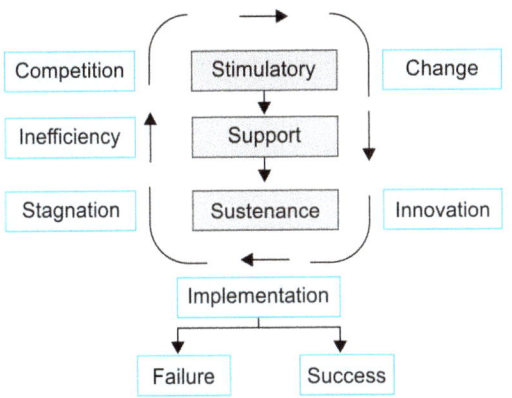

Flowchart 3.1.1: Entrepreneurship cycle—phases.

has to deal with competition, inefficiency, stagnation, change, innovation, and implementation **(Flowchart 3.1.1)**. Various skills contribute towards the clinical/business integration process—leadership, motivation, communication, support, change management, and teamwork. Mutual respect and trust amongst the members are vital for effective bonding and long-term sustenance of the practice.

REFERENCES

1. Ehrlich A, Kostecki J, Olkaba H. Trends in dermatology practices and the implications for the workforce. J Am Acad Dermatol. 2017; 77(4):746-52.
2. Werschler WP. (2008). Integrating dermatology and cosmetic dermatology practice: An expert interview with William Philip Werschler. [online] Available from: https://www.medscape.org/viewarticle/582738. [Last accessed January 2020]
3. Malpani A. Successful Private Practice—Winning Strategies for Doctors. New Delhi: UBS Publishers; 2004.
4. Russell J. The 7 Keys to a Successful Aesthetic Practice: Strategic Insights from IAPAM Members, Faculty, and Associated Industry Experts. Las Vegas, NV: IAPAM; 2009. pp. 1–17.
5. Viswanath V, Velaskar S. Establishing and managing a cosmetic practice. In: Viswanath V, Gopalani V (Eds). Cosmetic Dermatology: A Practical and Evidence Based Approach, 1st edition. New Delhi: Wiley; 2016. pp. 1067-70.
6. Jain MK, Gopalani V. Financial aspects of establishing and managing a cosmetic practice. In: Viswanath V, Gopalani V (Eds). Cosmetic Dermatology: A Practical and Evidence Based Approach, 1st edition. New Delh: Wiley; 2016. pp. 1042-8.
7. American College of Physician. (2010). Income distribution and partner buy-ins and buy-outs. American College of Physician. [online] Available from: http://www.acponline.org/running_practice/practice_management/. [Last accessed January 2020]
8. Dhepe N. Building and marketing an aesthetic practice. In: Viswanath V, Gopalani V (Eds). Cosmetic Dermatology: A Practical and Evidence Based Approach, 1st edition. New Delhi: Wiley; 2016. pp. 1061-3.

3.2 Involving Other Dermatologists in Building Your Team

Dipak Kulkarni

INTRODUCTION

There is a long tradition of private dermatology practice in India, where many stalwarts build individual clinics like one-man institutes with a massive goodwill, clientele, and fame. More and more doctors are attracted to private practice and they also prosper over a period of time. Every medical practice goes through three distinct phases in its life cycle.

GROWTH PHASE

In the initial phase, the doctor puts all his or her efforts to build the practice, exerts for long hours, tries new ideas, puts all other commitments in life aside, and develops goodwill as well as a monetarily successful practice.

PLATEAU PHASE

Practice is now stabilized but eating into all the available time in the day. There is little scope for further growth. The income rises only by increasing the fees or by adding more lucrative procedures. One has to keep the clinic often closed, to attend family functions, vacations, and conferences. One may have to curtail practice timings to suit the needs of the family, especially the kids. One foregoes many hospital attachments and visits to peripheral towns, to free the time and concentrate on one's own main clinic. It does not affect the income as such, as the practice is well established. But the growth is probably not happening now. Administrative work grows with growing income and it also eats into the valuable time.

DECLINE PHASE

Many patients find alternatives as they find this clinic busy and start turning to junior doctors. Some of the younger crowd prefers younger doctors as they can connect well with them. New technologies emerge which are sometimes available only with juniors. In addition, frequent absence of the senior doctor, for personal reasons, leads to the irritation of the clientele. So, the younger breadwinning patient population starts positioning this clinic as old, stale, and irrelevant to the modern times. Here the decline begins when in spite of the popularity, experience, and goodwill of the doctor, the patients stop coming to him. By this time, the second generation of the family may enter the profession, but sometimes, it is already late to sustain the crowd.

If you want to keep the clinic vibrant, and your practice growing relentlessly and aligned to the modern era, then you must think differently. It is a time to team up with juniors. There could be a nice synergy between the experience, financial power and goodwill of the senior, and the energy, hard work and fresh ideas of the junior member of the team. Many dermatologists are already using this style of practice very successfully. I have been using this model since 1999. Let us see its advantages.

- *Advantages to the senior member:* The practice can keep expanding in volume and money. New ideas and skill sets, which the juniors have gained from the institutes, can be incorporated into the practice, thus improving its quality. The junior member is likely to be academically fresh, trained in dermatosurgery or esthetic dermatology, and become an asset to the clinic. Academic work in the clinic, such as clinical meetings, conference presentations, and paper publications, can be enhanced. Juniors can help in computerization of the clinic, social media presence, and website design. The clinic can offer social service in the form of medical camps due to increased work force. The junior member can have a better connect with the younger crowd and help to satisfy their needs which the senior may be unaware of. This keeps the clinic relevant to the changing times.

The senior member remains a backbone of the clinic, as the practice is growing due to the initial hard work, experience and goodwill developed by him. He can also relax a little as he can take more leaves for conferences and personal reasons, without having to close the clinic in that period.

It is possible to open multiple clinics in various suburbs or towns with the help of junior members to increase the reach of the clinic in the community.

- *Advantages to the junior member:* Juniors can learn about challenges and nitty gritties of private practice and tricks to solve them. They learn the practical prescription writing, available medicine brands, techniques of patient conversations, financial management, and the skills which they will need in their own clinic in the future. They can learn this without having to invest in the initial part of their career, if they are part of such a group practice. They also can take some holidays for enjoyment, conferences, fellowships, marriages, and pregnancies without having to think about loss of clientele.

Due to rising estate rates and cost to set up a clinic, it is becoming more and more difficult to start one's own clinic and maintain it over a period of time. The above-mentioned arrangement gives juniors an opportunity to work like their personal private clinic and get very good remuneration, without having to invest in it.

- *Advantage to the patients:* The clinic can remain open for longer hours, more branches, more facilities, and lesser holidays. All this will benefit the patients.

WHY WAS THIS IDEA NOT POPULAR IN THE PAST?

Given the many advantages, one might wonder why teaming up with juniors was not practiced in the past.

In the past, people preferred building one-man institutions. Sharing of the goodwill was only with sons and daughters. Doctors were skeptical to share the experience, as they thought that the junior member will leave the clinic and start on his own after learning some skill set. In turn, junior doctors feared that they may be exploited by the senior members by forcing them to deliver hard work and paying poorly. Some juniors felt that this will delay their entry in private practice.

But with more demanding clientele in modern urbanized and prosperous India and more disposable money with them, we need to team up to remain relevant.

TYPES OF GROUP PRACTICE

- *Using juniors as employees or assistants:* In this scenario, the senior member holds ownership and decision rights and gives only a fixed salary to the junior dermatologist. This pattern is good if the junior person has just finished post-graduation and is inexperienced. He works as if he is doing a lectureship in a private institute. The junior is just an employee and does not get a sense of being a real independent consultant. Thus, he will always consider this job as a stepping stone. He will have no initiative to develop the workload in the clinic and will be less willing to take direct responsibility. But the senior will feel more secure that the goodwill is intact with him.
- *Juniors as associates:* I feel that this is a better arrangement and I have been personally using it for the last 20 years. After a tenure with a fixed salary, the junior member is allowed to put his (or her) name on the clinic's letterhead as well as the signboard. He accepts patients on his own name and consults them independently. This gives him a feeling of ownership, responsibility, and an urge

to develop the quantum of the work in the clinic. But the junior does not invest any capital. Whether to task him for administrative work or not depends on the clinic's policy.

To give stability to his income, ideally the junior should get income in two parts: (1) a part as a fixed income which he will get anyway for his presence in the clinic, even if few or no patients agree to consult him and (2) another part should come as a share of the consulting fees or procedure charges from the patients which he has independently handled. The share in the consulting charges is generally more than that of the procedures, as the clinic incurs more expenditure in procedures. The junior can remain associated with the clinic in one shift and practice elsewhere independently, if it is mutually suitable.

- *Franchisee-type peripheral clinic:* This arrangement is good where the senior wants to open a chain of the clinics. The junior is managing a branch either himself or with the team. He is using the brand of the original clinic. The junior may have to invest and may have equal or higher financial stakes than the second arrangement. The senior doctor will make a periodic visit to such a clinic for expert opinion and helping in administration.
- *Skill-based group practice:* When a particular junior trained in a special skill like hair transplantation or dermatosurgery visits the clinic regularly and takes share of the procedure fees.
- *Peer-to-peer group practice:* If a peer group of dermatologists of a similar age start a common practice at the outset, it is probably a better option to share capital, responsibilities, and time which will add up to the goodwill, patient base, and income for the clinic. But for this idea to be successful, none of the group members ideally should have an independent practice of his own.

RISKS OF INVOLVING JUNIORS

The most feared thing is when the junior member, after acquiring good skills in the clinic, will depart creating a manpower shortage in the clinic and more so, take away a chunk of the clientele. I think (from personal experience) that if you have given adequate respect, decent remuneration, and reasonable workload to any junior, they are unlikely to go hostile with you. Nobody is expected to stay as an associate or an assistant in one clinic for lifelong. So, one day he or she is bound to start his or her new clinic. If the junior considers you as role model, then he or she will quit without hurting your interests. The second risk is possible error and negligence at the hands of the juniors. If you train and orient them properly, then this can be minimized. It is worthwhile to have appropriate indemnity insurance to cover this because even if the senior does not form a team, he/she himself/herself can start committing mistakes due to old age or overwork.

It is worthwhile to have a legal notarized document of memorandum of understanding (MOU) with the junior doctor, especially when you have allowed him to work independently. Difficult patients and nonresponders should take a second opinion of the senior partner periodically.

Create an atmosphere in which the junior will feel to be important and respected in the clinic setup. If done properly, this point can retain these juniors for a long time.

Mishandling of instruments and repairs, ego issues between two juniors or with staff members, gross misbehavior or inappropriate patient handling, and financial misappropriation are some risks which you have to handle with your administrative skills. But these problems are to be managed anyway with other nonmedical staff members in a bigger clinic. So even if you do not form a team, you have to face them someday.

PREPARING YOUR CLINIC FOR GROUP PRACTICE

- Explain all your patients about the presence and availability of junior dermatologists in the clinic, their education, and proficiency. Urge them to take their assistance when the senior doctor is busy or absent.
- Computerization of the clinic is very useful for this type of practice as standardization is easy. The associate doctors get full access to the patient data when he or she interacts with the patient. The senior doctor also finds easy to monitor working of the juniors due to these gadgets. Website of the clinic is useful to promote all members of the team.
- Training program for the doctors is essential to impart similar ethos and treatment methods, conversational techniques, and procedural skills.
- Orient the nonmedical staff to adapt to this new environment.

DAY-TO-DAY WORKING AS WELL AS REMUNERATION PATTERN IN A SENIOR–JUNIOR MODEL

There are various ways in which a senior would delegate the work to the juniors and get it done from them. Let me explain one such way which is being practiced successfully in my clinic for the last 20 years.

Junior doctors join me basically for learning the nitty gritties of practice. They are initially getting oriented and only helping me in my OPD, when they are paid a fixed salary. Their initial job is to understand my working pattern and learn the computer setup in the clinic. They slowly develop good skills in conversation and counseling and also fine-tune their procedural skills. Once I get confidant about their proficiency, they are allowed to work independently in my clinic. We call them associates and not assistants and insist that the patient should also use a similar nomenclature for them.

Majority of the patients initially contact my clinic with a desire to consult me and only me. But once I am fully booked, the remaining patients are requested by our staff to consult any of the available junior dermatologist, instead. The patient is reassured that the junior is equally qualified and oriented to my clinical and therapeutic methods and the advice as well as the outcome should be similar to that of mine. In addition, the patients are told that if any diagnostic or therapeutic difficulty arises, then I will be called for a second opinion. Not all, but at least 30% of the patients who are anyway not getting an appointment with me due to nonavailability accept this proposition and are ready to consult some of the juniors in the team. The female junior doctors have an advantage, as many female patients opt for them without much resistance. In the initial years of starting this concept, there was tremendous resistance from the patients. But now slowly they have got used to it and the trend to consult the associates is growing. Almost two-thirds of the total workload in my clinic is managed by these junior associates. So, if you want to start this kind of practice, then you have to start sowing seeds much earlier to harvest the fruits later.

Some patients do come back complaining that they did not improve as the senior doctor had not examined them. Some reassurance, repeat examination, some change of treatment as well as hand holding are required. However at the end, we politely affirm that the treatment of the junior doctor was right but I am making minor modifications as the patient did not show response.

The fixed remuneration of a typical MD doctor is in the tune of ₹ 50,000. This figure depends on various factors such as educational qualification (MD/DNB/Diploma), hours of working, experience, and ability to give academic inputs. Once allowed to work independently, he or she additionally gets 25% of the consulting charges and 20% of the procedure charges. Fixed remuneration gives him stability and variable portion gives him additional incentive. Most full-time juniors fetch remuneration above 1 lakh, within few months after getting permission for independent practice.

We try to incentivize the doctor, if any additional activity is conducted by him for patient benefit.

CONCLUSION

If handled properly, group practice with juniors or peers can help you expand the scope of your practice, income, and fame. You can do more relaxed and academically oriented practice and keep the fame of the clinic intact for decades together.

3.3 Managing 120 Plus OPD with Cosmetic Practice

Anil Dashore, Shuken Dashore

INTRODUCTION

As your outpatient department (OPD) starts to grow, it becomes increasingly difficult to manage the patient load and give proper time for each consultation. The balance between giving your best to each patient and seeing many patients in a limited time is an art. The aim is to maximize the efficiency so that you can spend as much time with a patient as possible by decreasing the unnecessary time-consuming activities and delegate them to designated personnel. Managing a big OPD is not a one-person show; it is a well-oiled machine that works seamlessly. There should be redundancies for unexpected circumstances. In private practice, consultation for a patient does not just include treatment of the disease. Patient satisfaction comes from a doctor carefully listening to the complaints of the patient, understanding him or her empathizing with him or her and reassuring.

APPOINTMENT SYSTEM

An appointment system is a must when treating many patients. The system not only ensures that a patient who is coming from far away, like a village, will be sure that you are there in the clinic but also informs us what is the expected OPD for the day so that too many patients do not come at the same time. A walk-in system appears useful, but it discourages out-of-station patients and it becomes difficult to close the clinic on days of emergency. If people are taking leaves from their jobs to visit the doctor, they feel reassured if they have an appointment.

Ideally, a combination of two forms of patient consultation is the best. So we must keep around 85% of the slots for appointment and keep the rest 15% for walk-ins. The receptionist informs walk-in patients to take an appointment for the next visit. Otherwise, there may be a longer wait time. This way, both emergency visits and planned appointments can be included.

A disadvantage of the appointment system is that if there is a slight variation in the initial appointments, which can happen due to either the patient or the doctor being late the whole queue is disturbed. So, the authors suggest a variation of the appointment system. They recommend the use of a queue system in the clinic. The appointments are not for an exact time like 5:50 PM but for a slot like 5:00–5:15 PM which means that the patient needs to come at 5:00 PM and the consultation will happen between 5:00 and 5:15 PM. This appointment slot needs to be explained to the patient on the phone while the appointment is being given. Once the patient reaches the clinic, he or she is entered into a queue system that works on a first-come, first-serve basis. This system ensures that none of the patients is treated unfairly and the walking patients may also be adjusted.

RECEPTION

Reception is an important place in the clinic. It can make or break the reputation of the clinic and hence must be managed with utmost care and discipline. At least three people are required for proper workflow in a busy OPD. One person manages the cash and billing, the second person handles the phone and gives the appointments, and the third person manages the incoming patients. The prescription paper is prepared at the reception itself. The full name, address, age, and sex of the patient are noted down carefully on the prescription at the reception itself. This system saves a lot of time when seeing a lot of patients. After this, patient is directed for history-taking.

HISTORY-TAKING

The history-taking must be on a printed form and must be taken by an assistant doctor. The history must rule out diabetes, hypertension, and all other comorbidities. This will ensure that we know about the patient's habits (such as alcohol intake and smoking) before entering the chamber. This will help us choose a safer medicine for the specific patient. All previous medicines must be noted down on the history sheet, and the assistant doctor must note down the content of the brand names of medicines prescribed by other physicians (we are usually not familiar with the brand names of other specialty). This helps in two ways: (1) we have a concise note of all the medicines the patient is receiving and (2) it saves time in the doctor's chambers when the patient fiddles with bundles of old files to finally show what medication he is on presently. Also, the patient is satisfied that his previous papers have all been examined and a summary has been made for the same.

CONSULTATION

Inside the doctor's chamber, there are two assistants. One assistant writes the prescription and the other guides the patient. This is useful in a busy OPD as the doctor can dictate the medicines to the assistant. The doctor can then spend the extra time talking to the patient and listening to his story while the assistant completes the prescription. With proper posture toward the patient and proper eye contact, the doctor can build a faster rapport and inform the patient about the pathogenesis of the disease and explain the precautions regarding the various diseases and how to apply the creams, etc. The assistant can also type the prescription in case an electronic medical record (EMR) software is being used. When using EMR software, the doctor faces the screen and types, which this looks impersonal to many patients. Use of EMR software can sometimes take more time.[1]

After the prescription has been written, the doctor then checks the prescription and hands it over to the patient. The second assistant then escorts the patient to the pharmacy. After the patient purchases the medicines, he returns to the assistant doctor where he/she cross-checks the medicines to ensure that no mistake has been made while dispensing the medicine. The assistant doctor again explains the medicines to the patient. Thus, the medicines are explained three times to the patient, and this reduces the risk of a mistake, even in illiterate patients. Another advantage is that the sale of medicine increases from the in-house pharmacy. However, the patient must be free to purchase medicines from anywhere he wishes. He should not be coerced in any way to do the same. This also increases the trust in the doctor.

MANAGING PROCEDURES WITH A BUSY OPD

In case a procedure is advised, the assistant can guide the patient to the therapist, who then explains the procedure to the patient. An optional counselor can be employed who explains the pros and cons of the procedure advised including the pricing of the same. A predefined checklist must be made for each procedure which the counselor explains one by one. The counselor also ensures that the patient signs the consent form and he/she properly saves it in the clinic. A separate time of the day must be assigned for the procedures that will be performed by the dermatologist, and all such procedures must be posted then. Particular days of the week may also be defined for the same. In case the procedure is performed by a therapist, machine parameters must be written on the procedure requisition form by the dermatologist during the clinical consultation, e.g., for a case of fractional CO_2 laser treatment, something like "45 mj/pitch 0.8/points of shot 2" can be written on the sheet. This reduces the risk of choosing the wrong parameters by the therapist.

GIVING A NEGATIVE PROGNOSIS

Even in cases of negative prognosis, detailed examination has to be done, which includes investigations and biopsy, if needed. All efforts must be put to try to understand a disease. Any condition should be labeled untreatable only after confirmation and a legitimate attempt to treat the disease must be done, e.g., performing a biopsy in a case of lichen planus pigmentosus or cicatricial alopecia. As dermatologists, we deal with a lot of diseases that have a poor prognosis, but labeling diseases untreatable on the first visit will lead the patient not to believe the diagnosis. He/she will try to get a second opinion. Often, we see patients who have been denied treatment visit quacks who promise them complete cure. They waste time and effort on the disease only to realize that you were right all along. You need to build rapport with the patient before he/she can accept a diagnosis of no treatment. A simple investigation or biopsy goes a long way in establishing trust in you.

MISCELLANEOUS POINTS TO BE KEPT IN MIND

As commonly pointed out by many patients, mobile phone is probably the biggest distractor in a consulting room. Many patients talk about their previous doctors with disdain, as they were busy with their phones during the consultation. A patient may wait for hours for a 5-minute consultation with the doctor, and a phone call during the consultation makes him/her feel that his problems have not been given due importance. During consultation, the mobile phone should not be in the pocket nor should it be on the table. It should be in a drawer. Doctors must leave the habit of glancing at the phone with every Whatsapp notification.

A suggestion box must be placed outside the clinic. This allows an angry patient to complain to the doctor regarding a point he/she did not like and could not discuss face to face. This dissipates his/her anger at the clinic itself and prevents negative public reviews from being added online.

Many patients are afraid that doctors will not listen to their problems. They sometimes forget to ask something which they feel is important. They should be given the option of coming in the consultation room once or twice after the consultation in case they want to ask something else. This relaxes the patient and builds faith. A clinic email can also be given to the patient in case he/she has any further queries. Giving doctors their personal mobile number for WhatsApp consultations is not advised and now illegal. There are several advantages to the email. These can be screened by an assistant and all required information assimilated before looking for a solution. The patient is asked to attach a photo of his prescription along with the email which makes it easier for the doctor to solve the query.

In a big OPD, it is important to be attentive to how the patient describes his/her problem. The nonverbal communication plays a big role. In a case of tinea cruris, if the patient repeatedly says that he/she has uncontrollable itch, then the focus should be on giving a higher dose of antihistamine to calm down the itch. Although many of the dermatological treatments can be done via preset prescriptions, especially in EMR software, tailoring the prescriptions to the patient makes a lot of difference. This requires complete concentration toward the patient during the consultation. If a patient, who at first looks like a case of tinea corporis, does not complain of any itching, he/she must be looked again for a differential diagnosis like granuloma annulare or pityriasis rosea. An accurate diagnosis is what differentiates us from quacks, and hence a correct diagnosis is a must, no matter what is the OPD number.

Continuous electricity and internet connection is a must if online EMR software is being used for prescription. A 2-kw inverter is useful for the clinic lights, but the laser machines need an online UPS connection with at least 3–4 hour battery backup. The requirement of UPS can be read behind the laser machines themselves. If a machine writes "220 v 10 A," it means its usage is 2200 VA or 2.2 KVA. This machine will require a UPS of more than 2.2 KVA capacity. If multiple lasers are present in the clinic, and purchasing multiple UPS is not affordable, then a long power cable can be attached to one UPS, and different machines can be used on the same UPS one by one. This leads a hassle-free smooth-running clinic, which is ready for any situation.

CONCLUSION

Managing a big OPD needs planning and preparation for all situations. As problems cannot be solved when many patients are waiting, planning must be done for all case scenarios beforehand. Delivering a "WOW" experience to the patient is a challenge and needs a mind shift in the dermatologist and a trust in the staff to perform as a single unit.

REFERENCE

1. Hribar M, Read-Brown S, Reznick L, Chiang M. Evaluating and improving an outpatient clinic scheduling template using secondary electronic health record data. AMIA Annu Symp Proc. 2018;2017:921-9.

3.4

All in the Family: Practicing Dermatology with Family Members

Ankur Talwar, Suresh Talwar, Kshama Talwar

INTRODUCTION

We define family dermatology practice as medical practice where father, mother, son, daughter, son-in-law, or daughter-in-law are engaged in joint practice in various combinations by virtue of being from the same specialty. Usually, the place of practice is common as is the specialty and the name of the medical establishment. One is lucky to be involved in family practice. This has a lot of advantages and is a real fun to practice.

ADVANTAGES OF A FAMILY PRACTICE

- *Stronger bonds:* A family practice generally works at a fixed common time. Such common hours of working allow the family members to be together at work and also be together at home. This leads to development of stronger bonds (professionally as well as on the family front). With an increasingly busy schedule of each person in these modern times, it is harder for family members to spend quality time with each other. A common workplace allows you to be able to interact and stay in touch with each other.
- *Company:* This is a very important factor, which most individuals engaged in private practice does not have the luxury of. Doctors who work in corporate set ups have the luxury to interact with doctors of the same as well as other specialties. This helps to keep away the monotony of a routine working lifestyle. A family practice provides you the luxury of good company with whom you can share lighter moments which in turn help to ease the workload and prevent monotony from setting in.
- *Common equipment:* With ever-increasing advancements in medical technology, newer and costlier equipment and lasers have become the backbone of medical practice. The equipment that were once considered a luxury have increasingly become a necessity in modern practice. It may be very difficult for an individual engaged in solo medical practice to able to afford all such costly medical technology and then optimally utilize it. Much of such latest equipment require substantial initial investment. Similarly, if one of the family members is in another specialty, the

division of investment among different specialties may become a bone of contention. This is where family practice substantially scores over a solo practice. A family practice by virtue of using common equipment in the working area allows you to invest freely and keep abreast with the latest technologies. With the advantage of multiple working hands, it also leads to optimum utilization of the equipment. A faster return on investments furthers boosts you to invest in other available technologies as well, thereby establishing your center as one of the premier establishment of the city with all the latest available technologies.

- *Planning a vacation:* Often, doctors engaged in solo practice find it difficult to take a break from their practice at regular intervals. The main issue faced is that frequent breaks from the clinic lead to an interruption in the continuity of patient follow-up and care with the final result being decreased inflow of patients. Often, patients have a problem regarding the availability of doctors engaged in solo practice. This problem is obviated in family practice. Family members can plan their vacation according to the availability of other members working together. One can split the team of working family members; some can go now and some at a later date. The advantage here is that the continuity of a practicing center is maintained at all times. Patients will not suffer and chances of losing patients due to doctors' unavailability are also not there. Even patients, especially those coming from far-off places, come to realize over a period of time that they will receive treatment and care at the center at all but the rarest of occasions and that even if their original consulting doctor is not available, an alternative specialist would see them and their visit shall not go waste. Generally, if the patient is familiar with one doctor he may not mind taking consultation from another family member in his absence.

- *Sharing of knowledge:* With the advancements in medical field occurring at a stupendous rate, it is necessary to keep one abreast of all the latest developments occurring in their specialty. Although often desired, this sometimes becomes difficult with all the time lost in managing one's workplace and juggling with the work-life balance. This may upset your academic acumen. A family practice allows you the luxury of continually updating yourself from each other's experience and knowledge. It is like a readily available round table meet where you can discuss your problems and clear your doubts with each other anytime. Any one member, who has attended a conference or read an interesting medical article or come across an interesting case, may immediately share the same with other members, thereby updating the knowledge of others too.

- *Specialization in different sub-specialties:* With increasing expansion of each medical specialty, each medical field is growing beyond the defined horizons. Nowadays, no job is restricted to one particular specialty and specialists of one field are doing great jobs at tasks which were hitherto considered domains of another specialty. A doctor engaged in solo practice may find it nearly impossible to excel at all the subspecialties in a medical field. On the contrary, a family practice allows different members to choose their fields of interest and thereby work toward enhancing their skills in that particular field. Just as an example, in the author's family center, one member has special interest in cosmetic dermatology such as botulinum toxin and dermal fillers, another has a keen interest in dermatosurgical procedures while yet another has a liking for lasers and other light-based technologies. This allows each one to pursue his/her passion whilst excelling at his/her individual fields and providing the best patient care.

- *Better management and reduced stress*: A solo practice is often associated with increased stress. This may be due to a person's inability to divide the working hours between patient care and clinic management. Often, the management of clinic affairs extracts a lot of time from your working hours. This includes clinic maintenance issues, clinic staff issues, equipment maintenance, and hordes of other stuff which sound trivial but which when combined eat up a lot of your time. This may lead to increased stress and improper management. Division of work between family members is a great way of obviating this problem. Meeting once in a clinic during tea time helps in discussing clinic problems related to patients, staff, finance, and clinic maintenance. This avoids monotony and leads to better management. As an example, at the our center, one member is in charge of clinic staff-related problems, another member looks after clinic maintenance issues while another member is tasked with the responsibility of taking care of pharmacy-related issues. This is just an example of how division of labor eases the workload.
- *Collective responsibility:* It is a known truth that there are lesser lawsuits against doctors engaged in family practice as compared to doctors engaged in solo practice. On scratching beneath the surface of this truth, the most plausible explanation can be due to sharing of responsibility between different doctors. Doctors, like any human, are bound to commit mistakes; however, one's ego combined with insecurity often blinds us to our mistakes. A sharing of responsibility between different doctors of a center may help us see through one's mistake and take remedial measures. Often, a doctor may end up in a verbal argument with a patient over a trivial matter. The sharing of concerns of the patient with other doctors may help salvage the situation.

DISADVANTAGES OF A FAMILY PRACTICE

- *Forging individual identity:* Nothing grows under a banyan tree. This oft-stated proverb often holds good in the setting of family practice. The most experienced member gets the status of a senior doctor while relegating others to the status of junior doctors. As a result majority of the patients, medical representatives, and clinic staff accord greater importance to the senior doctor. This can get quite suffocating for junior doctors who may find it difficult to establish their own identity in the presence of an established stalwart. This differentiation can be bad for the confidence and self-respect of young graduates who are just starting out their careers. Each person wants his/her own space, respect, and dignity and it can be quite difficult to accord equal importance to everyone in a competitive world.
- *Managing the finances:* This can be a tricky situation in a family setting.

The sticky issue of division of finances between family members can lead to a lot of bad blood. Often, it is the senior-most person who is in charge of a center's finances. A young member of the family setup with his/her growing family may have certain greater financial needs as compared to the established patriarch whose children are more settled. This can lead to disharmony between the different members of the setup.

- *A professional center built on personal bonds*: It is often said that a single straw can bring down the whole tree. This proverb holds good in the setting of a family practice as well. This is essentially a professional setup, which however is built on the foundation of strong family bonds. If these bonds shake, the entire setup can come down. We have all heard stories of corporate empires collapsing due to difference of opinion between the members of a family. The same can be said about the family practice center which runs on the goodwill of the family name. If the family collapses, there can be very little margin to salvage the center from going down as well.
- *Lack of quality family time:* An unwanted corollary of family practice is the inability to completely detach oneself from one workspace even at home. Since the environment and family members at both the workplace and home are usually similar, the free time may seem like an extension of the working hours itself. Academic discussions and management issues from the workplace may carry over to the family home. Dinner table conversations often end veering to clinic-related issues. This may lead to a burnout and lack of enthusiasm toward going to the workplace.
- *Lack of a family vacation:* Due to division of responsibilities at the workplace and in order to maintain the continuity of a working center, the different family members may find it rather difficult to take a joint vacation. A family vacation is probably the best detoxification therapy for the mind which becomes a rare luxury for individuals in family practice.

SUGGESTIONS FOR A SUCCESSFUL FAMILY PRACTICE

Just like any successful business, family practice requires careful planning and active personal interventions from time to time. Each successful business is beset with its own set of unique problems that requires specialized solutions. Here are some tips to ensure a successful venture.

- *Division of workload:* The workload of a center should be appropriately divided so that any one person should not feel overburdened while at the same time giving any other member the feeling of being inconsequential. For workload division, it is essential to formulate an action plan first. Decide how to divide the work depending on the kind of clinical practice one is engaged in. For example, in a dermatology center, the workload can be divided into clinical dermatology, esthetic dermatology, and procedural dermatology. The next step would be to explore the interests of each of the practicing doctors involved. According to the individual skills and interests, the workload can be divided and each member can be assigned individual roles. Each person is blessed with different skillsets; hence, there must be optimum utilization of the individual skills to assign the specific tasks. Such division should

not be kept rigid and each member should have the liberty to explore areas beyond their boundaries. This also helps to ensure uniform distribution of patients, thereby ensuring that each member feels equally important in the setup.
- *Effective communication:* Effective communication in the workplace is paramount. The team leader needs to ensure this in a family practice setup as well—usually the senior-most member of the team. One member in the family setup needs to take up this unenviable position of acting as the team leader. Good communication helps eliminate misunderstandings and encourages a healthy work environment. There are two ways of establishing effective communication. The first means is by open meetings wherein the team leader usually addresses the entire team and discusses strategy and planning. The second means is by one-to-one communication wherein the team leader listens to the problems of individual members and then chalks out a solution collectively. Encouraging feedback from members and appreciating everyone's participation is key to the success of any business setup.
- *Establishing equal identity:* The family practice center usually runs under a common name. However, all members of the setup might not get equal importance and credit for their work. This needs to be carefully handled. The concept of senior and junior doctors in a center should be abolished. All clinic doctors should address each other by names. Consultation fees of all the doctors should be same, thereby giving the impression that all the doctors are equal in status. Effort should be made to keep distribution of patient load uniform between the doctors so that feelings of jealousy or incompetency do not set in. Usually, the senior-most and most experienced doctor gets a major chunk of the patient load. It becomes their responsibility to ensure that workload is divided equally. Some patients may say that they came to consult a particular doctor and that on their previous visit they were sent to a different doctor in the same center, which resulted in flaring-up of the disease. It is important not to get carried away while simultaneously trying to counsel and pacify them. Sometimes, a patient may enter a particular doctor's room and on seeing him/her, the patient says that he/she wanted to consult the other doctor. It is imperative to not let one's ego come in the way in such a scenario. It needs to be kept in mind that it is the collective success of the center that is important and not anybody's individual name or fame. If some patient wants to consult a junior doctor, seniors should feel proud and honored that juniors have established their place. Management of medical representatives (MRs) in a family setup is equally important. While meeting the MRs, it should be made clear to them that briefing all the doctors equally is very important and they should not focus on any single doctor. There should be no disparity in distributing whatever medical samples or gifts that these MRs generally present to the doctors. The team leader needs to convey the impression that junior colleagues are equally authorized to add or delete any product of any medical company. For staff management, delegation of equal power to all practicing family doctors is paramount. Each member should be equally authorized to

take any necessary measures to maintain the stature of the setup. While taking these measures, however, the senior member should always keep an eye on quality management and ensure that no malpractice occurs.
- *Financial management:* To avoid finance-related issues, there should be a joint account with equal financial powers being given to all the doctors. In fact, the senior doctor should always discuss financial planning with all the members and honor the suggestions given by any junior doctor. The requirements of individual members need to be kept in mind, and a sound financial planning strategy should be devised to ensure fair distribution of a center's profit.
- *Strong financial planning:* It is better to make a company with all the family members as directors. In a company, you are liable to pay income tax @25% rate of your total income. The salary of each director can be fixed (depending on individual need, investment, time devoted—all on mutually agreed terms), and the savings are kept as reserve for purchase of assets and equipment. Since all practicing doctors also serve as directors, everyone will try to work hard to increase the income of the company as their share also grows proportionately.
- *Involvement of other family members who are not in a medical field:* Effort should be made to involve all the family members in the setup even if they are not from the medical field. This leads to greater involvement of all members and nobody feels left out or an outsider in the family. A nondoctor family member can also be an asset in family practice. They can look after human resource management, marking attendance of staff, welfare activity of staff, looking after clinic promotion, laboratory services, pharmacy inventory, managing finances of clinic, etc. Management of a successful center is a full-time task in itself and instead of employing salaried managers from the outside world, having a family member who understands the requirements and limitations of a family center intricately can help the setup grow in leaps and bounds.

To summarize, family practice is a real fun enterprise. The minor issues which crop up in the initial stages tend to get resolved on their own with passage of time. Patience and mutual respect is the key to success.

BIBLIOGRAPHY

1. Rao BC, Prasad R. Principles of family medicine practice: lessons gleaned over a lifetime in practice. J Family Med Prim Care. 2018;7:303-8.

3.5 Lasers to Invest in Practice: Which, When, and How

Sanjeev Aurangabadkar

INTRODUCTION

In the current day and age in the 21st century, it is difficult to image a dermatology practice without lasers and energy-based devices. The past two decades have witnessed an exponential growth in procedural dermatology including but not limited to injectables, chemical and mechanical exfoliants, energy-based devices, and lasers. A certain sect of skin conditions immensely benefit from lasers (which hitherto had no acceptable medical alternative) such as epidermal and dermal pigmentary disorders, hirsutism, port wine stains to name only a few. The advent of pulsed lasers, the introduction of the theory of selective photothermolysis,[1] and more recently the concept of fractional photothermolysis[2] all have paved way to novel, light-based therapeutic options in dermatology practice. This has given dermatologists some serious fire power like never before. But as they say, with great power comes great responsibility! This laser power in the inexperienced or untrained hands can be disastrous. Laser usage requires sound understanding of physics, biological interactions of laser with tissue, and due diligence to achieve satisfactory results and avoid adverse effects.

One of the most important aspects before buying lasers is to build a good medical dermatology practice. This acts like a pillar or foundation to build up a laser practice as many conditions amenable to lasers can be picked out from the OPD. If need be and upon introduction of new technology marketing can be resorted to, to enhance the practice.

The buyer should learn basic laser physics, indications for lasers, different technologies, and complications. These can be learnt by attending either workshops, symposia, conferences, or established laser centers. The physician should be aware of the prevalence of different dermatological and esthetic problems in the community and then decide which laser would be most suitable for practice in that area. Patients' attitudes, paying capacity, and marketing opportunities need to be assessed. While the choice of a laser system depends on an individual situation, some general recommendations are outlined.

IMPORTANT DERMATOLOGICAL LASERS

- *Hair removal lasers:* Mainly long-pulse diode and Nd:YAG
- *Pigmentary lasers*: Q switched lasers, picosecond lasers
- *Scars and rejuvenation*: Ablative fractional lasers—CO_2 and Er:YAG lasers
- *Scars and rejuvenation*: Nonablative fractional lasers—Er:Glass 1540 nm
- *Vascular lasers*: Pulse dye lasers 585 nm and 595 nm
- *Therapeutic lasers*: Excimer laser and lamp 308 nm—for vitiligo, psoriasis, alopecia areata, etc
- *Intense pulsed light (IPLs)*: With different filters used for various indications

Once basic training is obtained, the suitability of a given machine should be judged as below.

LASER SPECIFICATIONS

Spot size, pulse duration, peak power, customization options, etc.—these are of utmost importance and are explained below:

- A large spot size is preferable for laser hair removal.[3] A large spot size allows deeper penetration and allows faster treatments during the laser procedure. A spot size of 10–18 mm is available in conventional laser hair removal (LHR) systems. Newer low-fluence high repetition rate hair removal systems have even larger spot sizes.
- High peak power and ultrashort pulse for Q switched laser, Gaussian versus top-hat beam profile. Top-hat beam profile is preferable for Q-switched lasers that can prevent uneven energy distribution over a given area, thus preventing "hot-spots."[4]
- Scan density, pattern of scan, pulse width, fluence, etc., for fractional lasers. The laser should preferably have variable scan density, adjustable and variable scan patters, changeable spot size of each microbeam, high power (e.g., min 30 W for fractional CO_2).[5]
- Correct wavelength of filters, variable on time and off time, the HP of IPL should have built-in cooling.

Often, the first laser to purchase is a hair removal device. Either this can be an intense pulsed light (IPL) system or a stand-alone laser. IPLs generally are cheaper to own (there are exceptions) and have the advantage of having other wavelengths that allow other indications to be treated which can improve the return on investment (ROI). But the catch is that most laser devices give better outcomes and in less number of sessions compared to IPL.[6] Among the lasers for hair removal, the diode laser has been the wavelength of choice and is considered the gold standard for hair removal. A variety of diode lasers are available, including small spot size, large spot size, linear scanning diode, low-fluence in-motion diode, etc. Based on the budget, service provider, efficacy, and reliability, any of them can be purchased. It is prudent to go through the published literature and seek peer opinion before purchasing a machine.

VARIOUS WAVELENGTHS USED IN LASER HAIR REMOVAL

- Alexandrite 755-nm long pulse
- Diode 810 nm
- Nd:YAG 1064-nm long pulse
- IPL 650–1100 nm
- Dual wavelength and triple wavelength lasers

As a general rule, longer wavelengths are preferred for treating darker skin types. Always prefer a device with a large spot size for hair removal as it helps complete treatments quickly. Adequate cooling is essential for performing LHR. It can be either air, contact, or dynamic cooling.

A successful LHR practice will allow one to generate enough funds for purchase of the next system which would ideally be a fractional ablative or nonablative laser for treatment of scars and for rejuvenation. Literature suggests that ablative fractional lasers (AFLs) are superior to nonablative ones, especially for acne scars.[7] The AFLs are versatile tools which can treat a variety of indications and can also be used for laser-assisted drug delivery. Acne scars are a huge problem and having a device to address this is very helpful in practice.

The next laser to purchase would be a Q-switched Nd:YAG (QSNY) laser as it is the gold standard for pigment removal and tattoos. Certain points to consider while buying a QSNY laser are as follows:

- High power system—at least 2 joules at 8 mm
- Large spot size of at least 10 mm
- Top hat-beam profile

- Expanded wavelengths of 660 nm QS, 595 nm QS and 300 µs quasi-long-pulse mode and fractional hand piece as an option
- High build quality and robustness of the system

The QSNY laser has many indications and as such is fairly cost effective, thus making it a sound investment. The laser is capable of treating epidermal, dermal, and mixed pigmented lesions, and tattoos. Laser toning and carbon laser peel done with this machine have opened new doors to address issues such as tan removal, melasma, post-inflammatory hyperpigmentation (PIH), and rejuvenation. The laser has a bit of a learning curve, and hence it is a good idea to learn the basics and get some hands-on experience under expert supervision prior to attempting therapy. Picosecond lasers which have even shorter pulse duration (10^{-12} of a second) are now available which can deliver higher peak powers than the QSNY laser. These systems, being very expensive, can be considered as an upgrade to the existing QSNY laser practice, especially for certain colors of tattoos, and in pico-toning mode used for rejuvenation, acne scars, and melasma.

Depending on the practice, adding an excimer 308-nm system would be the logical move as it can tackle common dermatological ailments such as vitiligo, psoriasis, alopecia areata, and prurigo nodularis. The systems tend to be portable and sturdy allowing from transport from one clinic to the other. The excimer is particularly useful in childhood vitiligo where whole-body exposure to UV rays is not recommended. They are cost-effective and have good ROI.

Pulse dye lasers (PDL) with a wavelength of 585 and 595 nm are the laser of choice for treating vascular lesions due to the selective absorption of these wavelengths in oxyhemoglobin.[8] PDL are particularly useful for conditions such as port-wine stains, hemangiomas, telangiectasias, venous lakes, and other conditions such as viral warts, rosacea and striae rubra. These highly specialized lasers tend to be expensive to own and maintain and hence tend to be available only at selected secondary or tertiary care centers. Unless one has a good referral base or has surplus funds, it may not be the best laser to invest in initially in practice.

Laser systems are available either as stand-alone or platform systems. Stand-alone systems tend to be of a single wavelength with one hand piece (HP) designed for specific purposes such as a long pulse alexandrite 755-nm laser for laser hair reduction. Platform systems have the ability to attach multiple hand pieces to the machine and have the ability to deal with various indications. The hand pieces could be a hair removal HP or an IPL HP for treating vascular lesions or even a near-infrared HP offering skin-tightening treatments, etc. At any given time, one or two HPs can be attached to the system and can be changed as desired. The software of the system recognizes the HP attached and the settings can thus be changed as needed. Each of these two systems has its advantages and disadvantages and these are enumerated in **Table 3.5.1**.

Buying a laser is one aspect but maintaining it is another. A proper purchase contract needs to be signed before buying expensive equipment which should include the warranty information, service details, spare parts costs, and annual maintenance contract amount. This will ensure peaceful ownership experience and avoid bill shocks. The author has published a model purchase contract which is published in the JCAS journal (Journal of Cutaneous and Aesthetic Surgery) and can be downloaded from[9] http://www.jcasonline.com/text.asp?2014/7/2/124/138363.

Table 3.5.1: Advantages and disadvantages of stand-alone and platform systems.

	Advantages	Disadvantages
Stand-alone lasers	• Tend to be robust-work horse systems • Dedicated machine for selective work • Ability to treat multiple patients simultaneously if more than one stand-alone system available in clinic	• Take up more space • More expensive to own multiple systems • More number of service visits if systems are of different make • Higher maintenance costs
Platform system	• Cheaper to own with ability to treat different indications • Takes up less office space • Less number of service visits needed • Probably lower maintenance costs • More easy to transport amongst different centers	• In case of breakdown of platform, all HPs may not work • Only one patient or indication can be treated at a time • HP needs to be used carefully as each HP tends to be expensive • Not as robust and perhaps less effective when compared to stand-alone systems

COST NEGOTIATION

The ultimate aim of a buyer of a laser system is to get the maximum discount possible as compared to the list price or quoted price. This will depend on the communication skills of the buyer, knowledge of the global and local pricing, discounts offered by the dealer/distributor, and approximate price paid by the other purchasers of the system. Try not to show the sales representative that you are interested in their system only; make them aware that you are looking at other competing systems. Never be in a hurry to buy a laser! Get quotes from different companies for the similar systems. This will allow better negotiation. Also, ask colleagues about the price paid by them. It is important to understand that all medical lasers depreciate as soon as they are sold. So getting the best price is more crucial. Always strike a balance between cost and quality while making a decision. This cost-quality equation has to be kept in mind while buying a laser system. It is also not practical to buy and own every new laser that is launched in the market. It is paramount to evaluate each technology in depth and choose only that system which will benefit the practice; only then will the money be well spent.

FUNDING

A doctor may have to take a bank loan to purchase the laser. Check the interest rates and required documents to procure the loan. The following is a rough checklist of the documents needed for procuring a loan for medical equipment:
- Quotation from the company
- Purchase contract
- Income tax returns
- Registration documents of the clinic
- Clinic building documents
- Medical council registration
- Personal documents such as identity, address proofs, taxation documents

Having a laser purchase contract on paper signed by the buyer and distributor is essential. Many distributors take a brief one page purchase order (PO) from the customer, but this is insufficient as full details of the deal are not mentioned. The purchase contract should include:
- *Advance:* Once a price is negotiated, and a contract is signed, an advance amount is sought by the company. Generally, this should not be more than 25% of the total amount. A proper receipt clearly stating the cheque number and the amount needs to be obtained.

- Clause for balance payment, with date of repayment; instalments, if any, need to be specified.
- *Dollar/foreign currency value*: Since many machines are imported, the price often depends on the price of dollar or other currency which are subject to market fluctuations. This should be properly discussed and proper understanding reached with respect to market fluctuations of currency.
- Check the cost of the machine mentioned and note if there is any undervaluation. *Do not undervalue the machine for any reason.*
- *Check if all costs are mentioned:* Taxes, customs, transportation, insurance while transportation, and instalment costs.
- *Warranty*: Warranty should include all parts of laser; check the fine print and see if there are any exclusion clauses. Check if the warranty is subject to any specification of laser room and associate devices such as vacuum evacuator or air conditioner. Check the frequency of servicing and need for distilled water replacement if any. Sometimes, the company or parent organization may offer an extended warranty or extra service that should be in writing and mentioned in the contract.
- *Clause on repair:* Check how many hours or days will it take to attend to breakdown? Rough estimate of time frame to repair or replace parts? Installation of a standby system while the machine is being repaired so that work will not be affected should be asked for.
- It is wise to sign a contract or agreement between the buyer and seller before purchase of a laser which covers key aspects of installation, after-sales service, and maintenance of the machine.
- Adequate training is essential; understanding laser physics and laser–tissue interaction goes a long way in getting the best out of the machine.
- The credibility of the dealer and company should be ascertained in order to be assured of after-sales service.
- Buying used machines and sharing of equipment to offset high initial investments are good options but even more care is required to ensure proper functioning and maintenance.

To summarize, some important points to consider while purchasing a laser system are given in **Box 3.5.1**.

Box 3.5.1: Points to consider while purchasing a laser system.

- The type of practice and the patient profile of the doctor
- Common esthetic problems seen in one's practice
- Choice of laser systems—single or platform
- *Laser company background*: Credibility, number of installations, customer satisfaction
- Stability of the laser system, cost of spares, consumables
- Warranty offered, AMC/ASV post-warranty, service back-up, availability of local service engineers, expected time taken to attend to problems if and when they may occur
- Educational and marketing material provided by the company
- Training provided by the company on the machine
- Visit to the factory/HQ of the parent organization to access the commitment and R&D
- Published articles in peer-reviewed journals on the laser technology to access the efficacy and side effects profile of a given system
- *Laser specifications*: Spot size, pulse duration, peak power, customization options

PRACTICE POINTS

- Meticulous planning of the type of machine, specifications, financial aspects, maintenance, and warranties is important.

CONCLUSION

Before taking the plunge, access your practice profile and decide what lasers are best suited for your practice. Do discuss with your peers and check evidence of efficacy and adverse effects. Always insist for a demonstration of the machine. Choose the right technology and choose the right company. Check the after-sales record and cost of maintenance and then finally purchase the machine. Ensure that a detailed laser purchase contract is made and signed by the two parties as this will allow a healthy and hassle-free relationship between the dealer and the doctor in the future.

REFERENCES

1. Anderson RR, Parrish JA. Selective photothermolysis: precise microsurgery by selective absorption of pulsed radiation. Science 1983;220:524-7.
2. Manstein D, Herron GS, Sink RK, Tanner H, Anderson RR. Fractional photothermolysis: A new concept for cutaneous remodeling using microscopic patterns of thermal injury. Lasers Surg Med. 2004;34:426-38.
3. Buddhadev RM; IADVL Dermatosurgery Task Force. Standard guidelines of care: laser and IPL hair reduction. Indian J Dermatol Venereol Leprol. 2008;74:68-74.
4. Aurangabadkar S, Mysore V. Standard guidelines of care: lasers for tattoos and pigmented lesions. Indian J Dermatol Venereol Leprol. 2009;75 (Suppl 2):111-26.
5. Goel A, Krupashankar DS, Aurangabadkar S, Nischal KC, Omprakash HM, Mysore V. Fractional lasers in dermatology—current status and recommendations. Indian J Dermatol Venereol Leprol. 2011;77:369-79.
6. Gan SD, Graber EM. Laser hair removal: a review. Dermatol Surg. 2013;39(6):823-38
7. Cho SB, Lee SJ, Cho S, Oh SH, Chung WS, Kang JM, et al. Non-ablative 1550-nm erbium-glass and ablative 10 600-nm carbon dioxide fractional lasers for acne scars: a randomized split-face study with blinded response evaluation. J Eur Acad Dermatol Venereol. 2010;24(8):921-5
8. Srinivas CR, Kumaresan M. Lasers for vascular lesions: standard guidelines of care. Indian J Dermatol Venereol Leprol. 2011;77:349-68.
9. Aurangabadkar SJ, Mysore V, Ahmed ES. Buying a laser—Tips and pearls. J Cutan Aesthet Surg. 2014;7:124-30.

3.6 Expansion Dilemma: Partnership Firm, Limited Liability Partnership or Private Limited?

Dipak Kulkarni

INTRODUCTION

Many of our dermatologist colleagues sense the need to expand their profession after developing an excellent reputation and goodwill. They often want to have a bigger setup or a chain of clinics in multiple cities. This requires a transformation from mere medical professionals to entrepreneurs. (Many young dermatologists understand this professional need earlier than the previous generation.)

But for expansion, certain aspects need careful consideration:
- *Financial resources or capital:* An individual doctor's personal wealth may not be sufficient to finance the expansion of the setup. Taking bank loan may prove expensive and there is higher liability. A

better alternative is to create a partnership firm or a company. So, the capital from more individuals can be pooled from doctor's family members, relatives, other dermatologist colleagues, personal friends, or simply known investors.
- *More number of administrative or technical (medical) hands*: A bigger setup cannot remain a one-man army. A team of doctors is needed for expansion including administrative help for the management of the clinic. Other nonmedical partners or directors can help in this regard.
- *Brand building:* Brand building is better done in the name of the firm rather than on the name of an individual doctor. More number of doctors can later work under the same brand and share goodwill. So, such a brand is essential for expansion.

Apart from brand building, continuation of the profession in a firm or a company has various advantages:
- One can start group practice with like-minded professional friends.
- One can share the profits with the non-medico family members.
- One can limit personal financial liability [only in limited liability partnership (LLP) or Pvt. Ltd].

There are many options available for expanding a dermatology setup:
- Sole proprietorship firm
- A simple partnership
- Limited liability partnership
- Private limited company

SOLE PROPRIETORSHIP FIRM

This is a single-owner business or profession. It is linked to the PAN number of the owner and is not a separate legal entity. The need for creating such a firm is only to create a current account in a bank in the name of that firm. The brand building can be done in the name of the firm. Otherwise, the income of the firm is clubbed with the doctor's personal income.

SIMPLE PARTNERSHIP OR PARTNERSHIP FIRM

This is the easiest way of associating with more persons. A mere *partnership deed* is enough to start the business. Registration of the firm with *Registrar of Firms* is beneficial to solve possible legal disputes within the partners or with any third party. All partners should be Indian citizens. A partnership firm in the for the purpose of taxation, is an independent financial entity with a unique PAN number. These firms are taxed (income tax) at flat 30% rate (plus 12% surcharge if income exceeds ₹ 1 crore).

A partner gets income from the firm in the following ways:
- Remuneration is distributed to partners (maximum total allowed is 90% of the first 3 lakhs of profit and 60% of the profit above 3 lakhs)
- Profit share
- Interest on capital, if mentioned in the deed

The ratios in which remuneration is paid and profit is shared, are mentioned in the deed. But simple, partnership is not an independent legal entity. The responsibility or liability of any dispute comes directly on the individual partners. If there is an outstanding payment or debt, the individual partners are liable and have to pay it from their personal assets. In addition, there is a principle of mutual agency, i.e., each partner is legally bound by any action taken by other partners or by his own action. So, this type of association is not very convenient in long term and for an expanding business. This model may be okay to run a pharmacy next to the clinic, where all partners are family members.

PRIVATE LIMITED COMPANY

To limit the liability to the individuals involved in the clinic expansion, it is a good idea to form a private limited company. One can pool the capital from individuals who become shareholders. Some of them become directors who run the actual operations. Each director should have a Director's Identification Number (DIN) and the company is incorporated after prescribed paperwork with the Ministry of Corporate Affairs.

A private limited company becomes a legal as well as a financial entity, reducing the legal and financial liability on shareholders. It has a perpetual existence, i.e., it does not perish if any major shareholder sells his holding or by death of a director. But shareholders cannot sell their holdings to general public.

The company has a flexibility of how much remuneration/salary/perks it can give to a director. (But obviously, if such remunerations are disproportionately high, then it can come on the radar of Income Tax Department.).

The shareholders will get the share of profit after tax, in the ratio of their capital contribution. A tax called dividend distribution tax is payable.

The formation and tax/legal compliances of a private limited company are more complicated and thus expensive than a partnership firm. DIN and digital signatures of directors need to be obtained. The expense of incorporation could be around ₹ 20,000-50,000. The yearly audit and appointment of a chartered accountant are mandatory. Reports of annual meeting and board meetings need to be recorded and submitted.

The income tax payable for private limited companies having turnover less than ₹ 250 crores is 25%. The company also needs to pay surcharge (taxable income exceeding ₹ 1 crores—7% of computed income tax; taxable income exceeding ₹ 10 crores—12% of computed income tax). Companies are liable to pay secondary and higher education cess at a rate of 1% of the amount of income tax over and above the applicable surcharge.

There is a concept of minimum alternate tax (MAT). If any profit making company is paying less tax (<18.5% of book profits) due to some incentives or schemes, such company has to pay MAT not clearly defined.

So, if an aggressive expansion is planned, especially using the money of nonfamily investors, a private limited company is a better option. It will reduce liability, still one can draw a decent salary from the company as a director.

But many dermatologists may find company formation a bit complicated and may not be ready for it. For them, a limited liability firm may be more convenient.

LIMITED LIABILITY PARTNERSHIP

This is a new kind of entity allowed in India by an act in 2008. The LLP combines advantages of private limited company and simple partnership.

There is no limit on the number of partners and some partners may not be Indian citizens. At least two partners should be called as designated partners, who would be required to obtain a "Designated Partner Identification Number" (DPIN) on the lines similar to "Director's Identification Number" (DIN) required in case of directors of companies. LLP is also incorporated after registration with the Ministry of Corporate fairs.

Table 3.6.1: Comparison of various business models.

Type of business	Simple partnership	Limited liability partnership	Private limited company
Independent financial entity with separate PAN and IT filing	Yes	Yes	Yes
Independent legal entity limiting the liability of partners/directors	No	Yes	Yes
Registering authority	Registrar of firms	Ministry of Corporate Affairs	Ministry of Corporate Affairs
Need for DIN/DPIN	Not needed	Needed	Needed
Governed as per	Partnership deed	Partnership deed	Memorandum of association or charter of the company
Owned by	All partners	All partners	Shareholders
Managed by	All partners	Designated partners	Directors
Liability	Totally on all partners	Limited liability on partners	Limited liability of directors and shareholders
Income tax	Flat 30%	Flat 30%	Flat 25% (up to ₹ 250 crores turnover), 30% beyond that
Surcharge	12% if income exceeds ₹ 1 crore	12% if income exceeds ₹ 1 crore	7% after ₹ 1 crore 12% after ₹ 10 crores
Cess	3%	3%	1%
Dividend distribution tax	No	No	Yes
Remuneration to managing people	Limited by government law	Limited by government law	No limit for remuneration to directors by law but may be on radar of IT if grossly out of proportion
Profit sharing	As per ratio mentioned in the partnership deed	As per ratio mentioned in the partnership deed	As per the share ratio to all shareholders
Perpetual existence	No	Yes	Yes
Cost of formation	Low	Higher	Much higher
Respect in the eyes of bank and investors	Low	Medium	Much better
How to leave the organization	If a partner leaves, the partnership deed needs to be rewritten and submitted	If a partner leaves, the partnership deed needs to be rewritten and submitted	A shareholder simply sells his holdings to any other shareholder and can quit

The remuneration, profit sharing, etc., is similar to a partnership firm and governed by the directives in the partnership deed. But no partner would be liable on account of the independent or unauthorized actions of other partners and there is no joint liability created by other partners. In addition, like a private limited company, LLP also enjoys the status of an independent legal and financial entity giving limiting liability on the partners. It also has perpetual existence. It is slightly cheaper to incorporate the LLP as compared to a private limited company. Accounts of LLP with turnover less than ₹ 40 lakhs do not need audit from a CA. Minutes of annual meetings or board meetings are not required.

In short, if the persons coming together for business are within one family, then simple partnership is better as the formation as well as fulfilling the tax compliances are much easier.

When people outside the family are involved, then either LLP or private limited company is suitable. LLP is easy and cheaper to form as well as operate and enjoys almost all the benefits of a private limited company. But in the eyes of a bank, while giving loan, a generally private limited company is considered more respectful (may be as LLP is a new concept).

If any member wants to leave a private limited company, it is easier. He/she can simply sell his share to any of the partners and be away. In LLP, if somebody wants to leave then the entire partnership deed needs to be amended and Ministry of Corporate Affairs has to be informed **(Table 3.6.1)**.

3.7 Building Bridges: Interspecialty Interaction in Practice

Sushil Tahiliani

INTRODUCTION

When I started as a medical student in 1973, our physiology professor once told us that, to be relevant as doctor in a rapidly changing world of medicine, one must specialize in a particular subject of medicine. Things have changed further and now we have a situation where dermatologists are getting to be superspecialists in various subspecialties of dermatology. Interaction between physicians belonging to various specialties of medicine is essential to have a two-way beneficial effect on interacting individuals/groups/organizations. This would lead to a better understanding of each other's view point with better management of patients. Better medical care of the patient should be the underlying reason for such interaction.

Advantages

- There is a lack of awareness in other faculties about the newer advances in dermatology—the doctors and their relatives are known to visit homoeopathic clinics for their hair-related issues just because the clinics are advertised as trichology clinics.

- A rapport based on better diagnosis and management increases cross references.
- There are lesser chances of medical negligence and litigations.

METHODS

- Reference specifying the exact reason for the same
- Surgical procedures where a joint effort would lead to better outcome
- Hospitalization for conditions such as toxic epidermal necrolysis (TEN), Stevens-Johnson syndrome (SJS), systemic lupus erythematosus (SLE) and immunobullous conditions—management jointly with intensivist/rheumatologist/endocrinologist/cardiologist/nephrologist, etc., depending on systems involved or comorbidities necessitating management by other specialties to reduce risk of management-related complications.
- Shifting the patient to management by other specialties. We diagnose systemic diseases due to cutaneous markers but patient may not need regular management by a dermatologist. Examples are cutaneous T-cell lymphoma (if lymph nodes are involved or when the cutaneous lesions become significantly infiltrated) or in a case of SLE/systemic sclerosis/dermatomyositis.
- Participating in multifaculty conferences/webinars, etc., as a faculty to emphasize dermatologist's viewpoint in a multisystem disorder and inviting other specialty consultants to "Dermatology Conferences" to enable dermatologists have a more complete approach toward diagnosis/management of diseases.
- Making other specialty doctors realize that skin lesions seen by us could have resulted from the treatment being given for internal ailments and in case of drug rashes with eosinophilia and systemic symptoms (DRESS)/drug hypersensitivity syndrome/erythema multiforme (EM), etc., the treatment may have to be altered. A patient of mine who had nonhealing ulcer due to hydroxyurea being prescribed for lymphocytic leukemia by an eminent hematologist, recovered only after the persistent convincing of the treating doctor to change the "culprit" drug.
- Getting another opinion for management strategy in cases such as polycystic ovarian syndrome (PCOS)/psoriasis (PsO) with psoriatic arthritis (PsA), etc.
- Making other specialties realize that acute eczema is not to be treated as acute infection like cellulitis.

Where and how it matters: Skin cannot be treated in isolation. Health of skin reflects health of human being concerned. Skin lesions could be indicative of a systemic disease involving any system of the body. Treatment of a skin condition could be dependent on comorbidities and drugs being used to treat such comorbidities.

Some examples:
- *Pediatrics*: Genodermatoses and syndromes
- *Endocrinology*: Diffuse alopecia, patterned baldness, acne, hirsutism, acanthosis nigricans (AN), and dryness of skin due to thyroid diseases.
- *Rheumatology*: Vasculitis, PsO, and connective tissue diseases (CTDs)
- *Emergency medicine*: SJS, TEN, severe angioedema with compromised vital parameters, and IV drug administration (Rituximab, Infliximab, and IVIg).
- *Internal medicine*: Erythema nodosum and fever with rash
- *Hematology*: CTCL and blood dyscrasias due to drugs used for a skin ailment. A patient being investigated for Behçet's

disease, was discovered to have eosinophilia (64% in a total count of 11,000/cmm). Hematologist diagnosed an eosinophilic leukemia. Patient is under remission with imatinib and thalidomide.
- *Oncology*: CTCL, nodules due to precocious cutaneous metastasis, squamous cell carcinoma (SCC)/malignant melanoma to grade the malignancy.
- *Gastroenterology*: Management of hepatitis accidently discovered during workup of a case or raised transaminases suspected to be due to drugs such as Methotrexate (MTX)/dapsone. We may also suspect gastrointestinal (GI) involvement in cases of EN/vasculitis/mucosal pigmented lesions since childhood, etc.
- *Plastic surgery*: In cases where benign tumors on esthetically critical areas need to be excised, correction of deformities developing as a sequelae to Hansen's disease, surgically correctable congenital malformations and nevi.
- *ENT (ear, nose, and throat)/oral surgeon*: Biopsy from mucosal lesions are not easily manageable by dermatologists.
- *Vascular surgeon*: Cases of venous insufficiency and arterial ulcers.
- *Psychological medicine*: In difficult psychocutaneous conditions such as "hesitation" lines, intractable trichotillomania, and severe neurotic excoriations. I had a patient with schizophrenia who was very aggressive and thought dermatologists were incapable and inefficient in managing his intractable generalized pruritus. I convinced him to get hospitalized for a couple of days for specialized investigations, parenteral therapy, and a meeting of a group of "experts" to find out the best way out to manage his "itch." That was how his condition was diagnosed and effective therapy introduced.
- *Laboratory medicine*: We can sensitize the pathologist/microbiologist about our specific requirements. For instance, I make my microbiologist look into my notes to know where to take scraping/smear from. A laboratory also has made packages for adverse drug reaction monitoring which makes the investigations cheaper for my patients.
- *Radiology:* We have to sensitize the radiologist about need to look for small subungual tumors (glomus), osteophyte in case of pincer nail, bone in relation to skin in cases of miliary osteoma cutis, etc.
- *Nutritionist*: Their role cannot be undermined. In cases of excessive hair loss, metabolic syndrome-related dermatologic issues, etc., they play a very important role in successful management.

Drawbacks and limitations: The patient feels that he/she is being sent to different consultants to increase cost of therapy and is being treated as a commodity. We have to counsel the patient in detail and convince him/her as to why the interaction is being arranged. I try to talk to the concerned doctor on phone in patient's presence. What is lacking and needs to be done is a group discussion to enable an integrated approach to patient management. Not uncommonly, I am called upon to see a hospitalized patient with no doctor being present at the time of my visit and no notes on the case sheet to know the purpose of referral.

Dermatology has evolved but the other specialities have not come to terms with these advances. It is difficult to get consultants from other specialities to understand the exact role we want them to play—they are woefully inadequate and are not sensitized to our medical viewpoint.

Most of us practice in a stand-alone clinic or use a cabin for fixed hours in a polyclinic. It may be difficult to send a patient to another consultant in a different location and get the patient back to us with required advice. Patient may not go to the referred consultant or may not get back to us. I have had many experiences of a patient with hyperandrogenism with Frank clinical signs and some biochemical evidence-being referred to a gynecologist/endocrinologist by me and the concerned consultant telling the patient that she only needs to change her diet/do some exercise. Patients diagnosed with Hurley's grade 3 hidradenitis suppurativa, who need "unroofing," are referred to an anesthesiologist for fitness for standby general anesthesia only to be told that they should be seeing a general surgeon for the job. One such patient landed up with a full-thickness skin grafting done for lesions in both axillae and being told that the perigenital and gluteal lesions were too extensive to be tackled with a similar surgery. The radiologists get flummoxed and lack experience to report X-rays in suspected cases of primary miliary osteoma cutis or pincer nail. USG probes to pick up diagnosis of soft tissue swellings of cutaneous/nail disorders are not available in tertiary care centers also.

To summarize, interspeciality interaction is the need of the day and more emphasis should be given to it not only in practice, but it should be a part of medical education curriculum. Keeping a list of consultants who understand their respective role as well as our role, will help in proper management of dermatology cases.

3.8 Role of Doctors as Assistants, Fellowship Training and Academic Work in Dermatological Practice

Venkataram Mysore

INTRODUCTION

Dermatological practice has evolved from a single doctor sit and treat arm chair clinic and is now practiced in large centers in several cities. This is due to introduction of procedural dermatology in the practice. It can be said that Dr PN Behl who was the father of vitiligo surgery in India is also the pioneer of practice in a large center which trained doctors, employed assisting dermatologists, was recognized for DNB and also performed academic work. This chapter outlines the relevance of such practice and also the challenges involved. The chapter will be dealt in three headings:
1. Need for assistants
2. Imparting training
3. Performing academic work in a private clinic.

NEED FOR ASSISTANTS

What are assistants? The assistants can be:
- Doctors
- Technicians
- Nurses

As practice grows in numbers, into multiple clinics, in procedures, assistants are needed. Doctors are necessary for consultations, performing procedures, and assisting surgeries. These assisting doctors are usually young aspiring doctors who wish to learn or young ladies who are uncertain of immediate future plans or young doctors looking some employment till they can plan their career.

There are some risks of employing young doctors:
- They usually do not stay for a long time and sooner or later move out. So while employing them would help meet the above needs, they should not be expected to stay for long, and also their level of expertise is low. Often they leave at very short notice throwing the system out of gear. Hence this should be expected and system should be ready to absorb this. Either there should be a written memorandum of understanding (MOU) or a bond, which however, may be difficult to enforce.
- Since they do not have much expertise, there can be an occasional problem with patients, particularly complications in procedures or dissatisfied patients. So, strict supervision is necessary. One needs to have standard operating procedures (SOPs) for all procedures.
- Poor communication with patients—often a disinterested doctor may communicate poorly with patients.
- There is generally a fear in the minds of doctors that such young doctors will soon open their clinics and will take away patients, while this may happen this is usually not a worry. Some centers have enforced a MOU with geographic and time limitation that the doctor should not practice for certain period (6 months) with in such distance of the center (5 km).
- *Taking away staff:* This can happen more often and has happened to many senior doctors, particularly in HT.

In my opinion, young doctors have their needs and often go over the most difficult period of their lives. So the senior doctor should take a generous view and be a guide, to overcome the above risks.

TRAINING

Training in procedural dermatology is not available in medical colleges. Now such training is available in many centers around India. This training can be in three ways:
1. Informal medium term observerships of 1–3 months
2. Short-term workshops of 1–3 days
3. Formal university recognized fellowship courses of 1 year.

From personal experience, it can be said that instituting such practice is a rewarding experience. It helps the senior doctor to maintain academic excellence, in addition to the students assisting in clinic work. The reputation of the center is enhanced. And it helps the larger objective of achieving satisfaction of passing on what you have learnt and nurturing talent.

ACADEMIC WORK

It is generally recognized that academic work is the domain of medical colleges. However, it is not necessarily true. Academic work can be done in private centers for the following reasons:
- Dermatology is a clinic-oriented day care specialty, not a hospital-oriented specialty.
- In procedural dermatology, documentation is of the highest order because of medicolegal requirements.
- Most procedures are introduced and available in private setups.

- Dermatology work, particularly if one employs assistants, allows time to be used for academic work.
- It is easy to establish an environment and space for such work in a large center.

Hence, several dermatologists have performed excellent academic work in private centers. And such publications in turn help the center to establish reputation and attract patients.

3.9 Interaction with Industry

BS Chandrashekar

INTRODUCTION

The interaction of pharma industry with medical professionals should have the highest ethical standards. The interaction should also meet the legal requirements and the applicable laws laid by the government authorities. The interactions of healthcare professionals with the pharma and laser industry should not be perceived inappropriate and unethical by the patient, the public, and the media. They should be based on professional ethics followed by both the parties. The exchanges between the two parties should benefit patients in the therapeutic area and medical professionals in continued medical education (CME) along with the patient education.

Pharmaceutical company representatives who approach healthcare professionals play an important role in delivering accurate, up-to-date information about the approved indications, benefits, and risks of pharmaceutical therapies. These representatives often serve as the primary point of contact between the doctors and the companies who research, develop, manufacture, and market life-saving, quality of life-enhancing medicines and medical devices.

The healthcare professionals should note that representatives who visit them receive training about the applicable laws, regulations, and industry codes of practice that govern the representatives' interactions with healthcare professionals.

The exchange of knowledge must be patient centered based entirely on a patient's medical needs and medical knowledge and experience of healthcare professionals. The ethics code should evolve on the standards and principles prevailing in that geographical region.

CORE PRINCIPLES OF INTERACTIONS

Promotional activities and materials provided to healthcare professionals must:
- Be accurate and not misleading
- Claim on product and activity only, whenever necessary, with proper substantiation
- Reflect the right balance between risks and benefits
- Be in concurrence with the requirements and regulations of the governing authorities

INFORMATIONAL BRIEFING BY MEDICAL REPRESENTATIVES

Briefing by medical representatives (MRs) in a hospital, clinic, or office setting should only comprise valuable scientific information about drugs and devices which may contribute to better patient care. This can happen on a working day including lunch breaks. It is seen as appropriate lunches that can be offered as business promotions to doctors and their staff as long as such briefings provide scientific and educational value. Such lunches should not be a part of recreation or entertainment. Guests and family members of medical professionals are to be excluded. Such interactions should always happen in the presence of a company representative.

PHARMA SUPPORT FOR CONTINUING MEDICAL EDUCATION AND CONFERENCES

Continuing medical education and conferences help healthcare professionals to learn insights and gather knowledge about the recent and updated medical information that contribute to patient care.

In these situations, financial support from pharmaceutical companies is appropriate. The company should have a separate budget for educational grants without restriction on the amount to be spent. The following regulations should be in place:

- Should not promote a particular drug or device.
- Financial support should be utilized by the organizers to reduce the overall registration fee of all participants.
- The company should respect the commercial support guidelines established by the accreditation council for CME.
- When a company sponsors the event, the responsibility and control lie with the organizers in selection of contents, facility, scientific deliberation, material, venue selection, etc.
- The company should not direct or advice regarding the inclusion or exclusion of faculty even if a request comes from the organizers.
- Monetary support should not be given for travel, lodging, or any other expenses for nonfaculty members attending the proceedings either personally or to the organizers. Funding is also not allowed to compensate for the time spent by the delegates.
- The company should not provide recreation, food, or entertainment directly at the CME events; however, the organizers can utilize the financial aid for lunches and dinner.

THIRD-PARTY EDUCATIONAL PROFESSIONAL MEMBERSHIP

This can contribute to improvisation of patient care. Financial support is acceptable.

All the other guidelines laid down for CME and conferences are to be followed.

Consultants

Consulting arrangements with healthcare professionals allow companies to obtain information or advice from medical experts on topics such as the marketplace, products, therapeutic areas, and needs of patients. Companies use this advice to ensure that the medicines and devices they produce meet the needs of patients. Decisions regarding the selection or retention of healthcare professionals as consultants should be made based on defined criteria such as general medical expertise and reputation, or knowledge and experience regarding a particular therapeutic area. Companies should continue to ensure that consultant arrangements are neither inducements nor rewards for prescribing or recommending a particular medicine or course of treatment.

It is appropriate for consultants who provide advisory services to be offered reasonable compensation for those services and reimbursement for reasonable travel, lodging, and boarding expenses incurred as part of providing those services.

Token consulting or advisory arrangements should not be used to justify compensating healthcare professionals for their time or their travel, lodging, and other out-of-pocket expenses. The following factors support the existence of a bona fide consulting arrangement.

- A written contract specifies the nature of the consulting services to be provided and the basis for payment of these services
- A legitimate need for the consulting services has been clearly identified in advance of requesting the services and entering into arrangements with the prospective consultants
- The number of healthcare professionals retained is not greater than the number reasonably necessary to achieve the identified purpose
- The retaining company maintains records and makes appropriate use of the services provided by consultants
- The venue and circumstances of any meeting with consultants are conducive to the consulting services. Activities related to the services are the primary focus of the meeting specifically. Resorts are not appropriate venues.

Though modest meals or receptions may be appropriate during company-sponsored meetings, companies should not provide recreational or entertainment events in conjunction with these meetings.

It is not appropriate to receive honoraria or travel or lodging expenses as a nonfaculty and nonconsultant healthcare professional attendee at company-sponsored meetings, including attendees who participate in interactive sessions.

Speaker Programs and Speaker Training Meetings

Healthcare professionals participate in company-sponsored speaker programs in order to help educate and inform other healthcare professionals about the benefits, risks, and appropriate uses of company medicines and devices. Any healthcare professional engaged by a company to participate in such external promotional programs on behalf of the company will be deemed a speaker. Company decisions regarding the selection or retention of healthcare professionals as speakers should be made based on criteria such as general medical expertise and reputation, knowledge and experience regarding a particular therapeutic area, and communication skills. Companies should continue to ensure that speaking arrangements are neither incentives nor rewards for prescribing a particular medicine or course of treatment or promoting devices.

It is appropriate for healthcare professionals who participate in programs intended to train speakers for company-sponsored speaker programs to be offered reasonable compensation for their time, considering the value of the type of services provided, and to be offered reimbursement for reasonable travel, lodging, and boarding expenses. Such compensation and reimbursement should only be offered when the speakers receive extensive training on the company's drug products, device, or other specific topics to be presented. Speaker training sessions should be held in venues and locations other than resorts.

Any compensation or reimbursement made to a healthcare professional in conjunction with a speaking arrangement should be reasonable and based on the current market value. Each company should, individually and independently, calculate the total amount of annual compensation it will pay to the healthcare professional in connection with all speaking arrangements.

While speaker programs offer important educational opportunities to healthcare professionals, they are distinct from CME programs, and companies and speakers should be clear about this distinction. Speakers and their materials should clearly identify and display the company that is sponsoring the presentation.

Healthcare Professionals who are Members of Committees that Set Formularies or Develop Clinical Practice Guidelines

Healthcare professionals who are members of committees that are set to develop clinical practice guidelines that may influence the prescribing of medicines often have significant experience in these fields. This experience can be of great benefit to companies and ultimately to patients. These individuals may be chosen as speakers or commercial consultants for companies. To avoid even the appearance of impropriety, companies should require any healthcare professional who is a member of a committee that sets formularies or develops clinical guidelines and also serves as a speaker or commercial consultant for the company to disclose to the committee the existence and nature of his or her relationship with the company. This disclosure requirement should extend for at least 2 years beyond the termination of any speaker or consultant arrangement.

Scholarships and Educational Funds

Financial assistance for scholarships or other educational funds to permit medical students, residents, fellows, and other healthcare professionals in training to attend *carefully selected educational conferences may be offered.* The selection of individuals who will receive the funds is made by the head of the department of the training institute. *"Carefully selected educational conferences"* are generally defined as the major educational, scientific, or policy-making meetings of national, regional, or specialty medical associations.

PROHIBITION OF NONEDUCATIONAL AND PRACTICE-RELATED ITEMS

The materials provided by the pharma companies to healthcare professionals for their use that do not refer to disease or treatment education—even if they are of minimal value (such as pens, note pads, mugs, and similar "reminder" items with company or product logos)—may foster misperceptions that company interactions with healthcare professionals are not based on medical and scientific issues. Such noneducational items should not be accepted by the healthcare professionals or members of their staff, even if they are accompanied by patient or physician educational materials.

Healthcare professionals should not accept items intended for personal benefits (such as floral arrangements, artwork, music CDs, or tickets to a sporting event). Payments in cash or cash equivalents (such as gift certificates) should not be accepted by the healthcare professionals either directly or indirectly, except as compensation for bona fide services. Cash or an equivalent receipt of any kind creates a potential appearance of conflict of interest.

It is appropriate to receive product samples for patient use.

Educational Items

It is appropriate for healthcare professionals to accept items from companies, permitted by law, designed primarily for the education of patients or healthcare professionals if the items are of value < ₹ 1,000 (Rupees one thousand only). For example, a skin model for use in an examination room is intended for the education of the patients and is therefore appropriate, whereas a DVD or CD player may have independent value to a healthcare professional outside of his or her professional responsibilities, even if it could also be used to provide education to patients, and therefore is not appropriate.

Items designed primarily for the education of patients or healthcare professionals have to be accepted on an occasional basis, even if each individual item is appropriate.

Independence and Decision Making

No grants, scholarships, subsidies, support, consulting contracts, or educational or practice-related items should be accepted by the healthcare professional in exchange for prescribing products or recommending a device.

WHAT WE NEED FROM THE PHARMA INDUSTRY AT THIS JUNCTURE?

- *More involvement from the industry:* Doctors should develop stronger collaboration with the industry with the objective of raising the quality of patient care and improving treatment outcomes.

The healthcare professionals should guide the pharma companies to take a more holistic approach that adds value beyond the product itself.

Healthcare professionals should call for industry assistance in many areas including online consultations, facilitating care at the bedside, individual patient follow-up, patient information services, and novel ways to enhance self-management.

- *Better services:* Good communication is seen as a vital aspect of patient care.

Communication technology that supports two-way understanding between the doctor and the patient is very interesting. The doctor should be smart enough to answer real patient questions and give useful guidance that reassures people.

Pharma companies should "provide digital information with good content. It has to be delivered in a fast and an easy way."

- *Information and education:* Life science companies have long been seen as a potential source of information.

Healthcare professionals should look for life science companies to take on a role as health educators, making information easily accessible to everyone—both professionals and patients.

Digital communication provides ways to do this in a relevant and timely fashion.

"Examples should be in the form of presentations of the newest studies, based on the drugs that they are talking about, the newest indications, the most frequent side effects, long-term safety, etc."

- *Help to improve adherence:* A key need for healthcare professionals is treatment-compliant patients. As healthcare professionals, we should know that many patients do not strictly follow their treatment regimen.

Development in consumer health-tracking apps should make us think that it may be possible to pursue a similar strategy for low-adherence situations.

- *More involvement with patients:* As medical professionals, we should positively value the trend of patient empowerment and face the challenges. In contrast to previous generation of patients who would accept any advice, today's empowered patients are more likely to question it, though they may be acting on poor quality or incorrect information gathered though online research.

Doctors should look at the industry to ensure that there is ready access to credible sources of information.

The pharma companies can help by providing authoritative, clear, and useful materials that healthcare professionals can share with their patients.

"Patients who are more informed tend to follow physicians' advice properly."

Partnerships with sales representatives: The way these relationships are built, however, will depend on the individual requirements of the healthcare professionals.

Technology has a key role in facilitating these new relationships by pharma companies with healthcare professionals. By connecting through face-to-face engagement, remote meetings, and self-guided multichannel communication, it is possible to respond to individual preferences of healthcare professionals while providing the same high-quality experience.

BIBLIOGRAPHY

1. Brax H, Fadlallah R, Al-Khaled L, Kahale LA, Nas H, El-Jardali F, et al. (2017). Association between physicians' interaction with pharmaceutical companies and their clinical practices: a systematic review and meta-analysis; 2017.
2. https://agnitio.com/6-things-marketing-doctors/. [Last accessed March 2020].
3. https://www.phrma.org/-/media/Project/PhRMA/PhRMA-Org/PhRMA-Org/PDF/A-C/Code-of-Interaction_FINAL21.pdf. [Last accessed March 2020].
4. The Principal Regulations namely, "Indian Medical Council (Professional Conduct, Etiquette and Ethics) Regulations, 2002" were published in Part–III, Section (4) of the Gazette of India on the 6th April, 2002, and amended vide MCI notifications dated 22/02/2003, 26/05/2004&14.12.2009.

SECTION 4
Hiring and Managing Staff

4.1 Staffing Needs of a Dermatology Center

BS Chandrashekar, Praveen Kumar SP

INTRODUCTION

Staffing is also called as human resource planning and consists of putting right number of people, right kind of people at the right place, right time, and doing the right things for which they are suited for the achievement of goals of the organization. Human resource planning has got an important place in the arena of healthcare industry. Human resource planning has to be in a systematic approach and is carried out in a set procedure.

- Staffing is done based on certain criteria which are as follows:
  - Type of organization, e.g., institute, teaching academy, hospital, clinic, etc.
  - Number of departments, e.g., clinical staffs, billing, pharmacy, accounts, etc.
  - Number and quantity of such departments
  - Employees in these work units
  - Illustrating the same with an example in **Table 4.1.1** considering four categories of dermatology centers based on inflow, ranging from 40 to 300 OPD (outpatient department) patients and working for 12 hours a day.

A SPECIAL MENTION ON MEDICAL COUNSELOR IN DERMATOLOGY CENTER

Responsibilities

- Assess patient through detailed conversations, interviews and observations to determine the appropriate testing or examination.
- Assess patient's mental and emotional stats/aspects.
- Create effective treatment plans that include counseling, medication, or other services.
- Work with your patient and develop goals.
- Regularly discuss the treatment plan with your patient to identify faults or room for improvement.
- Educate appropriate coping mechanisms to help patients through tough situations.
- Record the patient's progress and change their treatment plan when needed.
- Orient the patient about the hospital protocol and policies with respect to the flow of events.
- Counselors should put efforts to understand the socioeconomic status of the patient so as to smoothen their transaction in the hospital.
- Counselors play a major role making the patient to understand the fee structure of the treatment.

Section 4: Hiring and Managing Staff

Table 4.1.1: Four categories of dermatology center with criteria.

Sl no.	Department	Consideration criteria	Derma clinic (max 40 OPD's)	Derma clinic with (ranging from 40–70 patients)	Dermatology setup in a multispecialty hospital with range of 100–150 patients per day	Institute of dermatology where 200–300 patients come per day
1.	Consultants	Considering a doctor can see up to 5 patients an hour and work for 8 hours a day	1	2	3	10
2.	Procedures (including OT)	Considering an average conversion of 15% (from outpatients to procedures)	1	1 consultant	1 consultant +1 registrar	2 consultants + 3 registrars
3.	Receptionist (including procedure floor)	1 receptionist can handle up to 40 patients a day along with phone calls	1+1 reserve	2	4	12
4.	Billing	Considering a maximum of 70 bills per head	1	1	2	3
5.	Marketing	1 marketing manager and 1 executive			1	2
6.	Pharmacy	Considering 400 bills per day and a maximum of 60 bills per staff	1	2	3	7
7.	Technicians	Considering 6 patients per staff per day (45 patients per day)	1	2	3	9
8.	OT technician	Considering 2 OT cases per day	-	-	2	3
9.	Laboratory	Considering 20 samples a day	-	-	1	2
10.	Housekeeping	Considering area to be 10000 sqft, 1 HK required for every 2000 sqft of area	1	2	3	5
11.	Security	2 staffs, 1 for day and 1 for the night	1	1	2	2
12.	Accounts	Considering 1 accountant for every 50 employees we would require 2 accounts executives for an organization with 100 employees and 1 chief accountant	-	1	2	3
13.	Human resource (HR)	1 HR for 100 employees	-	-	1	1
14.	Counselors	1 counselor for every 40 patients	1	2	3	5
15.	Administration	1 admin for 100 employees	-	-	1	1
16.	Multipurpose worker	In case of a small setup we can have this category who would be handy (who would act as PRO + billing + accounts, etc.)	1	2	-	-
	Total		9	13	30	64

- They would also prepare a questionnaire and make the patient to answer the same pertaining to the specific conditions which patient would be suffering from.

Requirements
- Bachelor degree in psychology, social work, or counseling
- A minimum of 3 years of experience as a professional counselor
- Superb verbal and written communication skills
- Aptitude to empathize with clients and help them open up
- Good time management skills
- Proven experience in developing effective treatment plans
- Assess patients through detailed conversations, interviews, and observations to determine the appropriate tests or examination

QUALITIES AND ATTRIBUTES TO LOOK OUT IN A HOSPITAL STAFF DURING INTERVIEW

- *Pleasing personality:* A good hospital staff requires having a pleasing personality who is easily approachable, the personality being expressed not only in body language but also while speaking over the phone.
- *Highly organized*: Being organized in their work is another important requirement for a hospital job. There is so much information which needs to be passed on through each day; hence, to keep a track of it is of high importance. As we are dealing with the health of the patient, the health records, lab values, test reports and many other information have to be intact and the individual has to be well organized to carry out these tasks.
- *Time management*: Imagine a scenario where exactly at the same time, the phone is ringing, employees are asking for some urgent data, a courier person is there and a visitor is standing in a hospital reception or a doctor in emergency is treating a critical patient, and patients in OPD start asking for a doctor due to delayed OPD consultation. There are times when a staff may feel this situation to be panicky but with an efficient understanding of time management this can be handled easily. Hence you look out for this quality during the interview of a candidate.
- *Technical knowledge*: Knowledge and ability of the individual in that field to be assessed during interview before inducting the staff.
- *Empathy:* While empathy is considered a basic human quality, it is often missing from the workplace. In a healthcare setting, we often need to have this quality to larger extent to be successful in the job.
- *Up-to-date with technology:* Technological skills are important for the efficient hospital staff. A good staff needs to know how a computer functions and how internet works, including emailing. This is helpful as it will make their job easier and efficient.
- *Reliable:* Any hospital staff is required to be someone who can be trusted. A situation where if the phone is ringing and it is not answered leaves a bad impression about the organization. They need to cater to the patient's requirements and resolve the issue at its best so that the management does not have to look further ahead. They need to ensure that the entire job is done on time and that people can trust them with their information and data.
- *Strong communication skills:* Communicating the right information

to the concerned person is an essential job requirement of a good employee. When someone comes with a query to them, they are required to communicate the information with clear instructions. They also need to be clear to inform the employees about the message left or any other information is to be passed on. Communication not only signifies words but also the manner in which it is dealt with including a positive body language.

JOB DESCRIPTION OF CERTAIN POSITIONS IN THE ORGANIZATION

- *Medical counselor job responsibilities*:
  - Assess patients through detailed conversations, interviews, and observations to determine the appropriate testing or examination.
  - Diagnose patient's mental and emotional disorders.
  - Create effective treatment plans that include counseling, medication, or other services.
  - Work with your patient and develop goals.
  - Regularly discuss the treatment plan with your patient to identify faults or room for improvement.
  - Educate appropriate coping mechanisms to help patients through tough situations.
  - Record the patient's progress and change their treatment plan when needed.
  - To orient the patient about the hospital protocol and policies with respect to the flow of events.
  - Counselors put efforts to understand the socioeconomic status of the patient so as to smoothen their transaction in the hospital.
  - Counselors play a major role making the patient understand the fee structure of the treatment.
  - They would also prepare a questionnaire and make the patient answer the same pertaining to the specific conditions which patient would be suffering.
- *Requirements*:
  - Bachelor's degree in Psychology, Social Work, or Counseling.
  - A minimum of 3 years' experience as a professional counselor.
  - Superb verbal and written communication skills.
  - Aptitude to empathize with clients and help them open up.
  - Good time management skills.
  - Proven experience in developing effective treatment plans.
  - Assess patients through detailed conversations, interviews, and observations to determine the appropriate testing or examination.
- *Human resource manager job description*: Human resources management plays a vital role in the healthcare workplace in ensuring the delivery of healthcare services and facilitating optimal patient outcomes. In any healthcare setting, the Human Resource department fills a variety of personnel needs that both employers and employees encounter. The role of this department is to manage all aspects of operations that are personnel related.
- *Human resources management functions include*:
  - Hiring
  - Physician and nurse and hospital staff recruitment
  - Employee orientation
  - Personnel management

- Aid in finding counseling for employees
- Staff benefits and compensation management
- Claims handling
- Training and performance monitoring
- Professional development program
- Regulations education
- Workplace safety and sanitation
- Labor mediation
- Administration—employee meetings
- Staff morale and retention

▪ *Hospital administration manager (HAM) responsibilities include*:
- Supervising daily administrative operations
- Creating quarterly and annual budgets
- To be successful in this role, one should have a deep understanding of all administrative hospital procedures, from creating work schedules and communicating with doctors to budgeting and maintaining supplies stock
- Supervise daily administrative operations
- Monitor expenses and suggest cost-effective alternatives
- Create monthly, quarterly and annual budgets
- Prepare Management Information System (MIS) reports
- Develop and implement effective policies for all operational procedures
- Prepare work schedules
- Maintain organized medical and employee records
- Train new employees
- Ensure prompt ordering and stocking of medical and office supplies
- Answer queries from doctors, nurses and healthcare staff
- Stay up-to-date with healthcare regulations
- Resolve potential issues with patients

▪ *Requirements*:
- Knowledge of medical terminology and hospital industry
- Hands-on experience with database systems and MS Excel
- Solid understanding of healthcare procedures and regulations
- Basic accounting skills
- Familiarity with medical transcription
- Excellent organizational and time management skills
- Ability to supervise and train team members
- Problem-solving attitude.

▪ *Chief Operating Officer (COO) job purpose*:
- COO directly reports to the MD, providing overall management and oversight of Hospital Services. This position has overall responsibility for policy development, program planning, administration, and operation of assigned plan functions, programs, and activities. The position assists the MD in implementing the organization's strategic goals by partnering and regularly interfacing with the Chief Medical Officer, Finance Officer, health services, quality improvement, government relations and information technology. Plans, directs, and oversees a company's operational policies, rules, initiatives, and goals. Helps organization execute long-term and short-term plans and directives by implementing judgment, vision, management, and leadership.

- *Major Functions and Accountabilities Duties may include, but are not limited to, the following*:
  - Measures effectiveness and efficiency of operational processes both internally and externally and finds ways to improve processes.
  - Develops and implements growth strategies.
  - Acts as a liaison between company and client for quality assurance.
  - Provides mentoring to all employees, including manage.

4.2 Role of Counselors and Technicians

Venkataram Mysore, Vani Yepuri

INTRODUCTION

In recent decades, understanding of the health predominated problems has stopped being just a doctor's job. Counseling has become a cornerstone in providing quality services, especially in health care. The role of counselors in health care is gradually becoming important. In dermatological setting where esthetic practice is on the rise and where the patient awareness on the various treatment options available has increased, the role of counselors becomes more significant. Many patients put forth many queries, which a busy dermatologist may be unable to address and the patient may fell either let down or may be aggressive. Counselors can bridge this gap and devote time in responding to their queries.

WHAT IS COUNSELING?

The World Health Organization (WHO) defines counseling as a well-focused process, limited in time and specific, which uses the interaction to help people deal with their problems and respond in a proper way to specific difficulties in order to develop new coping strategies.[1]

Patients in any medical specialty are interested in short-term and focused interventions that can facilitate early recovery, rather than long-term therapies. These requirements are typically met by behavioral, cognitive, and cognitive-behavioral approaches.[2] The process of counseling represents a valid intervention made of a quality interaction between the counselor and the patient, characterized by the capacity of the counselor to empathize with the interior world of the patient. The main purpose of counseling is to help the patient amplify the vision of the specific situation and enable the proper potential in dealing with the conditions, in order to promote a better quality of service.

One other aim of counseling should be to identify the emotional problems early and prevent serious disturbance developing. Counselors do assessment and determine the mental state. They deal with the issues of the patients, spend time in educating the patients about the disease or treatment. They help patients to understand the risks or benefits related to a particular treatment or disease.

The range of these approaches for the patients is quite wide preparing the patient for the procedure, letting them know the outcome of the treatment, teaching them to cope with the side effects if happens, helping them to change unhealthy behaviors (weight control and smoking cessation), and dealing with their unrealistic expectations to make realistic.

Significance in Dermatology

Dermatology is a specialty where most of the conditions are chronic and require long-term treatment. Moreover, the time has changed from when a patient would leave from the doctor's cabin without asking anything further after being diagnosed and prescribed to a fully demanding patient who has multiple queries about the diagnosis and treatment options. Added to this, people turn on to google search for their problems, landing up before the doctor with their collected data. Due to paucity of time, the doctor may not answer all the questions. But again this may add to the mistrust or misconception already existing on the medical fraternity. Counselors can bridge this gap of doctor–patient communication.

Chronic diseases like psoriasis and eczema need prolonged treatment and also maintenance therapy. Patients follow the medication prescribed for some time, and then stop on clearance. They do not turn up for follow-up visits until any exacerbation. But they should understand that the treatment has to be continued in milder dosages and some moisturizers has to be continued for preventing relapse, thus follow-up visits are necessary. Good patient education is needed to hold the patient and also for better patient compliance. Good counseling helps in clearing patients' doubts and increases the faith of patient in the doctor as well as the clinic. This should include educating the patient about the pattern of illness, prognosis, the treatment options available, the need for adherence for treatment, the pros and cons, and follow-up at regular intervals. Since most of the treatments include topical medications in dermatology, creating awareness on the proper method, duration and amount of application increases the efficacy of the treatment and prevents in creating a dissatisfied patient. Also, relapse is common thing for many conditions. Keeping the patient well informed on the possibility of relapse, makes him/her accept it more easily. Good communication is important for compliance and outcome. For example, tinea infections are emerging resistant everywhere, added to this the steroid abuse. At the first visit, the patient should be educated about the adverse effects of the steroids when prescribed by a quack or by a relative and thus the importance of consulting a skin doctor instead of a pharmacist or a quack. The patient should be well communicated about the duration of treatment, the additional care to be taken like maintaining hygiene, keeping the areas dry, the method of application, and the need to continue treatment even after clearance for some time as suggested by the doctor to prevent relapse. Relapse always creates a negative impact on the doctor by the patient. And this type of patient education and good communication prevents relapse, increases compliance, and also prevents dissatisfaction if even relapse occurs.

Counselors can also be trained with basics of phototherapy like number of sessions required, how does it work, what are the intervals between sessions, what would be the protocol if a session is missed, or if there is long gap after the last session. The patient should be educated if one session is missed, dose may have to be reduced by 25%. If there is a long gap, the dosage might have to be reduced by 50%. It should also be communicated to the patient that slight erythema visible for less than 24 hours is normal with phototherapy, but erythema extending beyond 24 hours is to be considered and should be brought to the notice of the doctor.

Similarly, counseling an acne patient will ensure better compliance and result. Generally, in spite of a clear written prescription by a dermatologist on how the acne medications have to be applied, patients do not follow and end up with irritation or dryness or some redness on the face. Here the counselor should explain the acne patient that, the topical medication of acne may be little irritant or cause dryness. Hence it is important to apply a moisturizer for full face before applying the acne creams, more over the creams should be applied on the pimple without rubbing or spreading to prevent irritation.

Certain conditions like vitiligo have social stigma and patients generally feel discriminated or isolated. Proper counseling of the patient gives him/her the confidence to face the society. Educating the patient's attenders or relative also helps in spreading the awareness that vitiligo is noncommunicable disease and it is just lack of color at certain parts of the body.

Further there are certain skin conditions which are nontreatable, some are harmless even if not treated. Patient education on such conditions helps in alleviating the anxiety they have regarding their problem.

In this era of violence and consumer acts, where any patient turns up against doctor, it is mandatory to keep the patient well informed, well educated, and well communicated, which is likely to make the patient able to cope up with minor issues and prevent litigation issues.

Significance in Esthetic Dermatology

The increasing patient demand for esthetic procedures makes a dermatologist busy and exhausted that he may be unable to meet the queries of the patients to their satisfaction. But then writing or advising a procedure to the patient, without giving much information on the same is also not acceptable to an esthetic patient. Here comes the counselor who plays a major role in esthetic practice. In addition to patient education and counseling, they need to learn about esthetic procedures, maintaining hospitality, costs, complications, and rescheduling follow-up visits. A good hospitality to the patient in the first visit making him feel comfortable in the premises helps to keep the patient in synchronization. The counselors should expertise in pacifying a patient who faces some complication postprocedure.

The counselor should have minimum knowledge on the treatment done, its course of events, possible complications—minor as well as major which have to be communicated to the patient prior to the procedure. For example, indications of the different lasers, the number of sittings required, and the expected results which will be achieved. Counselor should know few general things like avoiding trimming of hair before or after the laser hair removal, importance of photoprotection, and all these has to communicated to the patient properly. It should be educated that laser hair removal is not permanent removal but is permanent reduction. Keeping the patient well informed makes the patient to accept the results easily and happily. Taking informed consents and explaining the consent form is one another major job of the counselor.

Patients can be tricky sometimes. They come for some treatment, get the treatment done, and while the treatment is done, the patient may take advantage by trying to get some other procedure done at the same sitting freely. The counselor should be aware of handling such instances and refuse in a very polite and informed manner that the patient accepts easily. It is also important to make the patient understand about the outcome of the treatment, the results achieved, and the need for follow-up in case of multiple sittings of a particular treatment. Either the doctor or the counselor should always under promise regarding the desired results which helps in preventing future hurdles.

It is important for a counselor to identify patients with psychosomatic disorders like body dysmorphic disorder, schizophrenia, or any other illness. This makes a doctor's job easy to handle them and can avoid advising any esthetic treatments to them. Similarly, it is a major job of counselor to counsel a patient with unrealistic expectations to realize and accept whatever results achieved.

Who is a Counselor?

The accreditation qualification for counseling varies from country to country. May western countries have long-term as well as weekend courses available, wherein one is trained to be called themselves as counselors. In US, one needs to hold a minimum of master's degree in counseling to be a licensed counselor. In most Asian countries, including India, counseling is not well established nor is the courses. There is no basic qualification required to be counselor. Any graduate with good rapport in regional language as well as English can be a counselor after proper training. A dermatologist can train his/her paramedical or nonmedical staff in counseling skills in an effective way of dealing with immediate and more simple problems of clients. This should include effective communication, patient–medical staff relationships, stress management, and psychological factors associated with health and illness. They can also be taught specific techniques for dealing with problems like pain or insomnia, or specific ways for managing personal and professional difficulties, like burnout or troubled communication.

TECHNICIANS

Technicians in dermatology are medical assistants who assist the dermatologist in procedures like chemical peels, lasers, or any other skin procedures. Their duties include minimal medical history taking, recording the vital signs, preparing the patient for the treatment, and helping the doctor during the treatment. They also need to take up certain administrative tasks like maintaining records, scheduling appointments, checking bills, etc.

There are certified esthetic technician courses available which train them with basics of anatomy and physiology, dermatology, medical terminology, computer applications, record-keeping, insurance processing, laboratory techniques, pharmacology, and medical law and ethics. Any nursing staff can serve the role of technicians in dermatology. Many national and international conferences organize workshops or certified courses wherein interested person or nurses can be trained. The technicians can perform some basic esthetic procedures and some laser treatments in a busy practitioners, clinic.

They should be well verse with the basics of these procedures and their outcome, they should be able to communicate the same to the patient adequately for better results. However, these have to be done under the supervision of a dermatologist to ensure patient as well doctor safety in medicolegal terms.

In a national conference, Kaur V presented results from a study that showed the difference in treatment outcome in acne patients with the intervention of a trained nursing assistant in the OPD. Forty patients with grade II acne vulgaris were included in the study. Patients were randomly divided into two groups—group A who had only dermatologist consultation and group B was counseled by a trained dermatology assistant following the dermatologist consultation. The results show that the percentage of patients showing no improvement was greater in group A (17.6%) as compared to group B (5.0%).[3] Also, a larger percentage of patients in group B reported good and satisfactory improvement. This study deduced that where there was additional nursing intervention, the outcome was better. Technicians and counselors can also serve similar purpose and help in bringing better outcome in daily busy practice of a dermatologist. Even career wise, there is increasing demand in the field. According to the US Bureau of Labor Statistics, opportunities as dermatology technicians are expected to grow more quickly by 2024.

Besides communication skills, counselors and technicians should be well groomed and appealing to the patients. They should be well mannered and polite in all circumstances. They should be aware of every aspect of the doctor, about the clinic, how the clinic works, and the clinic protocols. There should be proper coordination among themselves. This avoids miscommunication among the staff themselves and also with the patients.

At no point in time should they behave rudely or become impatient. Special training sessions should be arranged for the counselors and technicians by the doctor once in 6 months or yearly to keep them in track.

> **Advantages of Counselors and Technicians**
> - Save time of doctor—counseling and patient education
> - Help to build patient–doctor–staff relationship
> - Help in pacifying patients regarding any administrative or treatment issue of patient
> - Help in identify psychosomatic disorder patients, thus making the doctor cautious while treating them
> - Taking feedback from the patients
> - Can discuss and handle issues regarding cost of treatment which cannot be done by the doctor

CONCLUSION

Both counselors and technicians need patience, empathy, well-developed communication skills, good grooming, pleasant manners, and the ability to multitask often in a stressful environment. In circumstances wherein a dermatologist cannot afford to keep large number of staff, or in a small clinic setup, even one person either paramedical or a nonmedical can be trained such a way that he/she can serve dual role of technician as well as counselor. Hence counselor and technicians can be multitaskers when well trained. They should not behave rudely in whatever circumstances to the patients or relatives. But then a clinic should not depend on counselor entirely for the counseling job, the remaining staff or even the doctor should be ready to answer the patient whenever needed. It should be a multidisciplinary team-based approach for a good doctor–patient relationship which at the end benefits the doctor, the staff as well as the patient.

> **Qualities Required for Counselor and Technician**
>
> - Pleasant and patience
> - Good grooming
> - Well mannered and polite
> - Empathy
> - Hospitality—making patient comfortable, explaining everything properly
> - Good communication skills
> - Multitask
> - Knowledge on the procedures as well as every aspect of how clinic works
> - Ability to handle complicated patients
> - Ability to identify emotionally disturbed patients or those with unrealistic expectations
> - Ability to maintain patience even in worst situations
> - Always communicate with the doctor whenever needed

REFERENCES

1. Radoja D. The Role of Counselling in Medical Settings. ResearchGate; 2015. pp. 28-30.
2. Karademas, Evangelos (2009). Counselling Psychology in Medical Settings: The Promising Role of Counselling Health Psychology. European Journal of Counselling Psychology. 1.10.5964/ejcop.v1i1/2.9.
3. Kaur V. Nursing interventions in dermatology. Presented at 35th National Conference of Indian Association of Dermatologists, Venereologists and Leprologists, Chennai, India; 2007.

4.3 Time Management

Venkataram Mysore, Anuradha Jindal

"Productivity is never an accident. It is always the result of a commitment to excellence, intelligent planning and focused effort"
— **Paul J Meyer**

"Show me a physician with time to spare and I'll pinch you to stop you from dreaming"

INTRODUCTION

The workload on physicians is increasing, increased work load demands more efficient time management to maintain the balance between work and personal life. Time can be considered as fixed, nonrenewable natural resource, which cannot be replenished once it passes by. Adapting time management techniques can help utilizing the time a dermatologist has in hands, increase the output of practice without compromising on the personal life.

All physicians need to consider the following questions:
- Do you think you work too long?
- Have you ever been hours behind your schedule in a clinical day?
- Do you lag behind in keeping up-to-date with latest journals?
- Are you always late for meetings?
- Do you want to carve out more time for your family?
- Are you looking for ways to plan your work week better?
- Do you have trouble "getting it all done"?
- Do you feel stressed just contemplating what you need to do today or tomorrow?

If the answer to any of these is yes, tips in this chapter might help manage the same amount of time in better way. We as doctors are expected to attend to multiple tasks including patient care, family, personal, business, sports, research community, and sometimes arranging conferences. It is therefore no wonder that time is of the essence and most physicians seem to always lag behind.

Why do we need effective time management? So that we can manage practice and career effectively, utilize finite healthcare resources appropriately, to serve in administration and assume leadership roles, and at the same time find time for family and attend to other recreational interests in life.

Effective time management techniques can be grouped as follows:
- Managing routine work effectively and prioritizing tasks
- Making Standard Operating Procedures (SOPs) and protocols
- Multitasking or set shifting
- Organizing clinic for saving time during consultations
- Time saving in procedures
- Utilization of e-resources

MANAGING ROUTINE WORK EFFECTIVELY AND PRIORITIZING TASKS

The key element to understand is, time management is about behaviors, not time. It is about matching your behaviors with your true priorities and goals. Like any skill, it takes time to master.

Stephen R Covey, the famous American author, described a story of woodcutter who sawed 15 trees on first day, 18 trees on second day of work, 12 trees on day 3, on day 4 he worked an hour extra but still could cut only 12 trees. A man asked him "why do not you sharpen the saw". The lumberjack replied "I am too busy in cutting trees, I do not have time to sharpen my saw". As rightly said by Abraham Lincoln "Give me six hours to chop down a tree and I will spend the first four sharpening the ax". Simply throwing more effort at a situation does not work. It is time to stop, take stock, and sharpen the saw.

Time is a limited resource: As much as we would like to, we cannot add more hours to a day. The only solution to not having "enough" time is to make better use of the time we *do have—to sharpen the saw*. This involves making choices, in keeping with our priorities.

Time cannot be managed, we can manage ourselves.

Efficiency leads to creativity. Physicians need a healthy balance between organizational efficiency and creativity. The more they have of the former, the more time there is for the latter.

Pareto's principle—80/20 rule states that 80% of effective results, or rewards, are derived from about 20% of all energy. 80% of our work is routine, mundane. This 80% should not interfere with the really challenging and creative 20%. So manage the 80% in as less time as possible. It should be done quickly and efficiently. To finish 80% of common work at par, we should learn to prioritize, inculcate punctuality, multitasking, and work efficiently. How to learn to prioritize your tasks should be learned from Sherlock Holmes. He was excellent in criminology, psychology, history, poisons, and law. He was average in geography, medicines, and culture and was completely nil in entertainment, business, politics, and sports. He had no family life of his own but he was the master of his field. Learn what is useful, know what is needed, and adopt what is practical. Identify where you have natural talents, the work you enjoy is easier to do. Identify where you have no inclination; try to delegate, or hire or do when you have time. To cite an example, author does not like doing follicular unit extraction (FUE), which is usually managed by his co-doctors.

MAKING STANDARD OPERATING PROCEDURES AND PROTOCOLS

We should invest more time for management of clinic and protocols. It helps in better streamlining of the work. Teaching is an important tool for learning, by learning you will teach, by teaching you will learn more.

It is equally important to keep a close eye on the turnout of the clinic, not only financially but also patient's satisfaction, procedure results, and final outcome of procedures. The following tips will be useful for the same:
- SOPs—for everything—how to do peels, laser parameters for common procedures like tattoo removal, hair removal, platelet-rich plasma (PRP), intralesional injections, sclerotherapy, radiofrequency, etc.
- For pharmacist—how to dispense drugs, SOPs for application of scabicides, steroids, methotrexate, etc.
- For OT nursing staff—preoperative questionnaire, postoperative information.
- Feedback forms.
- A reminder through mail or sms can be sent to patients regarding their upcoming appointment.

MULTITASKING AND SET SHIFTING

Multitasking means doing multiple things at one time or a bit of everything at one time. Set shifting is better than multitasking. Set shifting means consciously and completely finishing one task, shifting your attention, and then focusing on the next task at hand. Giving your full attention to what you are doing will help you do it better, with more creativity and fewer mistakes or missed connections. Set shifting is a sign of brain fitness and agility. We should do multiple things but one after another. Planning and conceptualizing on multiple things at different times of the day. Execution should generally be one at a time unless you are getting someone else do them. Multitasking should not mean starting multiple things and tapering off on all of them.

Stamina to carry on the work with all the enthusiasm, consistently and persistently, ability to focus and concentrate, and use up-to-date and relevant technology to enhance efficacy are also important. We should know where to say "no" also, say no to what you do not want to do, and perform what you want to do. To focus more energy into productive work, we should avoid distractions, should not react to provocations, comments after seeing e-groups, google reviews or WhatsApp. Thinking about things which are not in your control is just merely wasting precious time of your day.

As the famous proverb goes, all work, no play makes jack a dull boy. Sadness and grey is not good for soul, it dulls the mind and hence hinders innovations and discoveries. Life is a balance of work and personal life. We work to live not live to work. Few hours in 24 hours should be dedicated to being happy, by spending quality time at home, having stress busters by means of internal and external devolution. Avoid overindulgence with work, delegate what can be done by others, and do only what cannot be done by others.

ORGANIZING CLINIC TO SAVING TIME DURING CONSULTATIONS

In a well-run enterprise, the team is running around like crazy people and the owner is relaxed.

In any enterprise that is not well run, the owner is running around like a crazy person and the team is relaxed.

Doctor is most vital part of the clinic, but he should not be the only part of the clinic. Make your clinic system driven, not doctor driven. Hiring counselors and nurses/

doctors as assistants definitely saves time of the doctor in charge of the clinic. Other things like questionnaires, videos, charts, and brochures will help keeping patients engaged without involvement of manpower and will also clarify usual patient's doubts and queries.

I will illustrate step by step how patients go about in our clinic:

Step 1: Patient is first seen by front office. Patient is asked if the problem is pertaining to hair, skin, or cosmetics. Relevant questionnaires and general tips for each have been prepared which are distributed to the patient. We have prepared our own videos of 5–7 minutes each, on educating patient on lasers, hair transplant, liposuction, etc. This keeps the patient engaged till the time there turn comes for second step, also saves doctors time in explaining basic things related to procedures and it also helps in priming the patient for the procedure they are looking for.

Step 2: Junior doctors take history, do examination and bedside OPD basis investigations like Wood's lamp, hair scan, dermoscopy, etc. Fellows also provide some information on management and clear patient's doubt to some extent.

Step 3: My role (Consultant). My role in the clinic is very refined. I try to extract any more relevant history, examine the patient quickly, and come to a final diagnosis. Then counseling is done about procedures, further investigations, and treatment. A junior doctor writes prescription in front while I enter the treatment chart in system simultaneously.

Step 4: Counselor explains the cost of the procedure as per protocol. All procedures are listed with rates as per categories A, B, and C. More information about treatments is provided by junior doctor or counselor and respective brochures are provided.

Booking for procedures is done by front desk, I have not talked about money with a patient for years!

Make a fixed protocol for prescriptions. Prescription explanation by pharmacist (we have 2). I do not explain about how to take drugs.

Patient will spend approximately 45 minutes to 1 hour in this whole process. Some patients may not like this, so we tell our patients prior itself that the complete evaluation of the disease will take around 45 minutes to 1 hour, most of the patients understand. But few patients may not like it. Like one hair patient came to my clinic and said "Doctor, I am here just for medicines, I do not want all these. I do not have time". I told him "sorry, please come when you have time. I cannot treat you in 2 minutes."

TIME SAVING IN PROCEDURES

Procedures are done by other staff, I do only hair transplantation (HT) and liposuction.

Nurses can do phototherapy, potassium hydroxide (KOH) smear, patch testing, PRP preparation, epidermal cell suspension, dressings, lasers with training, Microdermabrasion (MDA), and chemical peel. Doctor is one part of this chain. For example, in vitiligo surgery, the following things can be done by assistants with 3 months training:
- Preoperative cleaning, anesthesia. All dressings, suspension preparation, applying suspension
- Grafting needs training for more than few cases

System should run even if doctor is not there. Assistants and consultants should be available for help.

An efficient clinic is definitely born out of a good teamwork, hence a good setup requires more manpower. One counselor, two receptionists to manage appointments and calls, and other to manage OPD patients. Two junior doctors one of them allotted for taking history and other doctor for writing prescription. At least one pharmacist to dispense medicines. As drugs are explained by pharmacist in our clinic, we have two pharmacists. More manpower with properly designated tasks always adds more to the output of the clinic. A simple example, having a driver gives you about 90 minutes of work time or reading time or chatting with friends. There should be passion for the work. Time and money are instruments for your benefit, do not be their slaves. It is human tendency to spend effort and time on more insignificant tasks than those which are perceived as important, rather than those of true importance.

UTILIZATION OF E-RESOURCES

This is an era of e-communication, almost everything we do in our routine is in our phone or laptops, like various apps, presentations, emails, images, planning, dermoscopy, etc. But most of the patients would not appreciate if you are working or gazing into laptop or mobile while consulting. Moreover, the chances of making errors increases proportionately as our level of distraction increases. Mishaps do happen due to mobiles, for example, a doctor asked a resident (junior doctor) to temporarily stop the order for daily warfarin. Using her cellphone, the resident began to make the change via a computerized order entry system. Part way through, she received a text message from a friend about a party. She responded to the text, but forgot to go back and complete the medication order canceling warfarin. As a result, the man kept getting a high dose of warfarin leading to severe bleeding from his wounds.

Teledermatology is becoming popular among patients and doctors too as it saves time and gives personal undivided attention. Consultations can also be done through e-mails, video calls, and other available resources. Esthetic practice is amendable to e-consults for hair, liposuction, acne scars or any easily visible condition on body. But there are few limitations to e-consults, it is difficult to counsel the patient regarding the cost of the surgery, patients ask for quotation for procedures; multiple mails by few apprehensive patients.

Dermatologists have maximum time, very little stress, and little postpractice effects. I would like to end this chapter with few keywords:
- Organize your mind, organize your life
- Tame your emotion
- Focus and sustain attention
- Curb your impulses to act—think, plan
- Gather and mold information
- Shift from one task to another
- Connect the dots

SECTION 5
Finance and Planning

5.1 Investments for a Medical Practitioner (Esthetic Dermatologist)

Ganesh S Pai

INTRODUCTION

In today's world of private practice, it is essential to have cosmetology services included in a dermatology practice. Therefore, investments will essentially be confined to lasers and energy-based devices.

The cost of setting up a clinic is in itself an expensive proposition. Since the clinic is a fixed asset, it is a one-time investment and its costs will get absorbed over a decade of practice. But lasers bring up other issues, such as technology changes every 3–5 years; therefore, the costs have to be recovered along with substantial profit within this period of time. Bank loans have often to be arranged to procure equipment. This adds to the financial burden. Apart from this, a young dermatologist has precious little knowledge of the technical specifications of the machines, quality of service, running cost, and maintenance. It is therefore important to evaluate all these factors by enquiring about them at reputed centers of cosmetology owned by senior dermatologists.

Apart from the payback time, the cost of developing skills to run the business is important. At least 3 months of training and observership are required to handle a laser more efficiently.

Every 5 years, a process of reinvestment in equipment takes place and there are two reasons for it. The equipment may be worn out or the technology may be upgraded. In either case, one has to trade in the old machine for a new one from the supplier. A loyalty bonus is offered by all reputed companies when you buy the new equipment to replace the old. This makes it all the more important to approach reputed companies in the first place at the time of original purchase.

Good products from reputed companies will always cost more, but the good results achieved with their use go a long way in enhancing the reputation of a good dermatologist. With a set of poor tools, even the best carpenter cannot chisel a piece of wood into a work of art.

Many young dermatologists have invested in cheap-quality machines with the logic that they could not afford anything better. Such purchases have led to a gradual destruction of practice as the sum total of our reputation is patient satisfaction and their recommendation to new clients.

Generally, the level of investment should be three times the annual income after deduction of all expenses. Thus if the net income per year is ₹ 20 lakhs, the investment in lasers can be up to ₹ 60 lakhs. These 60 lakhs should be divided between two different wavelength technologies (i.e., two machines of ₹ 30 lakhs each). Under normal circumstances, the payback time of a laser should be 18-24 months factoring in depreciation. Since most lasers have a lifetime of 5 years, the last 3 years will ensure good profitability.

A marketing strategy has to be developed and an analysis of the patient load is a first step. Since cosmetic problems are centered around hair growth, pigmentation, and scars, this subset of clients is a must in the clinic. At least 20 new patients in this category must visit the clinic everyday to justify investments in lasers. Otherwise it better to wait for 3-5 years to have such a patient load.

A market analysis must include the financial capability of the patient and the place of practice whether it is a large city, a small city, small town, or a rural set up. Small cities often show the fastest growth and are underpenetrated by cosmetic dermatologists.

An analysis of the competition must be made. This includes cosmetology chains, corporate hospitals, and other dermatologists in the city. Developing right marketing mix and evaluating the economics is important. Two decades ago, the first purchase would often be a hair removal laser and the second would be for scars. Today, Q-sw lasers for pigment and radio frequency (RF) technology generate the fastest return on investment.

When your clinic is small and you as well as your organization is young, growth through creativity and direction will be quick. But as the clinic becomes larger in size a crisis of leadership can develop and unless growth is driven through direction, delegation, coordination and collaboration, investment will boomerang. Growth through direction would depend on that aspect of cosmetology which is the inherent strength of the center. There are three segments of cosmetology, namely devices, hair transplantation and liposuction, and injectables such as botulinum toxin and fillers.

Devices are both ablative and nonablative but are expensive to own. Different lasers and RF devices for hair reduction, scar reduction, pigmentation, skin tightening, and cryolipolysis would cost at least ₹ 1.50 crores.

Hair transplant and liposuction require much less investment but are procedures which require good skills and several hours of work on each client.

Injectables and fillers generate high income on a low financial base as recovery of investment on a vial occurs as the patient pays simultaneously with the end of the procedures.

Delegation and coordination involve setting up a good team of staff who seamlessly integrate different procedures. Collaboration with plastic surgeons, hospitals, and dermatologists is important to boost footfalls in the clinic.

Investment in traditional publicity or content marketing is the next dilemma. Posters, brochures, standees, and wall mounts are fine within the clinic but waste of investment if done outside. For example, leaflets only hold attention for a short period of time and are expensive. Content marketing is a better option as it is not static like traditional publicity but gives valuable information. It would contain articles, videos, and reviews by patients. With the use of multimedia, a different set of clients are attracted to the clinic. Educating the public with the description of cosmetology procedures simultaneously also serves as an advertisement.

My personal investment began with the purchase of an erbium laser from Germany in the year 1999. Subsequently in the year 2002, I added an 810-diode hair removal system; in 2005, I added a multi-platform system with erbium laser, Q-sw laser, and an IPL for vascular lesions. Thereafter every 2 or 3 years, a new laser of RF device was purchased involving Q-sw-1064, 532 laser as a stand-alone entity, long pulse ND:YAG laser, a fractional CO_2 laser, finally a Pico-Q-sw laser.

Essentially, each machine earned money to buy the next machine. Today, there are 10 machines of different technologies which offer complete solution for all cosmetic disorders.

A customised website and Instagram (social media) provide value to clients who can correspond to clear their doubts even before their first visit. A large number of people can be tapped including patients from foreign countries with the help of advertising in website and marketing media. Videos and photographs of patients should be properly uploaded for other potential clients to assess procedures.

We first have to be passionate about dermatology to succeed in cosmetology and must present ourselves a challenge of differential diagnosis every time we see a case. Investment in textbooks on lasers and cosmetology is the next logical step on completion of MD in dermatology. Money is a byproduct which will always follow when you invest in time to understand the physics and technical content in textbooks.

The French philosopher Francois Voltaire likened life to a game of cards. Each player must accept the cards given to him. But once those cards are in the hand, he alone decides how to play them to win the game.

If we superimpose Voltaire's statements on our practice, the cards are those of finance and location. Passion and attitude are the only two cards that we generate on our own. Somebody with good financial support from the family gets a headstart in life.

A youngster marrying into the family of a dermatologist finds the job quite easy. We always have a number of opportunities in our hand and we must decide whether to take a risk and act on them. I suggest that you follow the advice of Mark Twain, who said, "Take your mind out every now and then and dance on it. It is getting all caked up."

All machines will not necessarily succeed. Failure can occur because of undercharging the patient or outdated technology. As a case in point, my first machine was an Erbium YAG laser. The fees that I collected was twice the amount of what I would charge for a cautery, which meant that I had undercharged the patient. It was inexperience that led to this. By the time the laser broke down, 3 years had passed and spares were prohibitively costly. I had to give up on the machines as I did not have an annual maintenance contract. Moreover, the company had sold only three machines in India which meant that there was no local agent to service the machine. This is the reason why one must buy equipment from companies which are well entrenched in India and have sold many pieces of equipment that ensure there is prompt service and moderately priced spares.

The second machine which failed was 1450 diode meant for acne. The results were poor, sometimes leading to scarring. Finally, the company withdrew the product from the market.

At the end of the day business capability, marketing technique, and prudent investment alone can ensure that investment in lasers which in turn will lead to financial success, provided the passion persists and a dynamic attitude remains the driving force of a vibrant cosmetology center.

5.2 Professional Indemnity for Dermatologist

Omprakash HM, P Prasanna

BACKGROUND

Case 1

A middle-aged working male presents with psoriasis vulgaris involving 30% body surface area. It is also associated with arthropathy. It is a classic indication for oral methotrexate. All investigations done were normal, the patient counseled, and methotrexate started. The patient is regular for follow-up. His liver function test, renal function, and hematological workup are all normal during follow-up.

Suddenly, after 1 month the patient lands in the emergency department, with headache and loss of consciousness. The neurology department takes over the case and finds that he has intracerebral bleed due to pancytopenia. Probably methotrexate was induced. Despite best efforts, the patient succumbs.

The patient's family files a complaint of homicide and presses for compensation. The dermatologist now has to prove that it is not homicide, and there was no negligence of his part. Lastly, the compensation component includes loss of family revenue of the patient and damage charges. To defend this, the dermatologist has to pay for a good lawyer, frequently visit the court, and make arrangements for compensation.

Case 2

An engineering graduate, getting married in 6 months, wants his postacne atrophic immature scar corrected. Fractional resurfacing was done using a CO_2 laser. The patient develops postinflammatory hyperpigmentation and the scar correction is around 50%.

Postinflammatory pigmentation will resolve, but the impending marriage stresses the patient. Moreover, the scar correction results do not measure up to his expectation.

The patient files complaint using two clauses—mental agony and cosmetic procedure results not measuring up to his expectation.

This case highlights the professional service rendered by a qualified dermatologist, trained in the above procedure, but despite his best effort, has caused bodily injury.

Case 3

A busy clinic has good laser hair reduction practice. Many female patients are being treated by nurses under the supervision of a dermatologist. But unfortunately, one of the patients develops laser-induced burns.

Here, the claim is made against the nurse through the supervising dermatologist.

The above cases present common scenarios wherein a dermatologist should protect his practice and family revenue through a good professional indemnity. Misery can strike at any time.

SERVICE PROVIDERS

Professional indemnity cover is provided by (1) government agencies such as oriental, New India Assurance or National insurance company; (2) private players such as

Docklands. AMC (Association of Medical Consultants), ICICI Lombard, Bajaj Alliance; and (3) professional bodies such as IADVL trust.

When one approaches the above service providers, one has to ask a single important question:

Is the company Insurance Regulatory and Development Authority (IRDA) of India approved? One can check the approval status in the IRDA website.

Also, please check the financial status of the insurer and his service record. Finally, check their claim settlement history. Some insurers dodge settlement, which could be worse than the patient.

GOVERNMENT VERSUS PRIVATE INSURERS

Many government agencies are usually IRDA approved and are in business for decades. The insurance premium will be low, and they do cover lawyer fee and compensation component. The only problem is that the response of the government agencies could be slow, and cosmetic procedures might not be covered. The lawyer panel approved by the government insurance company could be bad in some cases. Many government agencies provide professional indemnity service, but it may not be cashless. The dermatologist may have to pay from his pocket and later claim the same from the insurance company.

Private players will charge a joining fee, in addition to the premium. They do cover cosmetic procedures. The lawyer panel could be good. Also, they cover your travel expenses to court, hotel stay, lawyer fee, and compensation. They do assist in out-of-court settlement of cases. They also handle defamation cases and provide services such as handling false social media posts about the dermatologist. But the premium could be very high. One plus point is that it is cashless. Interestingly, the private players act like middlemen and tie up with government agencies such as Oriental Insurance Company.

Lastly, the professional bodies such as IADVL tailor-make the indemnity. Here, the premium is very low. Cosmetic procedures may be covered partly. They may or may not be tied up with governmental insurers.

What should one look for before buying an indemnity policy?

- Policy document which has inclusion and exclusion list. This is called Proposal form with terms and conditions.
  - For a dermatologist, first one should see whether the common scenarios are covered such as drug reaction, missed diagnosis, and medication error. Second, cosmetic procedures such as nevi excision, phototherapy, cryosurgery, electrosurgery, laser therapy for acne scar, laser therapy for hair reduction, chemodenervation, fillers, chemical peels, and nail surgery are covered.
  - For special interest group liposuction, hair transplantation, thread lift, flaps.
  - For this, all insurers have inclusion list and exclusion list. A dermatologist has to read the policy document carefully and search for loop holes. He/she should request for a copy of terms and conditions every year. These conditions could change every year.
- Who is covered by the insurer and what is the policy name?
  - An individual dermatologist running a clinic can take a *"Professional indemnity individual"* policy. In the individual indemnity policy, he/she

can cover himself in his clinic and different places of visit such as nursing home and hospitals. By paying extra 7.5% of the basic premium, he can cover qualified staff (other dermatologists working with him) and unqualified staff (nondermatology staff) such as MBBS doctors, nursing aid, phototherapy technician, and lab technician.

- The hospital with a team comprising dermatologist, plastic surgeon, and anesthetist, who are specialists, along with nonspecialist such as an MBBS doctor, nurse, nursing aid, phototherapy technician, OT technician, and lab technician can take a policy called *"omission and error policy."*

    The point to note is that the dermatologist is considered a specialist. MBBS doctor, nurses, nursing aides, phototherapy technician, OT technician, and lab technician are called nonspecialist.

    The clinic is a place of day care. The hospital is place with minimum 10 beds with admission facility.

    In omission and error policy, the hospital takes the policy and covers the entire hospital team.

- *Places of practice*: The dermatologist has to notify the number of clinics or hospitals he/she visits so as to protect him/her comprehensively. You can ask for pan-India cover if you visit multiple states in the country.
- *Indemnity subclauses*: Does it cover (1) lawyer fee, (2) compensation of patient, (3) travel expenses of doctor to court, and (4) defamation clause if one is interested?
- *Insured amount*: The minimum amount insured should not be less than ₹ 1 crore. The premium calculated per lakh will be less in government or group insurance scheme. Some companies give 75% subsidized premium.
- Selecting claim AOY (any 1 year). This means the policy holds good for a year. In this year, the insurer can settle one, two, or three incidents. This is mentioned as 1:1, 1:2, and 1:3, respectively. Suppose you have opted for ₹ 1 crore insurance; if the clause is 1:1 then ₹ 1 crore amount will be settled for a claim. But if it is 1:2, then ₹ 1 crore will be split and only ₹ 50 lakhs will be paid for the first claim and another ₹ 50 lakhs for the second claim if both arise in the same year. 1:4 claim could be good in group practice or hospital taking omission and error policy. Choose the sum assured depending upon your practice risk profile.

    The premium for 1:4 is low. If you have a high-risk profile, then one can take 1:4 insurance, but the sum assured must be increased. By this, though the risk coverage is greater and premium is lower, your total sum assured will still be secured. For example, instead of taking ₹ 1 crore 1:1 insurance by paying ₹ 5,000–10,000 premium (depending upon the insurer—government or private), a high-risk profile dermatologist can take ₹ 4 crore 1:4 insurance by paying ₹ 12,000 minimum premium in some insurance schemes and still get ₹ 1 crore cover for all four events if they arise.
- *Does the insurance company help in porting the policy*: Some insurance company help you to switch policy to their company. They might charge extra fee for this.
- *Is the policy retroactive*: Retroactive date is the date when the risk is first incepted under the claim. Suppose you port your

policy from company "X" to company "Y"; does the company "Y" cover your indemnity for all the years you have been associated with the previous "X" company? Only private players such as AMC and ICICI Lombard offer this service with extra fee.

- *Revision of limits*: During a financial year if you want to increase your insured amount, this is called "revision of limits." During the correction of policy for new premium, your risk date might change. Please ask the service provider.
- *Runoff cover*: If an insured wishes to seek protection for an anticipated liability in excess of the available limit of indemnity for past periods due to different retroactive dates, the company may consider granting run-off cover based on the merits of each case. This service is provided by United India, Oriental Insurance Company, and National Insurance.
- *Endorsement*: Some companies give an additional document. This is called endorsement. In this, the local manager might add some missed or additional clauses or the dermatologist might later want to add additional staff name in the policy. This additional information is called endorsement. One has to take this endorsement and confirm the validity with a legal expert. Some local insurance managers, despite not having authorization, might cover procedures done by a dermatologist, mentioned clearly in exclusion list. In the endorsement, please check policy holder name, address, retroactive dates, and other matters such as additional procedures covered and staff covered. Take endorsement from the company every year. It is a must. The company has to provide this. Any changes in the policy have to be reflected for that financial year.
- *Additional rider*: An additional rider like coverage of qualified and unqualified staff can be covered by paying extra 7.5% of the basic premium, and maintain staff attendance and payslip according to "Shop and Establishment Act, and Labor Act".
- *What happens if you forget to renew your insurance*: Government insurers will issue you a new policy without the benefit of "risk coverage" for all the previous years. But private players have an option of reviving your policy with a "penalty" and covering the risk for previous years.
- What is the premium collected?

	Oriental, National, New India	ICICI	Bajaj	Dockland	AMC	DVL trust	National Insurance under IADVL
1:1	100 ₹/lakh	110 ₹/lakh	110 ₹/lakh	164 ₹/lakh + membership fee	190 ₹/lakh + membership fee	50 ₹/lakh	50 ₹/lakh
1:2	80 ₹/lakh	90 ₹/lakh	100 ₹/lakh				
1:3	70 ₹/lakh	70 ₹/lakh	80 ₹/lakh				
1:4	40 ₹/lakh	60 ₹/lakh	60 ₹/lakh				

Add 18% GST.

- What are the gray areas in professional indemnity pertaining to dermatologist?
  - A dermatologist can opt to cover himself under "specialist category physician (nonsurgical)." This option is good for a dermatologist who only consult and does not do surgical procedures.
  - But for a dermatologist who does surgical procedures, taking policy in the physician category may not suffice.
  - Many government agencies cover the dermatologist performing surgeries under "plastic surgeon" category. But we are not plastic surgeons.
  - All government insurance agencies clearly mention that "cosmetic procedures are not insured." But this exclusion list is ambiguous. Laser-assisted hair reduction, chemical peels, microdermabrasion, fillers, botulinum toxin chemodenervation, and hair transplantation are then excluded.
  - A controversy exists of cosmetic and noncosmetic procedure under the GST list of IADVL.
  - List of cosmetic or plastic surgery exclusions in terms and conditions of the policy not mentioned in many of the insurance companies—proposal form.
  - The Medical Council of India's syllabus prescribes that a dermatologist be taught all cosmetic procedures. So if a dermatologist's syllabus is different from that of a plastic surgeon, then the exclusion list of a plastic surgeon cannot be imposed on us. If this is highlighted to the insurers, then our specialist-dermatologist policy should cover all procedures. Thus, the bane of taking two different professional indemnity policies, i.e., (1) medical dermatology (2) cosmetic dermatology, can be avoided.

Seeing this loophole, private players have entered the market and are charging hefty premium and covering the above procedures.

CONCLUSION

With the introduction of "Consumer Protection Bill 2019," at the district level, the compensation awarded could be ₹ 1 crore. At the state level, it can be ₹ 10 crores and above this amount it goes to the national level. So opting for ₹ 1 crore professional indemnity, to begin with, makes sense. For a medical dermatologist, adverse drug reaction could be his nemesis. For a procedural dermatologist, anaphylaxis, sepsis, scaring, and failed outcome could mean trouble.

Also, apart from the consumer court a patient can opt to take his complaint to the civil court or state bodies such as grievance redressal authority and Karnataka Medical Council.

It is better to be safe than sorry.

5.3 Tax Planning for Dermatologists

Shashi Kumar BM, Sanjay Labh, Savitha AS

INTRODUCTION

The doctor's economic cycle begins late compared to other professions. Medical syllabus is so vast that doctors hardly get any time to know or learn about Taxation. Often, due to long and irregular hours of service, doctors socialize less with other professionals. Most of us either begin our career by assisting senior and well-established doctor or work with corporate chains of clinics. This results in delayed earning and delayed social life events such as marriage and kids. Therefore, doctors tend to compensate for this by hard work and neglect on tax planning. This chapter gives an overview of tax planning for dermatologists.

Doctors have to decide whether they want to set up their own practice or work in a hospital or do both. Some also want to start their own hospital, which means that they are getting into a business, which is a different ball game. They need to see the pros and cons of each option and decide which works best for them. If one feels that he is not financially savvy but good in medical skills, he can set up a small private practice and be a consultant doctor in hospitals. If you are a doctor setting up a new practice, you should devote time to the set up the practice and it should start before you finish your previous employment (if your current employer allows this), if any, so that you have a steady source of income. You need to calculate how much capital you will need for setting up a practice and consider things such as space required, where to set up the practice, cost of space, services offered, etc. List the revenue and expenses to find out what will be the status of cash flow. You should constantly upgrade your skills and offer innovative and honest services to patients or clients so that they will be satisfied with the treatment they are receiving.

TAX PLANNING

A Dermatologist with total income of more than ₹ 2.5 lakhs in a financial year must file an income tax return. The first step is to have a PAN number (Permanent Account Number). Total income means income earned from all sources such as salary, rental income, professional income, income from fixed deposits and savings accounts, and income earned from sale of any shares or property, called capital gains, etc. Renumeration received from a university or college towards examination duty has to be considered under income. Also, the amount received toward research grants, postmarketing surveys, etc., is to be included as income.

There are two ways to calculate income from your practice. Either consider it like a business activity and deduct actual expenses from actual receipts to calculate its profit and loss or pay tax on it or opt for presumptive taxation.

Once your income is calculated from all sources, the individual can reduce taxable income by claiming deductions under section 80 and pay tax on the remaining income as per prevailing income tax slabs and tax rates **(Table 5.3.1)**. Also, certain expenses may be

Table 5.3.1: Income tax slabs and rates: FY 2019–2020 (AY 2020–21).

Income slabs	General category (nonsenior citizens)	Senior citizens (60 and above years of age, but below 80 years)	Very senior citizens (80 years and above of age)
	Income tax rates		
Up to ₹ 2,50,000	Nil	Nil	Nil
₹ 2,50,001 to ₹ 3,00,000	5%	Nil	Nil
₹ 3,00,001 to ₹ 5,00,000	5%	5%	Nil
₹ 5,00,001 to ₹ 10,00,000	20%	20%	20%
Above ₹ 10,00,000	30%	30%	30%

Box 5.3.1: Allowable expenses under Income Tax Act, 1961.

- Consumable items
- Lab expenses
- Salary of staff
- Advertising expenses
- Audit fees
- Bank charge
- Computer repair and maintenance
- Consultant fee
- Postage and courier expenses
- Depreciation on equipment
- Electricity expenses
- Repair and maintenance
- Fee and subscription
- Clinic expenses
- Vehicle running and maintenance
- Printing and stationery
- Staff welfare expenses
- Telephone and mobile expenses
- Conveyance expenses
- Staff uniform expenses

claimed by a dermatologist for running his/her clinic and it is allowable expense under the Income Tax Act, 1961 **(Box 5.3.1)**.

COMMON TERMINOLOGIES

Cash book: A record of day-to-day cash receipts and payments. A record that shows cash balance at the end of the day or at best at the end of each month.

Journal: A journal is a log of all day-to-day accounting transactions.

Ledger: A ledger is where all entries flow from the journal; it can be used to prepare the financial statements.

Copies of bills: Photocopies of bills or receipts issued by you which are more than ₹ 25.

Original bills: Expenditure bills incurred by you which are more than ₹ 50.

Under Section 44AA, it is mandatory for the medical professionals to maintain the books of accounts for income tax purpose. The books of accounts and the other documents specified in sub-rule (2) and sub-rule (3) should be maintained for a period of 8 years from the end of relevant assessment year.

The additional registers which should be maintained by all doctors are as follows:
- Daily cash register with details of patients, services rendered, fees received, and date of receipt in Form No. 3C.
- Inventory as on the first and the last day of the previous year showing details of stock of drugs, medicines, and other consumables used.

Under Section 271A of Income Tax, the penalty for nonmaintenance of records or the books of accounts is ₹ 25,000.

Those who opt for a presumptive scheme are exempt from record keeping, but some basic bill book, receipt book, and bank statements must be kept for cross-validation.

TAX AUDITING

Tax audit refers to the independent verification of the books of accounts of the assessee to form an opinion on the matters related to taxation compliances carried out by the certified Chartered Accountant (CA). It is covered under Section 44AB of the Income Tax Act, 1961, and CA will report to IT department in Form no. 3CA/3CB and Form no. 3CD along with the income tax return.

Tax auditing is mandatory when gross annual receipts of dermatologists exceed ₹ 50 lakhs in a financial year or when gross receipts are under ₹ 50 lakhs but profit is lower than 50% and total income is more than ₹ 2.5 lakhs (i.e., total income is taxable). Basically, when the total income is taxable and profits are less than 50% of gross receipts.

ANNUAL RECEIPTS

The term "gross receipts" are not specifically defined in the income tax laws. However, all your receipts directly because of profession, must be considered. Other receipts such as royalty on authorships, guest lectures, and contributing articles, may not be included while computing gross receipts.

Under Section-271 B of the Income Tax the Act, the penalty for noncomplying with tax audit is ₹ 1,50,000 or 0.5% of gross receipt, whichever is lower.

Due date for filing IT:
- *Nonaudit case:* 31st July of the year
- *Audit case*: 30th September of the year

PRESUMPTIVE TAXATION

Presumptive taxation for doctors has been introduced effective from FY 2016–17. This scheme is available to individuals and HUF (Hindu Undivided Family). When clinic establishment is incorporated as a company, then profits cannot be presumptive. When an individual opts for presumptive taxation, one's income is presumed. Actual profit is not calculated. Here, profit is assumed to be 50% of gross receipts. However, only those who have annual receipts of ₹ 50 lakhs or less can opt for this scheme. If the annual receipts exceed ₹ 50 lakhs, a dermatologist should report them and deduct actual business expenses to compute profit (or loss). This profit may be less or more than 50% of receipts.

Dermatologists owning a pharmacy or inpatient bed should report as business and cannot take presumptive taxation for that portion of income. Presumptive tax will only be available to a doctor's income earned directly due to his/her profession. But a dermatologist can report a part of his/her income (professional income) as presumptive and balance income as business and can claim actual expenses, such as running any other business. In such a case, bookkeeping and audit rules may apply to the business activity, whereas presumptive activity may be exempt from these.

Advantages of Presumptive Taxation

- No need to keep books of accounts and no audit is required
- Savings in auditor professional fee
- No need to pay advance tax in installments; paying your entire tax dues by 15th March of the financial year will suffice.

ESTABLISHING A CLINIC

A dermatologist can start a clinic under sole proprietorship, partnership firm, limited liability partnership (LLP), or as private limited company. The advantages and disadvantages should be thoroughly discussed before incorporating clinic establishment **(Table 5.3.2)**.

Table 5.3.2: Difference between private limited company and proprietorship firm.

Point of difference	Private limited company	Proprietorship
Registration	The private limited company will be registered under the Companies Act, 2013 with the Ministry of Corporate Affairs	There is no formal registration required at all in proprietorship firm
Name of the business	It must be approved by the registrar of the company. It will end with words private limited company	There is no need for approval before using the name
Separate legal entity	It is a separate legal entity under the Companies Act, 2013	It does not have a separate legal entity and owner is personally liable for the liability of the business
Liability of owner (shareholder)	Liability of owner (shareholder) is limited to the extent of their shares (their ownership in company). Liability is limited to the extent percentage of their holding in company's ownership	Liability of owner is unlimited because an individual proprietor is the sole owner of his business
Minimum and maximum members	Minimum—2 members or owner Maximum— 200 members or owner	Minimum—1 member or owner Maximum—1 member or owner
Foreign ownership	In many sectors, it is allowed to invest in it under automatic approval route under the guidelines issued by central government	Foreign ownership is not at all allowed
Transferability of ownership	Ownership can be transferred to any third person or party by way of transfer of share	Ownership cannot be transferred unless sell of entire business
Existence	Independence of its member/owner and director	Dependence on the owner of business
Taxation	Its profit is taxed @ 30% plus surcharge and cess applicable as may be notified by government from time to time	Taxed as per the individual slab rate as applicable to proprietor
Legal compliance	Board and general meetings to be conducted. It has to file annual accounts and annual return with the registrar of the company every year. Also, income tax return has to be filed for it	Not required to conduct any annual meeting. No need for filing an annual report with the registrar of the companies. It files income tax return on the basis of income of the owner
Reliability	Books of account are audited by qualified auditor that show a true and fair view of actual position of financial strength of any company	Unless and until proprietorship is covered under audit provision books of account of income tax reliability of books of account of proprietor business is uncertain
Fund raising	In case of private limited company for expansion purpose, additional fund requirement can be fulfilled by further issue of equity share of a company	For any financial requirement has to be fulfilled by only bank loan/bank debt option only
Answerable to others	The owner who handles the day-to-day business of company by way of Board of Director is answerable to other investors/shareholders of company in case of any query raised by them	The owner is not answerable to anyone

Contd...

Contd...

Point of difference	Private limited company	Proprietorship
Succession	It has perpetual succession and an independent identity that is different from its shareholders. The company will still exist even if shareholders die or cease to be a member	It does not have perpetual succession if the owner dies or business or proprietorship automatically ceases to exist
Credibility	It has to comply with more stringent compliance measures as described by central government or any other authority	It does not require to comply with stringent compliance measure of any law; hence credibility is less compared to private limited company
Books of account	Books of accounts of any private limited company are required to maintain at the registered office of the company, so that they can be available for any member or shareholder at any time for verification	Books of accounts to be maintained if only required by law in force at a particular point of time. Otherwise not required to make it available to any person
Brand value	This form of business helps to create brand value of product or service in which the private limited company is dealing with	With this form of business it is going to hand to make brand value of product or service in which proprietorship is dealing with
Preferability	This form of business is preferable to developed business which wants to expand their business nationally or in the international (global) market since making brand value of a product or service is the main point of focus	This form of business is more preferable for startup, as at the initial stage, cost cutting is to the extent as required to sustain in market
Risk related to business loss	The liability of a shareholder (owner) is limited to the extent of holding of equity share in any company. His personal assets cannot be affected due to any loss in company due to a separate legal entity concept	The liability of owner is unlimited as proprietor is the sole owner of his business so any loss to business can also affect his personal assets
Marketing tool	This form of business provides you indirect marketing of your business	This will not be treated as a marketing tool of product or service provided by proprietor

Financial Planning

Financial planning is the process of determining ways to earn, save, and spend money and the amount an individual needs to earn, invest, and spend. Personal finance and financial planning have never been taught in our curriculum. So, many face difficulty in managing finances.

Common problems faced by dermatologists are with regards to personnel financial management are discussed below.

Doctors are so busy with erratic hours that they do not have the time or inclination to spend time on managing finances. The below points help the dermatologist in better planning:

- Separate out personal and professional expenses.
- Create a budget.
- Create an emergency fund.
- Get insurance cover for self and family so that personal goals and professional expenses get paid off in case of unfortunate events.
- Make financial goals such as children's education and retirement plans and work toward achieving them by investing properly and reviewing investments regularly.

Dermatologists should take the following steps to ensure that their finances are in a good condition:

- They should not be tempted to splurge once they start earning money. Some of them feel that they missed out the opportunities to have fun as they spent many years studying and started to earn well much later in life. They splurge on fancy vacations, new cars, eating out, etc. It is important to keep a check on expenditure and concentrate on savings and investments.
- Invest wisely! Starting a clinic with all expensive lasers is not advisable. Instead, build practice steadily and upgrade in phases.
- They should ensure that they have adequate life cover and disability insurance cover so that the financial needs of family and profession are taken care of in case of unfortunate events.
- Decent indemnity coverage is must. There should be a minimum of ₹ 50 lakhs for practicing clinical dermatologists and ₹ 1 crore for aesthetic dermatologists.
- In some cases, practice is the biggest investment doctors have—nurture, save, and grow. A chain of clinics is also worth trying.
- Good physical health is as important as finance.
- They should have a proper investment plan. Always keep an alternate source of income apart from profession. They should invest in a variety of assets including equity, mutual funds, and debt so that their investment portfolio is diversified and they get optimum returns and long-term capital appreciation.
- Pay off education loans taken and only then go for home loan or loans for buying property to set up the clinic.
- Invest time and money in upgrading their skills, learning about latest trends, and networking with other doctors and professionals in the healthcare business.
- Ensure part of earning for upgrading the clinic.

5.4 Creating a Business Plan in Practice

Krupa Shankar DS

INTRODUCTION

A business plan is a formal written document containing business goals, the methods on how these goals can be attained, and the time frame within which these goals need to be achieved. It summarizes the operational and financial objectives of a business and contains the detailed plans and budgets showing how the objectives are to be realized. It is the road map to the success of the business.

All financial thinking is done in a 3–5-year frame time. This is the frame for equipment loan from authorized lenders such as banks and also the life of most equipment we use.

Some financial acumen is needed for every practice, as the other choice is to join a corporate set-up with full-time financiers who will inevitably demean and victimize clinicians.

A medical practice cannot be treated as merely a business transaction because the stock in trade is trust. All businesses need this, but in medicine the need is all the time, with every patient, and there is no room for let up over a period of time. Success in medicine is measured in terms of how trustworthy you are as opposed to how much you accumulate; once the running costs are covered and your living and continuing education costs are met, all else is hot air.

Doing a thorough job with few patients a day is to be preferred to chasing gee whiz numbers such as 50 patients a day. A very large low-paying patient population carries a higher risk of misbehavior and litigation.

LOCATION

Location is an important issue when people would walk in by looking at the board and marquee. Few things to keep in mind while deciding the location of the clinic is commute to the clinic. Time is money for doctors, so we should make sure we are not wasting awfully lot of time in traveling to-and-fro from the clinic. Locality and neighborhood of the clinic also matter; some patients might not prefer to visit a doctor in a substandard neighborhood or also may be in a too posh neighborhood thinking that it might be too expensive. The key to establish a good clinic practice is the visibility of the clinic. Hoardings should be used to guide the patient to the location; prescriptions can display a map on the backside which can be used by the patients or patient's referrals in future.

As of today, most people will look up the internet to reach you, and some still come in by word-of-mouth recommendation or referral from a general practitioner (GP) or a specialist.

Parking space is an important issue; however, if you locate yourself in a very crowded locality tell your patients in advance to use cabs and reassure them that such services are easily accessed in your area. If there is a metro station nearby, please name it in your confirmatory SMS. Please train your secretary to do this.

While taking an appointment, ask the patient as to where they he/she is located and ask your secretary to look up on Google maps to estimate the time required to reach your clinic and add 50% to the estimated time and book an automatic future SMS on a site like way2sms.com so that an alarm will ready the patient at the time appropriate for departure from his or her home or office. This will prevent you from having to open your door again and turn on the computer for the patient who leaves 15 minutes before the scheduled appointment for a 1-hour journey.

Meet all the other specialists and GPs in your area and hand them your card. If they say that they refer all their patients to an existing specialist, show your respect for that specialist, indicate your friendship with him or her, and close by saying you now have a choice when one of you is full up or out of town, if you locate your practice in a relatively remote urban area, offer your services on weekends and keep time for your family and personal work on 1 or 2 weekdays.

Get yourself a website, no matter how basic, with location, appointments, phone number, address link to Google maps, your qualifications, services offered, timings, and holidays. Employ a secretary exclusively to speak on the phone.

ACCREDITATIONS AND REGULATORY FULFILLMENTS

These will be attended to by the owner if you are in a polyclinic or hospital where you own your department with a memorandum of understanding (MOU)/contract not to duplicate your services with the owner. If you operate in a stand-alone clinic, different states have different regulatory requirements. For example, in Karnataka you first enroll with a medical waste management company, practice segregation and disposal of medical waste, train your staff in it, and then apply to the Pollution Control Board for clearance. With their certificate, you apply for Karnataka private medical establishment registration. Karnataka Private Medical Establishments Act (KPMEA) registration is mandatory and entails certain physical requirements such as two toilets in your facility, one each for men and women. Read the rules before you buy or rent a place. Similar rules may exist elsewhere. Also, check for rules regarding locating your services in a residential area. Some areas permit and some do not. The problem with residential areas is parking space used by your clients obstructing the residents and constant movement of strangers. Some cities demand that you have a trade license from the corporation.

REVENUE STREAMS

Consultation is your first and constant revenue stream. A free consultation renders you into a state of elementary failure and forces you to offer and promote procedures when one may not be really needed. Space patient visits based on the approximate time to recovery and charge accordingly—1 week for zoster, 10 days for cellulitis, 1 month for scabies and tinea, 3 months for melasma, and so on. Always fix a follow-up visit for a procedure patient no matter how trivial the procedure.

Esthetic treatments that go beyond a prescription should at first be addressed with a prescription that will be the sheet anchor of maintenance forever or prolonged but stated periods, such as topical retinoid, sunscreens, or minoxidil. This session is also used to detail the procedure or procedures if multiple, cost or package cost, conditions and caveats for rebates if any, display of before-after pictures, exposure to testimonials from happy clients, and time for the client to have his or her questions answered. Use the time to align patient expectations to deliverables. For example, in scar revision, show a before and after picture and point out how the scar is no longer the center of attention, but still visible to the discerning or fault-seeking eye.

As per procedures, there are two revenue streams—diagnostic and therapeutic. Diagnostics include skin biopsy, patch test, skin prick test, KOH mount, Tzanck smear, urethral and cervical smears, blister fluid smears, patch test, photo patch test, and dermoscopy. Therapeutic streams include peels, microneedling, microdermabrasion, intense pulse light, platelet-rich plasma (PRP) therapy, electrosurgery, radiofrequency, ablative and nonablative, and cold steel surgeries. All procedures that breach the skin with the exception of intramuscular injection need a clean room; and flaps, grafts, vitiligo surgery, hair transplant, and liposuction (if trained and certified) need an operation theater and appropriate instruments. The instruments needed for surgery and their maintenance are detailed elsewhere. Nonablative lasers need to be housed in a separate room with intense pulse light and targeted phototherapy, and ablative lasers are best used in the OT. All procedures need to be billed, or else the resentment of doing something free will prevent you from doing it. In major hospitals, 60% of the revenue come from laboratory and pharmacy and the remaining from 15–25 other specialties. Pharmacy is a revenue stream, and there are guidelines on how to hire a pharmacist and on space allocation and other regulatory issues. If you dispense directly, the patient will hold you responsible for all the costs accrued in case of therapeutic failure or delay. Given the proliferation of labs, offering a high rent collection room in your clinic may be a better idea. This can be renewed annually depending on the National Accreditation Board for Testing and Calibration Laboratories (NABL) accredited lab that pays you the highest. The choice of services depends on space and readiness of clientele to travel for repeat procedures at regular intervals, with phototherapy being the most challenging. A price list is also a regulatory requirement.

Streamline informing the patient and educating him/her about procedures with handouts or recorded video lecture/lecture demo in order to prevent wear-out. Videos should be between at least 90 seconds and 10 minutes in length at most. Once the patient has read the handout or seen the video, ask him/her if any more questions need to be answered.

OWNERSHIP MODELS

Most practices are privately owned, but given the cost of real estate and the limited services an individual dermatologist can offer, it may be better to form a group as a limited liability partnership with the space divided by time so that each doctor gets 8 hours a day and the center provides nearly 16 hours of access. Case files can have a password-protected access system that permits sharing if and when needed. As dermatology subspecialties grow, it may be better for different subspecialists to be housed under one roof.

An ordinary partnership is a weak system and prone to collapse; a private company involves adherence to company law but offers many perks in the long run. It permits you to get on board only those you want to. As of now, only very large hospitals can afford to be listed in public limited companies with shareholders, with the downside of the institution being answerable to the shareholders to the detriment of patients.

ITEMIZING AND BILLING SERVICES

The rates can be listed as per the anatomical area treated, small/medium/large or whole body on an excel sheet in documents, with a shortcut folder on the desktop. It may not be possible to remember all prices off-hand and if you refer to a list, then the patient knows that there is a method to your pricing which is not arbitrary or opportunistic. Please mention the fee when a patient calls for an appointment. This eliminates a lot of heartburn and anxiety to both you and your patients. If all services are prepaid, please mention that too. That will prevent patients who wander about and spend their time to socialize with doctors for free services from eating into your time. Train your secretary in how to do this. The other way is for him or her to have a preset SMS message which can be sent as soon as the patient completes taking an appointment.

Pricing procedures are done by checking with your colleagues in your town, if not forthcoming, from a friend in another town, or one of your seniors. Your teachers in medical school will be clueless, as most services offered there are highly subsidized and are not the primary source of income of the institute. The rule of thumb in many lending and project report writing agencies is 1:5 in 5 years. For example, if a laser is ₹ 10 lakhs, you expect to earn ₹ 50 lakhs in 5 years which boils down to ₹ 3,333 per day, of which two-third takes care of establishment, assistance, AMC, EMI, power, water electricity accessories such as stabilizer, AC, UPS, upgradation, and reinvestment corpus and the rest will be your fee of which you will keep 70% after tax. This is the very least you can afford to charge per procedure; as the numbers build up, so does the profitability, albeit with a marginal raise in other costs. The formula is capital cost x 5 divided by 1500@ 300 working days per annum.

For example, if a laser costs ₹ 40 lakhs, you need to earn ₹ 2 crores in 5 years from it, i.e., ₹ 13,333 per day. If you miss 1 day, it doubles, if 2 days it becomes 3 times, and so on. Similar calculations can be arrived at for every piece of equipment and cost center.

A personally endorsed strategy is to start with electrocautery and a CO_2 laser as it requires some skill, and hence the competition is likely to be less from nondermats. Once you see your revenue stream stabilize, you can plan for the next revenue stream or cost center.

Taking the CO_2 laser example, if the machine costs ₹ 10 lakhs and you have averaged at ₹ 3,333 per day over a 6-month period, then you can consider the next large investment.

Maintain a separate register of excel sheet for each equipment; after 3–5 years in practice, as things ease out, you do not need to micromanage.

A cost center is a part of an organization to which costs may be charged for accounting purposes. The consultation chamber is a basic cost center. The other cost centers are a minor OT/esthetic procedure room which has a couch, cautery and radiofrequency, electrosurgery, a dental chair for Botox and fillers, refrigerator for patch and prick test allergens, a peel cupboard, mirror for patient, and wash basin. A laser room for light and nonablative therapies containing diode, long-pulsed Nd:YAG or multiple wavelength laser for hair reduction, Q-switch Nd:YAG, nonablative radiofrequency, intense pulse light device; optionally, it may also contain LED panel or mask, low level laser light for wound healing and hair treatment.

Please remember to choose your equipment based on the indications covered, rather than completing the list of all technologies available in the market or competing with peers under pressure from the seller.

A hair reduction laser, CO_2 laser, and Q-switch Nd:YAG will cover almost all laserable indications.

There are companies which have platforms on which all of these are mounted. The advantages are bundled cost and space saved. The disadvantage is loss of all wavelengths if one breaks down and limitation of one patient at a time in a multiuser environment. Items which earn more are few in number. Items which are more in number earn less per procedure.

Methods of being payed in a group practice: All payments need to be in white with cash payments at the counter with proper receipts issued and collated at the end of practice each day with your practice software. Card payments are on the rise and will become the norm in a few years, so get a swipe machine right away. In a stand-alone proprietorship practice, you still need the swipe machine. Also be ready to accept through Paytm, BHIM, UPI, Google Pay, and a few other apps on your phone as well as account transfer which many patients do in minutes if your instructions are clear as follows:

You may kindly pay my fees as follows:

Please remit consultation fee of ₹ xxxx- favoring Dr ABCDEFG to
Your name/clinic name:
Current/SB account number 12345678910
Bank_____
Branch _____
City _____
IFSC Code: ABCD 987654321 (used for IMPS, RTGS and NEFT transactions)

To summarize, the key elements to keep in mind when starting a new setup are as follows:
- Location
- Accreditation
- Revenue streams
- Ownership models
- Itemizing and billing of services

SECTION 6: Marketing: Ethics and Means

6.1 Ethical Marketing: Best within Limits

Rohit Batra

INTRODUCTION

Medical profession and especially dermatology has seen a lot of transformation in the last decade. A practice confined to a small chamber with a waiting room has now moved to swanky clinics with multiple procedure rooms and an array of lasers and other gadgets. A one-man show has now evolved into a full dermatology and Esthetics Pvt Ltd industry.

Running a clinic today not only requires a dermatologist's clinical acumen but also a business sense. Lasers are added to practice considering not only their clinical results but also return on investment (ROI).

The growing demand of dermatology and esthetic services has lured many business houses to enter the industry and the concept of multiple clinics by many. Entrepreneurial dermatologists with various funding houses have brought in the concept of marketing in a big way.

Everyone wants to excel. A new dermatologist today want to start an esthetics practice and even those who are inclined toward clinical dermatology or dermatosurgery, hair transplant, etc., want to carve a niche for themselves quickly.

Though "word of mouth" still rules today but with the sharp penetration of internet through social media platforms such as Facebook and YouTube, and search engines such as Google, a reconfirmation has become a bitter truth.

As per the Code of Medical Ethics Regulations, 2002 published by The Medical Council of India—*soliciting of patients directly or indirectly, by a physician, by a group of physicians or by institutions or organizations is unethical. A physician shall not make use of him/her (or his/her name) as subject of any form or manner of advertising or publicity through any mode either alone or in conjunction with others which is of such a character as to invite attention to him or to his professional position, skill, qualification, achievements, attainments, specialties, appointments, associations, affiliations or honors and/or of such character as would ordinarily result in his self-aggrandizement.*

A medical practitioner is, however, permitted to make a formal announcement in press regarding the following:
- On starting practice
- On change of type of practice
- On changing address
- On temporary absence from duty
- On resumption of another practice
- On succeeding to another practice
- Public declaration of charges

The code also states that:

"A physician should not contribute to the lay press articles and give interviews regarding diseases and treatments which may have the effect of advertising himself or soliciting practices; but is open to write to the lay press under his own name on matters of public health, hygienic living or to deliver public lectures, give talks on the radio/TV/internet chat for the same purpose and send announcement of the same to lay press."

It further adds that:

"An institution run by a physician for a particular purpose such as a maternity home, nursing home, private hospital, rehabilitation center or any type of training institution, etc., may be advertised in the lay press, but such advertisements should not contain anything more than the name of the institution, type of patients admitted, type of training, and other facilities offered and the fees."

Thus, the above-mentioned rules need to be followed by the physicians, institutions, and organizations while advertising or marketing.

Adding a new service, treatment modality can also be advertised as per the latest amendments of the council.

The Code does not state anything about the online media but the legal experts are of the opinion that the same rules apply to the various online platforms.

As per the current understanding of the Code and information available from the medical council, a medical professional can do marketing ethically by following the below-mentioned principles:

- Avoiding his/her own photograph on any sort of advertisement be it print/online/hoarding, etc.
- Avoiding tall/false claims about himself/herself or any sort of procedures performed at the clinic.
- A physician cannot advertise on his/her own but the rules do not apply on companies for profit (*it is always prudent to form a company in case one intends to advertise extensively*).
- Avoid advertising cases, especially before and after images (*it is better to form a marketing strategy on patient information and awareness and not on procedure results*).
- One can easily advertise about adding new services/technology in their practice as there is no specified time limit till when they can continue advertising it (*thus, one can easily market a new procedure in their practice for a couple of months*).
- Informative videos and healthcare tips can be posted without soliciting new patients and can make you a brand.
- Talk shows on radio and TV or print media can help you market your clinic and services without coming under the shade of marketing (*a good public relations firm can help you get those slots at a reasonable price*).
- Online marketing has come up in a big way and presence of your clinic through social media page has become a necessity not only to get new patients but also to retain the existing clientele (*keep adding your patients to your community to keep a connect and repeat visits*).
- News about clinic, social initiatives, recognitions, and awards can be shared with public (*any opportunity for publicity should not been missed*).

Marketing has become an evil necessity for practices big and small, old and new. As more and more medical professionals, corporate hospitals, and business houses are entering the esthetics industry, competition is becoming fastly voracious. A scholar dermatologist who enters private practice studying medicine and dermatological procedures for over a decade might get a shock of their life when they have to compete against the might of "ayas", "atra", "ichfeel", etc.

A medical professional should try and stick to the rules laid down by the medical council, as various cases of unethical marketing by the doctors in past have resulted in stringent punishments such as removing names for a period of 15 days from the medical register.

We have to accept that marketing has become a necessity in today's dermatology and specially esthetic practice. We do have a marketing team to take care of the day-to-day needs. We keep innovating and experimenting to make people aware and informed about the various treatments and latest technologies our clinic offers for best results. Various marketing activities we do on regular basis are:

- Articles, case studies, latest news, and interviews about various treatments are published in various newspapers and magazines. Though media contacts are helpful and sufficient in most cases, a dedicated public relation marketing team or advisor is required to scale up things.
- A dedicated social media manager or a team is a must nowadays and daily postings, offers, and public education initiatives go a long way in creating a dedicated community and increasing your brand value and patient footfall in clinic. Various platforms such as Facebook, Instagram, and Twitter are just a few where we promote our services. A dedicated YouTube channel also helps to spread the word about various skin diseases, treatments, and procedures done in clinic. It helps a prospective patient make an informed decision and also existing patients can be asked to watch the channel to get more information about their diseased condition.
- Carry bags, stationary items such as pens, key chains, and coffee mugs can be used for clinic's branding and help spread the word about the clinic to patient' friends and family.
- Skin care range comprising few moisturizing creams, cleansers, sunscreens, etc., can also help in making a brand. Such cosmeceuticals neither require drug licenses nor a licensed pharmacy for dispensing. It helps in making your clinic brand a household name.
- Organizing skin camps and public lectures in association with various institutions and public societies help in making people aware about your clinical and professional skills. People from various walks of life and various strata further strengthen our social standing and help in professional work.
- Interdisciplinary forums through discussions and round table meets help in marketing amongst peers from various medical specialties and generate cross referrals.
- Bulk sms, e-mail marketing, and WhatsApp media pushing is routinely being used to reach existing patients as well as selected data of neighborhood population to carry out various activities such as making them aware of offers, addition of new technology at the same time, and wishing them during festive season.

The whole idea behind ethical marketing is to be in news—legally. One must add disclaimers regarding result variations and should not disguise public. Patients should not be solicited by showing unrealistic results.

6.2 Traditional Marketing in Practice

Rajat Kandhari, Tanay Tulsaney

INTRODUCTION

The way clinical operations have transformed today is a testimony of the impact of medical marketing. From the first contact with the patient to the right diagnosis and treatment, the whole scenario has evolved immensely.

Healthcare marketing primarily revolves around improving awareness and educating patients by approaching them via different media, in comparison to any other sector non-governed by the stringent and ethical laws of healthcare in India. A few decades ago, the word "marketing" was considered a "taboo" in the medical profession, while today it seems to have become a necessary evil. In the current scenario, it is indeed a boon for a medical practitioner to acquire and entrepreneurial skills and set a part of the budget for marketing efforts alone. While it has become important to increase awareness and educate our patients, it is our duty as medical professionals to protect and respect the sanctity of our profession. Generating awareness about a certain cause or symptoms of a condition needs an unfiltered medium, and it is sometimes confusing to decide which aspect of brand marketing should one focus on, traditional marketing or digital marketing.[1]

WHAT IS TRADITIONAL MARKETING?

Traditional marketing refers to a conventional mode of marketing that we all are familiar with, which helps us reach out to a "semi-targeted" audience via offline advertising and/or promotional means. Traditional marketing typically comprises:

- *Word of mouth:* Sharing reviews, opinions, and suggestions about a certain practitioner or a group of practitioners was and even currently is recorded as the primary and possibly, the most reliable source of publicity. "Word of mouth" allows one to candidly share one's experience about the doctor or services offered at a particular clinic/hospital.
  - *Advantages:* Low cost, gives long-term value, helps in earning the trust of the patients.
  - *Disadvantages:* Lack of control. Good or bad, one cannot stop the word from spreading.
- *Print media:* The print media (magazines, newspapers, etc.) emerged as a communication channel purveying to a larger audience with a solid standpoint. This medium can be most helpful in targeting the local population or a specific stratum of society. Even in today's digital age, some people may still rely on print media as they consider it a source of authentic information. Similarly, high-end magazines (e.g., vogue, cosmopolitan) with educative dermatological content can enable the reach to luxury consumers as they recognize these magazines as a more reliable information providers than something random they come across on the internet. Although, there is no doubt that print ads work great if executed in the right manner, without consistency,

print advertising fails to give favorable results. Moreover, whether one chooses to advertise in a major magazine or a local newspaper, the investment involved is usually high and needs to be done over a long period of time in order to make this an effective exercise. Further, the actual number of readers actually seeing your ad will be lesser than the number of magazines in circulation.
- *Advantage:* High recall value.
- *Disadvantage:* Multiple exposures are required, so the lead time can be longer.

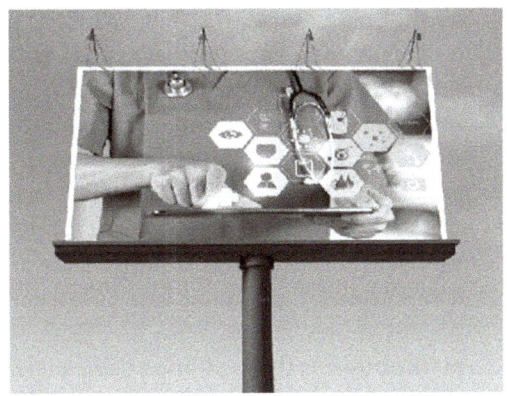

Fig. 6.2.1: Use of billboards for distributing educational content.

- *Broadcast*:
  - *Radio*: The impact of radio broadcasting has been huge. Faceless heroes of radio are capable of disseminating educational information about various conditions and treatments vis-a-vis branding your medical practice very effectively. This can be done through a 60 seconds small advertisement or by participating in a talk show.
    - *Advantages:* Reasonable cost and broad reach.
    - *Disadvantage:* Many listeners do not pay enough attention to radio advertisements.
  - *Television commercials*: Television has been celebrated as the means of enhancing the credibility of your esthetic or medical practice and invoke emotions which other mediums usually fail to do. We have seen a lot of commercials backing pharmaceutical products, focusing on the science behind the product built and focusing on further educative content.
    - *Advantage:* Helps in building a reputation at a regional or national level.
    - *Disadvantage*: Relatively expensive and may need multiple exposures to grab the attention of the audience.
- *Billboards:* Publishing the educative content on billboards and hoardings contributes to the majority of educative content being distributed to a mass audience **(Fig. 6.2.1)**.
  - *Advantage:* One of the most rewarding forms of marketing for targeting a specific geographical area.
  - *Disadvantage:* Very brief exposure to the viewers.
- *Direct mail:* The direct mail can be a good source of communication where your message is directly delivered to the audiences through catalogues, postcards, etc. This method may be employed in a "direct" manner, wherein actual personalized mail can be delivered directly at the doorstep or "indirectly" via newspaper leaflets or brochures. These methods are particularly useful to suggest a new clinic/branch opening, a change in address or to a few loyal patients for a special offer or trial for a new technology. "Brochures" or "leaflets" in the newspaper also appear to be a commonly employed and are an effective

method of communication. While the cost of investment in this form of marketing is low, it requires for the delivery of brochures to be "regular" for it to have a real impact, i.e., actually becoming noticeable and bringing the patient to the clinic. In our opinion, the "quality" of the brochure is also of critical importance as it represents your brand and an extension of your services. With this form of marketing, it is difficult to actually gauge *how many* of your brochures reach the readers, are they *actually noticed*, and do they make a *lasting impact*.

Mostly, a combination of direct mail and telemarketing is considered to be more result oriented **(Fig. 6.2.2)**.

- *Advantage:* Pamphlets and brochures are helpful in educating the patients and informing them about the availability of various dermatological services.
- *Disadvantage:* Pamphlets can be easily discarded and disregarded. Tracking the delivery is difficult in both the cases (emailers and pamphlets).

- *Telephone (telemarketing, SMS marketing, etc.):* Telemarketing and SMS marketing are nowadays common tools of healthcare marketing **(Fig. 6.2.3)**. But here again, a multimedia channel approach may prove to be more beneficial as telephonic communication can only provide a limited information to the audience, etc.
  - *Advantage:* Allows direct communication; therefore, the patient's doubts and queries can be addressed in a better way.
  - *Disadvantage:* Training the staff is time consuming. If the calls are not handled properly, it can portray a poorly managed practice.

- *Internal marketing*: Internal marketing in one's practice enables your patient to "know" you and your services before they enter your chamber in the clinic. Internal marketing may be in various forms:
  - *Standees and posters:* These may be provided by pharmaceutical companies elaborating upon a certain product or may be designed as per the services of the clinic. Standees may also be used to introduce a new branch, a new doctor to the practice, a new service, or even a special offer.
  - *Televison*: One may employ the use of a television in the waiting area in order to educate patients regarding

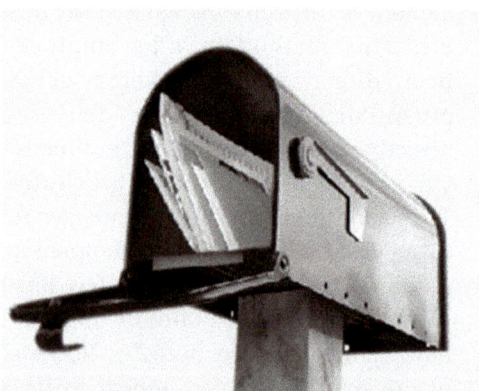

Fig. 6.2.2: Direct mail enables direct delivery of communication to the target audience.

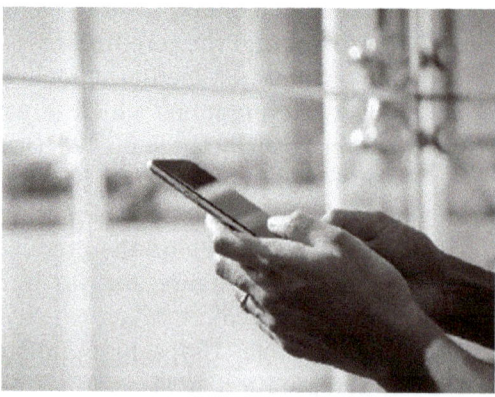

Fig. 6.2.3: Telemarketing and SMS as a means of communication with your target audience.

services available in the clinic and even how they are done, "about" the doctors and the clinic, elaborate upon your "vision" statement and your "core" values. Also posting some of your "before" and "after" results and video testimonials from happy patients will help in educating patients. This method is particularly useful in practices with good footfall as more patients coming into the clinic allows for more viewership. In our opinion, this form of internal marketing is easy and very effective in generating awareness and queries.

- *In clinic staff:* From the moment your clinic connects with a patient on the phone till the patient walks out of the clinic, it is your duty to provide a "pleasant experience" and this particularly holds true for an esthetic practice. Regular "staff training" and "grooming" goes a long way in directing this process. Having a designated smart tablet elaborating upon your services or having a "counselor" talking to the patients regarding a certain service or procedure helps in "breaking the ice" many a times, as the patient may find his/her comfort zone outside your chamber and is able to discuss the procedure and its costing with ease with the counselor. At the same time, keeping your employees happy is of key importance as that translates into smiling faces, a positive work environment, better patient retention, positive "word of mouth", converting enquiries, inspiring patient referrals, and so much more. Of course, the aforementioned is easier said than done as it requires time and commitment to execute proper trainings for the staff in between a busy practice.
- *Advantages:* Low cost and high return on investment.
- *Disadvantage:* It is a continuous and ongoing process. Do not expect immediate changes and the results can be inconsistent to start with.

In the age of digitalization, the aforementioned mediums still play a crucial role. One can still impart valuable information to existing and potential patients through brochures, pamphlets, explanatory charts, posters, handy booklets, and so on.

Implementation of correct traditional marketing revolves around the proper sales funnel, which comprises utilization of the four P's of marketing: Product (a good understanding of your service, e.g., laser hair reduction), Price (the overall cost, i.e., how well you understand the costing by your competitors and how you place your own), Promotion (how you market your service to your target audience, e.g., educating the target audience regarding the safety, effectiveness, and the advantages of the laser hair reduction over other conventional methods of hair reduction), and Place (placing your service to the right audience at the right time to increase chances of converting prospects to customers or clients).

While the aim of traditional marketing is to provide time, place, and possession utility leading to better customer satisfaction,[2] it has certain advantages and disadvantages.[3]

Advantages of Traditional Marketing

- *Faster results*: Correct placement and targeting of your ads may produce results that are faster or more effective compared to digital marketing methods that can take several weeks to produce effects.

- *Durability and longevity of traditional means of marketing*: Offline materials are often more durable than the online ones.
- *The level of trust*: Trust is typically higher with traditional marketing, e.g., paying for services and offers online on fraudulent sites may lead to mistrust with the actual organization.

Disadvantages of Traditional Marketing

- *Difficulties in measuring*: It is challenging to accurately measure your return of investment with traditional marketing when one compares it with digital marketing means.
- *High costs*: In most cases, this deters a new organization or a practice to employ these methods of marketing.
- *Static*: Lack of interaction with your target audience, and thereby a lack of understanding them.
- *Customizations*: It is difficult to target "specific" audiences with traditional marketing. One may generate interest in this segment of the population although to target a specific subset of individuals is challenging.
- *Inability to make changes*: While using traditional methods of marketing in the form of static text or advertising commercials to promote a product or service in the event that changes are desired in the content, it may not be possible to incorporate these fast enough once the processing has begun.
- *Pricing options*: As compared to the digital medium wherein certain websites and portals mention pricing and offers with proper explanations, it is often difficult to explain complex pricing in traditional marketing.

While the above-mentioned methods and strategies seem worthy of exploring for a budding esthetic or medical practice, as a practicing physician one must be well versed with the stringent regulations laid down by the Medcial Council of India (MCI). The MCI Code of Medical Ethics Regulations 2002,[4] amended on October 8, 2016, states that a *medical practitioner is permitted to make a formal announcement in press regarding the following:*

- *On starting the practice*
- *On change of type of practice*
- *On changing the address*
- *On temporary absence from duty*
- *On resumption of another practice*
- *On succeeding to another practice*
- *Public declaration of charges*

Printing of self-photograph or any such material of publicity in the letterhead or on sign board of the consulting room or any such clinical establishment shall be regarded as acts of self-advertisement and unethical conduct on the part of the physician. However, printing of sketches, diagrams, and picture of human system shall not be treated as unethical.

HOW TO MARKET A NEW PRACTICE

As one starts their individual practice, the first thing to do is to reach out to as many people as possible. This is where marketing comes into play. Having a professional marketing agency as your partner can be really handy. In terms of budget, start slow but be steady. Constant efforts are required to be in the eyes of your target audience.

Among the traditional marketing methods, *announcement* of a new practice is always a good idea through direct mailers at least in the area of practice. Further, one may contemplate putting brochures in the newspaper or in the clinic delineating the list of services offered by the clinic or in a folder where the patient may also store his/her prescription **(Fig. 6.2.4 and Box 6.2.1)**.

It may also be worthwhile investing in a sign board listing the services inside the clinic, close to the reception area or around the entrance, if space permits.

Figure 6.2.4 and Box 6.2.1: Inside of a brochure, outlining the services available at your clinic. The outside of the brochure could have your clinic name/logo, website, address, and phone numbers.

Meeting doctors around the area of work from other specialties and letting them know that you are starting a practice and are offering a set of services which they may keep in mind for referring patients. Moreover, use of telemarketing and use of internal marketing methods are good tools to start with, particularly if one is keen to promote "offers" or "discounts." However, this may vary for different practices and on where you might want to place your practice (brand) in the eyes of your potential patients. As the practice picks a little pace, one is certain of the areas one may want to focus on (e.g., lasers, injectable, pure clinical dermatology) and the target audience. Use of digital platforms such as Google AdWords, Facebook, Instagram,

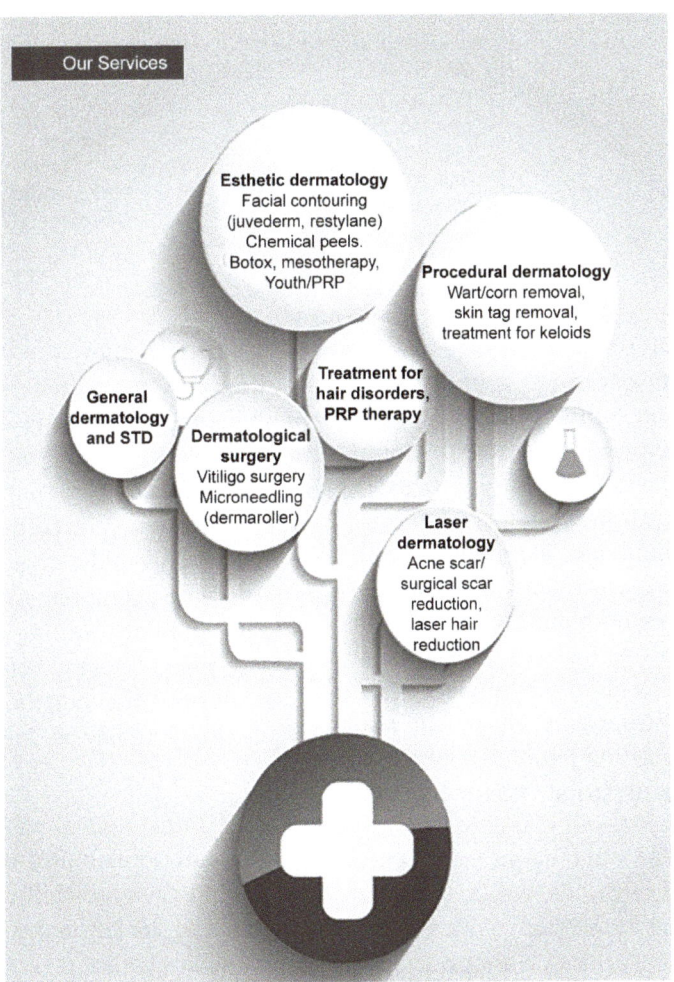

Fig. 6.2.4: Inside of the folder listing the services offered by the clinic. (PRP: platelet-rich plasma; STD: sexually transmitted diseases)

Box 6.2.1: Inside of brochure listing, services available.

Dermatology and dental services

General dermatology	Esthetic dermatology	Hair care
• Acne • Pigmentation • Hair fall • Vitiligo • Psoriasis • Eczema • Urticaria • Fungal infections • Nail diseases *Laser clinic* • Laser hair reduction • Acne scar reduction • Stretch mark reduction • Wart and corn removal • Skin tag removal • Mole removal • Tattoo reduction • Laser toning • Laser peel • Carbon peel • Other skin disorders	• The facecraft program • Cheek augmentation • Chin enhancement • Lip enhancement • Smile line reduction • Botulinum toxin (Botox) • Skin tightening • Chemical peels • Hydralift treatment • Vampire facelift (PRP) • Thread lift • Mesotherapy • Microdermabrasion *Dermatological surgery* • Skin biopsies • Wart and corn removal • Skin tag removal • Ingrown toenail surgery • Vitiligo surgery • Microneedling • Acne surgery	• Platelet-rich plasma (PRP) • Mesotherapy • Hair transplant *Cosmetic surgery* • Blepharoplasty • Tummy tuck • Male breast surgery • Breast augmentation • Liposuction *Dental services* • General dentistry • Braces • Root canal therapy • Implant dentistry • Smile designing and makeover • Gum therapy • Child dentistry • Oral surgery

and YouTube along with the traditional methods to help carve out a path ahead in terms of brand building, visibility, and ultimately more patients enquiring about your practice. Having a clear "vision" from the start of what you want to focus on, what you want your brand to be like, and your core values goes a long way in terms of planning your marketing methods and the road ahead. One would also need to get their visiting cards, brochures, and posters in place. Even if you use these internally, these will help to educate the existing patients about your specializations and various treatments that you provide.

Marketing is an ongoing process; hence once your practice builds, you may utilize certain marketing tools which work for you, e.g., announcement of a new branch opening/new technique/new equipment in the clinic. Moreover, you may continue your brand building exercise which engages engages your patients with you on a day-to-day basis, e.g., letting them know you are orating at a particular conference or publishing a paper/book and enhance credibility. More than anything, this builds "trust" in preexisting patients and promotes visibility for new, potential patients. Setting aside a regular, ongoing "budget" for marketing is crucial and as per your requirement, this may either be a "steady" input or may be "incremental".

THE RIGHT MIX

Planting and nourishing a healthcare structure is a big responsibility and are aided by a mix of traditional and now digital marketing strategies. It is important for the practitioner to understand the differences

Table 6.2.1: Differences between traditional marketing and digital marketing.

Traditional marketing	Digital marketing
Unidimensional communication with little customer/patient interaction	Multidimensional communication with active communication with consumers/patients
Involves greater costs	Cost of campaigning is on the lower side and one can invest in different segments, e.g., AdWords, search engine optimization, social media, etc.
Campaigns tend to be rigid with little room for change or improvement	Strategies have room for facilitating editing and adjustments
Tough to "target" a specific audience	Larger "scope" as the reach is more and directed to a target audience
Results are fast and impactful	Takes time to reap results
Brand building and trust building are easier—the "connect" with the customer/patient may be more impactful	Building trust over online platforms may take some time, however the "connect" with the customer/patient tends to develop over time
Longevity and durability are higher	Longevity and durability is lesser

between traditional means and digital methods of marketing before making investments in either **(Table 6.2.1)**.

CONCLUSION

The debate between traditional and digital marketing seems to be an ongoing one. While the popularity of digital marketing strategies gain ground, traditional marketing is still here to stay. How people consume information will always be individualistic in nature. Consequently, a multichannel strategy may turn out to be more effective than only choosing to communicate through a single medium, e.g., the elderly may still consider newspapers as a more reliable source of information while the younger generation wants everything at their fingertips because their lifestyle patterns are such.

Be it traditional or (now mostly) digital platforms, we as healthcare practitioners must understand that we choose this profession as our calling and not as a business opportunity. The whole essence of marketing a practice lies in a true representation of the practice, and a heartfelt and fact-based communication to the masses, in an ethical manner. One should never forget that marketing should not be done in a manner which is misleading in a direct or indirect way.

Under the strict and well-defined guidelines of what can be marketed and what cannot be, a sincere attempt of a practitioner to make the best use of his services will create a better and ethical impact both ways, leading toward the betterment of the practice vis-a-vis making it convenient for our patients.

REFERENCES

1. Shriram M. (2017). Traditional marketing vs. digital marketing. [online Available from https://yourstory.com/mystory/e09309421c-traditional-marketing. [Last accessed January, 2020].
2. Islamoğlu AH. Pazarlama Yönetimi (6. Baskı). Istanbul: Beta Basın Yayın Dağıtım AŞ; 2013.
3. Todor RD. Blending traditional and digital marketing. Bulletin of the Transilvania University of Brasov. Economic Sciences. Series V. 2016;9(1):51.
4. https://www.mciindia.org/documents/rulesAndRegulations/Ethics%20Regulations-2002.pdf.

6.3 Digital Marketing: Website as a Marketing Tool

K Feroz

INTRODUCTION

The challenge most often faced by a self-employed medical practitioner or a medical entrepreneur is that he/she needs to don multiple hats to run the show. However, a basic understanding of all aspects of running a business is also a core area, which will put us in good stead. In today's era, where connectivity is ubiquitous, we cannot ignore the technological invasion in the marketing space.

According to a recent report by the market research agency, Kantar IMRB, the number of internet users will reach 627 million by the end of 2019. Over 78% are regular internet users, which means they have had accessed the internet in the last 30 days. Another interesting finding is that 290 million of these users are from rural India and 97% use their mobile phones as one of the devices to access the internet. These figures, when combined with the common knowledge that today, people engage in an online research prior to making any purchasing decisions, invariably point to the need of having an online presence. This indirectly implies that even prior to consulting a doctor, patients go for an online search and research too.

A dermatologists' clinical credibility and word of mouth publicity may not work as effectively, as it used to, especially in a world which is becoming extremely individualistic and technology dependent in every aspect of life.

Digital marketing includes the promotion of products or brands via the Internet, social media, mobile phones, and electronic billboards, as well as via television and radio channels. In this chapter, we limit the coverage to the use of websites as a digital marketing tool.

WHY DO I NEED A WEBSITE?

With digital transformation shaping up the IT strategy of businesses across the world, we cannot overlook its importance in marketing as well. Marketing success these days largely depend on your digital presence or otherwise online visibility. A website is one of the basic and the most important components of any contemporary business today. An online presence is no longer optional for healthcare providers, as patients are constantly seeking health information and searching for new doctors online.

Medical websites help the users find necessary information regarding medical services, doctors, and facilities, as well as educate the patients about certain health issues.

A website is the perfect reflection of your brand intended to attract a wider audience and inform them about the specific types of services provided.

A good website has the following benefits:
- Your website appears on searches, which helps in brand recognition and possible patient conversion.
- Good content can establish your credibility and expand your market share.
- It provides better user experience for your customers to book appointments and share feedback.

- It supports marketing campaigns and customer service.

WHO SHOULD DEVELOP YOUR WEBSITE?

The choice of your website developer is crucial in creating the perfect website. A good website not only pleases the eyes of the visitors, but also ranks high on search engines. The developer should have a good esthetic and industry sense to come up with a suitable design that meets your vision as well as your needs. You may demand to see the website developer's portfolio and customer references before awarding your work to them.

Website development and Search Engine Optimization (SEO) are not a onetime job and hence the developer should continuously work and collaborate with you. So choose someone whom you can trust, someone who is easily accessible, understands you and your business well, and is a thorough professional.

A good website development team will ensure that your website is:
- Attractive and user friendly
- Available almost all the time
- SEO friendly
- Secured and safe from hackers
- Optimized for fast rendering in browsers
- Responsive (mobile friendly)

TYPES OF WEBSITES

Based on the ease with which one can change the contents of the website without depending on the developer, a website can be classified as static, dynamic, or content management system (CMS).
- *Static website*: One cannot edit the contents of the website without changing the code. You will have to depend on your website developer every time you need to change the content.
- *Dynamic website:* These are customized websites where you will have administrative rights to edit the contents such as your profile, images, and appointments.
- *CMS:* These are generally dynamic websites created using frameworks such as WordPress. You can manage the contents as and when required with ease.

WHAT SHOULD BE ON YOUR WEBSITE?

Your website is the digital gateway to your business. The name must be short, simple, and easy to remember. A name that represents you or your mode of practice. The website should have an esthetic design, a simple layout, attractive, and easy to navigate through. Ensure that you link pages in such a way that a website visitor will be able to track their steps back to the homepage if they need to. Please take care not to use jarring colors or overcomplicate things by using a variety of stylistic web design aspects. Limit animation and use of flash and multimedia to places where these are needed. This will increase your website's speed making it easier for your visitors to access information easily. Content is the most important part of any website. The content should be informative, precise, and easy to comprehend. Highlight your main functional areas and various treatment facilities and services offered. Posting fresh and unique content at frequent intervals keeps your website engaged and increases hits.

Ideally, as a medical practitioner, your website should have the following content:
- *Compelling information* about you, your credentials, and your services, i.e., a brief profile, pictures of your staff, your center and certifications, if any.
- *Online booking (appointments)*: One can provide the web audience with a quick

and easy way to make an appointment with the doctor at their convenient date and time.
- *Photo gallery*: Always remember to put visuals wherever necessary and in context with the data. These images can include before-after pictures of treated patients, good results or video testimonials, but with the consent of the patient and privacy protection. Patient identifying information such as tattoos, identity cards, and tags, should never be displayed on a public domain without proper consent.
- *Contact us*: Include all the basics (address, phone number, email address, etc.) on your home page and even on a separate *contact us* page as well. Always mention the clinic timings and contact timings clearly and visibly.
- *Clinic locator*: Consider including extra features such as a Google Map of your clinic's geographic location.
- *Testimonials from patients*: One of the most important ways to promote your healthcare business is to get feedback on the quality of service you provide. Make sure you act on any suggestions to improve the business and acknowledge feedback in a proactive way, including negative comments. By responding in a positive way, you will encourage people to leave open and honest comments, which will help your business develop. We may not be able to satisfy all our patients, and nowadays it is quite common that people respond or react on social media or websites. Place a control mechanism in place, so that only the testimonials you approve can be seen by public who visit your website.
- *Blogs, health tips, FAQs, informative news, events, etc.*: Ensure that you have a reservoir of information via a blog which can help give your clients up-to-date information on the goings on of the field that you are in. Other things to add in your blog can include updated information on what is going on in their community and the latest in medical discoveries, short videos on health education, information about your achievements, news, FAQs regarding various procedures, current common seasonal diseases, precautions to be taken with basic home care, etc. A physician can regularly write blogs with interesting articles on various medical topics. Adding a blog can be a great way to educate, share information, and engage patients, while improving your website's ranking in search results.
- *Social media links*: Social media is a powerful way of promoting businesses and attracting clients. It is interactive and can be shared. Make sure your posts encourage action and can be shared with others to spread the news. Social media is great for advertising promotions, holding competitions, and sharing information to a wider audience. Create a page for your clinic on social networks such as Facebook, Twitter, Instagram, and make sure to provide a link of these pages on your website.

IMPORTANCE OF MOBILE RESPONSIVE SITES

With the increased use of smart phones and tablets to surf the internet, it is crucial to have a mobile-friendly website. The website must be designed in such a way that it renders well on any device. Websites that are not mobile optimized do not appear favorably in Google results when searched on mobile devices. Google automatically ranks websites without mobile optimization lower because it considers them to be less user friendly.

SEARCH ENGINE OPTIMIZATION

Search engine optimization is the most vital tool for good visibility on the Web.

The essentials for the SEO-friendly website are:
- It needs to have a light design to allow quick page loading speed.
- Your website host should also provide fast page loading speed and minimum downtime.
- Your domain name should be relevant to your business and the content of your website.
- The URLs should have keywords in them but must also be relevant to the content of the page.
- Your website should be keyword optimized.

All these tips and tricks will help you rank higher in search engines and foster trust between your practice and clients.

WHAT NEXT?

Once you have a web presence, the next step is to promote your website to appear at the top on most popular search engines. SEO is one such activity. You can give paid ads on search engines so that you appear on the top. Your payment to search engine providers will be based on the clicks your website attracts. This is called pay-per-click (PPC).

With more and more people getting hooked on Social Media, promotion via Social Media Marketing (SMM) is a profitable option. You can use your profile pages with regular updates to promote your brand. Social media platforms also offer paid campaigns and promotions.

Chatbots that engage customers by providing responses to their queries without any manual intervention is a new trend that uses the power of Artificial Intelligence in your website.

CONCLUSION

Technology is evolving at a great speed. Digital transformation is redefining the way business is done. Big Data Analytics, Artificial Intelligence, Blockchain, and Internet of Things (IoT) make things easier, faster, and wiser. The new developments also make way to new challenges, such as security issues. But to stay ahead, one must be aware of and adopt the latest digital trends.

ACKNOWLEDGMENT

Ashfaque KP (Bluecast Technologies, Dubai-Kochi), Dr Soumya J, Dr Rakhesh SV, Dr Manish Gautam, Dr Venkataram Mysore, Dr Ramesh Bhat M, Dr Ashique KT, Surender (Health Connect Digital, Bangalore-Singapore), Athul (JKL Info Solutions, Kannur), Dr Hazeena C, and Aazim Feroz.

BIBLIOGRAPHY

1. Anderson E. Online promotion a must for hospital marketing professionals. Employ tactics to ensure your website is working to build your brand. Profiles Healthc Commun. 2007;23(2):1-3.
2. Auinger A, Brandtner P, Großeßner P, Holzinger A. Findability and usability as key success factors. Proceedings of the International Conference on e-Business (DCNET/ICE-B/OPTICS). DCNET/ICE-B/OPTICS; 2012. pp. 237-50.
3. Chen CY, Shih BY, Chen ZS, Chen TH. The exploration of internet marketing strategy by search engine optimization: a critical review and comparison. Afr J Bus Manage. 2011;5:4644-9.
4. Diaz JA, Griffith RA, Ng JJ, Reinert SE, Friedmann PD, Moulton AW. Patients' use of the internet for medical information. J Gen Intern Med. 2002;17(3):180-5.
5. Doulgeris J. (2012). How the pros market medical practice websites. [online] available from: http://www.physicianspractice.com/blog/how-pros-market-medical-practice-websites. [Last accessed January, 2020].
6. Finch T. Marketing your medical practice with an effective web presence. J Med Pract Manage. 2004;20(3):143-7.

7. Hasan L, Abuelrub E. Assessing the quality of websites. Applied Computing and Informatics. 2011;9(1):11-29.
8. Kantar Imrb. (2018). 21st edition ICUBE Digital adoption & usage trends. [online] Available from https://imrbint.com/images/common/ICUBE%E2%84%A2_2019_Highlights.pdf. [Last accessed January, 2020].
9. Labow K. Taking a traditional website to patient portal technology. J Med Pract Manage. 2010;25(4):240-2.
10. Larsen B. 7 easy steps to create your medical practice (internet). 2019 (cited 2020 January 6). [online] Available from: https://blog.evisit.com/7-easy-steps-to-create-your-medical-practice-website. [Last accessed January, 2020].
11. Narsaria R. (2015). Creating a Website for your Medical Practice. [online] Available from https://doctors.practo.com/creating-a-website-for-your-medical-practice/. [Last accessed January, 2020].
12. Radu G, Solomon M, Gheorghe CM, Hostiuc M, Bulescu IA, Purcarea VL. The adaptation of health care marketing to the digital era. J Med Life. 2017;10(1):44-6.
13. Rothschild MA. Marketing your practice on the internet. Otolaryngologic Clinics of North America 2002;35(6):1149-61.

SECTION 7: Medicolegal Aspects in Practice

7.1 Informed Consent

KHS Rao

INTRODUCTION

The concept of consent arises from the right to self-determination[1] of each individual with respect to taking decisions affecting his or her well-being. Legally, consent is a contract. Two or more persons are said to consent when they agree upon the same thing in the same sense.

Consent in the medical context involves mutual communication between doctor and patient with an expression of choice, permission, or authorization by the patient for the doctor to act or not to act in a particular way. Consent is more important in esthetic surgery than in conventional medical practice as the intervention is desire or demand-based rather than therapeutic.

Treating a patient without permission amounts to physical assault, which is legally called "battery", a punishable offence.[2] Taking consent is also an ethical obligation arising out of the principle of patient's autonomy.[3,4]

> Written consent is mandatory even for a minor surgery or cosmetic procedure.[5]

LEGAL LIABILITY

Insufficient or lack of informed consent is a frequent cause for medical malpractice litigation.[6,7] In cases of alleged medical negligence, the complainant has to prove that there was medical error or that standard care was not provided or that there was negligence on the part of the doctor. When it is difficult to do so, the easier option for the complainant is to allege improper or inadequate informed consent,[8] in which case it is for the doctor to prove[9] that the patient was adequately informed before taking consent.

Lack of documentation of the informed consent process, incompletely filled printed forms of consent,[5] blanket consents, and consents taken as a ritual in a casual manner are likely to go against the doctor in case of litigation.

Failure to take consent before doing any surgical intervention is a "professional misconduct" and is liable for disciplinary action by the State or Indian Medical Council.[10]

> Obtaining patient's signature on a dotted line as a ritual cannot constitute a proper consent and can be contested legally.[11]

Validity of Consent

There are three criteria for a consent to be valid:

1. It should be given by an adult. In case of minors, one of the parents or legal guardian can give it. In case of persons, aged between 12 and 18 years, the law is

not clear. It is preferable to take assent of the teenager as well as consent of a parent.[11]
2. It should be voluntary, i.e., free from compulsion, pressure, inducement, influence, or misrepresentation of facts.
3. Individual giving consent must be of sound mind and must be in the right state of mind at the time of giving consent.

Informed Consent[12-19]

Doctors are legally bound to provide adequate information and disclose all material risks before administering treatment or performing any procedure, so that the patient can decide to undergo the procedure or otherwise. It may not be possible or practical to disclose all side effects of drugs or very rare complications of surgery or anesthesia. In fact, such a move may create a sense of scare rather than helping the patient to take a decision.

There is no clear enunciation of the level of disclosure that can be considered adequate. Two standards[20,21] have been mentioned—(1) what a reasonable patient would want in a similar situation; (2) what a reasonable doctor would provide in a similar circumstance.

In case of litigation, there being no clarity of what constitutes a truly informed consent, judicial forums have to decide whether the information provided was adequate based on the circumstances of the particular case. In other words, no doctor can be 100% sure that the informed consent taken is foolproof.

In general, the following information has to be provided:
- *Procedure* or treatment details and the benefits thereof.
- *Alternative* options including "no treatment" and its benefits and consequences.
- *Risks* involved in both options, if possible with approximate quantification.[5]
- *Complications* that can arise and their expected frequency.
- *Outcome* expected which should be realistic.
- *Duration* of treatment and *downtime*— including average number of sittings, top-up procedures, etc.
- *Expenditure* involved (approximate).

A mnemonic "*PARCODE*" may be helpful in quickly recalling the components of the information to be discussed with the patient.[11]

Components of a Proper Informed Consent

- Written consent should be signed by both the patient and doctor.
- An uninterested third person should sign as witness.
- There is no prescribed fixed format for a consent form. It should be customized for each procedure.
- The contents should be in simple terms without technical jargon and in a language that patient can understand.
- It should be clearly mentioned that adequate opportunity has been given to seek additional information or clarifications.
- Consent taking should be preceded by adequate disclosure of material information.
- Consent should be taken a few days earlier to the day of procedure, and not on the day of the procedure or weeks prior to it.
- Consent is procedure specific. Consent taken for one procedure does not hold good for doing another or additional procedure.[22]
- Consent is person specific. If consent is taken by Dr A, procedure can only be done by Dr A and not by Dr A's assistant or Dr B.

- Consent is purpose specific. Consent taken for a diagnostic procedure cannot hold good for a therapeutic procedure.[23]
- If anesthesia is to be used, consent form must mention the type of anesthesia, anesthesiologist's name, and his or her endorsement that possible side effects of anesthesia have been explained to the patient. Alternatively, there can be a separate consent.[24]
- Specific consent is necessary for photographing the patient for documentation, scientific, academic or research purpose, or for follow-up. Specific consent must be taken, if the identity of the patient is likely to be revealed while publishing.
- Specific mention in the consent form is a must, if a new procedure or equipment is being tried out along with associated risks.
- In case a printed form is used, all blank spaces must be filled.
- There must not be any cuttings, overwriting but corrections under signature are acceptable.
- Consent form must indicate the place and date.[25]
- Patient retains the right to revoke the consent at any time.
- Denied consent also needs documentation as "informed refusal of consent"
- No kind of surety, guarantee, or money back policy can be a part of the consent.
- *Consent form should mention at the end*: "I have read and understood everything that is stated above. I have been given adequate time to think and decide. I have been given enough opportunity to seek clarifications and all my questions have been addressed satisfactorily. I hereby give my voluntary consent."

Some tips:
- Audio-visual recording of the consent process is not mandatory but may be useful.
- Consent taken well ahead of surgery suggests that time has been given to patient to think.
- If consent taken is several weeks old, it is preferable to take consent again on the day of surgery.
- It is useful that some part of consent is in the patient's own handwriting.
- Witness signature is important. If no one is there from patient's side, a hospital staff can be a witness.
- If consent form is more than one page, patient should sign on all pages.

CONCLUSION

Disclosing adequate information and taking an informed consent before performing any plastic or cosmetic surgery or procedure is mandatory. Insufficient and improper informed consents have resulted in judicial decisions going against doctors. It is important to note that informed consent is not a protective shield against litigations arising out of alleged medical error, negligence, or failure to provide standard medical care.

CONFLICT OF INTEREST

None.

REFERENCES

1. Mallardi V. The origin of informed consent. Acta Otorhinolaryngol Ital. 2005;25(5):312-27.
2. Trehan SP, Sankhari D. Medical Professional, Patient and the Law: The Institute of Law and Ethics in Medicine, 2nd edition. Bangalore: National Law School of India University; 2002.
3. Francis CM. Autonomy and Informed Consent, Medical Ethics, 2nd edition. New Delhi: Jaypee Brothers Medical Publishers (P) Ltd; 2004.
4. Rao KHS. Ethics, Etiquettes and Legal Issues, Management Issues for a Dermatologist, 1st edition. New Delhi: Jaypee Brothers Medical Publishers (P) Ltd; 2009.
5. Kapoor L. Informed consent in aesthetic surgery. J Cutan Aesthet Surg. 2015;8:173-4.

6. Vila-Nova da Silva DB, Nahas FX, Ferreira LM. Factors influencing judicial decisions on medical disputes in plastic surgery. Aesthet Surg J. 2015;35(4):477-83.
7. Therattil PJ, Chung S, Sood A, et al. An analysis of malpractice litigation and expert witnesses in plastic surgery. Eplasty. 2017;17:e30.
8. Park BY, Kwon J, Kang SR, et al. Informed consent as a litigation strategy in the field of aesthetic surgery: an analysis based on court precedents. Arch Plast Surg. 2016;43(5):402-10.
9. Bastia BK, Kuruvilla A, Saralaya KM. Validity of consent—a review of statutes. Indian J Med Sci. 2005;59:74-8.
10. Indian Journal of Medical Ethics. (2002). Indian Medical Council (Professional Conduct, Etiquette and Ethics) Regulations, 2002, published in Gazette of India, No.14, Part III, Section 4 dated 6.4.2002. [online] Available from http://ijme.in/articles/the-indian-medical-council-professional-conduct-etiquette-and-ethics-regulations-2002/?galley=html [Last accessed December, 2018].
11. Rao KHS. Informed Consent: An Ethical Obligation or Legal Compulsion? J Cutan Aesthet Surg. 2008;1(1):33-5.
12. Sacchidanand SA, Bhat S. Safe practice of cosmetic dermatology: Avoiding legal tangles. J Cutan Aesthet Surg. 2012;5(3):170-5.
13. Goldberg DJ. Legal issues in dermatology: Informed consent, complications and medical malpractice. Semin Cutan Med Surg. 2007;26:2-5.
14. Rao KHS. Safer practice of dermatosurgery. Indian J Dermatol Venereol Leprol. 2008;74:S75-7.
15. Goldberg DJ. Cosmetic dermatology: legal issues. Dermatol Clin. 2009;27:501-5.
16. Nejadsarvari N, Ebrahimi A. Different aspects of informed consent in aesthetic surgeries. World J Plast Surg. 2014;3(2):81-6.
17. Srinivas P. Consumer Protection Act and Dermatological Practice, a Dermatologists' Perspective of Medical Ethics and Consumer Protection Act: An IADVL Book, 1st edition. 2007.
18. Goldberg DJ. Medicolegal issues for the dermatologist. Semin Cutan Med Surg. 2000;19:181-8.
19. Sharma A, Arora S. Current Scenario of Informed Consent in India. [online] Available from http://knowledgeisotopes.com/blog/wp-content/uploads/dlm_uploads/2016/02/AS_Whitepaper-Informed-Consent_230216-2-1.pdf [Last accessed December, 2018].
20. Reisman NR. Medicolegal issues in plastic surgery. [online] Available from https://plasticsurgerykey.com/medico-legal-issues-in-plastic-surgery/ [Accessed December, 2018].
21. Weinmeyer R. Lack of standardized informed consent practices and medical malpractice. Virtual Mentor. 2014;16(2):120-3.
22. Shah AK. Newer implications of medicolegal and consent issues in plastic surgery. Indian J Plast Surg. 2014;47:199-202.
23. Nandimath OV. Consent and medical treatment: The legal paradigm in India. Indian J Urol. 2009;25(3):343-7.
24. Kumar A, Mullick P, Prakash S, et al. Consent and the Indian medical practitioner. Indian J Anaesth. 2015;59:695-700.
25. Sharma R. Informed consent in clinical practice and research: ethical and legal perspective. International J Healthcare Biomedical Res. 2014;3(1):144-51.

7.2 An Overview of Laws and Acts Applicable to Medical Professionals in India

Manjunath R

INTRODUCTION

Doctors belong to one of the most educated layers of our society. Yet, the legal awareness of doctors in India is surprisingly at a very low level.[1-3] When we hear about "Legal Education and Legal Awareness", we think that it is for law students and lawyers. The truth is that every person in our society needs basic legal education. Doctors are going to need it more than anyone else. Medical professionals in India are facing a multitude of problems. Patients are increasingly becoming aware of their rights and are always ready to take the doctors and hospitals to courts for treatment failures and complications. General public are ready to indulge in physical violence against hospitals and medical professionals for deaths in the hospitals even if they are caused due to road traffic accidents. Statutory bodies and governments are going overboard to please the general public with stringent provisions in the laws even when such provisions violate the fundamental rights of the doctors themselves.

In these testing times, it is essential for doctors and hospitals to have a reasonably good awareness of our laws to—(1) safeguard themselves and their rights, (2) safeguard their patients and the patients' rights, and (3) carry out their duties in accordance with the laws of the land.

The following are a few of the laws which are essential for the clinical establishments and medical professionals in India.

CODE OF MEDICAL ETHICS 2002[4]

The Medical Council of India has laid down certain regulations for modern medical practitioners regarding their professional conduct, etiquette, and ethics.[4] A copy of this is given to all modern medical graduates at the time of their registration at the medical councils, which needs to be signed and submitted. Hence, these regulations are binding on all modern medical practitioners. They need to be followed in letter and spirit.

These regulations define—(1) duties and responsibilities of medical professionals to the general public, to their patients, to the paramedical personnel, and to one another, (2) unethical acts, (3) misconduct, (4) punishments and disciplinary actions, and (5) formats for prescription and medical certificates.

FUNDAMENTAL RIGHTS[5]

The Constitution of India has given certain fundamental rights to all citizens of India.[5] They are: right to equality, right to freedom, right against exploitation, right to freedom of religion, cultural and educational rights, and right to constitutional remedies. Any violation of any of the fundamental rights, even if such violations are committed by governments and statutory bodies, can be successfully challenged in the High Courts and the Supreme Court.

It is surprising that the Indian medical communities have not defended this right as often as they should have been. As a consequence of this apathy, the statutory bodies and the governments have always felt free to ignore the fundamental rights of the doctors while framing the rules and regulations for medical profession.

In 2015, the Government of Karnataka legislated an act making it mandatory for MBBS graduates to undergo 1 year of mandatory rural service after internship to be eligible for registering their MBBS degree at the Karnataka Medical Council.[6] This was challenged at the High Court of Karnataka stating that it violated the rights of the doctors. The High Court of Karnataka has stayed the execution of the above-mentioned legislation.[7] As a result, the medical graduates of Karnataka can now register their MBBS degree at the Karnataka Medical Council by submitting an affidavit, without having to undergo the 1 year rural service that was to be imposed by the Government of Karnataka.[8]

CONCEPT OF MEDICAL NEGLIGENCE AND THE REMEDIES AVAILABLE TO THE ALLEGED VICTIM

Medical professionals in India are in the midst of a highly litiginous atmosphere. The patients are alleging medical negligence for any shortfall in treatments and their outcomes. Under Indian law, the remedies available to a person seeking redress for alleged medical negligence are: (1) suit for damages under the Civil Procedure Code, (2) complaint for negligence under the Criminal Procedure Code, (3) redressal under the Consumer Protection Act, and (4) Medical Council of India for disciplinary action.

However, it is essential for the medical professionals to know that medical negligence is established only if the following three criteria are established: (1) existence of legal duty, (2) breach of legal duty, and (3) damage caused directly by the breach of such duty.

Medical professionals should also know that mere complaint alleging medical negligence is not going to form a basis for action against medical professionals. There are legal guidelines for the courts and the police to follow before they can initiate any action against the medical professionals.[9,10]

CONSUMER FORUM

The consumer forum is the most easily accessible forum for the victims of alleged medical negligence. The fees are nominal, there is no need to hire a lawyer and the decisions are faster. Hence, there is a spurt in the number of consumer forum cases against medical professionals. Therefore, it is essential for the medical professionals to know about The Consumer Protection Act, 1986 and Rules, 1987.[11] However, even the consumer courts need to follow the defined criteria and guidelines for establishing medical negligence.

THE KARNATAKA PRIVATE MEDICAL ESTABLISHMENTS ACT, 2007[12] AND THE CLINICAL ESTABLISHMENTS ACT, 2010[13]

For the promotion and monitoring of private medical establishments in the State of Karnataka, the Government of Karnataka has enacted this legislation. All private medical establishments in the state of Karnataka need to register under this act.

A similar act is centrally enacted—The Clinical Establishments (Registration and Regulation) Act, 2010.[13] This Act is applicable to all States, which do not have a Medical Establishments act of their own.

VIOLENCE AGAINST MEDICAL PROFESSIONALS AND CLINICAL ESTABLISHMENTS

Violence against medical professionals and establishments has become a daily affair in India. There are legislations providing for strict actions against those involved in violence against medical professionals and establishments in many States.[14-16] Karnataka government has issued standard operating procedures to police personnel regarding what is to be done in case of such violence[17] (**Appendices 7.2.1 and 7.2.2**). Key aspect of this Act is that any offence committed under Section 3 of the Karnataka is that the act shall be cognizable and nonbailable (**Appendix 7.2.1**). However, despite the Act, incidents of violence against the medical professionals and medical establishments are on the rise in the State. There appears to be a lack of understanding on part of the local police in handling incidents of violence against medical professionals and medical establishments. To ensure clarity in this regard, the standard operating procedures (SOPs) were issued (**Appendix 7.2.2**).

However, these laws and SOPs have not been able to deter the perpetrators of such attacks.[18] The situation is so dismal that even the judiciary has indirectly legitimized violence by proclaiming that if doctors cannot face violence, they are unfit to work. In such a scenario, all medical professionals need to be well aware of how to identify, prevent, and fight against these violent incidents.[19]

RTI ACT AND CLINICAL ESTABLISHMENTS

Clinical establishments come under the ambit of Right to Information (RTI) Act of 2005 regarding provision of medical records to patients and their relatives. A decision by the Central Information Commission (CIC) makes it mandatory for all private hospitals to maintain daily reports of medical records of patients and provide them the information.[20] However, medical establishments need to consider the merits of each case with respect to patient confidentiality before giving out medical records under RTI Act.

QUACKERY: RIGHTS AND DUTIES OF MEDICAL PROFESSIONALS

According to the Indian Medical Association (IMA), some 10 lakh quacks practice in India. These include compounders, assistants to doctors, laboratory technicians, medical store owners, and Vaidyas. Quacks constitute 57% of persons practicing modern medicine in India. Dermatology is one of the most favorite specialties of the quacks. Each and every doctor needs to play an active role in the fight against quackery by identifying quacks, collecting evidence against them, and reporting them to the associations and authorities.

DRUGS AND COSMETICS ACT OF 1940

This act regulates the manufacture, sale, and distribution of medicines in India. A registered practitioner of modern medicine can dispense medicines to his/her patients without a license under the Drugs and Cosmetics Act of 1940, provided he/she is supplying drugs to his/her own patients, not running an open shop, not selling across the counter, purchasing medicines from a licensed manufacturer or distributor, and is maintaining all relevant bills and records.[21]

REFERENCES

1. Varghese AM, Vaswani VR, Kumar BK, et al. Awareness and Attitude of Medical Negligence and Medical Ethics among Interns and Resident Doctors. Int J Curr Microbiol App Sci. 2016;5(11):532-5.

2. Rao GV, Hari N. Medicolegal knowledge assessment of interns and postgraduate students in a medical institution. IAIM. 2016;3(10):105-10.
3. Haripriya A, Haripriya V. Knowledge about Medical Law and its Negligence among Doctors: A Cross-sectional Study. Int J Sci Res Pub. 2014;4(5):1-3.
4. Indian Medical Council. (2002). Indian Medical Council (Professional Conduct, Etiquette and Ethics) Regulations, 2002. [online] Available from https://www.mciindia.org/documents/rulesAndRegulations/Ethics%20Regulations-2002.pdf. [Last accessed December, 2018].
5. Know India. The constitution of India, Part III, Fundamental Rights, Articles 12 to 35. [online] Available from http://knowindia.gov.in/profile/fundamental-rights.php. [Last accessed December, 2018].
6. Department of Parliamentary Affairs and Legislation. (2015). The Karnataka Compulsory Service Training by Candidates Completed Medical Courses Act, 2012, (Act 26 of 2015). [online] Available from http://dpal.kar.nic.in/ao2015/26%20of%202015%20(E).pdf. [Last accessed December, 2018].
7. High Court of Karnataka Daily Orders of the Case Number: WP 25391/2016 for the date of order 28/04/2016.
8. Karnataka Medical Council. (2016). Affidavit for registration. [online] Available from http://karnatakamedicalcouncil.com/userfiles/file/Affidavit%20for%20rural%20service.pdf. [Last accessed December, 2018].
9. Wikipedia. (1957). Bolam v Friern Hospital Management Committee. [online] Available from https://en.wikipedia.org/wiki/Bolam_v_Friern_Hospital_Management_Committee. [Last accessed December, 2018].
10. Supreme Court of India. (2005). Jacob Mathew vs State of Punjab & Anr on 5 August, 2005. [online] Available from https://indiankanoon.org/doc/871062/. [Last accessed December, 2018].
11. Department of Food and Civil Supplies Department (Rajasthan). (1987). The Consumer Protection Act, 1986 & Rules, 1987. [online] Available from http://food.raj.nic.in/Docs/18C.P.Act.pdf. [Last accessed December, 2018].
12. Government of Karnataka. (2007). The Karnataka Private Medical Establishments Act, 2007, (Karnataka Act No 21 of 2007). [online] Available from http://dpal.kar.nic.in/pdf_files/21%20of%202007(E).pdf. [Last accessed December, 2018].
13. Advocate Khoj. (2010). The Clinical Establishments (Registration and Regulation) Act, 2010. [online] Available from https://www.advocatekhoj.com/library/bareacts/clinical/index.php?Title=Clinical%20Establishments%20(Registration%20and%20Regulation)%20Act,%202010. [Last accessed December, 2018].
14. Government of Karnataka. (2009). The Karnataka Prohibition of Violence against Medicare Service Personnel and Damage to Property in Medicare Service Institutions Act, 2009. [online] Available from http://dpal.kar.nic.in/pdf_files/1of2009(E).pdf. [Last accessed December, 2018].
15. The Andhra Pradesh Gazette. (2007). Andhra Pradesh Ordinance against the Violence on Doctors and Medical Establishments. [online] Available from http://medind.nic.in/jal/t08/i1/jalt08i1p54.pdf. [Last accessed December, 2018].
16. Government of Maharashtra. (2010). The Maharashtra Medicare Service Persons and Medicare Service Institutions (Prevention of Violence and Damage or Loss to Property) Act, 2010. [online] Available from http://www.lawsofindia.org/pdf/maharashtra/2010/2010MH11.pdf. [Last accessed December, 2018].
17. Medical Dialogues. (2017). Standard Operating Procedure to deal with violence against Medical Professionals laid in Karnataka. [online] Available from https://medicaldialogues.in/standard-operating-procedure-to-deal-with-violence-against-medical-professionals-laid-in-karnataka/. [Last accessed December, 2018].
18. Kapoor MC. Violence against the medical profession. J Anaesthesiol Clin Pharmacol. 2017;33(2):145-7.
19. Nagpal N. Incidents of violence against doctors in India: can these be prevented? Natl Med J India. 2017;30(2);97-100.
20. Indian Kanoon (2015). Prabhat Kumar v/s GNCTD, Delhi; CIC/SA/A/2014/000004. [online] Available from https://indiankanoon.org/doc/117751905/. [Last accessed December, 2018].
21. Schedule K (1945) Drugs and cosmetics Rules, 1945. [online] Available from http://www.mogsonline.org/pdfs/shedule_k.pdf. [Last accessed December, 2018].

APPENDIX 7.2.1: KARNATAKA VIOLENCE ACT

KARNATAKA ACT NO. 1 OF 2009
(First Published in the Karnataka Gazette Extraordinary on the Second day of March, 2009)

THE KARNATAKA PROHIBITION OF VIOLENCE AGAINST MEDICARE SERVICE PERSONNEL AND DAMAGE TO PROPERTY IN MEDICARE SERVICE INSTITUTIONS ACT, 2009

Arrangement of Sections

STATEMENT OF OBJECTS AND REASONS

Sections
1. Short title and commencement
2. Definitions
3. Prohibition of violence
4. Penalty
5. Cognizance of offence
6. Recovery of loss for the damage caused to the property
7. The provisions of this Act shall be in addition to other laws.

STATEMENT OF OBJECTS AND REASONS

In order to prevent violence against Medicare Service personnel and damage to property in medicare service, institutions, it is considered necessary to enact a law.

Hence the Bill.
(LA Bill No. 3 of 2009, File No. DPAL 21 Shasana 2008)
(Entry 1 and 6 of List II of the Seventh Schedule to the Constitution of India.)

KARNATAKA ACT NO. 1 OF 2009

(First Published in the Karnataka Gazette Extraordinary on the Second day of March, 2009)

THE KARNATAKA PROHIBITION OF VIOLENCE AGAINST MEDICARE SERVICE PERSONNEL AND DAMAGE TO PROPERTY IN MEDICARE SERVICE INSTITUTIONS ACT, 2009

(Received the assent of the Governor on the twenty-sixth day of February, 2009)

An Act to prohibit violence against medicare service personnel and damage to property in medicare service institutions and for matters connected therewith and incidental thereto.

Whereas it is expedient to prohibit violence against medicare service personnel and damage to property in medicare service institutions and for matters connected therewith and incidental thereto;

Be it enacted by the Karnataka State Legislature in the Fifty-ninth year of the Republic of India, as follows:

1. **Short Title and Commencement:** (1) This Act may be called the Karnataka Prohibition of violence against medicare service personnel and damage to property in medicare service institutions Act, 2009.

    (2) It shall come into force at once.

2. **Definitions:** In this Act, unless the context otherwise requires:
    (a) "Medicare Service Institutions" means all institutions, providing medicare services to people, which are under the control of State or Central Government or Local Bodies, etc. including any private hospital having facilities for treatment of the sick and used for their reception or stay, any private maternity home where women are usually received and accommodated for the purpose of confinement and antenatal and postnatal care in connection with child birth or anything connected therewith; and any private nursing home used or intended to be used for the reception and accommodation of persons suffering from any sickness, injury or infirmity whether of body or mind, and providing of treatment for nursing or both of them and includes a maternity home or convalescent home, etc.
    (b) "Medicare service personnel in relation to a medicare service institution" shall include:
        (i) Registered Medical Practitioners, working in Medicare Institutions (including those having provisional registration);
        (ii) Registered nurses;
        (iii) Medical students;
        (iv) Nursing students;
        (v) Paramedical workers employed and working in Medicare Service Institutions;
    (c) 'Offender' means any person who either by himself or as a member or as a leader of a group of persons or organization commits or attempts to commit or abets or incites the commission of violence under this Act;
    (d) 'Violence' means activities of causing any harm, injury or endangering the life or intimidation, obstruction or hindrance to any medicare service personnel in discharge of duty in the medicare service institution or damage to property in medicare service institution;

3. **Prohibition of violence:** Any violence against medicare service personnel or damage to property in a medicare service institution is prohibited.
4. **Penalty:** Any person who commits any act in contravention of Section 3, shall be punished with imprisonment for a period of three years with fine which may extend to fifty thousand rupees.
5. **Cognizance of offence:** Any offence committed under Section 3 shall be cognizable and non-bailable.
6. **Recovery of loss for the damage caused to the property:** (1) In addition to the punishment specified in Section 4, the offender shall also be liable to a penalty of twice the amount of purchase price of medical equipment damaged and loss caused to the property as determined by the Court trying the offender.
   (2) If the offender has not paid the penal amount under subsection (1), the said sum shall be recovered under the provisions of the Karnataka Land Revenue Act, 1964 (Karnataka Act 12 of 1964) as if it were to be an arrears of land revenue.
7. **The provisions of this Act shall be in addition to other laws:** The provisions of this Act shall be in addition to and not in derogation of the provisions of any other law, for the time being in force.

The above translation of the ಕರ್ನಾಟಕ ವೈದ್ಯೋಪಚಾರ ಸಿಬ್ಬಂದಿಯ ಮೇಲೆ ಹಿಂಸಾಚಾರವನ್ನು ಮತ್ತು ವೈದ್ಯೋಪಚಾರ ಸಂಸ್ಥೆಗಳ ಆಸ್ತಿಗೆ ಹಾನಿ ಮಾಡುವುದನ್ನು ನಿಷೇಧಿಸುವ ಅಧಿನಿಯಮ, 2009 be published in the official Gazette under clause (3) of Article 348 of the Constitution of India.

Rameshwar Thakur
Governor of Karnataka

By order and in the name of the Governor of Karnataka

GK Boregowda
Secretary to Government
Department of Parliamentary Affairs and Legislation

ಸರ್ಕಾರಿ ಮುದ್ರಣಾಲಯ, ವಿಕಾಸ ಸೌಧ ಘಟಕ, ಬೆಂಗಳೂರು.

APPENDIX 7.2.2: STANDARD OPERATING PROCEDURE (SOP)—DIRECTOR GENERAL OF POLICE (DGP) KARNATAKA TO HANDLE VIOLENCE AGAINST MEDICAL PROFESSIONALS AND HOSPITALS

GOVERNMENT OF KARNATAKA
POLICE DEPARTMENT

Office of the
Director General and
Inspector General of Police
Karnataka State, Bengaluru
Date: 18-05-2017.

No.L&O/MISC-13/2017-18

STANDING ORDER NO. 1018.

Sub: Standard Operating Procedure (SOP) to deal with violence against Medical Professionals and Medical Establishments.
******

Incidents of violence against Medical Professionals and Medical Establishments are on rise in the State, even though 'Karnataka Prohibition of Violence against Medicare Service Personnel and damage to property in Medicare Service Institutions Act' was enacted in 2009 to prevent such violence. There appears to be a lack of understanding on the part of the local police in handling of incidents of violence against Medical Professionals and Medical Care Establishments in the State. To have clarity in this regard this Standard Operating Procedures (SOP) to handle violence against Medical Professionals and Medical Care Establishments is issued.

Karnataka Prohibition of Violence against Medicare Service Personnel and Damage to Property in Medicare Service Institutions Act - 2009:

The Act prohibits violence against Medicare service personnel or damage to property in a medicare service institution. The Act defines a medicare service personnel as any registered medical practitioner, working in medicare institutions (including those having provisional registration, registered nurse, medical student, nursing student and paramedical worker) employed and working in medicare service institution.

The Act defines a Medicare Service Institution as any institution providing medicare services to people, which are under the control of State or Central Government or local bodies, etc. including any private hospital having facilities for treatment of the sick and used for their reception or stay, any private maternity home where women are usually received and accommodated for the purpose of confinement and antenatal and postnatal care in connection with child birth or anything connected therewith; and any private nursing home used or intended to be used for the reception and accommodation of persons suffering from any sickness, injury or infirmity whether of body or mind, and providing of treatment for nursing or both of them and includes a maternity home or convalescent home, etc.

The Act further defines 'violence' as an activity of causing any harm, injury or endangering the life or intimidation, obstruction or hindrance to any medicare service personnel in discharge of duty in the medicare service institution or damage to property in medicare service institution. 'Offender' is defined as any person who either by himself or as a member or as a leader of a group of persons or organization commits or attempts to commit or abets or incites the commission of violence under this Act. Section 3 of the Act prohibits any violence against medicare service personnel or damage to property in a medicare service institution. Offences under the Act are cognizable and non-bailable with imprisonment for a period of three years with fine up to fifty thousand rupees.

Nature of violence against Medical Professionals and Medical Care Establishments:

Violence encountered against Medical Professionals and Medical Care Establishments can broadly be categorized as follows:
1. Verbal abuse by the attendants of the patients.
2. Creating scary situations by the mob.
3. Intimidation
4. Assault on Medical Professionals and Medical Care Establishment staff.
5. Ransacking of the Medical Care Establishment.
6. Preventing Medical professionals from discharging his/her duties.
7. Creating problems/nuisance to the outpatients and inpatients.
8. Entering the restricted areas like Operating theaters, Intensive Care Units, Documentation office and other areas in the Medical Care Establishment.
9. Damaging the property and documents.
10. Refusal to take dead body by the attendants and to pay the bills.
11. Directly or indirectly putting pressure on the Medical Professionals and Medical Care Establishment staff/extortion.
12. Snatching the medical records/documents
13. Forcing the Medical Professionals to treat unrelated treatment.
14. Revengeful act by the patients or their attendees.
15. Unnecessary intervention of media and pressure groups.

Precautionary and Preventive Measures to be taken by the Police:

1. Police personnel at the police station level shall have contact numbers and addresses of all Medical Professionals/Medical Care Establishments in their jurisdiction.
2. Under the new beat system, the Beat Officer shall have such numbers and addresses in his beat area.
3. Police Stations incharge shall form a WhatsApp Group of the Medical Professionals along with beat officers so that there can be regular exchange of information pertaining to any incident of violence.
4. A WhatsApp group at SP/DCP level may also be considered with the Medical Professionals/ Medical Care Establishments of the respective jurisdiction.
5. Sensitization of Police personnel about the provisions of the Karnataka Prohibition of Violence against Medicare Service Personnel and Damage to Property in Medicare Service Institutions Act, 2009.

Response by Police:

In case of violence against Medical Professionals and Medical Care Establishments, response of the local police shall be as follows:

1. Once Police Control Room/Mobile Police/Police Station/Higher Authorities receive information of such a violence, responsible police personnel shall immediately reach the place.
2. Immediate protection shall be provided to the Medical professionals/Medical Care Establishment staff/property and other patients.
3. Police personnel on reaching the place, should first disperse the mob from the Medical Care Establishment and control the situation. This is necessary as there are other patients in the Medical Care Establishments as well as doctors attending to them who would be disturbed unless the mob is dispersed. The police should therefore reach the spot with adequate force to do so.
4. In case of death of a patient, the dead body should not be allowed to be kept in the Medical Care Establishment by the agitators as that would instigate further disturbance. The police personnel should talk to the relations/attendants of the concerned patients to shift the body out of the Medical Care Establishments.
5. Immediate steps shall be taken to shift the dead body to mortuary in event of death of a patient.
6. Registration of case under the existing Karnataka Prohibition of Violence against Medicare Service Professional and Damage to Property in Medicare Service Institutions Act 2009 shall be taken up.
7. Protection shall be provided to the Medical Care Establishment till the situation settles.
8. If the attendants of the patient do not have faith on the Medical Care Establishment about their competency in curing of the patient, the attendants of the patients should be asked to shift the patient to any other establishments instead of making a scene in the medical establishment.
9. Any violence at the Medical care establishment shall be brought to the notice of Dy. Commissioner of Police/Superintendent of Police immediately.
10. In case of complaint against doctor by the patient or his relatives, Hon'ble Supreme Court's guidelines shall be followed. In case of deviance, disciplinary action shall be taken against concerned Police Officers.

Relying on Hon'ble Supreme Court Judgments in this connection, the Hon'ble High Court of Madhya Pradesh in its judgment in Dr BC Jain v/s Moulana Saleem on 28-02-2017 has laid down the following guidelines:

I. That, all allegations relating to negligent conduct on the part of a Government Doctor for which a prosecution u/s. 304-A IPC and/or its cognate provisions or under such other law involving penal consequences is sought, the same shall be enquired into by a Medical Board consisting of at least three doctors, constituted by the Dean of any Government Medical College, upon the request of the Police, Administration or the directions of a Court/Tribunal/Commission, within seven days of such requisition.
II. The doctor so selected by the Dean of the Medical College concerned to sit on the Medical Board, shall not be inferior in seniority and experience to that of an Associate Professor.

III. The doctor against whom such negligence is alleged, shall be given an opportunity by the Medical Board to give his reply/explanation in writing and if the doctor so desires to be heard personally, he shall be given such an opportunity by the Medical Board. However, if the Medical Board is of the opinion that the request for personal hearing is with the intent of procrastinating the proceedings before the Board, it may, for reasons to be recorded, waive the opportunity or a personal hearing and proceed to decide the case on the basis of the documents/treatment record and give its finding.
IV. The Medical Board shall endeavor to complete the exercise within sixty days from the date on which it is constituted and upon completion of the enquiry, submit the report to the Police, Administration or the Court/Tribunal/Commission, as the case may be.
V. The police shall not register an FIR against such a doctor in the absence of the report of the Medical Board referred here in above and also, only when the report by the Medical Board has held the doctor prima facie guilty of Gross Negligence and not otherwise.
VI. If a complaint case has been preferred U/s. 200 Cr.P.C, there shall be no order u/s. 156(3) Cr.P.C unless the complaint is accompanied by the report of the Medical Board adverted to in guideline I with prima facie finding of Gross Negligence on the part of the Doctor. However, if the complaint is not accompanied with a report of the Medical Board, the Court may ask the Police to enquire into the case u/s. 202 Cr.P.C. The police, if so directed by the Court, shall approach the Dean of the Medical College for the constitution of the Medical Board and thereafter place the report of the Medical Board before the Court concerned.
VII. If the opinion of the Medical Board is one of Gross Negligence on the part of the doctor, the Court concerned shall direct the police to seek sanction u/s. 197 Cr.P.C from the State Government. The State Government shall, within thirty days from the date of such request for sanction, either grant or refuse the same, which the police shall convey to the Court concerned. Thereafter, the Court concerned shall either dismiss the complaint case against the doctor by exercising jurisdiction u/s. 203 Cr.P.C or issue process u/s. 204 Cr.P.C and try the case in accordance with the law.

All the Commissioners of Police and District Superintendents of Police shall ensure compliance of above instructions.

(RUPAK KUMAR DUTTA, IPS)
Director General and
Inspector General of Police
Karnataka State, Bengaluru

To :
1) All the Addl. DGPs in Karnataka State.
2) All the Commissioners of Police—Bengaluru/Mysore/Belgaum/Hubli-Dharwad/Mangalore cities.
3) All the Inspector-Generals of Police in Karnataka State.
4) All the Dy. Inspector-Generals of Police in Karnataka State.
5) All the Superintendents of Police in Karnataka State.

7.3 Malpractice and Related Issues

Subodh P Sirur

In clinical practice, the one thing that is dreaded is a threat of allegations of medical negligence or a notice from a court of law for alleged medical negligence. Therefore, we, as doctors, need to be conversant with the basic principles of law so that we are better equipped to handle any such threat. In law, malpractice is known as professional negligence. Thus, in the context of doctors, malpractice is called as medical negligence.

Dermatologists, for a fairly long period of time, have not been facing allegations of medical negligence. The reason could be the relatively low incidence of morbidity and mortality associated with the ailments handled by dermatologists. However, the addition of esthetic procedures by dermatologists to their therapeutic armamentarium and an increased awareness among patients, has led to a definite surge in the number of cases where allegations have been raised against dermatologists. A lack of effective communication can result in unrealistic expectations and thus trigger allegations of medical negligence and litigation.

WHAT IS MEDICAL NEGLIGENCE?

Every doctor is expected to exercise a duty of care while treating patients. This duty of care can be a duty of care in deciding whether to undertake to treat a patient presenting to the doctor; a duty of care in deciding what line of treatment is to be administered to the patient, and thirdly a duty of care in administration of the treatment.

Duty of care in deciding whether to undertake to treat a patient: A doctor is not bound to treat every patient who presents to him or her for treatment. However, in case of an emergency, this freedom to refuse to treat a patient is either limited or nonexistent. If the patient's ailment is not within the scope of the said doctor, then the doctor would have to refer the patient to a doctor who is an expert in that field. In the field of dermatology, there are a set of doctors who practice only clinical dermatology, some others whose focus of practice is largely esthetic dermatology and some who practice a mix of clinical dermatology and esthetic medicine. Therefore, if a patient desirous of having a hair transplantation surgery presents to a dermatologist who is exclusively into clinical dermatology, such a dermatologist would refer the patient to one who is trained and skilled in performing hair transplantation.

Duty of care in deciding the line of treatment: The second important duty of care is in deciding the line of treatment to be administered to the patient. Treatment based on standard protocols and evidence-based medicine should be the preferred line of treatment. In cases where there is a departure from the standard protocols, there should be adequate medical justification for the line of treatment adopted in that particular scenario. The medical records should also reflect the justification for the departure from the accepted professional practice protocol. A previous history of drug allergy, pregnancy, other comorbidities also determine the line of treatment to be administered.

Duty of care in administration of the line of treatment: The third important duty of care is in the administration of the chosen line of treatment. If certain investigations are required to be carried out before administering certain drugs such as methotrexate or biologicals, then it is imperative that the investigations are done prior to administration of such drugs. It cannot be dispensed with on grounds of financial stringency of the patient. Failure to do a preprocedure assessment for correct patient selection and ruling out contraindications (relative and/or absolute) for such procedures can amount to medical negligence. It is essential to ask during preprocedure assessment wherever recommended, questions such as a history of keloidal tendency and that of herpes simplex infection. Performance of a chemical peel without priming (wherever it is recommended) leading to any complication can also bring out a charge of medical negligence.

ESSENTIAL INGREDIENTS OF MEDICAL NEGLIGENCE

A failure of any of the above-mentioned duties of care resulting in loss or injury or death of the patient, can result in a finding of medical negligence. A court, before making a finding of medical negligence, will look for the presence of the following ingredients:
- Existence of a duty of care
- Breach of such duty of care
- Loss or injury or death of the patient
- Causal relationship between the breach of duty of care and the loss or injury or death of the patient.

Therefore, if a doctor fails in the duty of care toward a patient, which results in some loss or injury or death of the patient, court will hold that doctor liable for medical negligence. If there is no relationship between the loss or injury or death of the patient and the breach of duty of care, then there cannot be any liability for negligence. For example, if a patient is taken up for a procedure and reacts adversely to a test dose of lignocaine and subsequently develops cardiac arrest, the doctor is not liable for the adverse reaction. However, if the doctor does not identify the reaction in time and take all appropriate steps to treat the adverse reaction, then the doctor can be held liable for negligence. Therefore, an occurrence of a drug reaction by itself would not indicate medical negligence.

Accepted professional practice: Further, if despite the doctor adopting a standard and accepted professional practice protocol, the patient develops some morbidity or even mortality, by itself it will not indicate negligence on the part of the doctor. So, if a patient with Stevens–Johnson syndrome is treated as per accepted professional practice but the patient develops loss of vision (a known complication), the doctor cannot be held liable for negligence.

Two schools of thought: If there are two or more schools of thought on the modality of treatment for a clinical condition, the courts would be slow in holding a doctor liable for medical negligence if a doctor chooses one of the modalities to the exclusion of the other. If there are "pro-steroid" and "no steroid" schools of thought in the treatment of toxic epidermal necrolysis and if the dermatologist adopts one over the other, the courts will not hold the dermatologist liable simply because one of the modalities was adopted to the exclusion of the other. It is important that both the accepted professional practices are current.

Error of judgment: Similarly, an error of judgment by itself would not result in a finding of medical negligence. Error of diagnosis, such as psoriasis and psoriasiform skin lesions and lichen planus and lichenoid skin lesions, is not indicative of failure of duty of care. However, in cases which do not follow the expected natural course of the provisional diagnosis of the ailment need to be reassessed after a certain and reasonable period of time and investigations such as a skin biopsy should be performed to arrive at a conclusive diagnosis. Failure to do so can make the doctor liable for medical negligence.

SAFEGUARDS AGAINST LITIGATION

It is important to remember that medical records form an important piece of document evidencing the treatment administered to a patient. Therefore, proper documentation is an important tool to prevent and handle the risk of litigation alleging medical negligence. A consent should be obtained in all appropriate cases after having informed the patient about the nature of the ailment or the procedure to be performed; the risks and complications associated; the various options or modalities of treatment available as also the adverse consequences of not undergoing the recommended treatment. Further, regular updating of knowledge in the field is important because a clinical approach based on standard protocol accepted by medical professionals is a valid defense in case of alleged medical negligence. It is not feasible to eliminate entirely the risk of litigation despite all appropriate safeguards. However, the risk can definitely be minimized as also the litigation or legal action can be better handled with better safeguards in place.

DISCLAIMER

The information in this chapter is for information purpose only and it is not expected that decisions in specific legal cases should be taken purely on the basis of the above information. It is to be noted that some laws may be modified, repealed or new laws are enacted from time to time. The decisions of the courts can have a bearing on our clinical practice. Such decisions can be reviewed or reversed by the higher courts. Therefore, a reference should be made to the latest rules, regulations, laws, and binding precedents of the courts on the subject.

7.4

Quackery

Putta Srinivas, Rajesh Buddhadev

"Quackery is the legitimate offspring of ignorance and can only be abridged by elevating the standards of medicine and disseminating a correct public statement."
—**Charles K Winston and Paul E Eve (1851)**

DEFINITION

Health quackery is defined as the promotion and commercialization of unproven and often dangerous health products and procedures.[1]

BRIEF HISTORY

Quackery refers to unproven or fraudulent medical practices, often through the sale or application of "quack medicines." The word "quack" derives from the archaic Dutch word "quacksalver", meaning "boaster who applies a salve." A closely associated German word, "Quacksalver", means "questionable salesperson." In the middle ages, the word quack meant "shouting." The quacksalvers sold their wares on the market shouting in a loud voice.[2]

Quack medicines were especially prevalent in the British Empire for centuries, including in the American colonies. Following the American Revolution and the War of 1812, American products began to dominate the domestic market. The American term for quack medicine was "snake oil", a reference to sales pitches, in which outrageous claims of medicinal successes were made.

The snake oil was used for inflammation. Original Chinese snake was made with the fat from Chinese water snakes. However, the snake oil marketed in US contains mineral oil, beef fat, red pepper, and turpentine but no snake oil. Cocaine was used as local anesthetic agent, during dental surgeries. Opiates were used for crying babies to put them to sleep.[2]

TYPES OF QUACKS

Quacks can be categorized into three types: (1) charlatans, (2) cranks, and (3) health hucksters.[3]

Charlatans

"One who is not what he or she claims to be."[4] Charlatans are deliberate fakers and they exploit people without feeling guilty. They want and do whatever they like, and they are blind to the conscience and totally indifferent to the feelings of others. They are health predators, who charm, manipulate ruthlessly go ahead with their deception, leaving a trail of broken hearts, shattered expectations, and empty wallets.[3]

Cranks

They are delusional individuals who sincerely believe in themselves and their nostrums. However, they are likely to be honest and they exhibit generosity and selflessness. They defend themselves blindly and vehemently and they are often paranoid and counter scientific criticism as persecution done with vengeance. Usually charlatans are cautious and limit their claims and they try to escape from law and regulations; on the contrary, cranks do not accept their limitations and are more dangerous to society.[3]

Health Hucksters

They are business persons and use marketing techniques to promote their secret remedies without any scientific evidence of efficacy and safety, which any responsible business person or health professional will do. They idealize entrepreneurialism and exploit the potential offered by public interest in areas in which modern science provides slow and long-term and sometimes limited solutions for which general public feel difficult to follow, like reducing obesity, improving color and complexion, etc.

They do not have any ethics and on the other hand they expect buyers to be aware "caveat emptor" (meaning thereby "without a warranty, the buyer must take the risk"). *"They operate with a principle that if people are not aware and intelligent enough to identify useless health remedies, they are foolish enough to survive in modern economic society which is called as social Darwinism."* Vigorous business promotion and showmanship are hallmarks of health hucksters and they continuously use celebrities like movie stars, models, sportsman, and women who are usually adored by common people to promote their health remedies/drugs. Presently, it is prevalent in almost all sectors of life, but unfortunately more so in the dermatology field.[3]

Quackery can be also classified as medical quackery, nutritional quackery, and device quackery.

Medical Quackery

It pertains to the malpractice in the medical profession where pseudo doctors, claim to be experts and competent in treating diseases. Their intention is always to make profit at the expense of deceiving people; they capitalize on the hope, ignorance, and fear of people.

Nutritional Quackery

Any form of fake or unclassified claims of nutritional value or impact. Some of the most popular and profitable hoaxes that go on in the form of dietary supplements, herbal remedies, weight loss products, energy boosters, and which do not have any scientific evidence. More often than not, these products become detrimental to one's health, contradictory to what its label tells.

Device Quackery

It pertains to the claims or information about the products that are "too good to be true." They deceive the customers by exaggerating about the quality, efficiency, and try to justify the cost or lower its price along with quality.

WHY QUACKS ARE SUCCEEDING AND FLOURISHING?

It was expected that as the medical sciences progressed, as many diseases became curable and quality of health of people improved remarkably as reflected by increase in life expectancy, decrease in infant mortality rate (IMR) and maternal mortality ratio (MMR), will lead to gradual elimination of quackery. But surprisingly it is not so and on the contrary, quackery is booming!

In spite of advanced state of medical science, many people with health problems turn to dubious methods. Faced with the prospect of chronic suffering, deformity, or death, many individuals are tempted to try anything that offers relief or hope. The terminally ill, the elderly, and various cultural minorities are especially vulnerable to health frauds and quackery. Many intelligent and well-educated individuals resort to worthless methods, procedures with the belief that anything is better than nothing.[5]

The success and survival of quackery has multiple reasons and is composite in nature. There are psychological, sociocultural, educational, and economic factors.[6]

- Quacks listen spare more time, show concern with sympathy, take care and establish rapport and a cordial relationship which is their trump card, however, it may not be true every time and many a times they show rigid attitude also when asked a question or query.[7]
- Various studies have revealed that whenever humans are not able to get benefits of science and technology, they revert and look toward quacks. Quacks exploit the dimension that science and modern medicine cannot.
- Appeal of the quack is not unlike that of a gambler, the quack offers a *"get well quick"* temptation akin to the gamblers inducement to *"get rich quick."*[6]
- *Lack of suspicion*: Many a times people believe that if something is printed or broadcast, it must be true or otherwise its publication or broadcast would not be allowed and are attracted by promises of quick, painless, or drugless solutions to their problems.[5] The mass media-both print and electronic media provide much false and misleading information in advertisements, news reports, feature articles, and books, and on radio and television programs. News reports are often sensationalized, stimulating false hopes, and by creating fear psychosis by misleading and false propaganda. The most unfortunate aspect is that the producers of print and electronic media escape from responsibility by putting a disclaimer and also claim that they are providing entertainment and have no ethical duty to check the claims. In India, there is a need of more stringent advertisement rules and regulations and strict penalty, which is not there unfortunately.
- *Desperation*: Whenever people faced with a serious health problem or beauty-related issues that doctors cannot solve, become desperate enough to try almost anything that arouses hope. Many victims of cancer, arthritis, multiple sclerosis, and acquired immunodeficiency syndrome (AIDS) are vulnerable in this way. Some squander their life's savings searching for a "cure." Many people suffer from chronic aches, pains, or other discomforts for which medicine cannot offer clear-cut diagnoses or effective treatment. The more persistent the condition, the more susceptible the sufferer may be to promises of a "cure." Fears of social unacceptability or growing old, wrinkles, loss of hair and sensory acuity, and decreased sexual potency can also lead people astray.
- *Alienation*: Some people have deep antagonism toward scientific medicine, but are attracted to methods represented as "natural" or otherwise unconventional. They may also harbor extreme distrust of the medical profession, the food industry, drug companies, and Government agencies.[5]

HEALTH QUACKERY HAZARDS

There are three categories:
1. *Direct health hazard*: These are harmful effects of using unsafe and unscientific medicines.
2. *Indirect health hazards*: These are not directly due to the medicines, as they have

no proven therapeutic value, but they cause severe and sometimes irreparable indirect damage, like stoppage of modern medicines by patients suffering from diabetes, hypertension or cancer patients. "Penelope Dingle" incident in Australia *is a classic example of indirect health hazard.*

"Penelope Dingle Incident in Australia"
Penelope Dingle was an Australian woman, 45 years old, who died of colorectal cancer on 25th August 2005. She was treated by homeopath Francine Scrayen with homeopathy alone and forbade Penelope to take even pain killers for her extremely painful condition. Penelope at last sought medical help, but by then it was far too late.

3. *Economic hazards*: Usage of ineffective and useless medicines or procedures may not cause any direct damage, however, in the process it will have wastage of hard earned money of not just the individual but also overall public expenditure on health-related issues.

DERMATOLOGY AND QUACKERY

Quackery in treatment of skin diseases is not new and quackery has no boundaries. Quackery in dermatology has become that much easier as it is accessible directly and anything and everything can be blindly applied basing on assumptions and imaginations.

Advances in medical science and technology, lasers, acne scar/cosmetic surgeries, chemical peels, hair transplant surgeries led to development of different sub-specialities, especially dermatosurgery, esthetic medicine, and medical cosmetology. There is an enormous increase in awareness about beauty, appearance, and to look young in all sections of society and among all age groups. Unfortunately, there are many gray areas in statutory regulations which are not updated. This has led to mushrooming of many chains of cosmetology centers, esthetic centers, and hair transplant centers.

Quacks and quackery in relation to dermatology can be divided in to six basic categories as follows:

1. *Quacks with no qualification whatsoever*: One who sees, prescribes allopathic medicines, and performs procedures which only a qualified dermatologist can do.
   - Beauty parlors/salons/who are not qualified as per laws to treat any medical skin conditions without knowledge of any skin pathology or physiology which can cause certain skin changes and still they treat it with various peels/lasers, etc. and may end up with short- or long-term complications.
   - In many institution or so called skin clinics, under the name of a doctor, unqualified staff/technicians who performs certain esthetic procedures without direct supervision of a qualified dermatologist is another form of quackery.
2. Practitioners of Indian medicine- Ayurveda, Yoga and Naturopathy Unani, Siddha Homeopathy, commonly called AYUSH, who are not qualified to practice modern medicine (allopathy), but are practicing modern medicine in dermatology.
3. Practitioners of so called integrated medicine, alternative system of medicine, electrohomeopathy, indo allopathy, etc. terms which do not exist in any act.
4. *Those dermatologists themselves, who train*: Practitioners of Indian medicine

(*Ayurveda, Siddha, Tibb,* and *Unani*), Homeopathy, Naturopathy, commonly called AYUSH, who are not qualified to practice modern medicine (allopathy), beauticians and salon workers and provide them certificates of training. This types of practices, in turn, produce more quacks and they use these certificates as their qualifications.

5. *Training of quacks by eminent dermatologists and certain training institutions— those dermatologists themselves, who trains*: Dentists, gynecologists, and other specialists (with PG diploma/degree) provide them certificate of training. These types of practices, in turn, produce more quacks and they use these certificates as their qualifications.

6. *Pharmacist and chemist-based quackery*: A big issue in India today: Why? As they:
   - Dispense by themselves: Schedule H/H1 medicines without a genuine prescription by a qualified allopathic practitioners
   - Redispense by themselves without a fresh prescription, which in long run harms the skin and produces harmful adverse/side effects also.
   - Remember, a prescription is not only advice for patient's recovery, but it also is a legitimate order for the sale of controlled drugs and pharmaceutical product; thereby functions as a regulatory tool for consumption of pharmaceutical products at retail level.

There is acute lack of awareness amongst state governments, the legislature(s), judiciary, and even doctors themselves regarding the threat the nation's health from quackery and about non-entitlement of practitioners of Indian medicine who are practicing modern medicine.

Having *not* succeeded to take advantage of ambiguity in State Medical Acts and Drugs and Cosmetics Act and rules, some practitioners of *Ayurveda, Siddha, Unani* and *Tibb,* commonly called Ayush, have concocted a fake name like integrated medicine and practice modern medicine (allopathy) under its garb. The Government has clarified that they have not recognized integrated system of medicine and currently there is no proposal to develop integrated system of medicine by Government of India. Even Central Council of Indian Medicine (CCIM) in their letter dated 5-12-2008 has announced that the term "Integrated System of Medicine" has not been defined in their Act and it is not one of the approved systems of medicine in India. The practitioners of Integrated System of Medicine are quacks and should be treated like them.

Then there are a variety of fake medical degrees like electrohomeopathy, indo allopathy, etc. who call themselves alternative system of medicine and under this guise practice modern medicine. Alternative system of medicine is not recognized by law. Since they are a danger to the nation, there is a need to take action against such quacks wherever we find them. In fact, practitioners of *Ayurveda, Siddha, Unani,* and *Tibb* keep jumping from their original system of medicine to integrated or alternative system of medicine just to keep practicing modern medicine under different façade. If required, they are not averse to concoct a new system of medicine just to avoid detection.

PRESENT LEGAL STATUS OF DEALING WITH QUACKERY

- *Beauty clinics*: Quack is an unqualified person. He/she cannot practice modern scientific medicine. As per Section 15(2)

of Indian Medical Council (IMC) Act, 1956, and clause 1.1.3 of IMC, (Professional Conduct, Etiquette, and Ethics) Regulations 2002, an unqualified person, i.e., quack, cannot practice modern medicine.
- Doctors with BHMS-homeopathy BAMS-ayurvedic, and BUMS-Unani.

Nowadays, it is very common that many homeopathic doctors with BHMS, ayurvedic doctors with BAMS, and Unani doctors with BUMS, claiming as skin specialists and dermatologists, are treating and prescribing allopathic drugs for skin diseases. Some of them are getting trained by bogus illegal institutions and with fake certificates are claiming themselves as dermatologists, cosmetologists, and estheticians, trichologists, etc.

Now it is well settled in law that prescribing allopathic medicines by homeopaths, ayurvedic, and Unani doctors is unlawful and amounts negligent act.[8-22]

Legal References

Honorable Supreme Court of India, in the case of Poonam Verma versus Ashwin Patel and also in case of Dr Mukhtiar Chand versus State of Punjab, held that:

"The right to practice modern scientific medicine (allopathic medicine) or Indian system of medicine cannot be based on the provisions of drug rules and declarations made there under by State Governments. Indeed the right to practice a system of medicine is derived from the Act under which a medical practitioner is registered."

In pursuance of the above judgments "a person having obtained qualification in particular system of medicine can practice medicine in that system of medicine only. If a person having qualification in alternative medicine or ayurvedic medicine or homeopathy or Unani and found practicing modern medicine, he/she is liable for disciplinary action by the authorities of AYUSH. If a person having qualification in other system of medicine and prescribing drugs of modern medicine, he/she is liable for prosecution as per the provisions contained in Drugs Act/Drugs Rules."

Government of India has issued Government Notification vide Memo No. 8914/L2/97-1 dated, 17-3-1997, implementing the Supreme Court judgment in Poonam Verma versus Dr Ashwin Patel, the judgment of Honorable Supreme Court in Dr Mukhtiar Chand and Others versus State of Punjab and others.

Quack

Quack is an unqualified person. He/she cannot practice modern scientific medicine. As per Section 15(2) of IMC Act, 1956 read with clause 1.1.3 of IMC Regulations, an unqualified person, i.e., quack, cannot practice modern medicine. In case a quack is found practicing modern medicine, police complaint shall be given and the procedure laid down in police manual shall be followed. An aggrieved/affected person may file a criminal complaint before competent magistrate. The procedure laid down in Section 200 of Criminal Procedure Code (CrPC) shall be followed.
- The State Government's authorities have the power to control or abolish or eradicate the quackery/unethical/unregistered/unauthorized modern medicine practice. The concerned state authorities are: (1) The District Collector, being the District Magistrate. (2) The Superintendent of Police/Deputy Superintendents of Police of the concerned district/subdivision. In the case of cities, the Commissioners of Police. (3) The District Medical and

Health Officers of the district concerned as per the provisions contained.
- There are several Central/State Acts, like Indian Medical Degrees Act, 1916, IMC Act, 1956, several notifications of Medical Council of India (MCI), and Notification of State Government in the year 1997.
- State Medical Councils have to take appropriate action against quacks/unqualified persons, whenever complaints have been received. State Medical Council Law has to address letters to the police authorities and District Medical and Health Officers to take action as per law.
- The authorities concerned in the districts to eradicate or control quackery are concerned police authorities or the District Medical and Health Officers.

FIGHTING AGAINST QUACKERY[1]

Professional bodies like concerned associations, e.g., IADVL (Indian Association of Dermatologists, Venereologists and Leprologists) shall actively oppose quackery and fraudulent medical practices. Dermatologists should educate patients and their attendants. They should also disseminate this information by educating the people and through print and electronic media.

Prevention of quackery—to deal with quackery, we have to focus attention on multiple factors responsible for its existence.
- First is to educate the people about the accurate factual information about the health and specific conditions, including the areas where people are more concerned like, beauty, color improvement, hair fall, baldness, lasers, chemical peels, esthetics, etc. Quacks are always agile, they sense quickly and rush to exploit the people's real concerns. We shall also make them aware about the real facts about the false and extravagant claims of quacks. These educational and awareness programs will tackle the aspect of "ignorance" which is one of the major factors for survival of quackery.
- Second factor is the emotional aspect, which makes the patient feel that "something is better than nothing" and gets attracted toward quacks. These types of patients with emotional immaturities and variations, need an extra degree of support, care, and sparing extra time, and thorough and meaning full discussion with patients and attendants will go a long way in preventing them from getting attracted by quackery.
- Dermatology and all subspecialty services should reach all the areas particularly semiurban and rural and tribal areas to meet the needs of people and very crucial to reduce the public receptivity to quackery.[6] There are about 10,000 dermatologists in our country for a population of 1.3 crores. There is a dire need to interact and conduct awareness programs not only to general practitioners but also to sister medical organizations, Indian Medical Association (IMA), associations of other specialties and super specialties, nurses, and paramedical associations.
- *Law enforcement*: Vigilance and proactive approach of medical associations and creation of special task force groups to tackle the menace of quackery and approach statutory authorities for effective law enforcement.

Unauthorized and Unqualified Hair and Cosmetology Centers

In the last two decades, innumerable number of cosmetic clinics/centers have come up in all major metros and cities, just to exploit the people's desires, expectations particularly with regard to "beauty and appearance." If we go through especially the Sunday edition of any newspaper of any language we will find innumerable advertisements of these cosmetology or beauty centers with attractive catchy titles. But if we check carefully, they will not mention about the names and qualifications of experts who are doing the cosmetic/esthetic procedures. They do not engage the services of either dermatologists or plastic surgeons, who are the actual, qualified physicians to perform all these procedures.

Typically they offer discounts and festival offers and sometimes bumper offers of cars, two-wheelers, and TV's total worth of ₹ 1,000,000–1,500,000 for booking and making initial payments.

Most of them take permission from municipal authorities for running a salon, but later gradually start doing cosmetic procedures and sometimes surgeries, without obtaining any permission or license from health authorities.

Court Orders "Cosmetic Clinic" to Pay ₹ 100,000 Compensation plus Refund of ₹ 95,000 and Additional ₹ 20,000 toward Cost of Litigation

Brief facts of the case: In 2015, one consumer resident of Pernem in the state of Goa, known diabetic, approached a cosmetic clinic for transplantation of 6,000 strands of hair for ₹ 140,000. He developed, after first session of transplant of 500 hair, headache, giddiness, and diarrhea and having paid the full amount, he underwent a second session but subsequently developed boils in the head and unsteadiness of his legs.

He approached the consumer forum and forum held that there was complete negligence and gross deficiency of service. The entire conduct of the clinic in the matter so far has been *totally unethical, unprofessional, highly casual and unconcerned*, and regardless toward complaint and his health the quorum stated, in its order.

The forum directed the cosmetic clinic in Calangute to pay a compensation of ₹ 100,000 for harming a consumer with "illegal activities of hair transplant."

The quorum also observed that the opposite parties *did not have a license to operate the said cosmetic clinic. The directorate of health services informed that the clinic has not taken any license to operate under the Goa Medical Practitioner's Act, 2004 and Rules 2011, as a health clinic.*

"Based on the above three letters from the Food and Drug Administration (FDA), directorate of health services from Panaji, Campla, and from the letter of the primary health center, Candolim, it is clear that the *Opposite Party No. 2 Mrs Leema George, who is the incharge of Opposite Party No. 1, that is the Looks Cosmetic Clinic, is doing illegal business and cheating people and making wrongful gains for herself at the cost of the clients who come to her Looks Cosmetic Clinic also known as Looks Health Services,*" the order stated.[23]

Unauthorized and Illegal Diplomas/Degrees

We find many MBBS, BDS, and other doctors claiming as dermatologists, cosmetologist, esthetician, etc. by dubious certifications by attending a course of few days to few months and being awarded by these diplomas and degrees.

Examples:
- **PGDCC**: Postgraduate Diploma in Clinical Cosmetology given by ILAMED
- **PGMT**: Postgraduate Diploma in Medical Trichology given by ILAMED

- *PGDCC*: Postgraduate Diploma in Clinical Cosmetology given—Germany
- Diploma in Practical Dermatology
- MSc Clinical Dermatology
- MSc Dermatology Skills and Treatment, University of Hertfordshire
- Masters in Clinical Dermatology
- Diploma in Clinical Dermatology (UK).

Fellowships: Advanced Fellowship in Cosmetic Dermatology, Mahatma Gandhi University, Jaipur

Unfortunately, sometimes reputed medical journals also print advertisements endorsing unrecognized postgraduate diplomas, fellowship, and certificate courses of dermatology, cosmetology, and esthetics conducted by private institutions and hospitals for MBBS/BDS and other ineligible doctors.

Various judgments of Indian Courts make it amply clear that any postgraduate medical course conducted under any title (diploma, postgraduate diploma, certificate, fellowship, etc.) become illegal unless it is recognized by MCI and/or the central government.

According to the MCI ethics code regulation 7.20, a physician should not claim to be a specialist unless he/she has a special qualification in that branch. Practicing a specialty, without having a qualification in that branch, amounts to flouting regulation 7.20 of the ethics code.

In 2008, the Madras High Court quashed *a State Government Order (GO) which had allowed a certificate course in diabetology without the prior permission of MCI.*

The judges reasoned that the executive power of every state should be exercised ensuring compliance with the laws made by parliament and any existing law applied in the state. *Therefore, the GO was ruled unconstitutional and preventable in view of Entry 66 of List I of the constitution. The judges clearly stated that no course in medical education by any name could be started without the permission of MCI and the Central Government.*

Factories Awarding Unauthorized and Illegal Diplomas in India

There are many unauthorized and illegal certificates of diploma, degree or fellowship awarded by private and non-MCI recognized institutions like, ILAMED, LEMED, Cosmetica India Academy, and Facial Aesthetics in Rajasthan.

Legal Status

In 2011, the Madras High Court declared 11 postgraduate diploma courses conducted by Tamil Nadu, Dr MGR University as illegal since they were being conducted without the prior approval of MCI or the central government. Justice N Paul Vasantkumar said *"The University is not empowered to grant permission to any institution or medical college to conduct any PG diploma course in medical science without prior approval of the MCI Act, 1956."* The judge also pointed out that according to the MCI ethics code regulations, 2002, a physician is supposed to suffix only recognized qualifications. *The Honorable Judge said that "Without such recognition, if any person is allowed to suffix PG diploma in medical sciences along with MBBS degree, the general public will definitely get an impression that the physician is a specialist. Special status can be claimed by any physician only after getting an approved PG diploma and not half-baked diploma courses offered by the university."*

So, the legal status of these unauthorized institutions, ILAMED, LEMED, etc. is crystal clear and well settled in law that they are not only completely unauthorized but also illegal.

Quackery—In Hair Transplantation

Throughout India there are multiple hair transplantation centers established and some have chain of centers and in majority of them hair transplantation is not done by dermatologists or plastic surgeons, who are the actual eligible experts, but unfortunately by MBBS, BDS, nonallopathic doctors, and sometimes by so called technicians. They take permission from municipal authorities for hair saloon services, but gradually start doing hair transplantation surgeries also, for which permission from health authorities is mandatory.

Death of a Final-year Medico in Chennai in June 2016 after Hair Transplantation

A final year medical student in Chennai, 22-year-old Santosh was shy of his slight baldness and decided to go for a hair transplant procedure last month. But 2 days after the surgery, he was dead. The MBBS doctor, the doctor at Advanced Robotic Hair Transplantation Center who performed the procedure, was not a surgeon equipped with either a dermatology or plastic surgery degree—a basic qualification in the field. Moreover, the Dr Hariprasad Kasturi, the anesthetist was not present throughout the procedure after administering anesthesia—another basic requirement ignored. Later, when the parents lodged complaint and on verification by authorities, it was found that, the hair transplant center Advanced Robotic Hair Transplantation Center had *obtained a license only to run a hair salon which too expired 2 months* before. Although they had qualified doctors one of them was trained in China, there was no infrastructure to tackle any complication. The center has no sterile place or an operation theater. The authorities have sealed the center. The drug controller has recovered a huge stock of medicines kept without license.

The health department is recommended using a tough law to regulate such centers dealing with surgical procedures including hair and wart removal, often masquerading as beauty parlors, spas, and hair treatment centers.

Later Tamil Nadu Medical Council has acted firmly and an anesthetist has been barred from practice for 6 months. An MBBS doctor, an MBBS graduate from a Chinese university, has been barred for a year.

Google, Facebook, and YouTube Medical Quackery

The new dimension of medical quackery is the spread of inaccurate, unscientific, and deliberately false content at high speed and making even educated people to believe them, unsuspectingly (Goebbels' propaganda). If one goes into YouTube and searches for treatment of melasma, one gets the wide range of suggestions from lemon face pack, turmeric, tomato, papaya face packs to lasers, and promoted and recommended by self-styled experts from nonmedical individuals to all varieties of nonallopathic doctors. The most shocking is, for dog bite it is well-established scientifically that active and passive immunization as well as wound treatment are gold standards throughout the world, but treatment recommendations in YouTube consist of a range of treatments from banana, garlic, homeopathy, and ayurvedic to lasers also.

The consequences of such treatments will be disastrous to the individuals and society.

In South Africa, the country's President in the late 1990s and 2000, came to believe that AIDS is nonexistent and a hoax and Government policies were framed accordingly, which has led to an estimated, more than 330,000 deaths as per the researchers.[24]

Amazon Medical Quackery

Quacks are always agile and take advantage of patient's eagerness.[25] Amazon websites are hawking a universe of dangerous, pseudoscience health products—to cure human immunodeficiency virus (HIV) infection to bleach enemas for autism.

That is according to an investigation by *UK's Sun newspaper*, which accuses the main internet giant of profiting off people's desperation and illness by selling unproven, snake oil products.

If one looks for treatment of acne and melasma on Amazon, you will find a range of products including unscientific and unproven products from attractive cosmetic products to "do yourself" physical modalities and instruments.

The main reason why Amazon sells such products is that though these products are recommended and promoted for medical purpose, but technically fall in the category of "dietary supplements" or "cosmetics" which are very loosely regulated by FDA or our Indian regulatory authorities.[26]

SUMMARY WITH KEY MESSAGES AND PEARLS

- Medical quackery is a malpractice in the medical profession where pseudo doctors claim to be experts and competent in treating diseases.
- Quacks always try to make profit at the expense of deceiving people; they capitalize on the hope, ignorance, and fear of people.
- Health quackery hazards are direct health hazards, indirect health hazards, and economic hazards.
- Quackery in dermatology became much easier as skin is accessible directly and anything and everything can be blindly applied basing on assumptions and imaginations.
- In a Land mark judgments, Honorable Supreme Court of India, in the case of Poonam Verma versus Ashwin Patel and also in case of Dr Mukhtiar Chand versus State of Punjab, has given judgment that "A person having obtained qualification in particular system of medicine can practice medicine in that system of medicine only. If a person having qualification in alternative medicine or ayurvedic medicine or homeopathy or Unani and found practicing modern medicine, he/she is liable for disciplinary action.
- Government of India has issued Government Notification vide Memo No. 8914/L2/97-1 dated, 17-3-1997, implementing the Supreme Court judgment in Poonam Verma versus Dr Ashwin Patel.
- As per Section 15(2) of IMC Act, 1956 read with clause 1.1.3 of IMC Regulations, an unqualified person, i.e., quack cannot practice modern medicine.
- The State Government's authorities have the power to control or abolish or eradicate the quackery/unethical/unregistered/unauthorized modern medicine practice. The concerned state authorities are: (1) The District Collector, being the District Magistrate. (2) The Superintendent of Police/Deputy Superintendents of Police of the concerned district/subdivision. In the case of cities, the Commissioners of Police. (3) The District Medical and Health Officers of the district concerned as per the provisions contained.
- Types of quacks and quackery:
  - Quacks with no qualification whatsoever
  - Practitioners of India medicine Ayurveda, Yoga, Naturopathy, Unani, Siddha and Homeopathy, commonly called AYUSH, who are not qualified to practice modern medicine (allopathy), but are practicing modern medicine in dermatology.
  - Certain dermatologists themselves are training practitioners of Indian medicine with qualifications of BHMS, BAMS, BUMS, BYNS which is not only un-ethical but illegal.
  - Training of quacks by certain unauthorized, unrecognized and illegal training institutions training Dentists, gynecologists, and other specialists in dermatosurgical procedures.

- **Prevention of quackery**
  - Educate the people about the accurate factual information about the health and specific conditions
  - Patients with emotional immaturities and variations need extra degree of support, care, sparing extra time, and thorough and meaningful discussion with patients and attendants
  - Dermatology and all subspecialty services should reach all the areas particularly semiurban and rural and tribal areas to meet the needs of people and very crucial to reduce the public receptivity to quackery
  - Law enforcement—vigilance and proactive approach of medical associations and creation of special task force groups to tackle the menace of quackery and approach statutory authorities for effective law enforcement.
- **Legal status of unauthorized and unqualified hair and cosmetology centers**: The Consumer forum of Goa state has given judgment that Hair and Cosmetology centers are doing illegal business and cheating people and making wrongful gains for herself at the cost of the clients.
- **Legal status of unauthorized and illegal diplomas/degrees**: Various Judgments of Indian Courts, make it amply clear that any postgraduate medical course conducted under any title (diploma, postgraduate diploma, certificate, fellowship, etc.) become illegal unless it is recognized by MCI and/or the Central Government.
- **Legal status of centers awarding unauthorized and illegal diplomas in India**: There are many unauthorized and illegal certificates of diploma, degree or fellowship are awarded by private and non-MCI recognized institutions like, ILAMED, LEMED, Cosmetic India Academy, Facial Aesthetics in Rajasthan. In 2011, the Madras High Court declared 11 postgraduate diploma courses conducted by Tamil Nadu Dr. MGR University as illegal since they were being conducted without the prior approval of MCI or the central government. Justice N Paul Vasantkumar said "The University is not empowered to grant permission to any institution or medical college to conduct any PG diploma course in medical science without prior approval of the Medical Council of India Act, 1956."
- **Legal status—hair transplantation**: Death of a final year medico in Chennai in June 2016 after hair transplantation and the doctor at ARHT Transplant center who performed the procedure, was not a surgeon equipped with either a dermatology or plastic surgery degree—a basic qualification in the field and later Tamil Nadu Medical Council has acted firmly and, Dr Hariprasad Kasturi, an anesthetist, has been barred from practice for six months. An MBBS graduate from a Chinese university, has been barred for a year.

REFERENCES

1. American College of Physicians. Health quackery. Philadelphia, PA: American College of Physicians; 1989.
2. Quackery, Workman Publishing. Credit: available from https://www.sciencefriday.com/segments/medical-cures-that-did-more-harm-than-good/ [Last accessed December, 2018].
3. NCAHF. (2001). Some notes on Quackery. [online] Available from https://www.ncahf.org/articles/o-r/quackery.html [Last accessed December, 2018].
4. Stanford Libraries. Webster's II New Riverside University Dictionary. Boston, MA: Riverside Pub. Co.; 1984.
5. Quackwatch (2005). Vulnerability to Quackery. [online] Available from https://www.quackwatch.org/01QuackeryRelatedTopics/quackvul.html [Last accessed December, 2018].
6. Bernard NW. Why people become the victims of medical quackery. Am J Public Health Nations Health. 1965;55(8):1142-7.
7. Datta R. The World of Quacks: A parallel Health Care system in Rural West Bengal. IOSR J Human Soc Sci. 2013;14(2):44-53.
8. Poonam verma vs. Ashwin Patel & Ors. 1996 AIR 2111, 1996 SCC (4) 332.
9. Dr Mukhtiar Chand & Ors vs. The State of Punjab & Ors. 1998.
10. Martin F D' Souza vs. Mohd. Ishfaq; 2009
11. Shiva Kumar Gautham (Dr) vs Alima; 2006
12. Kanaiyalal Ramanlal Trivedi vs Dr Satyanarayan Vishwakarma; 1997.
13. Jalaluddin Khan (Dr) vs. India Sen Verma 2009 (4) CPJ 89: 2009 (3) CPR 208 NCDRC.
14. SN Namboodri (Dr) vs Haneeefa, 1998 CPJ 389 (Ker.SCDRC).
15. Khairaiti Lal vs Kewal Krishna,1998 (1) CPJ 181: 1998 (1) CLT 637: 1998 (1) CPC 153 (Punj. SCDRC).

16. Manpreet Kaur vs Veena Ghumber (Dr) 2005 (2) CPJ 63: 2005 (1) CPR 656 (Punj SCDRC).
17. Sher Singh (Dr) vs Billu Khan, 2007 (4) CPJ 295: 2008 (1) CPR 45 (NCDRC).
18. Arun Dewangan (Dr) vs Madhu (Preti Chandei) 2009 (2) CPJ 315: 2009 (2) CPR 389 (NCDRC).
19. RR Singh AVV (Bom) vs Pratibha P Gamre, 2012 (2) CPJ 534 (NCDRC).
20. Alok Kumar (Dr) vs Devlal, 2013 (4) CPJ 31 (NCDRC).
21. PN Thakur (Prof) vs Hans Charitable Hospital, 2007 (3) CPJ 340: 2007 (3) CPR 157 (NCDRC).
22. Azizul Haq Khan (Dr @ Lallan) vs Shyamapati 2009 (2) CPR 61: 2009 (2) CPJ 49 (NCDRC).
23. The Times of India 5th August 2017.
24. UNDARK (2018). Social media algorithms help charlatans spread autism cures, vaccine disinformation, and AIDS denialism through online videos. Who's really to blame? [online] Available from https://undark.org/article/aids-denialism-quackery-facebook-youtube/ [Last accessed December 2018].
25. Yuong JH. American Health Quackery: Collected Essays of James Harvey Young. Princeton, United States: Princeton University Press; 1972.
26. Julia Belluz@juliaoftorontojulia.belluz@voxmedia.com

7.5 Medicolegal Cases in Dermatology

Venkataram Mysore, Saloni Katoch

INTRODUCTION

The legal scenario in dermatology is constantly evolving and keeping abreast with legal issues pertaining to one's field of medicine is now becoming the need of the hour. Dermatologists face lower malpractice rates as compared to other specialists but with an increasing number of dermatosurgical and esthetic procedures, the potential for problems and their legal consequences continues to increase. Hence, it is very essential that dermatologists educate themselves about the legal aspects of practicing medicine and the basic concepts of malpractice litigation.

CIVIL LAW AND NEGLIGENCE

The Supreme Court of India states that every doctor has a duty to act with a reasonable degree of care and skill. A doctor cannot guarantee cure and cannot be accused of negligence if the patient is not completely cured despite working in a manner best suited to the patient and adopting the right course of treatment.

According to Supreme Court ruling, doctors can be sued in Consumer Courts, for any service charged by them. As the medical profession has been brought under the Consumer Protection Act, 1986, patients can file a complaint in:
- The District Forum, if the value of services and compensation claimed is less than ₹ 20 lakh.
- The State Commission, if the value of the goods or services and the compensation claimed is not more than ₹ 1 crore.
- The National Commission, if the value of the goods or services and the compensation is more than ₹ 1 crore.

ELEMENTS FOR CAUSE OF ACTION IN NEGLIGENCE

A dermatologist may be sued for malpractice based on negligence if an act of omission or commission in breach of one's duty causing harm to the patient has to be committed. The burden of proof generally lies with the patient who files a complaint. There are four basic elements that need to be established for this:

1. Duty owed to the patient
2. Breach of the duty owed
3. Causation
4. Damages

Duty Owed to the Patient

It is the duty of a dermatologist to provide a standard of care as other dermatologists in good standing so as to protect the patient from unreasonable risk or harm. Standard of care is a way in which majority of the physicians in a similar medical community would practice. A dermatologist and a plastic surgeon performing a cutaneous laser surgery will be held responsible for an equal standard of care toward the patient, failure of which would result in a breach of duty. The standard of care can also be seen as a pragmatic concept varying from case-to-case based on the testimony of an expert physician; hence, a dermatologist must have the knowledge and skill ordinarily possessed by a specialist in the field and should use care and skill ordinarily possessed by a specialist in the field in a similar locality under similar circumstances. When there are two or more recognized methods of diagnosing or treating a condition, a physician does not fall below the standard of care even if using one method results in less effective outcomes than the others.

Breach of Duty Owed

Failure to provide a standard of care expected from a competent dermatologist in good standing will amount to breach of duty owed to the patient. In simple words, when a doctor does not perform an action that he or she has a duty to do, results in breach of duty. An example of this would be failure to obtain a proper informed consent by not informing the patient of risks involved in a treatment.

The doctrine of informed consent implies that a physician should obtain consent before treating or operating on the patient. It states that it is the duty of the doctor to discuss the risks, benefits, and alternative modalities of treatment with the patient. The aforementioned discussion should be documented preferably in the presence of a witness. The informed consent forms an essential part of the doctor–patient relationship and forms a basis of protection for both.

Causation

Causation refers to the breach of duty causing injuries or damage to the patient. For example, prescribing a sulfa drug to a patient with history of sulfa drug allergy due to failure of the doctor to check the same with subsequent development of Stevens–Johnson syndrome.

Damages

Damage to the patient may be economic in nature or noneconomic (emotional). The patient must show damages caused by breach of the physician's duty, if there are no damages caused then it is unlikely that the patient will have a viable case of negligence against the doctor. An example of this would be the following case:

A patient underwent cryotherapy for warts over the face with development of hypopigmented spots as a postprocedure sequelae. The patient was counseled regarding the same and explained that the spots will repigment. Unsatisfied, the patient sued the treating doctor in the Consumer Court, the first hearing of which was scheduled a few months later. At the time of hearing, the hypopigmented spots had repigmented completely. The case against the doctor was dismissed as there was no breach of duty and there were no damages to the patient.

Another important point to note from the above example is that occurrence of a complication is not the same as medical malpractice. A cordial doctor–patient relationship with efficient communication and counseling regarding management of a postprocedure complication will lessen the likelihood of a lawsuit. The best defense against a complication-based malpractice case is to adhere to the standard of care which requires that an informed consent explaining the reasonable risks of the procedure must be obtained from the patient.

All four elements of duty owed, breach of duty, causation and damages need to be established to sustain a prima facie case of negligence. The occurrence of complications may lead to a cause of action based on negligence but the plaintiff will not succeed if there has been no breach of duty on the doctor's behalf. The complainant by presenting best available evidence in medical science and an expert opinion must prove his allegations against the doctor. In some situations, the principle of "res ipsa loquitur" or "the thing speaks for itself" can be invoked where the occurrence of the accident itself is proof of negligence.

CRIMINAL LAW AND NEGLIGENCE

The liability in civil law is based on the amount of damage that the patient has suffered, criminal law on the other hand takes into account the degree of negligence and the amount of damage. A doctor cannot be held criminally responsible unless he/she acts in complete disregard for the patient's life and safety in an incompetent and negligent way amounting to a crime against the state. Section 304A of the Indian Penal Code of 1860 states, that whoever causes the death of a person by a rash or negligent act not amounting to culpable homicide shall be punished with imprisonment for a term of two years, or with a fine, or with both. The Supreme Court has stated that any conduct falling short of recklessness and deliberate wrong doing should not be the subject of criminal liability.

MEDICOLEGAL CASES IN DERMATOLOGY

1. **Public interest vs. Patient confidentiality: Disclosure of communicable venereal disease to partner**

   A patient accused a hospital in southern India of disclosing information about his HIV-positive status which was detected incidentally when he tried to donate blood. He claimed that he was socially cast out, had to leave his hometown, and his wedding was cancelled. He claimed compensation for the same and charged the hospital with breach of medical ethics. The Indian Supreme Court ruled in favor of the hospital and stated that any individual with a communicable venereal disease has a legal and moral duty to inform his or her potential spouse and in failing to do so and knowingly transmitting HIV infection is punishable with fines and imprisonment. The court stated that when there is a health risk to others, public interest overrides patient confidentiality and hence disclosing a patient's HIV status to his or her fiancé does not violate medical ethics.

2. **Deficiency in service: Excess dosage of steroids and lack of supportive care**

A patient developed skin rashes after consuming Chinese food, she was diagnosed to have vasculitis by a physician and was prescribed intramuscular (IM) injections of a long-acting depot preparation of steroid (Depo-Medrol) twice daily along with another oral steroid. As the patient did not improve on outpatient treatment, she was admitted to a tertiary care center, a referral was given to a dermatologist who diagnosed the case as that of toxic epidermal necrolysis (TEN). He stopped the Depo-Medrol injections which had been administered for 6 days and prescribed prednisolone 120 mg/daily in divided doses and topical ointments, the patient continued to deteriorate and was shifted to another hospital in a different state by an air ambulance where she died of septic shock and multiorgan failure 10 days later. The husband of the deceased accused the treating doctors of negligence by prescribing dosages of steroids in excess of recommended, lack of supportive care advised for a patient of TEN, and abysmal nursing care. Aggrieved by the dismissal of his complaint by the national commission, the complainant filed a civil appeal in the Supreme Court. A complaint for criminal negligence was also filed which was dismissed by the apex court.

The Supreme Court observed that the dose of corticosteroids, Depo-Medrol in particular at 120 mg/day was excessive. Depo-Medrol is a long-acting steroid with prolonged immunosuppressive action and the maximum recommended dose is 40–120 mg at 104-week intervals as mentioned by the drug manufacturer. A dermatology expert also stated that depot preparations were meant for chronic conditions and not for acute diseases like TEN and should not be administered twice daily. No supportive, symptomatic and emergency care was given to the patient. The treating dermatologist accepted that the same was necessary for a patient of TEN. The opinions of experts both in favor and against the use of steroids in TEN was placed on record. The pro-steroid group supported the use of steroid in TEN at a preliminary stage but with caution.

The court stated that the physician instead of referring the patient of a skin rash to a dermatologist prescribed excessive dosage of a long-acting steroid without confirming the diagnosis and without foreseeing its implications like immunosuppression. In doing the aforementioned the doctor was negligent in his actions. The court also stated that no doctor has the right to use a drug beyond the maximum recommended dose. The dermatologist after taking over the treatment also added excessive dose of oral steroids and did not ensure aggressive supportive care and monitoring of vitals and was held negligent in his duty toward the patient. The court found the doctors and the tertiary care institute guilty of dereliction of duty and awarded the complainant a record compensation.

3. **Informed Consent: A must before doing procedures**

A homeopathic doctor suffering from alopecia universalis underwent bio-fiber implantation over her scalp and developed a pustular reaction 2 years later for which she was treated and the hair implants were removed. She stated that the treating dermatologist had assured her that the procedure will be successful and that any side effects or deficiencies were not discussed with her.

The state commission dismissed the appeal as the patient had signed a consent form before the procedure which stated that she had clearly understood the pros and cons of hair implantation and had been given instructions and restrictions to follow after the procedure. The commission also stated that complications may arise during or after the procedure which the patient had understood and that the doctor cannot be held negligent in her services because the hair implantation was not successful for the complainant.

4. **Nurses and technicians operating lasers**

   A patient undergoing laser hair reduction with long-pulsed neodymium-doped yttrium aluminum garnet (Nd:YAG) laser accused the treating dermatologist and the hospital of being negligent by escalating the fluence of the laser and by allowing a nurse to do the procedure which led to development of pigmentary changes over her neck after undergoing the laser session.

   The state commission stated that the doctor did not breach his duty by increasing the fluence of the laser as this was done keeping in view the requirement for laser hair reduction in a systematic manner and was within the set limits. The complainant did not produce any expert evidence to prove that the pigmentary alterations were permanent in nature and had already improved at the time of her presentation. The complainant herself was found to be negligent in following the postprocedure medication and protocol which could have caused the pigmentary changes.

   The state commission dismissed the appeal as the fluence of the laser was determined by the treating dermatologist and only the laser machine was operated by the technician who was a staff nurse and had undergone certified training to operate the laser machine.

5. **Doctor cannot be held negligent only because something has gone wrong**

   A 17-year-old patient suffering from bipolar disorder on sodium valproate 500 mg was given lamotrigine 100 mg/daily as an additional medicine to her by her treating psychiatrist. The complainant stated that the patient after starting this new drug developed itching, skin rashes, and fever for which the psychiatrist prescribed paracetamol. The patient further developed difficulty in breathing for which she was referred to a physician. The physician stopped lamotrigine and sodium valproate and started methylprednisolone 4 mg/daily despite which her condition deteriorated and admission in a nursing home was advised under a dermatologist. The dermatologist diagnosed the condition as Stevens-Johnson syndrome (SJS), the patient being critical, died a few days later due to septicemia and noncardiogenic pulmonary edema.

   The patient's father accused the treating psychiatrist of negligence by prescribing lamotrigine along with sodium valproate due to which the patient developed SJS. The complainant accused the physician of negligence by prescribing a steroid which led to further deterioration of her condition and the dermatologist and the nursing home were accused of not providing adequate care needed for an SJS patient which led to the patient's demise. The district forum ruled in favor of the complainant, holding the doctors and nursing home responsible of professional carelessness and negligence. An appeal against this was made in the state commission and the observations made were as follows:

Neutral experts from the field of psychiatry, dermatology, and medicine were examined. The psychiatry expert agreed that the treatment given to the patient for bipolar disorder was approved and within therapeutic limits. The expert also stated that a severe drug reaction is idiosyncratic in nature. The dermatology and medicine experts stated that withdrawal of suspected drug and systematic application of steroid may prevent SJS from progressing to TEN. No proof of negligence was found against the dermatologist and the nursing home as the patient was admitted in an intensive care unit with monitoring and supportive therapy. The commission dismissed the case and stated that a doctor cannot be held negligent only because something has gone wrong.

6. **Misleading and misguiding advertisements: Nonspecialists claiming to be trichologists**

A 17-year-old Sikh boy visited a reputed homeopathic clinic claiming to have specialists in trichology for hair fall after seeing their advertisement in a widely circulated national newspaper. The advertisement of the clinic stated that the specialists could detect hair fall even before the patient could realize it by using cutting edge video microscope technology. After visiting the clinic, the patient and his father claimed that they were assured that his hair loss will be cured. The patient was started on homeopathic medication and laser comb sessions for the same. After no improvement despite treatment for three years and losing his scalp and eyebrow hair, the patient accused the clinic and treating doctors of deficiency in service.

The homeopathic expert in the above case stated that the homeopathic treatment given to the patient was correct but laser comb sessions are not a part of homeopathic science and medicine. The district forum also stated that the treating doctors were not specialists in the science of hair loss as claimed in the advertisements and hence were guilty of medical malpractice. The forum held that big advertisements in newspapers and magazines were misguiding and the doctors seemed to be more like salesmen. This was found to be against the professional conduct of homeopathic doctors and a compensation was awarded to the complainants on basis of deficiency in rendering service and unfair trade practice. An appeal against the above order was made in the state commission, which upheld the decision of the district forum.

7. **Delay in diagnosis: Failure to refer a patient in time**

An 8-year-old child with fever, cough and cold was treated by a general physician and was given an oral sulfa antibiotic, paracetamol and antihistamine. The fever did not subside with the medication and the patient developed blisters in the mouth with swelling of lips and a skin rash over the body. The general physician made a diagnosis of measles and referred the patient to a pediatrician who after examining the child confirmed the diagnosis of measles. As the child continued to deteriorate with blisters developing over the body, admission was advised in a hospital. Treatment for measles was continued for over 36 hours following which an ENT referral was made. The ENT surgeon diagnosed the case as that of SJS and started treatment accordingly, a dermatologist was also given referral who confirmed the diagnosis of SJS and advised management accordingly. An ophthalmologist was also given a referral for eye complaints. The child recovered but with permanent damage to tear gland of the eyes and impairment of vision.

The patient's father complained that because of negligence on part of the treating doctors, the child will have to lead a disabled life with permanent vision impairment. He claimed that the ailment had been wrongly diagnosed as measles and the delay in diagnosis and management of SJS had led to permanent disablement in the child. The state commission held the pediatrician negligent in his conduct and dismissed complaints against the treating physician, ophthalmologist, and the hospital. Aggrieved, the complainant appealed in the national commission against the above order. The ENT surgeon and dermatologist were not accused of negligence as they had made the diagnosis of SJS in time and started appropriate therapy. The national commission ruled in favor of the complainant and held the doctors and the hospital negligent with regard to diagnosis and treatment of the child and directed them to pay a compensation for the same.

8. **Test dose mandatory before giving local anesthesia**

A 26-year-old lady, beedi roller by profession, reported for removal of a wart from her left thumb to a dermatologist. Since she had undergone a surgery under spinal anesthesia 6 months back, the treating doctor did not administer a test dose before injecting local anesthesia. The patient complained of severe pain while the local anesthetic was being injected, the doctor stopped the procedure immediately and prescribed some anti-inflammatory and analgesic drugs. The patient reported 2 days later with a black discolored patch at the site of injection and pain and swelling of the left thumb for which medicines were prescribed again. The patient's condition deteriorated further as she developed fever and swelling of the left hand with inability to move it. She was given a surgery referral and advised admission. As there was no improvement, she was referred to a tertiary care hospital where a diagnosis of cellulitis was made. A surgery under general anesthesia was done with skin grafting. The patient lost mobility of her left thumb and was hence unable to earn her daily wages. She held the dermatologist responsible for the suffering that she had undergone and filed a complaint with the consumer forum.

The doctor responded by stating that the patient developed Nicolau syndrome, an arterial vasospasm that cannot be predicted even with a test dose of the anesthetic. Testimonials by a surgeon and another dermatologist supported the above and they added that wart removal was a minor surgery.

The state forum observed that Nicolau syndrome was not mentioned in the case sheets submitted by the doctor or the tertiary care center. There was no mention of a test dose before injecting the anesthetic either. No medical literature was produced regarding xylocaine injection causing Nicolau syndrome or that by administering a test dose the complication could have been avoided.

The commission ruled in favor of the complainant by stating that the dermatologist was negligent in not administering the test dose and that a surgery under spinal anesthesia a few months back is no reason to avoid the same. The failure of the doctor to depose for a long time was also considered relevant. The patient was awarded compensation for undergoing severe pain, a surgery under general anesthesia, and developing disability.

9. **Burden of proof lies with the patient**
A male patient was diagnosed to have balanoposthitis and genital warts after history of an extramarital exposure and treated accordingly with oral medications and weekly podowart application by a dermatologist. Despite continuing treatment for a few months, the patient complained that he did not have any improvement and visited another doctor who did a biopsy and made a diagnosis of squamous cell carcinoma. The patient had to undergo penile amputation as the carcinoma was invasive. The patient accused the skin specialist of negligence by failing to do other medical tests like a biopsy and not being able to diagnose his cancer in time.

The dermatologist stated that a biopsy had indeed been written in the patient's prescription after 2 months of treatment but the patient had not submitted these despite having submitted all the other prescriptions. The doctor pleaded that the patient had also visited other homeopathic doctors and that his diagnosis and treatment were according to standard medical practice and hence there was no negligence on his behalf.

A committee of experts stated that the treating doctor should have referred the patient to another expert if there was no improvement despite treatment and the next logical step would have been to do a biopsy. The district forum observed that the patient had filed prescriptions of all months except the ones in which the doctor claimed to have had advised for a biopsy. Medical literature submitted by the respondent showed that cancer could also arise from a long standing condyloma acuminata of the anogenital region and hence the diagnosis and treatment given by the doctor were in accordance with current medical standards. The forum concluded that there is appropriate material to show that a biopsy was suggested by the dermatologist but the patient deliberately did not bring those prescriptions on record. The case was dismissed by the forum on the account that a doctor cannot be held negligent just because a line of treatment does not work effectively.

10. **Consumer court can check exaggerated value of claimed compensation**
A 29-year-old female patient visited a dermatologist with complaints of pigmented patches over her face. A diagnosis of melasma was made and laser was advised by the doctor. The patient claimed that the laser was done by the doctor's assistant despite her insistence that the doctor does the procedure. The patient stated that after the laser she developed burnt marks over her face and a cream was given to her for one weeks' time for the same. The patient found no improvement in the postlaser pigmentation and hence more creams were advised which according to her made the spots turn even more dark. She was then advised a chemical peel, done again by the assistant of the doctor following which she alleged that her chin was left burnt. The complainant accused the doctor of negligence and held her responsible for marks on her face and

mental agony due to loss of potential matrimonial matches.

The state commission found the claimed compensation of ₹ 5,00,000/-, highly exaggerated in comparison to the expenditure of ₹ 10,000/- made by the complainant toward her treatment. She also did not provide a breakup of the amount claimed like past expenses, future expenses, physical strain, and mental agony. The commission was unable to accept the arguments and hence dismissed the complaint. The patient was given the liberty to file a fresh complaint in the district forum after making the claimed amount reasonable.

11. **Medical professionals are entitled to get protection so long as they perform their duties with reasonable skill and competence and in interest of the patient**

A patient consulted a dermatologist for treatment of unwanted hair over the upper lip and chin. She was counseled regarding laser hair reduction with long-pulsed Nd:YAG laser and the number of sessions that would be needed. The energy of the laser was gradually increased as the patient underwent the laser sessions. In the 11th session the fluence of the laser was escalated further to target thin hair, after which the patient developed a few blisters over the treated areas. Medication was prescribed for the same by the treating dermatologist but the blisters gave rise to keloids. The patient was advised intralesional steroid injections for the keloids but found no improvement after one and a half years of treatment. The patient accused the dermatologist of negligence for failing to analyze her skin type properly and administering high laser energy for a longer duration causing her physical and mental trauma. The patient appealed in the district forum and was granted a compensation for the same. The dermatologist appealed against the above order in the state commission. The state commission observed that the patient signed a consent form explaining the procedure of laser hair reduction, number of sessions required, and risks associated with it. It also stated that the patient failed to get an expert on record to prove that the laser energy and duration used were excessive and beyond the set guidelines recommended by the manufacturer and that the doctor was negligent in treating the side effects that developed. Medical literature on laser hair reduction also mentioned that a test patch is not feasible in all cases and hence is not to be recommended as a mandatory requirement.

The state commission dismissed the case by stating that the dermatologist prescribed a fluence that was within the set limits and the patient developed side effects of the laser treatment despite standard accepted medical guidelines being followed. The commission also stated that a medical professional may not be held negligent if he or she after assessing the gravity of illness takes a higher element of risk to redeem the patient out of his or her suffering but does not achieve the desired result. It also emphasized that it is the bound duty and obligation of the civil society to ensure that medical professionals are not unnecessarily harassed or humiliated so they can perform their duties without fear and apprehension.

CONCLUSION

Medical negligence claims usually arise when a dermatologist fails in his or her duty to provide a "standard of care" to the patient. The patient may also appeal against negligent supervision and training of technicians and staff, deceptive advertising, and inadequate informed consent. If all four elements of negligence are proven then the complainant will be awarded compensation for physical injuries, economic losses, and noneconomic afflictions like pain and suffering.

A cordial doctor–patient relationship, tactful and empathetic handling of the patient, counseling regarding treatment modalities along with their risks and benefits, shared and informed decision making, documentation and maintenance of records, proficiency in skills, keeping oneself updated with the latest developments in the field of dermatology, and adhering to the established standards of care and treatment are the best safeguards against litigation.

A medical malpractice claim can cause a lot of professional and personal stress to a doctor. This medical malpractice stress syndrome can be effectively managed by proper counseling, education, knowledge about medical law and previous litigated cases, addressing one's fears, support from colleagues and family, paying attention to one's health, and adequate prevention by always keeping the patient's best interest in mind.

BIBLIOGRAPHY

1. Goldberg DJ. Cosmetic dermatology: legal issues. Dermatol Clin. 2009;27(4):501-5.
2. Goldberg DJ. Legal considerations in cosmetic laser surgery. J Cosmet Dermatol. 2006; 5(2):103-6.
3. Goldberg DJ. Legal issues in dermatology: informed consent, complications and medical malpractice. Semin Cutan Med Surg. 2007; 26(1):2-5.
4. Goldberg DJ. Medicolegal issues for the dermatologist. Semin Cutan Med Surg. 2000; 19(3):181-8.
5. Michaels BD, Del Rosso JQ, Momin SB. Avoiding the legal "blemish": medicolegal pitfalls in dermatology. J Clin Aesthet Dermatol. 2009; 2(12):35-43.
6. Mudur G. Indian Supreme Court rules that HIV positive people inform spouses. BMJ. 1998;317:1474.
7. Murthy KKSR. Medical negligence and the law. Indian J Med Ethics. 2007;4(3).
8. Source of medicolegal cases: www.indiankanoon.org.
9. Torres A, Konda S, Nino T, de Golian E. Medicolegal issues. Clin Dermatol. 2016;34(1): 106-10.

7.6 Esthetic Procedures: Whose Domain it is?

— Putta Srinivas

Beauty is how you feel inside, and it reflects in your eyes. It is not something physical.
—Sophia Loren

HISTORY

The history of beauty is as old as mankind itself and throughout history people have tried to improve their attractiveness and to enhance their beauty.[1] Appearance is the most public part of the self and therefore men and women both try to improve their (apparent) imperfections with the intention to increase their self-perception and quality of life. *Ancient Indian surgeon, Sushrutha, around 500 BC performed reconstruction of damaged nose by rotation flap from the forehead and that's why he is known as Father of Plastic surgery.*

ESTHETIC: DEFINITION

The noun *Esthetic* is often found used in its plural form. In the plural form, *esthetics* can refer to the theory of art and beauty—and in particular the question of what makes something beautiful or interesting to regard. As a plural noun, *esthetics* can also be used as a synonym for *beauty*.

INTRODUCTION

Nowadays, every person irrespective of age and gender wants to look beautiful or handsome, conceal their actual age and appear young, and to be attractive. Once the basic needs are achieved, the next thing they would like to poses is beautiful physical appearance.

In today's world, with exposures to smart phones, internet, and social media, the desire to look beautiful and feel good is raging among people from all walks of life. They are quite confident about what they want.

Particularly since the last two decades there is greater consciousness of physical appearance, and there is mushrooming of health centers, chain of cosmetic centers with very attractive and tempting titles, just to catch people and exploit the desires of people to look beautiful. But unfortunately, these esthetic centers are focusing more on business and profits, and not giving importance for providing quality service by employing qualified and experienced experts. Since beauty has become one of the basic human needs, it turned out to be a big market which is booming in India.

The factors responsible for increased concern for appearance are the huge growth in the use of social media, increased use of the rating of images of the self and the body, for example, through social media "likes", and through self-monitoring apps and games, the popularity of celebrity culture, "airbrushed" images, and makeover shows, economic and social trends such as people retiring later, while having to compete in cultures that value youth and youthful appearance.[2]

India's beauty and wellness market which was ₹ 41,224 crores in 2012-2013 has nearly doubled to ₹ 80,370 crores in 2017-18[3] and growing very fast and trends are similar to European and American markets.

CURRENT SCENARIO IN INDIA

With increased awareness regarding appearance and beauty many medical and nonmedical persons are claiming as estheticians taking advantage of desire of the people and lack of statutory regulations and regulatory authorities.

CLASSIFICATION OF ESTHETIC MEDICAL PROCEDURES

Esthetic medical procedures should be supported by scientific evidence and/or have local medical expert consensus that the procedures are well established and acceptable.

These procedures can be classified into noninvasive, minimally invasive, and invasive.

Many countries, like in UAE, Malaysia, and Singapore, have recognized the importance of esthetic procedures and have framed guidelines on esthetic medical practice to ensure safety of these procedures. They have clearly defined classification of procedures, the eligibility criteria to perform, national registry to get registered to do the esthetic procedures and regulatory committees under countries' medical council:[4]

- *Noninvasive procedures*:[4] This is defined as external applications or treatment procedures that are carried

out without creating a break in the skin or penetration of the integument. They target the epidermis only. This procedure also includes superficial chemical peel, microdermabrasion, intense pulse light.
- *Minimally invasive procedures*:[4] This is defined as treatment procedures that induce minimal damage to the tissues at the point of entry of instruments. These procedures involve penetration or transgression of integument but are limited to the subdermis and subcutaneous fat; not extending beyond the superficial musculoaponeurotic layer of the face and neck, or beyond the superficial fascial layer of the torso and limbs. This procedure includes medium depth chemical peel, botulinum toxin injection, filler injection excluding silicone and fat, superficial sclerotherapy, lasers for treating skin pigmentation, lasers for skin rejuvenation (including fractional ablative), laser for hair removal, skin tightening procedures (radiofrequency, ultrasound, infrared up to upper dermis).
- *Invasive procedures*:[4] This is defined as treatment procedures that penetrate or break the skin through either perforation, incision or transgression of integument, subcutaneous and/or deeper tissues, often with extensive tissue involvement in both vertical and horizontal planes by various means, such as the use of knife, diathermy, ablative lasers, radiofrequency, ultrasound, cannulae and needles. This procedure includes laser for treating vascular lesions, chemical peels (deep), ablative skin resurfacing lasers, hair transplant, phlebectomy, ultrasound devise.

Eligibility to do the esthetic procedures.

STATUTORY STATUS OF ELIGIBLE SPECIALISTS IN INDIA

In India, Medical Council of India/National Medical Council is the regulatory authority for all levels of medical education, undergraduate, postgraduate, and super specialty courses. The postgraduate course which deal with esthetic procedures is MDDVL. Acne surgery, cryosurgical procedures, chemical peels skin grafting procedures, keloid treatment, nail surgeries, laser procedures, laser hair reduction, laser scar revision, laser pigment removal cosmetic surgical procedures, are in the syllabus of postgraduate course of DVL (Dermatology, Venereology, Leprosy).

As per the "Guidelines on Esthetic Medical Practice by Ministry of Health, Malasyia, and also Dubai to perform, noninvasive, minimally invasive procedures, as mentioned above, the core specialists eligible are dermatologists.[5,6]

Another specialty which deals with esthetic procedures is plastic surgery. Plastic surgery is a super specialty course dealing with reconstructive surgery, performing operations to repair or replace skin which has been damaged, or to improve people's appearance. The field of plastic surgery is quiet vast, breast augmentation, reconstruction with breast implant, with flap surgery, rhinoplasty, lip surgery, cheek surgery, ear surgery liposuction fat filling scar revision surgeries, replantation surgeries (micro surgery), endoscopic plastic surgery, face lift, flap transfer, skin grafting, acute burn care, trauma, tendon transfer, nerve repair, hair transplant.[7]

SUMMARY

The exciting field of esthetic medicine is a new trend in modern medicine. Patients not only want to be in good health, they also want to enjoy life to the fullest, be fit and minimize the effects of normal aging. Indeed, patients are now requesting quick, noninvasive procedures with minor downtime and very little risk. As a general rule, the needle is increasingly replacing the scalpel.[6] In India, as per the existing regulations dermatologists are eligible for noninvasive and minimally invasive esthetic procedures and it is the plastic surgeons who are eligible to perform invasive esthetic procedures.

Unfortunately, many individuals and institutions, with the sole intention of making quick money, are training MBBS, BDS, BHMS, BAMS, BUMS graduates, and giving certificates which are neither approved and recognized by MCI nor registered with State Medical Councils, but are accredited by certain foreign associations like International Society of Aesthetic Physicians and World Society of Interdisciplinary Anti-Aging Medicine.

Hence there is also need that Ministry of Health, Government of India, should constitute a task force to frame the guidelines on healthcare professional requirements, qualifications and experience, training course requirement, medical devise safety regulations, and constituting regulatory bodies to supervise all aspects to ensure public safety.

REFERENCES

1. Krueger N, Luebberding S, Sattler G, Hanke CW, Alexiades-Armenakas M, Sadick N. The history of aesthetic medicine and surgery. J Drugs Dermatol. 2013;12(7):737-42.
2. Archard D, Montgomery J. Nuffield Council on Bioethics: Cosmetic Procedures; 2017. p. 18.
3. Sethi D. Trade & Technology Expositions – Wellness Industry. KPMG Report; 2016.
4. Ministry of Health, Malaysia—Guidelines on Aesthetic Medical Practice for Registered Medical Practitioners, pages 8 and 9.
5. Medical Council of India: Syllabus of Postgraduate Degree/Diploma Syllabus Training Programs, MCI; 2006. pp. 43-52.
6. National Board of Examinations. Available from http://www.natboard.edu.in/notice_for_dnb_candidates/dermatology.pdf [Last accessed January 2020].
7. Medical Council of India: Standard Assessment Form of Plastic Surgery—2020-2021 (pages 5,6 and 16-8).

7.7 Safe Medical Practice

Venkataram Mysore, Ashwini L Hirevenkangoudar

INTRODUCTION

Modern health care is complex and error prone. Healthcare errors and adverse effects lead to unexpected events. Safe medical practice is, therefore, very important but yet underemphasized. This chapter highlights some aspects of a safe medical practice and measures for reducing the occurrence of errors.

Safe medical practice encompasses several aspects of medical practice such as:
- Safe patient relations
- Safe hygiene practices
- Safe documentation practices
- Safe prescription practices
- Safe surgery operation theater (OT) practices
- Safe waste disposal protocols

- Safe staff practices
- Safe doctor relations
- Safe adherence to law, Medical Council of India (MCI)

Several aspects of these have been emphasized in other chapters of the book. This chapter seeks to provide an overview.

SAFE PATIENT RELATIONS

Proper communication with the patient in a language of patient's interest, counseling about the condition and treatment options help in improving patient's experience as well as building-up of trust in you. Cultivate better bedside manner. Always tell the truth, allow sufficient time for each encounter, watch your body language, give patients freedom with a patient portal. These should be done not just by the doctor but by all staff in the facility.

SAFE HYGIENE PRACTICES

Maintaining cleanliness, use of sterilized instruments, clean linen, hand washing after examination of patients prevent in transmission of infection to other patients as well as yourself. This would also include proper waste disposal.

SAFE DOCUMENTATION PRACTICES

Documentation is recording and managing data. Proper documentation of relevant history, prescription, use of proper informed consent forms for all procedures and specific medications, printed post-procedure instructions is essential. Documentation of photos helps for further references like assessing the improvement. It ensures that your patients get the right care at the right time.

SAFE PRESCRIPTION PRACTICES

Be clear about the complaints (rationale) for prescribing, take into account the patient's treatment history before prescribing, other comorbidities and drug history, patients' ideas, concerns and expectations. Select effective, safe, and cost-effective medications, write the name of the medications in capital letters and mention how to use along with the duration of the medications. Explain regarding common adverse effects that the patient might experience. Lastly, prescribe within your knowledge, skills, and experience.

SAFE SURGERY OT PRACTICES

Strict asepsis must be maintained. Maintain a sterile environment in OT complex, instruments, sterile surgical barriers such as scrubbing, draping and painting of the surgical area to be maintained. Regular fumigation of OT complex should be carried out.

SAFE WASTE DISPOSAL PROTOCOLS

Healthcare establishments have a duty of care towards the environment and public health. This includes waste handling, treatment, and disposal activities. Healthcare waste is categorized as infectious waste, pathological waste, sharps, pharmaceutical waste, radioactive waste, cytotoxic waste, waste with heavy metal content, and noninfectious waste or general wastes. Proper color-coded waste disposal bags should be used for all purposes.

SAFE STAFF PRACTICES

Staff needs to well groomed, decently dressed and have a positive attitude while communicating with patients. Maintain confidentiality of the patients. The staff should have proper knowledge of different procedures to guide the patients. Hire well-trained, qualified, credible nursing staff.

SAFE ADHERENCE TO LAW, MCI

Always display your registration certificate and degree certificate in your clinic. Avoid negligence, malpractice, unethical, and irrational practice for personal gain at all times. Always keep a check on incentives offered by medical representatives.

DOCTOR RELATIONS

- *Need to get together and develop rapport*: Doctors need to gather socially which helps in developing good rapport, referral of patients, in treating rare or difficult cases and also in exchanging views.
- *Referrals to and from*: Referral is transfer of care for a patient from one doctor to another by request. Referrals should be by written document, addressing a specific specialist. It should be thorough and proper. Phone calls to the referring doctor while referring helps in conveying the condition of the patient patient, discussing about the condition helps in building trust with the patient as well. When a patient is referred to you, return your feedback, so that the doctor has a follow-up of the condition and adequate measures are taken for the same. No commissions should be received for referral cases. In cases of emergency, necessary measures need to be taken before referring the patient to higher center.
- *Jousting*: It means criticizing or commenting regarding the treatment that the patient has undergone so far before consulting you. For example, who gave you this scar? This could have been avoided! Or that the treatment was wrong, instead say, the treatment did not work for your condition. Patients get disheartened about the treatment and lose faith in doctors, leading to criticism of doctors that harms their reputation. This in turn leads to more medicolegal cases. Patient can quote you in a court of law. The other doctor can also sue you. Educated patients may get the wrong impression about the jousting doctor as well. So it should never be practiced.

One important way of enforcing these practices is by implementing protocols, standard operating protocols (SOPs), and checklists.

PROTOCOLS

They help in maintaining the uniformity and chances of missing out on something are reduced. For example, protocols for clinic—first line, second line, third line of treatment protocols and follow-up protocols especially in sexually transmitted disease (STD) and leprosy clinic. Protocols for surgery—before any procedure, protocols for pharmacy—proper dispensing of medicine and checking of expiry date and concentration.

CHECKLISTS

It is an organized way that reduces medical errors. They standardize and improve the clinical practice. Checklist creates a great sense of confidence in patients that the process is completed accurately and thoroughly.

Credentialing and privileging: Have a list of privileges and credentials. Privileging is a process of authorizing a specific scope of practice for patient care. Credentialing is a quality aspect of a person's background. Having a list of privileges and credentials helps in standardization and patient care.

CONCLUSION

In today's times, medical practice should not only be effective, but also ethical. Building the relation with the patient, being up-to-date in knowledge, proper documentation, adopting proper protocols are essential to ensure safe practice.

7.8 Code of Medical Ethics

Putta Srinivas, Nayeem Sadath Haneef

INTRODUCTION AND HISTORICAL BACKGROUND

Ethics is defined in Oxford English Dictionary as *"moral principles that govern person's behavior or conduct of activities."*[1] Medical ethics is a *"combination of moral principles and values that are applied to take judgments in medical education, practice and research."*[2]

Medical ethics is of utmost importance as medical profession is distinguished from other professions by a special moral duty of care to save lives and to relieve suffering. All the great religions of the world have prescribed moral codes of conduct for doctors based on divine instructions as mentioned in their respective holy books, be it the Vedas, Bible, Koran, or others like those of Buddhism.[2] In the ancient recorded history, concerns for the patient's welfare and the appropriate behavior of the physician were noted in the *"Code of Hammurabi"*, a code of ethics dating back to 2000 BC. Ancient Indian scriptures like *"Charaka Samhita"* and *"Sushruta Samhita"* (600 BC) also mention medical ethics in the form of eligibility criteria for being medical students and teachers, counsel on behavior with patients and their relatives, and pointers that can be used by us when dealing with such issues as brain death and organ transplantation.[3] Two millennia ago, Greek great Hippocrates gave the *"Hippocratic Oath"*, which established the doctor as a selfless caregiver.

Ethics in modern medicine can be traced back to 1803 when Thomas Percival, a physician based in England, coined the terms medical ethics and medical jurisprudence in his book on medical ethics, which subsequently became widely used reference on medical ethics for quite long.[4] Mass murder of concentration camp prisoners as a result of cruel experimentations by the Nazi Germans during World War II leads to formulation of *"Nuremberg code"* in 1947, mainly dealing with the absolute need for informed consent for human experimentation.[5] Within a month of this development, medical associations of 27 countries founded a global physicians' association, namely, *"World Medical Association (WMA)"* based at Geneva. The WMA, in its second General Assembly in 1948 announced a modernized version of Hippocratic Oath, *"The Declaration of Geneva"*, which binds the physician with the words, "the health of my patient will be my first consideration." In 1949, WMA adopted the *"International Code of Medical Ethics"* urging physicians to act in patients' best interest when providing medical care.[5]

A subject-specific *"Code of medical ethics for dermatologists"* was published in 2005 by American Academy of Dermatologists, based on Principles of Medical Ethics and *Current Opinions of the Council on Ethical and Judicial Affairs of the American Medical Association (AMA)*.

TECHNICAL PRINCIPLES OF CODE OF MEDICAL ETHICS

Code of medical ethics is based on the following four basic principles:[4]

1. *Respect for autonomy*: Respect the patients' ability to take decisions on behalf of themselves, after being informed thoroughly about the risks and benefits involved in the chosen therapeutic or diagnostic intervention.
2. *Beneficence*: The practitioner should act in "the best interest" of the patient with the intent of doing good to the patient (including constant updating of knowledge and skills).
3. *Justice*: Doctor should treat equitably and distribute scarce resources fairly and wisely.
4. *Nonmaleficence*: Above all *"do no harm."*

Based on these above principles, various codes of medical ethics have been formulated as described here.[5]

WMA Declaration of Geneva[5]

Adopted by the 2nd General Assembly of the WMA, Geneva, Switzerland, September 1948 (amended in 1968, 1983, 1994, 2005, and 2006)

At the time of being admitted as a member of the medical profession:

- *I solemnly pledge* to consecrate my life to the service of humanity;
- *I will give* to my teachers the respect and gratitude that is their due;
- *I will practice* my profession with conscience and dignity;
- *The health of my patient* will be my first consideration;
- *I will respect* the secrets that are confided in me, even after the patient has died;
- *I will maintain* by all the means in my power, the honor and the noble traditions of the medical profession;
- *My colleagues* will be my sisters and brothers;
- *I will not permit* considerations of age, disease or disability, creed, ethnic origin, gender, nationality, political affiliation, race, sexual orientation, social standing, or any other factor to intervene between my duty and my patient;
- *I will maintain* the utmost respect for human life;
- *I will not use* my medical knowledge to violate human rights and civil liberties, even under threat;
- *I make these promises* solemnly, freely and upon my honor.

WMA International Code of Medical Ethics[5]

Adopted by the 3rd General Assembly of the WMA, London, England, October 1949 (amended in 1968, 1983, and 2006)

Duties of Physicians in General

- *A physician shall* always exercise his/her independent professional judgment and maintain the highest standards of professional conduct.
- *A physician shall* respect a competent patient's right to accept or refuse treatment.
- *A physician shall* not allow his/her judgment to be influenced by personal profit or unfair discrimination.
- *A physician shall* be dedicated to providing competent medical service in full professional and moral independence, with compassion and respect for human dignity.
- *A physician shall* deal honestly with patients and colleagues, and report to the appropriate authorities those physicians who practice unethically or incompetently or who engage in fraud or deception.
- *A physician shall* not receive any financial benefits or other incentives solely for referring patients or prescribing specific products.

- *A physician shall* respect the rights and preferences of patients, colleagues, and other health professionals.
- *A physician shall* recognize his/her important role in educating the public but should use due caution in divulging discoveries or new techniques or treatment through nonprofessional channels.
- *A physician shall* certify only that which he/she has personally verified.
- *A physician shall* strive to use healthcare resources in the best way to benefit patients and their community.
- *A physician shall* seek appropriate care and attention if he/she suffers from mental or physical illness.
- *A physician shall* respect the local and national codes of ethics.

Duties of Physicians to Patients

- *A physician shall* always bear in mind the obligation to respect human life.
- *A physician shall* act in the patient's best interest when providing medical care.
- *A physician shall* owe his/her patients complete loyalty and all the scientific resources available to him/her.
- Whenever an examination or treatment is beyond the physician's capacity, he/she should consult with or refer to another physician who has the necessary ability.
- *A physician shall* respect a patient's right to confidentiality. It is ethical to disclose confidential information when the patient consents to it or when there is a real and imminent threat of harm to the patient or to others and this threat can be only removed by a breach of confidentiality.
- *A physician shall* give emergency care as a humanitarian duty unless he/she is assured that others are willing and able to give such care.
- *A physician shall* in situations when he/she is acting for a third party, ensure that the patient has full knowledge of that situation.
- *A physician shall* not enter into a sexual relationship with his/her current patient or into any other abusive or exploitative relationship.

Duties of Physicians to Colleagues

- *A physician shall* behave toward colleagues, as he/she would have them behave toward him/her.
- *A physician shall not* undermine the patient–physician relationship of colleagues in order to attract patients.
- *A physician shall* when medically necessary, communicate with colleagues who are involved in the care of the same patient. This communication should respect patient confidentiality and be confined to necessary information.

American Academy of Dermatology Code of Medical Ethics for Dermatologists (2005)[6]

American Academy of Dermatologists published a specialty specific "code of medical ethics for dermatologists" in 2005, based on Principles of Medical Ethics and *Current Opinions of the Council on Ethical and Judicial Affairs of the AMA*. This code includes various guidelines under nine broad categories, namely, physician–patient relationship, personal conduct, conflicts of interest, maintenance of competence, relationships with dermatologists, nurses, other allied health professionals, relationship with the public, general principles of care, research, and academic responsibilities, and lastly community responsibility.

INDIAN MEDICAL COUNCIL (PROFESSIONAL CONDUCT, ETIQUETTE, AND ETHICS) REGULATIONS, 2002 (AMENDED UP TO 8TH OCTOBER 2016)[7]: EXCERPTS, IMPLICATIONS, AND CONTROVERSIES

The Medical Council of India (MCI) has prescribed regulations relating to the professional conduct, etiquette, and ethics for registered medical practitioners in 2002, under the Indian Medical Council Act, 1956, with approval from the Government of India. The following are excerpts of the regulations, authors' comments (*in italics*) on their potential implications and controversies surrounding these regulations:

Chapter 1: Code of Medical Ethics

Declaration

At the time of making an application for registration, each applicant is required to submit a signed declaration pledging to serve the humanity with impartial, humane approach while upholding the dignity and nobility of the medical profession.

Duties and Responsibilities of the Physicians in General

- *Character of physician [doctors with qualification of Bachelor of Medicine and Bachelor of Surgery (MBBS) or MBBS with postgraduate degree or diploma or with equivalent qualification in any medical discipline]*:
  - A physician shall uphold the dignity and honor of his profession.
  - The prime object of the medical profession is to render service to humanity; reward or financial gain is a subordinate consideration. Physician shall keep himself pure in character and be diligent in caring for the sick.
  - No person other than a doctor having qualification recognized by MCI and registered with MCI or State Medical Council(s) is allowed to practice.
  - Modern system of medicine or surgery. A person obtaining qualification in any other system of medicine is not allowed to practice modern system of medicine in any form.
- *Maintaining good medical practice*:
  - Physicians should serve the patients with devotion and practice methods of healing founded on scientific basis, and continuously improve medical knowledge and skills.
  - Membership in allopathic medical societies for advancement of the profession.
  - A physician should participate in Continuing Medical Education (CME) programs, for at least 30 hours every 5 years.

Comment: Many of the State Medical Councils link this requirement of credit hours to renewal of registration once in 5 years. The need for renewal of registration with the State Medical Council once in 5 years or re-registration of doctor belonging to other state in new State Medical Council is itself controversial, as MCI rules indicate that name of any doctor registered with any State Medical Council is automatically entered in Indian Medical Council and hence such doctor can practice anywhere in India lifelong.

- *Maintenance of medical records*:
  - Every physician shall maintain the medical records pertaining to his/her indoor patients for a period of 3 years from the date of commencement of the treatment in a standard proforma.

Comment: The guidelines mention only indoor patients but not outdoor patients' records.
- If any request is made for medical records either by the patients or authorized attendant or legal authorities involved, documents shall be issued within the period of 72 hours.
- A registered medical practitioner shall maintain a Register of Medical Certificates giving full details of certificates issued.
- Efforts shall be made to computerize medical records for quick retrieval.
- *Display of registration numbers*:
  - Every physician shall display the registration number accorded to him by the State Medical Council or MCI in his clinic and in all his prescriptions, certificates, and money receipts given to his patients.
  - Physicians shall display as suffix to their names only recognized medical degrees or such certificates or diplomas and memberships or honors, which confer professional knowledge or recognize any exemplary qualification or achievements.
- *Use of generic names of drugs*: Every physician should prescribe drugs with generic names legibly and preferably in capital letters and he/she shall ensure that there is a rational prescription and use of drugs.

Comment: Prescribing generic names legibly and in capital letters may help in reducing the cost of medicines by curbing recommendation of costly brands by doctors. But in India, there is no guarantee of quality control of such medicines. Also, the pharmacists or salesmen may indulge in profiteering as they can choose a brand or manufacturer to suit their needs. With respect to dermatology, it may be noted that use of irrational combination of topical corticosteroids and antifungal agents has led to outbreak of recalcitrant or resistant dermatophyte infections.

- *Highest quality assurance in patient care*: Every physician should aid in safeguarding the profession against admission to it of those who are deficient in moral character or education. Physician shall not employ in connection with his professional practice any attendant who is neither registered nor enlisted under the Medical Acts in force and shall not permit such persons to attend, treat, or perform operations upon patients wherever professional discretion or skill is required.
- *Exposure of unethical conduct*: A physician should expose, without fear or favor, incompetent or corrupt, and dishonest or unethical conduct on the part of members of the profession.
- *Payment of professional services*: The personal financial interests of a physician should not conflict with the medical interests of patients. A physician should announce his fees before rendering service and not after the operation or treatment is under way.
- *Evasion of legal restrictions*: The physician shall observe the laws of the country in regulating the practice of medicine and shall also not assist others to evade such laws. He should be cooperative in observance and enforcement of sanitary laws and regulations in the interest of public health.

Chapter 2: Duties of Physicians to their Patients

- *Obligations to the sick*:
  - Though a physician is not bound to treat each and every person asking his services, he should be ever ready to respond to the calls of the sick and the injured. A physician advising a patient

to seek service of another physician is acceptable; however, in case of emergency a physician must treat the patient. No physician shall arbitrarily refuse treatment to a patient.
- Medical practitioner having any incapacity detrimental to the patient or which can affect his performance vis-à-vis the patient is not permitted to practice his profession.
- *Patience, delicacy, and secrecy*: Patience and delicacy should characterize the physician. Confidential information about patient's illness should never be revealed unless their revelation is required by the laws of the State or in order to protect a healthy person against a communicable disease to which he is about to be exposed.
- The physician should neither exaggerate nor minimize the gravity of a patient's condition.
- Once having undertaken a case, the physician should not neglect the patient, nor should he withdraw from the case without giving adequate notice to the patient and his family. Physician shall not willfully commit an act of negligence.
- When a physician who has been engaged to attend an obstetric case is absent and another is sent for and delivery accomplished, the acting physician is entitled to his professional fees, but should secure the patient's consent to resign on the arrival of the physician engaged.

Chapter 3: Duties of Physicians in Consultation

- Unnecessary consultations should be avoided.
- In every consultation, the benefit to the patient is of foremost importance.
- Utmost punctuality should be observed by a physician in consultations.
- All statements to the patient or his representatives should take place in the presence of the consulting physicians, except as otherwise agreed.
- Physician can make subsequent variations in the treatment, if any unexpected change occurs, but reasons for the variations should be discussed or explained.
- When a patient is referred to a specialist by the attending physician, a case summary of the patient should be given to the specialist, who should communicate his opinion in writing to the attending physician.
- A physician shall clearly display his fees and other charges on the board of his chamber and/or the hospitals he is visiting.

Chapter 4: Responsibilities of Physicians to Each Other

- A physician should consider it as a pleasure and privilege to render gratuitous service to all physicians and their immediate family dependents.
- In consultations, no insincerity, rivalry, or envy should be indulged in.
- When a physician has been called for consultation, the consultant should not take charge of the case. The consultant shall not criticize the referring physician. He/she shall discuss the diagnosis treatment plan with the referring physician.
- Whenever a physician requests another physician to attend his patients during his temporary absence from his practice, the other physician should accept only when he has the capacity to discharge the additional responsibility along with his/her other duties.
- The medical officer or physician occupying an official position should

avoid remarks upon the diagnosis or the treatment that has been adopted by other physician.

Chapter 5: Duties of Physicians to the Public and to the Paramedical Profession

- Physicians, as good citizens, should advice on public health issues and play their part in enforcing sanitary or public health laws and regulations.
- Physicians should enlighten the public concerning quarantine regulations and measures for the prevention of epidemic and communicable diseases, and also notify public health authorities.
- Physicians should recognize and promote the practice of different paramedical services such as, pharmacy and nursing.

Chapter 6: Unethical Acts

A physician shall not aid or abet or commit any of the following acts, which shall be construed as unethical.

- *Advertising*:
  - Soliciting of patients directly or indirectly, by a physician, by a group of physicians, or by institutions or organizations is unethical. A physician shall not make use of him or her (or his or her name) as subject of any form or manner of advertising or publicity through any mode either alone or in conjunction with others, which is of such a character as to invite attention to him or to his professional position, skill, qualification, achievements, attainments, specialties, appointments, associations, affiliations or honors, and/or of such character as would ordinarily result in his self-aggrandizement. A physician shall not give to any person, whether for compensation or otherwise, any approval, recommendation, endorsement, certificate, report or statement with respect of any drug, medicine, nostrum remedy, surgical, or therapeutic article, apparatus or appliance or any commercial product or article with respect of any property, quality or use thereof or any test, demonstration or trial thereof, for use in connection with his name, signature, or photograph in any form or manner of advertising through any mode nor shall he boast of cases, operations, cures or remedies, or permit the publication of report thereof through any mode. A medical practitioner is, however, permitted to make a formal announcement in press regarding the following:
    + On starting practice
    + On change of type of practice
    + On changing address
    + On temporary absence from duty
    + On resumption of another practice
    + On succeeding to another practice
    + Public declaration of charges.
  - Printing of self-photograph, or any such material of publicity in the letter head or on sign board of the consulting room or any such clinical establishment shall be regarded as acts of self-advertisement and unethical conduct on the part of the physician.
- *Patent and copyrights*: A physician may patent surgical instruments, appliances, and medicine or copyright applications, methods, and procedures. However, it shall be unethical, if the benefits of such patents or copyrights are not made available in situations where the interest of large population is involved.

- A physician should not run an open shop for sale of medicine for dispensing prescriptions prescribed by doctors other than himself or for sale of medical or surgical appliances. It is not unethical for a physician to prescribe or supply drugs, remedies, or appliances as long as there is no exploitation of the patient. Drugs prescribed by a physician or brought from the market for a patient should explicitly state the proprietary formulae as well as generic name of the drug.
- *Rebates and commission*: A physician shall not give, solicit, or receive nor shall he offer to give solicit or receive, any gift, gratuity, commission or bonus in consideration of or return for the referring, recommending or procuring of any patient for medical, surgical or other treatment, or for diagnostic tests.
- All the drugs prescribed by a physician should always carry a proprietary formula and clear name. Prescription of secret remedies is prohibited.
- *Human rights*: The physician shall not aid or abet mental or physical trauma or torture in clear violation of human rights.
- Practicing euthanasia shall constitute unethical conduct. However, on specific occasion, the question of withdrawing life-supporting devices even after brain death shall be decided only by a team of doctors and not merely by the treating physician alone.
- *Code of conduct for doctors in their relationship with pharmaceutical and allied health sector industry*:
  - A medical practitioner shall not receive any gift, cash, or monetary grant from any pharmaceutical and allied healthcare industry and their sales representatives. A medical practitioner shall not accept any hospitality or travel facility inside the country or outside, including rail, road, air, ship, cruise tickets, paid vacations, etc. from any pharmaceutical or allied healthcare industry or their representatives for self and family members for vacation or for attending conferences, seminars, workshops, CME program, etc. as a delegate.
  - A medical practitioner may carry out or participate as researchers, treating doctors, or consultants in research projects funded by pharmaceutical and allied healthcare industries, provided all the legal requirements for the medical research, including ethical committee clearing, humane treatment of human volunteers, and experimental animals are fulfilled. Physician should maintain his professional autonomy and patient safety during such participation.
  - A physician shall not indulge in endorsement of any drug or appliance, except in scientific journals for academic purpose only.
  - Any deviation from the above guidelines is punishable with censure, removal of name of the physician from Indian Medical Register or State Medical Register (for a period ranging from 3 months to more than 1 year).

Chapter 7: Misconduct

The following acts of commission or omission on the part of a physician shall constitute professional misconduct rendering him/her liable for disciplinary action:
- If he/she commits any violation of the MCI regulations.
- Failure to maintain the medical records of indoor patients for a period of 3 years or refusal to provide the same within 72 hours when solicited.

- Failure to display registration number in clinic, prescriptions and certificates, etc.
- Abuse of professional position by committing adultery or improper conduct with a patient.
- Conviction by a Court of Law for offences involving moral turpitude or criminal acts.
- Sex determination test undertaken with the intent to terminate the life of a female fetus, unless there are other absolute indications for termination of pregnancy as specified in the Medical Termination of Pregnancy Act, 1971.
- Signing professional certificates, reports, and other documents, which are untrue, misleading, or improper.
- Contravention of provisions of the Drugs and Cosmetics Act and regulations made there under. Accordingly,
  - Prescribing steroids or psychotropic drugs when there is no absolute medical indication;
  - Selling schedule "H" and "L" drugs and poisons to public except to his patient in contravention of the above provisions shall constitute gross professional misconduct by the physician.
- Performing or enabling unqualified person to perform an abortion or any illegal operation for which there is no medical, surgical or psychological indication.
- Issuing certificates of efficiency in modern medicine to unqualified or nonmedical person.

Comment: It is unfortunate that few dermatologists themselves are irresponsibly indulging in providing "certificate courses" for nondermatologist candidates. This is not only unethical, but also creating undue competition for our own fraternity.

- Contributing lay press articles and interviews regarding diseases and treatments for advertising himself or soliciting practices (writing in lay press or delivering public lectures, talks on the radio or TV or internet chat on matters of public health, and hygienic living are allowed).
- An institution run by a physician for a particular purpose such as a maternity home, nursing home, private hospital, rehabilitation center or any type of training institution, etc. may be advertised in the lay press, but such advertisements should not contain anything more than the name of the institution, type of patients admitted, type of training and other facilities offered, and the fees.
- Use of an unusually large signboard and writing anything other than doctor's name, qualifications obtained from a university or a statutory body, titles, and name of specialty, registration number including the name of the State Medical Council under which registered. The same should be the contents of prescription papers. It is improper to affix a signboard on a chemist's shop or in places where the physician does not reside or work.
- *Disclosure the secrets of a patient except*:
  - In a court of law under orders of the presiding judge;
  - In circumstances where there is a serious and identified risk to a specific person and/or community; and
  - Notifiable diseases.
- Refusal on religious grounds alone to give assistance in or conduct of sterility, birth control, circumcision, and medical termination of pregnancy when there is medical indication.
- Failure to obtain written consent before surgery or procedure.

Comment: Not obtaining written informed consent specific to the procedure concerned is the most common mistake, which lands the doctors into medicolegal problems.

- Publishing photographs or case reports of patients without their permission, in any medical or other journal in a manner by which their identity could be made out. If the identity is not to be disclosed, the consent is not needed.
- In the case of running of a nursing home by a physician and employing assistants to help him/her, the ultimate responsibility rests on the physician.
- Use touts or agents for procuring patients.
- Claiming to be specialist unless he has a special qualification in that branch.
- In vitro fertilization or artificial insemination undertaken without the informed consent of the female patient and her spouse as well as the donor.
- *Research*: Clinical drug trials or other research involving patients or volunteers as per the guidelines of Indian Council of Medical Research (ICMR) can be undertaken, provided ethical considerations are borne in mind. Violation of existing ICMR guidelines in this regard shall constitute misconduct. Consent taken from the patient for trial of drug or therapy, which is not as per the guidelines, shall also be construed as misconduct.

Chapter 8: Punishment and Disciplinary Action

Apart from above-mentioned clauses, the MCI and/or State Medical Councils are in no way precluded from considering and dealing with any other form of professional misconduct on the part of a registered practitioner. Upon receipt of any complaint of professional misconduct, the appropriate Medical Council would hold an enquiry within 6 months and give opportunity to the registered medical practitioner to be heard in person or by pleader. During the pendency of the complaint, the appropriate council may restrain the physician from performing the procedure or practice, which is under scrutiny. Professional incompetence shall be judged by peer group as per guidelines prescribed by MCI. If the medical practitioner is found to be guilty of committing professional misconduct, the appropriate Medical Council may award such punishment as deemed necessary. Any person aggrieved by the decision of the State Medical Council on any complaint against a delinquent physician, shall have the right to file an appeal to the MCI within a period of 60 days from the date of receipt of the order passed by the said Medical Council.

RELEVANCE OF MCI CODE OF ETHICS IN TODAY'S PRACTICE

Regulations on MCI code of conduct was issued in 2002 and periodically updated. However, many experts opine that perception of the society, administrators, and policy makers about the medical profession has changed drastically.

Introduction of Consumer Protection Act in 1986, and with bringing of the medical profession within the Consumer Protection Act purview, has dramatically changed the relationship of patient and doctor to that of consumer and service provider. The society generally expects the doctors to be service oriented with humanity, but paradoxically the law deals with doctors as consumer service providers. People when go to a doctor, are expressing that they have full faith and confidence, but when things does not happen as per their expectations, they are treating doctors as villains, without understanding the risk factors and limitations of modern medical science and variations of human response to different treatment methods. Consequently, the patients and their attendants are taking law into their hands and physically assaulting doctors and hospitals. Another aspect is that certain individuals are blackmailing doctors and lodging false complaints or filing cases in consumer courts.

Hence, there is growing feeling among medical profession that Code of Medical Ethics is fixing their responsibilities whereas it is silent about protecting their interests. There is an immediate need to make Code of Medical Ethics more relevant, and shall be updated and shall incorporate changes to protect the interests of doctors also keeping in view the changed circumstances.

REGISTRATION OF DOCTORS: INDIAN MEDICAL REGISTER OR STATE MEDICAL REGISTER

The doctors of modern medicine can register their MBBS, Doctor of Medicine (MD) or Master of Surgery (MS), Doctorate of Medicine (DM), or Master of Chirurgiae (MCh) either with Indian Medical Register maintained at MCI New Delhi or State Medical Register maintained at concerned State Medical Councils. There are certain gray areas where there are elements of ambiguity. When a doctor is registered in Indian Medical Register, it is expected that he should be eligible to practice in any state, anywhere in India; however, it is not so. As per the existing regulations, even if a doctor is registered in Indian Medical Register, still he has to register with concerned State Medical Council and State Medical Register to be eligible to practice in that particular state. This double registration is becoming an area of controversy. There is a need to remove this double registration and ambiguity.

REGISTRATION OF FOREIGN FACULTY WHO PERFORM SURGERIES OR PROCEDURES DURING CONFERENCES OR CME OR WORKSHOPS

It is mandatory that all the foreign doctors to register with concerned State Medical Council, to be eligible to perform on patients surgeries or procedures for live demonstrations during workshops or CME or conferences. The concerned State Medical Council will register them for a minimum period of 3 months during which he can do surgeries or procedures and without such registration, foreign doctors will not be eligible to touch the patients. There is one gray area, that State Medical Council can only register the foreign qualifications, which are recognized by MCI (in reciprocation), but cannot register foreign qualifications, which are not recognized by MCI, and such foreign faculty cannot perform surgeries or procedures. In reality, these rules are not strictly followed by both the organizers and foreign faculty also. However, when an unfortunate incident takes place there will be utter chaos and blaming of each other.

SIGNBOARDS AND ADVERTISEMENTS—NEED TO CHANGE IN CURRENT SCENARIO[7]

The MCI code of ethics 7.13 mentions about the size of signboard and specifies about what matter board should contain. However, there are revolutionary changes in publicity, advertisements, and professional promotion methods, with advent of internet, YouTube, and net-based promotional agencies like Justdial, Practo, etc. These changes in media and advertisements are being used effectively not only by business houses but also by many professional experts. Nowadays, every person looks into these sites for help, guidance as well as opinion generation. With such revolutionary changes, particularly when every professional experts, are using them for their advantage by effective presentation and professional promotion, it is unrealistic to put a bar on doctors from using them.

It is high time that the MCI code of medical ethics should be reviewed and guidelines should be framed for promotion of professional activities of doctors on net-based agencies like Justdial, Practo, and also in print and electronic media, etc. Also there is a need to review regarding the contents of signboards to include facilities that are available and services that are offered. We have to also keep in view the fact that now patient is a consumer and doctor is a service provider and naturally service provider should be allowed to put in signboards, what facilities and services that are available.

Another angle of advertisements is surrogate advertisements by nonallopathic doctors, chain of clinics of homeopathic, and ayurvedic doctors, just to circumvent code of ethics and has become a big menace misleading innocent people and exploiting them just for monitory benefit. Surrogate advertisements by pharma companies are another problem, as evidenced by recent advertisement by a leading pharma company of corticosteroid and antifungal combination cream disguised as plain antifungal (miconazole) cream for treatment of tinea infection.

There is an essential and urgent need to curb the menace and represent to law commission and Government of India to prevent surrogate advertisements.

Can a dermatologist put a board as cosmetic dermatologist or dermatosurgeon or cosmetic surgeon?

Thanks to very rapid advances in science and technology, the scope of dermatology has changed beyond imagination. There were times when one can start dermatology practice with a simple hand lens and a thermal cautery machine. Now one has to have to at least one or two lasers and other dermatosurgical and cosmetic equipment, which may in total need minimum ₹ 1–2 million.

The specialty of dermatology now has developed into subspecialties like dermatosurgery, cosmetic surgery, or medical cosmetology. The curriculum of postgraduate courses and mandatory equipment required as per MCI, includes three types of lasers, cryosurgeries, acne surgeries, vitiligo surgeries, nail surgeries, fillers, dermabrasion, chemical peels, and all dermatosurgical and cosmetic procedures.

However, unfortunately these advances are not reflected in the nomenclature of postgraduate qualifications, which still is by nomenclature of dermatology, venereology, and leprology (DVL). Consequently, people are asking the dermatologists, are you a cosmetologist? Are you cosmetic surgeon? Are you esthetic surgeon?, etc. To overcome the nomenclature issues and to counter the propaganda of nonmedical persons claims, many dermatologists are displaying in signboards and letterheads that they are cosmetic dermatologist or cosmetologists or cosmetic surgeon or dermatosurgeon, etc.

As per MCI Code of Ethics 2002, Regulation 1.4.2, physicians shall display as suffix to their names only recognized medical degrees or *such certificates or diplomas and memberships or honors, which confer professional knowledge* or recognize any exemplary qualification or achievements.

When one has basic postgraduate qualification in dermatology, and subsequently by having hands on training in workshops or CMEs acquiring skills and by getting experience in cosmetic surgery or dermatosurgery or esthetic surgery, we feel dermatologist can certainly claim and display as member of Association of Cutaneous Surgeons of India (ACSI), Cosmetology Society of India (CSI), etc. and as cosmetic dermatologist or cosmetologists or cosmetic surgeon or dermatosurgeon, etc.

CHANGE OF NOMENCLATURE OF POSTGRADUATE COURSE OF DVL TO DVL AND DERMATOSURGERY/COSMETIC SURGERY

Another aspect is that, after representation of concerned professional associations, basing on scientific advances, MCI has changed the nomenclature of many postgraduate courses. The nomenclature of PG course of TB and CD (tuberculosis and chest diseases) has changed to pulmonary medicine or pulmonology; similarly nomenclature of PG course of radiology has changed and separated to radiodiagnosis and radiotherapy. It is high time that the professional bodies like Indian Association of Dermatologists, Venereologists, and Leprologists (IADVL), in public interest, to protect the common people from exploitation by unqualified persons, and nonmedical persons, who claim as cosmetic surgeons or cosmetologists, or esthetic surgeons, and to protect the interests of genuinely qualified dermatologists, should represent to MCI to modify nomenclature of postgraduate course to include cosmetic surgery or dermatosurgery. For example, the nomenclature of MD DVL should be changed to that of MD DVL and dermatosurgery or cosmetic surgery.

CODE OF ETHICS: HOSPITAL INDUSTRY

All over the world, code of ethics applies to all professions more so to medical profession. However, code of medical ethics applies to individual doctors only but does not apply to nursing homes, hospitals, corporate hospitals, and chain of clinics and cosmetology centers. They all come under the control of local health and municipal administration, who give them permission. But in reality, there is not much of monitoring on them due to factors like huge work load, shortage of staff, administrative bottle necks, and political interference, consequently there will be lack of action on erring hospitals or centers.

These days hospitals, particularly corporate hospitals, are established under the category of health industry, and by taking huge loans in hundreds of cores of rupees from banks and financial institutions, and they are administered professionally and run as pure business in terms of profit and loss every year. When these hospitals are run as business, naturally ethical values are taking a back seat.

LEGAL IMPLICATIONS OF CODE OF MEDICAL ETHICS

Doctors' behavior in medical education, practice, and research is measured against the above-mentioned code of medical ethics. Any deviation from the same is likely to lead to punitive action against the errant doctors such as removal of name from Indian Medical Council Register. Such deviation may also result in breach of doctor-patient trust leading to litigation by patients, especially in the current era of Consumer Protection Act.[8]

REMEDY AND PREVENTION OF LEGAL IMPLICATIONS OF CODE OF MEDICAL ETHICS

In practice, ethical decision making can be facilitated by adopting the following simple steps:
1. After thorough consideration of technical facts, moral parameters, and legal constraints determine whether the issue at hand is an ethical one.
2. Consult authoritative sources to see how physicians generally deal with such issues.
3. Consider alternative solutions.
4. Discuss your proposed solution with those whom it will affect.
5. Make your decision and act on it.
6. Evaluate your decision and be prepared to act differently in future (in case of objections arising from factual errors, faulty reasoning or conflicting values, etc.).

SUMMARY

Attitude of the society toward medical profession and the outlook of doctors toward their own profession are undergoing tremendous changes with rapid change in socioeconomic status, especially in countries like India. Even then, the medical profession should be viewed differently.

From time to time, various codes of medical ethics have been formulated to uphold the nobility of medical profession. The Indian Medical Council Regulations 2002 are also a step in the same direction, despite some of its fallacies. Following code of medical ethics in letter and spirit is the need of the hour to retain the status of this profession as a noble, fulfilling but yet exciting profession. Doctors should adopt a more humane approach toward patient care. Ethical principles of medical research enshrined in the ethical guidelines of ICMR and WMA declaration of Helsinki should be followed more honestly.[2] The need for a comprehensive overhaul of undergraduate curriculum with regard to ethical and legal medical practices was long felt.[9] Fortunately, this seems to be moving in right direction with the new MCI curriculum for undergraduates, which may hopefully succeed in achieving the highest ethical standards expected out of the doctors of future generations.

SUMMARY WITH KEY MESSAGES AND PEARLS

- Medical ethics is a *"combination of moral principles and values that are applied to take judgments in medical education, practice and research."*
- Several codes of medical ethics have been prescribed including Code of Hammurabi, Hippocratic Oath, Charaka Samhita, Sushruta Samhita as well as the modern day International Code of Medical Ethics, Indian Medical Council (Professional Conduct, Etiquette and Ethics) Regulations, and AAD code of medical ethics for dermatologists.
- Code of medical ethics is based on the four basic principles of respect for patient's autonomy, beneficence (patient's best interest), justice, and nonmaleficence (do no harm).
- Indian Medical Council (Professional Conduct, Etiquette and Ethics) Regulations (2002; amended up to 8th October 2016) deal extensively with duties and responsibilities of physicians toward patients, society, professional colleagues and pharmaceutical companies as well as professional misconduct and its punishment.

- Following the code of medical ethics, such as Indian Medical Council (Professional Conduct, Etiquette and Ethics) Regulations, in letter and spirit is the need of the hour to retain the status of medical profession as a noble and fulfilling profession, devoted to service of humanity.
- However, in the Indian context, there is an urgent need to further amend these regulations to address the modern day concerns such as violence against doctors by patients/attendants, spurious/false consumer forum litigations against doctors/hospitals, double registration/re-registration of degrees in multiple states, surrogate advertisements by nonallopathic medical systems, surrogate advertisements by pharma companies, unnecessarily stringent restrictions on advertisement/display of dermatologists' qualifications (basic and additional) in the modern era of internet and internet based media, competition to dermatologists from unqualified practitioners/beauty clinic chains, etc.

REFERENCES

1. Kamdar BC. Dermatological practice & medical ethics. In: Srinivas P (Ed). A Dermatologists' Perspective of Medical Ethics and Consumer Protection Act: An IADVL Book, 1st edition. Kolkata: IADVL-Printco; 2007. pp. 57-66.
2. Ramana KV, Kandi S, Boinpally PR. Ethics in medical education, practice, and research: An insight. Ann Trop Med Public Health. 2013;6: 599-602.
3. Pandya SK. History of medical ethics in India. Eubios J Asian and Int Bioeth. 2000;10:40-4.
4. Boyd KM. Medical ethics: principles, persons, and perspectives: from controversy to conversation. J Med Ethics. 2005;31:481-6.
5. Kuroyonagi T. Historical transition in medical ethics—challenges of the World Medical Association. J Med Assoc J. 2013;56(4): 220-6.
6. American Academy of Dermatology. (2014). Code of Medical Ethics For Dermatologists. [online] Available from: https://www.aad.org/Forms/Policies/Uploads/AR/AR%20CODE%20OF%20MEDICAL%20ETHICS%20FOR%20DERMATOLOGISTS.pdf [Last accessed December, 2018].
7. MCI Code of Medical Ethics- IMC (Professional Conduct, Etiquette and Ethics) – Regulations 2002; amended up to October 2016.
8. Srinivas P. Consumer Protection Act and dermatological practice. In: Srinivas P (Ed). A Dermatologists' Perspective of Medical Ethics and Consumer Protection Act: An IADVL Book, 1st edition. Kolkata: IADVL-Printco; 2007. pp. 7-14.
9. Eckles ER, Meslin EM, Gaffney M, et al. Medical ethics education: Where are we? Where should we be going? A review. Acad Med. 2005;80: 1143-52.

7.9 Out-of-Court Settlement: Why, When, and How

Venkataram Mysore, Subodh P Sirur, Satish Bhat, KHS Rao

INTRODUCTION

It is generally accepted that medicolegal cases have increased several folds over the last few years. Generally, a medical practitioner is taken by surprise and does not know how to react, when the notice hits him/her. Every practitioner should expect a medicolegal case at some point and be prepared, if it indeed happens. This is particularly so in the prevailing situation in India, where healers are often treated as predators. It can be said that, in the authors' opinion, the situation changed drastically, after a TV reality show exaggerated the death of a renal transplant recipient who had succumbed to toxic epidermal necrolysis. The patient was a doctor's wife working as a therapist abroad and was compensated with several crores.

WARNING SIGNS OF A MEDICOLEGAL SITUATION

The most important part of being prepared is to recognize a potential medicolegal case early. Here are some tips to recognize a potential legal situation:
- When something has gone adverse in a case, results are not as anticipated or a complication has happened.
- Patient is unhappy either for above reasons or over payment issues.
- Relatives argue in reception over different issues.
- Request for a patient's records. This should not be ignored; patient records cannot be refused, but should be handed over only to the patient or an authorized person. An acknowledgment is to be taken for having received the documents. Whatever documents are requested should be handed over, without any modification.
- Doctor bashing happens in the media: whether conventional (print/online) or social media.

It should be noted that in cosmetic surgeries, such issues can arise months or even years after surgery as results are often delayed and doctor may not remember all facts of the case. Hence, proper documentation is vital.

PROCESS OF LAW IN NEGLIGENCE

At this stage, it is important to understand the process of law for medical negligence. An outline is presented here as this is dealt in detail in other chapters:
- *Step 1*: Patient sends a notice. The claim officially begins with the issuance of a legal notice. The legal notice outlines what the claimant wants, and gives a time frame for reply. The letter also serves as a warning that you will be taken to court, if you do not comply with the demands in the legal notice within the said time frame.
- *Step 2*: Doctor decides whether to defend or settle.
- *Step 3*: If doctor decides to defend, he responds to notice.
- *Step 4*: If patient is unsatisfied with the reply, and is convinced there is a deficiency of service and negligence, the patient files a case and court serves a summons. Even at this stage, doctor can choose to settle if he/she wishes or to respond to summons and defend.

On the occasions where the reply by the doctor answers the queries/allegations satisfactorily, with facts and information that the patient may not have revealed to their advocate, the patient's advocate may advise the patient to drop the matter there itself.
- *Step 5*: Once matter is in court/consumer forum, a notice is sent to the doctor, who responds to the same and the proceeding starts. The process is usually long, with arguments and counterarguments by the two parties. The onus is on the patient to prove negligence. Evidence is presented and witnesses are called and they can be cross-examined. The ensuing judgment can then be followed by a review or appeal. Out-of-court settlement is possible at this stage also.

If both the parties agree on an out-of-court settlement, the memorandum of settlement detailing the terms of settlement and the settlement, is executed with formal approval of the court.

RESPOND OR TO DEFEND

There are two choices in every claim on how to respond, settle the case out of court, or defend to trial. This is not a decision to be taken lightly; if the doctor settles too easily, it is a sign of panic, and he will be regarded as a soft target; if he defends then he has to follow the long process and pay for the costs. *This decision needs a proper consultation with a lawyer, with all the factual information, which will include a copy of the patient's records, preferably in consultation with another medical expert. The medical expert is consulted to give an impartial opinion as to whether there is any deviation from accepted guidelines of care.*

However, in India, doctors tend to be secretive and often do not wish to consult another doctor, which is not recommended.

WHY OUT-OF-COURT SETTLEMENT?

Not all cases reach judicial and quasi-judicial authorities but there is no data available on the number of matters that get settled out of court. Some cases do get settled after a legal notice is issued or even after a threat of legal notice or a threat of filing of a consumer complaint or a criminal complaint. No doctor wants to get entangled in litigation. There are certain factors, which would favor an out-of-court settlement whereas there would be other factors, which would not favor such a recourse. A balanced decision should be taken based on the facts and circumstances of the matter after consultation of the defense team and the medical experts in that field.

There are several concerns about the process of adjudication that cross the minds of the affected Doctors, as well as their immediate well-wishers, which may make them initially inclined to think of a settlement:

- The whole trial process is stressful—time consuming, may drag on for years. *The author is aware of an incident where a case of death after angioplasty got dragged on for several years as the patient was a judge and therefore the case was taken right up to the Supreme Court. The anesthetist and cardiac surgeons in the case came under immense stress, with a possible adverse judgment dangling over them.*
- Prohibitive costs of defense.
- Frequent visits to the court affect practice; this may involve traveling to another place where the court is located. Though it is not mandatory that the doctor attends each hearing after having appointed a duly authorized representative or a lawyer, it is in the interests of the doctor to do so.

An example for this is:
  - *In a case, the patient, in a claim for compensation for poor results after hair transplantation, said he bought a laser machine for hair growth on doctor's advice, and included the cost of the machine in the compensation claim. The doctor had not advised the machine, but what had happened was that the patient had sought advice on the machine and the doctor had written on the back of a prescription, the name of the website of the machine, for the patient to study and get more information. Doctor could claim that this was just for education of the patient and not a prescription and hence escaped any adverse outcome in court.*

- Even if facts are in favor of the doctor, the lawyer has to present them properly—often the lawyer may not be fully aware of the medical aspects, and hence close coordination is essential between the two. This consumes considerable time and expense.
- Often media gets into the issue, and adverse publicity affects the reputation and the practice of the doctor.

- Lastly, a doctor does not basically like the idea of standing in trial.
- Often patient complains in several agencies—Civil Court, Criminal Court, Medical Council, Women's Commission, Human Rights Commission, etc. It is difficult to fight in so many different agencies for an individual doctor.

A decision regarding "out-of-court settlement" should preferably be taken after involving the local medical fraternity—whether the Indian Medical Association (IMA) or any other medical association or an expert group related to the Doctor's area and after due consideration of all facts as outlined above. The decision should not be taken as a reaction to the pressure created by the impending proceedings, as this is the very impression that the patient's lawyer wants to create, to have an upper hand in the negotiations that would inevitably happen, if the matter does proceed for a settlement. The approval for a settlement should be seen as an option agreed to by the doctor and his/her lawyer, out of compassion for the patient more than anything else. It should be emphatically conveyed in no uncertain terms, that the doctor is more than willing to fight the case, else most of the benefits that the doctor gets from a settlement may be lost.

A Peer group, which gives the accused doctor moral support, and ensures the decision for settlement is not taken out of pressure, but rather on genuine grounds is of great help to the doctor. In the personal experience of one of the authors as the convener of the Medicolegal Cell of an Association of Specialist Doctors (AMC Mangalore), a group of 10 odd doctors committed to the cause have been meeting at least one evening a week, for the last 6–7 years. This gives a strong sense of support to all members of the association that their colleagues are available in the event of any matter, any time during the progress of their matter with the authorities.

The most accepted scenario in which an out-of-court settlement is recommended by all experts is when there is an "indefensible case." Classic examples include:
- Mop in the abdomen
- Operating on the wrong side of the body
- Injury to an organ/structure during the course of the surgery—ureter during a gynecological procedure.

There is no way such cases can be defended in court, by even the most brilliant lawyer. By having an out-of-court settlement, there is an additional benefit for the medical fraternity, besides the benefits to the patient and the doctor involved. Only a case that goes for trial, and is adjudicated finally, makes its way to law books, literature, and journals, and can be used as a "Case Law" or a precedent. By having an out-of-court settlement, the fraternity is avoiding a Case Law with a higher compensation amount, which the judgment may have.

WAYS OF SETTLING

- The most common way, which is not often realized, is in the clinic, before patient serves a notice, when there is a warning sign as mentioned above. As soon as patient is noticed to be unhappy, the physician identifies the potential of the situation and takes preventive action. This may be in the form of free treatment, procedures to correct the problem, or even refund of the cost of treatment.

In esthetic dermatology, there can be several examples:
- In cases of laser hair removal, additional sessions can be offered in cases of lack of response.

- In case of hair transplantation, additional touch up sessions can be done to correct lack of density.
- In some cases, refund or partial refund of treatment cost may be done. For example, in one case, patient said, doctor, I have got only 50% of result, so please refund 50% of costs, I do not want to go to court.
- A patient who underwent botulinum toxin treatment was unhappy over lack of results. Since he was from another country, he could not come for a touch up session. He threatened the doctor to complain to medical council, to take him to court and report media. Doctor counseled him about need for touch up session, and arranged a treatment with a doctor whom he knew. The condition improved and the case was settled.

Note: Offering free treatment or refund of fees carries the risk of being taken as an admission of guilt on the part of the doctor. Such allegations have been the grounds for claims for compensation in some cases. If such a course is found to be desirable then it is essential that the patient is counseled and explained that the refund of fees or free treatment is way of good will and in no way indicates admission of negligence or deficiency of service. It is preferable to have this in the written form. Refund of fees or free treatment can be part of the terms of the settlement.

It is advisable to ensure proper documentation in all such cases, as to why refund or additional sessions are being done with the consent signed by patient, in presence of a witness. All guidelines of care are to be followed thoroughly.

- This can also be done after a notice is issued, with involvement of the lawyer as mentioned above. At this stage, it is preferable to involve a lawyer or a mutual friend and ensure proper documentation.

Documentation of settlement: The document should state the details of settlement, compensation provided, with specific confirmation that the patient will not pursue the case in any court, and will not indulge in any action on social media or visual or print media adverse to the doctor. It should also mention among other points that the doctor does not admit any lack of duty of care in the management of the patient or any deficiency of service on the part of the doctor or his staff, nurses, and others.

MAKING THE DECISION TO FIGHT

When not to Settle?

Just as there are reasons to settle, there are also reasons to fight.

- The doctor believes there is no negligence, and hence no liability, patient is being unreasonable.

  For example, the first author successfully fought a case in consumer court, where he believed he was fully correct in every way and decided to fight just to get the experience of a trial. The attitude was, "if I cannot fight this case, how will I fight case which may be difficult." Of course, he was aided by the fact that documentation was perfect with signatures by patient about 10 places for every aspect in hair transplantation. The patient had claimed lack of results after hair transplantation and blamed the doctor for poor outcome. The author produced an informed consent document in which the patient mentioned that he does not want to take any drug after hair transplantation to prevent future baldness, and the court agreed that "patient was negligent, not the doctor."

- *The doctor is of the opinion that there is a liability on his part, but the demands of the patient are unreasonable.*

In the personal experience of one of the authors, a lawyer sent a legal notice to his treating dermatologist for a side effect of a drug. The financial compensation sought was not in commensurate with the alleged loss or injury suffered by the lawyer. Three rounds of discussion did not yield any fruitful outcomes. It was suggested not to settle the matter, if the demand for compensation was unreasonable and excessive and that no further negotiations were possible under such circumstances. Few days later, the lawyer voluntarily agreed to the initially offered compensation as settlement of the matter.

It is always preferable that the discussion on settlement is initiated by the complainant or his lawyer. Very often, when the discussion is initiated by the doctor or his defense team, it is presumed that the doctor has been negligent and is therefore willing to settle the matter. The negotiating power of the doctor and his team could then be compromised. A statement for settlement can also be made before the court where the matter is being heard. However, it should be made abundantly clear that the defending doctor does not admit any negligence or deficiency of service.

There are occasions where criminal complaints have been filed or verbal threats of filing complaints before different judicial and quasi-judicial authorities are made and the doctor is intimidated into making a payment as compensation. Compensation should not be paid unless there is a memorandum of settlement.

For example, the first author is aware of a case where a chemical peel resulted in pigmentation. The patient behaved aggressively in the clinic with a group of four well-built individuals. The doctor panicked and went to the nearby police station. The concerned inspector offered to mediate the case, and the case was settled with a payment of ₹ 25,000 to the patient, even though the pigmentation was temporary and could have been easily treated and hence the doctor was not at fault. This was clearly a case of intimidation.

Further, if the doctor has a professional indemnity insurance, payment of amount of settlement should not be made without the concurrence of the insurance company in writing. If a promise is made or money is paid as compensation as an out of court settlement without the written concurrence of the insurance company then the insurance company will not entertain a claim under the policy for reimbursement of such amount.

It is notable that cases of "out-of-court settlement" do not get reported and the information regarding such settlement or the terms of settlement does not come in public domain.

POINTS TO REMEMBER

- Out-of-court settlement is an option, which should be exercised in appropriate cases.
- It can help a doctor to avoid the protracted trial process.
- It should not be pursued in an overenthusiastic manner by the doctor, as it may be interpreted as an admission of guilt/negligence/deficiency of service.

- It should be done only after proper consultation with experts, both in law and medicine.
- A memorandum of settlement should be entered into between the doctor and the patient/legal representative of the patient as the case may be. Such a memorandum of settlement can be filed before the court/forum where the matter is pending following which the court/forum will close the matter.
- Inform the insurance company, if one has a professional indemnity policy about the possibility of having an "out-of-court settlement" and take their written concurrence for such a course.

7.10 Healthcare Professionals and Consumer Protection Act, 2019

Atulkumar K Shah

INTRODUCTION

Healthcare service is a procedure performed on a person for diagnosing or treating a disease (https://medical-dictionary.thefreedictionary.com/health+care+service). Trained, semitrained, and unskilled personnel get involved in this exercise in the healthcare organizations or healthcare institutions. The National Accreditation Board for Hospitals and Healthcare Providers (NABH) wing of Quality Council of India (QCI) has even come out with concept of small healthcare organizations (SHCO). The dictionary of modern medicine goes on to further define healthcare service as "a business entity that provides inpatient or outpatient testing or treatment of human disease or dysfunction; dispensing of drugs or medical devices for treating human disease or dysfunction." So the commercial angle is already added to these services which from time immemorial were considered humanitarian services, and physician to be compared to the supreme.

शरीरे जर्जरीभूते व्याधिग्रस्ते कलेवरे।
(sharIrE jarjarIbhUtE vyAdhigrastE kalebarE |)

औषधं जाह्नवीतोयं वैद्यो नारायणो हरिः।।
(auShadham jaanhavItOyam vaidyO nArAyaNO harih ||)

The Consumer Protection Act (COPRA), 2019 that finally got through both houses of Parliament and received assent of the President of India on 9th August, 2019 shall come to be known as Act No. 35 of 2019 (http://egazette.nic.in/WriteReadData/2019/210422.pdf). There were discussions, articles, and comments on exclusion of healthcare services from the draft bill and series of social media messages brought relief among healthcare professions, which was short lived, only till the act came in prints.

SERVICE IN CONSUMER PROTECTION ACT, 2019

Definition of services in the subsection 42 of Section 2 in Chapter 1 states that "service" means service of any description which is made available to potential users and includes, but not limited to, the provision of facilities in connection with banking, financing, insurance, transport, processing, supply of electrical or other energy, telecom, boarding or lodging or both, housing construction, entertainment, amusement or the purveying of news or other information, but does not include the rendering of any service free of charge or under a contract of personal service;...."

In some previous draft, there was inclusion of word "Health Care" in the list that includes banking, finance, etc. The same was removed from the above subsection, presumably after representation from healthcare providers. The author agrees with many legal experts who feel that the fact that healthcare services are not explicitly excluded from this definition and the existence of phrase "not limited to" keeps the window open for inclusion of healthcare services under ambit of COPRA 2019. In view of this legal language interplay, the original Supreme Court judgment prevails and is summarized here.

VP Shantha Judgment of 1995 in Supreme Court

Delivered on 13th November 1995, Justice SC Agrawal for himself and Justice Kuldip Singh and Justice BL Hansaria; wrote following conclusions: "...... *(1) Service rendered to a patient by a medical practitioner (except where the doctor renders service free of charge to every patient or under a contract of personal service), by way of consultation, diagnosis and treatment, both medicinal and surgical, would fall within the ambit of 'service' as defined in Section 2(1)(o) of the Act.* **(Old Act – emphasis inserted)**

(2) The fact that medical practitioners belong to the medical profession and are subject to the disciplinary control of the Medical Council of India (MCI) and/or State Medical Councils constituted under the provisions of the Indian Medical Council Act would not exclude the services rendered by them from the ambit of the Act. **(Old Act – emphasis inserted).......**" https://indiankanoon.org/doc/723973)

Poonam Verma Judgment of 1996 in Supreme Court

In this Hon'ble Apex Court defined Medical.... "Negligence as a tort is the breach of a duty caused by omission to do something which a reasonable man would do or doing something which a prudent and reasonable man would not do".... The definition involves the following constituents: (1) a legal duty to exercise due care; (2) breach of the duty; and (3) consequential damages. The COPRA also got amended on these lines in 2002 and the negligence of medical professional came within the expression of "deficiency in service." Thus, when doctors do not perform duties to the best of ability and with proper care and caution, it is deficiency as per COPRA (https://indiankanoon.org/doc/611474].

With legal interplay of these apex court judgments, consumer forums and commissions were now given the responsibility to decide what a due care in any circumstances is, and was there deficiency in that due care, and if there was any deficiency, was there any damage. The new COPRA 2019 has not made any changes to these legal responsibilities but added several other points.

WHAT IS MORE IN CONSUMER PROTECTION ACT, 2019

1. A patient can file his complaint with a commission at a district or state where he resides, or where he works and not

necessarily where the doctor or the hospital in question that provided health care; exists.

2. Consumer commissions can refer matter to mediation cell, during hearings, or if parties so pray or probably even before they take-up the matter. The rules for this part of the act are awaited. It, however, seems that this step is a good initiative to reduce burden on consumer fora. Section 74 in Chapter 5 of the Act talks about establishing district, state and central mediation cells. However, once route of mediation is chosen, further appeals cannot be made.

3. Pecuniary jurisdiction of the District Commission has been raised to claims worth ₹ 1 crore and less. The name of this district authority is elevated from forum to commission. The pecuniary limit for State Commission will be up to ₹ 10 crore and for National Commission beyond ₹ 10 crore. Healthcare personnel and organizations will have to rush to purchase matching professional indemnity cover.

4. Additional product liability clause in the Act will put responsibility on healthcare personnel and organizations to make sure that the quality of medicines, consumables and metal/nonmetal implants is proper. Entire Chapter 6 of the Act is dedicated to product liability. Section 83 states that "....A product liability action may be brought by a complainant against a product manufacturer or a product service provider or a product seller, as the case may be, for any harm caused to him on account of a defective product." Patient will be free to ask for additional compensation for harm caused by defective products, use of which was decided by healthcare service provider. Many consumer forum complaints may come up against healthcare service providers not for deficiency or negligence, but for faulty products used.

5. An Advisory Council is to be formed at different levels. The highest one will be termed as Central Consumer Protection Council (CCPC). There will also be State Consumer Protection Council and District Consumer Protection Council. In addition, there will be Central Consumer Protection Authority (CCPA) headed by Chief Commissioner that shall regulate matters relating to violation of rights of consumers, unfair trade practices and false or misleading advertisements which are prejudicial to the interests of public and consumers and to promote, protect, and enforce the rights of consumers as a class.

6. Subsection (11) of Section 2 of Chapter 1, defines deficiency as "....any fault, imperfection, shortcoming or inadequacy in the quality, nature and manner of performance which is required to be maintained by or under any law for the time being in force or has been undertaken to be performed by a person in pursuance of a contract or otherwise in relation to any service and includes:
    (i) Any act of negligence or omission or commission by such person which causes loss or injury to the consumer; and
    (ii) Deliberate withholding of relevant information by such person to the consumer";

    This addition, the author feels, will have effect on medical consent. Additionally the new Act speaks of filing complaint against unfair contracts. Since medical consent is also considered as contract, new avenue will open up. Again complaints against unfair contracts cannot be filed with

District Commission, and healthcare providers shall have to respond to such happening at state and national commissions only.

7. Subsection (18) of section 2 of Chapter 1, defines "endorsement", in relation to an advertisement, as:
   (i) Any message, verbal statement, demonstration; or
   (ii) Depiction of the name, signature, likeness or other identifiable personal characteristics of an individual; or
   (iii) Depiction of the name or seal of any institution or organization, which makes the consumer to believe that it reflects the opinion, finding or experience of the person making such endorsement;

   Further Clause (1) defines Advertisement as "......any audio or visual publicity, representation, endorsement or pronouncement made by means of light, sound, smoke, gas, print, electronic media, internet or website and includes any notice, circular, label, wrapper, invoice or such other documents;

   It is likely that the rules under new National Medical Commission Act 30 of 2019 (http://egazette.nic.in/WriteReadData/2019/210357.pdf) may add on aspect of advertisement, so there will be legal interplay between Code of Ethics 2002, till they are repealed, rules under NMC Act and rules under COPRA 2019.

   Section 89 warns that "...Any manufacturer or service provider who causes a false or misleading advertisement to be made which is prejudicial to the interest of consumers shall be punished with imprisonment for a term which may extend to two years and with fine which may extend to ten lakh rupees; and for every subsequent offence, be punished with imprisonment for a term which may extend to five years and with fine which may extend to fifty lakh rupees..." Only solace is that complaint attracting this section can be filed only by the central authority. Endorser will also be punished on the same lines with fine of up to ₹ 10 lakh and 1 year ban on further endorsements, repeat offence attracting fine up to ₹ 50 lakh and 3 year ban on endorsements.

8. Penalty for noncompliance of the orders of the district, State or National Commission is made strict. Section 72 reads that "...(1) Whoever fails to comply with any order made by the District Commission or the State Commission or the National Commission, as the case may be, shall be punishable with imprisonment for a term which shall not be less than one month, but which may extend to three years, or with fine, which shall not be less than twenty-five thousand rupees, but which may extend to one lakh rupees, or with both." And

   "...(2) Notwithstanding anything contained in the Code of Criminal Procedure, 1973, the District Commission, the State Commission or the National Commission, as the case may be, shall have the power of a Judicial Magistrate of first class for the trial of offences under subsection (1), and on conferment of such powers, the District Commission or the State Commission or the National Commission, as the case may be, shall be deemed to be a Judicial Magistrate of first class for the purposes of the Code of Criminal Procedure, 1973." (Act 2 of 1974)

9. There may be possibility of filing of complaint electronically as has been stated in Section 35. Further clarification on the procedure and web porter shall be available when respective rules are announced. The act seems to be silent as to within what time limit the first complaint can be filed after the cause of action has aroused, probably the rules shall specify it; however after filing the complaint, the admissibility or rejection shall have to be stated in 21 days. If no communication comes in 21 days the complaint will be considered as admitted. There may be possibility of video conferencing for hearings and appeals. Rules are awaited.
10. The limitation period for appeal to higher commission is fixed at 30 days as per subsection (3) of Section 73. State and National Commissions may condone reasonable delay as per this subsection. The period of appeal shall be 45 days if the subject matter is on facts of law as per Section 41, but after depositing 50% of amount of compensation if ordered so by lower commission. No appeals shall be entertained if compromise was reached through mediation. The act says that a complaint has to be disposed of within period of 3 months after the opposite party had received the notice, unless some analysis or testing of commodities is required in which case it is within 5 months.

Reader can refer to judgments of National Consumer Disputes Redressal Commission (NCDRC) in cases of medical negligence to have a feel of what direction the Consumer Commissions are heading to. All in all it appears to be a settled opinion now that healthcare services continue to remain under ambit of COPRA 2019.

SECTION 8: Doctor–Patient Interface

8.1 Hand-holding (Mentoring) in Healthcare Practice

Rakesh Bharti, Rabinder Kant Sikri

INTRODUCTION

Holding one's hand always shows affection and provides lot of mental satisfaction to patients in their distress. The traditional concept of hand-holding in practice is now better known as *mentoring in practice* which is totally *patient oriented*.

Mentoring is the key to the development of healthcare practice and can play an important role in advancing the quality of care to all humanity. Mentoring is defined as a process whereby an experienced, knowledgeable, and empathetic person guides another individual in the development and reexamination of their own ideas and learnings. Therefore, mentoring is all about lending a hand. All of us require hand-holding and close monitoring from time to time, but it becomes very important when one feels demotivated due to their health conditions.

Mentoring is more than "giving advice" and disclosing your experiences during practice. It is all about motivating and empowering the patient to identify his/her own issues/goals and further facilitates them to find ways to resolve (not by doing it for them or expecting them to do it the way I did it) by understanding and respecting different ways of handling the situation. Mentoring is not counseling or therapy though the mentor may help the mentee to access more specialized avenues of help if it becomes apparent that this would be the best way forward.

KEY FOCUS AREAS

The focus of mentoring in healthcare practice must be around the followings areas:
- Social communication and interaction
- Relationships
- Pre- and postdiagnostic support
- Managing stress and anxiety
- Anger management

If we put all above areas in one basket, then psychology, "a study of human mind and behavior," plays a vital role for mentoring

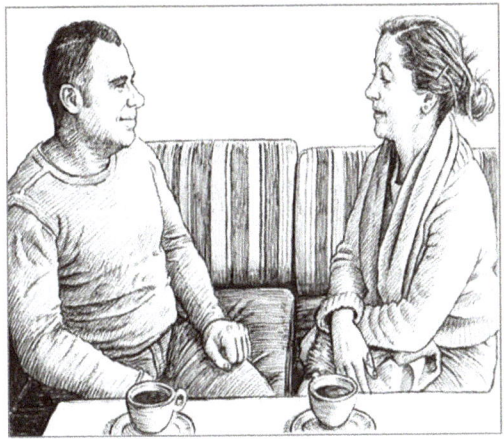

in healthcare practice. This will cover all psychological reasons why and how patient have acted in such behavior during pre- and postdiagnostic stage. Mentoring in practice is rather more powerful tool in our hands as compared to physically holding hands of a patient. This is one of the important keys which will facilitate to open locks of misunderstandings and provide win–win situation such as:

- Prevent unnecessary litigation
- Making friends for ever
- Achieve real objective of doctor (service to weak society)

KEY PRINCIPLES

Mentorship comes in many flavors and each practitioner should follow the key principles for achieving the best results during mentoring in practice. Further, we always underestimate the power of a touch, smile, kind word, listening ear, honest compliment, and smallest act of caring, all of which have a lot of potential to turn around the life of a patient. Benefits from this act of humanity are too large but the key summary is as follows:

- *Relationship is priority*: For effective mentorship to achieve results there needs to be baseline chemistry between a doctor and patient. At best, role of relationship between two must be as *common people* instead of titles such as boss and subordinate.
- *Great stress reliever:* Our skin gets more sensitive when cortisol is rushing through our bloodstream, therefore, have a significantly larger *impact of stress*. Mentoring during practice decreases the level of stress hormone called cortisol.
- *Boosts love and bonding*: Oxytocin is the hormone responsible for love and bonding. Oxytocin strengthens empathy and communication between patient and doctor, which is proven to be a contributing factor for *long-lasting* and happy relationships.
- *Character versus expertise:* Practitioners have a lot of *competency* and expertise in their field but mentoring must go beyond competency and focus on facilitating shaping the patient's character, values, self-awareness, empathy, and capacity for respect.
- *Devotion—patient versus organization:* In any organization of health care, we all want to retain good doctors and relevant staff. The success of an organization is directly linked to trustworthy and devoted doctors. But during mentoring in practice; devotion toward patient has an upper hand than the organization. The best doctor always avoids overriding the dreams of their patient and creates *high level of trust.*
- *Relieves pain:* While enduring pain, patient have the natural reflex to tighten their muscles. It is always easier to experience the *relieve of pain* during mentoring in practice.
- *Fights fear:* The human brain always responds to sudden stimulation using adrenaline; this stimulation gets our blood pumping and releases high levels of cortisol throughout our body. During these moments, mentoring during practice plays an important role *to fight fear.*
- *Safe heart:* Besides relieving stress, mentoring (hand-holding) lowers blood pressure, which is one of the major contributors to heart disease. When we are with our patient, we are not just easing stress and improving our relationships but we provide a comfortable sensation that facilitate toward safety *of our heart.* The power of a warm touch goes beyond the health benefits to the heart.

- *Sense of security and comfort:* Simply mentoring is a source of sense of security for the patient. The security that the doctor provides to the patient during mentoring turns around the *behavior* and way of thinking of patient such as insecurity disappears and allows patient to conquer obstacles and achieve desired results.

IMPORTANCE OF MENTORING (HAND-HOLDING)

So let's try to understand how emotionally and psychologically important is mentoring in day to day practice. Once the practitioner follows the above principles in practice, then it is important to know the mind-set of the patient which is primarily as "I do not demand a lot of my doctor's time. I just wish that he should understand my situation for at least 5 minutes and commit or provide his whole mind just once to diagnose my ill health. Without such understanding, I consider myself totally alone with ailment."

Readers, please try to recall, how many doctors you can remember respectfully as good professionals, when sitting on the other side of the table. We are sure you must have few names in your memory, of those doctors, who were "Good," not only as clinicians but also as human beings.

Presently, in the competitive environment, time has always a prime choice in practice. During the busy schedule of daily practice, most of the doctors may fail to notice what is right in front of them, we may be more concerned about those waiting for their turn in your waiting area. In order to see more and more patients, we ignore the time and concerns of the patient sitting in front of us. We use our clinical skill passionately (It is a different matter that in the process we may miss some important points of history or even miss physical signs) and dispose of the patient. Key incidents from our personal experiences as a patient/attendant and a doctor, which shall explain the importance of hand-holding (mentoring) during healthcare practice, is acknowledged below—*one step in mentoring is the beginning of a long journey.*

Incident 1

After superannuation from public sector bank, my (Sikri) parents made surprise visit to my residence during July 1986. One early morning, my father could not walk properly and was feeling a lot of discomfort. Immediately I called a very senior dermatologist and fixed an appointment. I reached the doctor's cabin along with my brother (a doctor himself), while my father was still following us slowly writhing with pain and discomfort, entering the cabin. Senior dermatologist well known for his competency in profession could quickly gauze the situation. He asked me to show the lesions. On seeing them and coming to know the agony of my father, which has been there for the last 1 day (father did not tell the family thinking not to trouble the busy son, a doctor, i.e., my brother), the dermatologist was slightly annoyed. He started rebuking us for ignoring the ailing father and delaying the treatment by 24 hours. Passionately, he diagnosed him as a patient of herpes zoster and prescribed the medicine. The perfect display lasted only for few minutes and the prescription was in our hands, even before my father could sit in front of the doctor. My father was not comfortable with the doctor and was not satisfied with his attitude at all. He refused to take the prescribed medicine. His point of view was "no interaction of the doctor with him— the patient". We were forced to approach another doctor (less reputed and not that senior), who also diagnosed the same disease and prescribed same medication but after mentoring (hand-holding) with the patient. An example of a good doctor (holding hands) and an OK doctor (not showing empathy for the patient) was in front of our eyes. Despite his reputation, the senior dermatologist could never become our family's physician. The example underlines the importance of the fact *that mentoring is above competency during practice.*

Incident 2

Another practical experience, I (Bharti) still recollect the name of Dr Alex Abraham, a well-known neurophysician. My mother was fighting her life's battle against Gullain–Barré syndrome. On strong recommendation of my senior faculty and assurances of personal attention, I visited the said doctor posted as the head of neurology in a premier hospital. While wheeling in my mother to the ICU of that premier hospital, right at the door, four doctors surrounded my mother and me. One was asking the history, other was drawing blood samples, another was examining her reflexes and consciousness, etc. But Dr Alex was nowhere to be seen. My perception before reaching there was that at that critical time, Dr Alex should have come personally and examined my mother. Feeling cheated to my perception, I was irritated and my first encounter with the situation was not comfortable. I could not control my emotion and shouted "where is Dr Alex, why do not you guys call him first, I am a doctor and she is my mother."

Suddenly a hand touched my shoulder and one short statured doctor introduced to me, "I am Alex Abraham." This was the beginning of a journey of my understanding the value of hand-holding in my professional domain. The next 7 days of my mother's life and my interaction with Dr Alex engrave long-lasting impression on my brain. Despite his clinical skills, his busy schedule and fighting a losing battle always kept me on my toes. I was not very happy with the treatment offered to my mother and even sought a second opinion from one of the premier institute of the country, Postgraduate Institute of Medical Education and Research (PGIMER), Chandigarh, which was on different line of treatment. The imminent occurred and I lost my mother.

Losing a mother is the biggest trauma for any human being. The assuring guidance offered by Dr Alex through the entire hospital procedure like shifting of dead body and clearing of dues at leisure was truly heartwarming. The dissatisfaction can be rubbed off by *this type of "hand-holding."*

Incident 3

This is about a lady patient who was suffering from systemic lupus erythematosus (SLE), a chronic disease, and her return to my clinic after a gap of 7 years or so.

She had been my regular patient since 2001, when she first came with a photoallergic drug reaction. After few months, she came back with a discoid patch and after complete diagnostics, she was diagnosed as a patient of "Discoid lupus erythematosus (DLE)." She was unlucky enough to progress to SLE. (The risk of progression to SLE in patients with DLE was demonstrated to be higher than previously reported, the reported rates were 16.7% progression within 3 years of diagnosis in one study and 17% progression within a mean time of 8 years in a second study.) One day during the discussion about her disease, inadvertently I informed her that her ailment was lifelong. Actually my plain speaking words crushed her so much that she did not want to live.

While putting the record straight, my words were not adequate/relevant (as I recollect from her communications on returning after 7 years). "Not appropriate" is a milder expression, actually my words or plain speaking hurt her so much that when she went back home, she started cooking the idea of signing off her life prematurely. Thanks to a better doctor who could hold her hands at the right time, that she lived on. After 7 years or so another doctor referred her to my clinic. *On retrospection, I realize that hand-holding is a continuous phenomenon and it is not a onetime process.*

CONCLUSION

"Only wearer knows where the shoe pinches," this saying no more remains a proverb when the doctor himself becomes a patient. During enhancing the capability of a good medical practitioner, one must learn the concept and principles of "Hand-holding." This is beyond the learnings of your own medical science. Hugs to untouchables of society like those suffering from stigmatized diseases like leprosy, HIV/AIDS, vitiligo can immediately bring life to semi-comatose, depressed souls (as patient) sitting in front of you.

To sum up, in the words of 20th century theologian Henri Nouwen, who wrote the book, "Out of Solitude". When we honestly ask ourselves which person in our lives means the most to us, we often find that it is those who have chosen to share our pain and touch our wounds with warm and tender hand.

Holding hands is an ongoing process and all practitioners must adapt and implement the concept of *"Mentoring in Health Care Practice."*

ACKNOWLEDGMENT

The authors humbly acknowledge the help of Dr Prateek Bhatia (Assistant Professor, Pediatric Hematology, Department of Pediatrics, Advance Pediatrics Center, PGIMER, Chandigarh-160012) in giving finer inputs to the manuscript.

BIBLIOGRAPHY

1. Broyard A. The New York Times Magazine; Doctor Talk to me. August 26, 1990:17.
2. Epstein RM. Mindful practice. JAMA. 1999;282: 833-9.
3. Fitzpatrick TB, Eisen AZ, Wolff K, Freedberg IM, Austen KF. Dermatology in General Medicine, Textbook and Atlas. New York: McGraw-Hill; 1987. pp. 470-1. pp. 652-4.pp. 1956-7.
4. Grönhagen CM, Fored CM, Granath F, Nyberg F. Cutaneous lupus erythematosus and the association with systemic lupus erythematosus: a population-based cohort of 1088 patients in Sweden. Br J Dermatol. 2011; 164(6):1335-41.
5. Gunderman R, LeLand B. Touch creates a healing bond in health care. 2016;27(2):143-8.
6. Langer EJ. Mindfulness. New York: Addison-Wesley Publishing; 1989. pp. 35-41.
7. Wieczorek IT, Propert KJ, Okawa J, Werth VP. Systemic symptoms in the progression of cutaneous to systemic lupus erythematosus. JAMA Dermatol. 2014;150(3):291-6.

8.2 Handling Celebrity Patients

Jaishree Sharad

INTRODUCTION

A celebrity patient is a patient who has an elevated social status and fame and is influential in the society, e.g., an actor, model, director, producer, musician, sportsman or a politician. Handling a celebrity patient is challenging for the clinician as well as the staff. A celebrity generates attention from each and every staff member, the people in the building, or neighborhood as well as media personnel. Some key points to remember while dealing with a celebrity patient are:

- *Maintain their privacy:* Right from the time an appointment is set, the staff should be trained not to leak out any information regarding the patient's appointment and contact details. Also, allot a time when no other patient is around. However, if sometimes they have to suddenly come in during routine hours, have a separate entrance for the celebrity patient, so that other patients do not see him or her. If there is no extra entrance, take your regular patients into treatment rooms and keep the reception and passageway empty until the celebrity enters the clinic and is taken to the respective treatment room.

  Keep a separate offline database for celebrities and avoid using online apps which will give away details of the celebrity. Alternately, you can use an alias name if you want to keep online records. Both you and your staff should keep the patient's profile and procedures strictly confidential.

- *Follow standard protocols:* Do not change the protocol to match the taste of the celebrity. Make sure you take an informed consent and photographs before doing any esthetic procedures. Let them know (if needed in writing) that you will keep their photographs confidential.
- Communicate well and understand what their needs are. They can often be very finicky about that one fold under the eye or that one wrinkle or dent which you may not be able to treat. Or the melasma that you may not be able to get rid of. Be very clear right in the beginning as to what is possible to treat and what is not or what is the approximate percentage of improvement they should expect. Also tell them the downtime and when actually to expect to see results. Be brutally honest about all the possible side effects. Even if they say they never bruise, you must reiterate the possibility of bruising with injectables. Even bruising becomes a big issue for them. So they must be mentally prepared. Give them every pretreatment and post-treatment instruction in writing apart from explaining to them personally. Have your assistant or nurse present when you are doing any explanation should the celebrity turn around and say he was not informed about something.
- It is better to under promise and over deliver in these patients. Giving them high hopes in pursuit of impressing them or not losing them to your competitor is the worst thing you can do to your own

practice. Do not tell them what they want to hear. Tell them what you want them to understand.
- Do not expect them to be a friend, just be friendly instead. It may seem exciting to party with celebrities but resist the urge to be in their friend circle. You want patients who can rely on you and value your work. Overfriendliness kills the respect and the adulation for a doctor. Besides, their expectations increase and they do not respect your time and effort. Barging in without an appointment, wanting all the attention at a time when the clinic is full of patients becomes a common affair in such cases. In such situations, you either end up upsetting the celebrity or the regular patient. Hence, it is better to have clarity.
- *Do not ask for favors or endorsements:* Even if you manage to gain their trust and confidence, do not ask them to endorse you or promote you on social media or anywhere for that matter. Remember this kind of publicity will disappear as quickly as it appears.
- When celebrities come to you, you are in a superior position and you must command that respect. Secondly, celebrities always value discretion as much as quality work. Abstain from taking any selfies or photographs with the celebrity or talking too much about their work. Avoid asking for any personal favors. Abstain from unnecessary praise or buttering. Train your staff equally well and let them treat the celebrities as they would treat every patient. In fact, train your staff in such a way that they treat every patient as a celebrity.
- Avoid offering free treatments. Charge the standard price that exists. Celebrities demand more time, attention, and sometimes even give you more stress. Cutting your costs will surely not do you any good.
- Be ready to face media queries. Professionals from print and digital media may try and ask you leading questions. Never disclose why the celebrity has come to you. Keep it as simple as "No comments." It is unethical to discuss any patient's profile, leave alone celebrities.
- One should also refrain from any kind of gossip regarding the patient even with friends and family. Teach your staff the same.

Understanding their needs, communicating with clarity, prioritizing their treatments in such a way that the regular patients do not get affected, and maintaining privacy are the ways to handle celebrity patients.

8.3 Managing an Angry/Difficult Patient

Apratim Goel, Zeba Chhapra

The terms cosmetic dermatologists, cosmetic surgeons, and cosmetologists apply to those dermatologists and other specialists who treat patients for cosmetic problems. Since a cosmetic patient is very different from a normal dermatology outpatient, there is an inherent risk of dealing with situations that leave the patient unsatisfied and angry and the doctor with a lawsuit.

Who can run into such a situation? Well this cannot be predicted. Even the most qualified, skilled, and professionally correct doctors can have a complication leading to such a situation in their practice.

Just as we prepare strategies to deal with procedural complications, it is wise to consider how you and your staff will deal with problematic patients. We cannot control everything, but the less left to chance, the smoother becomes our day. 15% of the clinical interactions with patients are perceived by doctors as "difficult".[1] There are several factors that make the doctor–patient interaction challenging. Understanding the reason behind these challenging interactions can help reduce the frequency of such difficult encounters.

UNDERSTANDING DIFFICULT PATIENTS

Difficult patients are those who are demanding, unreasonable, pessimistic, poorly compliant, or sometimes even delusional. However, in some situations, their anger may be for a valid reason which could be a mistake on the part of the treating doctor or clinic. Hence, they may act out of frustration.

Some of the examples being:
- Disease not cured or results lesser than promised
- Expensive treatment or unaffordable
- Unwanted, unexpected side effects
- Long waiting hours

The main issue with difficult patients is the difference of perception between their expectations and reality. As dermatologists, it is our duty to understand our patients and gauge their expectations and plan management accordingly. Our role is to gauge how much they are expecting and set real expectations. Any disconnect in this interaction leads to a difficult patient. We engage with the patient by using empathetic, nonjudgmental, and effective strategies.[4,5]

Here are a few examples of difficult patients and how to manage them:
- *The checklist patient*: This patient will come to you with a long list of concerns. Sit comfortably at eye level to the patient. Listen attentively. Start conversation positively, compliment the patient for their efforts of making the list. Tactfully let the patient know that all concerns may not be dealt together in one consultation as it may consume more time than average. You can also do this by informing the patient to prioritize their concerns and assuring them that all unattended concerns will be dealt with in the next consultation. Keep the conversation patient-centered.[2] Practice patient-centered engagement by reading the patients information and concerns prior to meeting to increase familiarity with the patient. Offer to mail the details of the treatment information that they would like to know.
- *Patient demanding immediate results*: Many dermatological and cosmetic concerns are chronic or unpredictable in nature, but such patients want immediate, fast acting treatments to suit their immediate desires.
  Example: Patient demanding an endless supply of clobetasol or demanding intralesional steroids for every acne lesion. The patient demands for potent medications or treatments without considering its side effects. Inform about the safety profile of a slow but steady treatment. Rather than outright telling the patient that there is no "cure" for their concern, explain to the patient the

difference between an acute and chronic condition and that their concern can be cured but may have relapses. Sometimes, patients find it difficult to choose treatment options if there is no cure. Explain to the patient by giving examples, just like a seasonal cold can be cured but cannot be promised to never return, some chronic dermatological concerns can be treated. This way the patient would be aware that it is up to the patient's compliance of treatment when the problem relapses and whether to be ready for it.

- *Pessimistic patient*: This patient has negative feelings about treatments to come, will cite side effects of medications provided, and would have also experienced problems with other dermatologists. Listen carefully to this patient. Showing empathy can go a long way in building a long-term doctor-patient relationship. Encourage the patient enthusiastically for a fresh start. Start with treatments that will show maximum result, particularly treatments which they have not tried before or show photographs of your patients who have responded to their concerns and then move to slow and steady long-term plan, once they have gained trust in you. Pessimistic patients are more worried about side effects of the medications or procedure advised than the benefits of the treatment. The reason for this is also—mistrust, misunderstanding, worry, or confusion with too many medications. Understand the patients worry and explain the side effects clearly in written. Make the patient comfortable to trust and understand the advised treatment.
- *Manipulative patient:* This patient will try to make others guilty by using rage, threat, or legal action to get what they want.

Examples:
- Threats to put negative feedback on social media
- Threats to sue
- Bribes staff

Managing such patients: Understand the patient's problems, assess how genuine and reasonable the demand is. Sometimes, you must learn to say "NO." Telling the patient, you will not cater to their demands, will give them a firm message that you cannot be manipulated. Saying no can be difficult if you have not done it before as you would do anything to retain a patient. It is however, important to take the decision to not treat a patient if the patient is abusive, manipulative with you or your staff, and makes unreasonable demands.

- *Delusional patient*: Special attention should be given to psychiatric comorbidities. Personality disorders (PDs) typically manifest in late adolescence or early adulthood and are estimated to affect approximately 15% of the general population. PDs such as dependent, histrionic, and borderline PDs occur more often in women, whereas antisocial, narcissistic, and obsessive-compulsive PDs occur more often in men.[3] Devote more time to such patients. Start the consultation with a clear mind and on a positive note, show empathy and interest by body language. Dermatologists should screen for body dysmorphic disorder (BDD) patients by asking patients with none or minimal flaws in their appearance—how much time they spend in a day thinking about their perceived flaw. It cannot be dismissed by telling them that they look fine. Focus on their concerns and disabilities rather than their appearance and help them accept a psychiatric referral. Apart from dermatologic treatment, treatment with serotonin reuptake inhibitors such as fluoxetine, citalopram, and sertraline along with cognitive behavioral therapies are effective.[6]

- *Angry patients due to specific reasons*: Situations such as long waiting hours, administrative issues such as billing errors, scheduling errors, unforeseen side effects with medications or lasers, and technician-caused side effects with treatments done in clinic. In the event of a difficult situation, the patient's emotion should be the center of your attention. Patient is bound to be angry and it is important to listen, apologize, and assure the patient you will review the situation and make sure it will not happen again. The dermatologist is the head of the clinic and must take up responsibility even for the action of their staff. Do not hesitate in offering a sincere apology, if you try to hide or minimize your or your staff's action due to pride or shame, it will only aggravate the patient's rage. Identify the cause of the patient's anger, how the error occurred on your part, and look at your systems—do not blame the patient. Offering a complimentary treatment such as a chemical peel or carbon laser would be a nice gesture. Sometimes the angry patient is not willing to listen to anything. Hear them out and let them vent out their frustration. Be empathetic toward them. You can involve your senior staff to get in touch easily with them so that they are heard and not felt neglected at any point. Note to document everything immediately. After the angry patient calms down, they are more receptive to listening. Offer a complimentary treatment and immediately follow it up with an email stating the same. This establishes you as genuine and maintain your reputation.

PAYMENT ISSUES

Difficult patients may do the treatment and not pay for it or ask for credit and never return. Always ask for payment before starting the procedure.

There may be cases where the patient may not be satisfied with the result and ask for refund. Explain the procedure performed and expected outcome with variability in each patient. In such a case, you can refuse to refund the amount as the procedure has been performed.

However, if you have taken advance payment for some procedures and the patient does not wish to continue with the treatments, the balance value of treatments not performed can be refunded.

HANDLING DIFFICULT PATIENTS WHO CALL AT ODD HOURS

You may categorize some of your patients as VIP and may take the decision of answering their calls at odd hours too as their job profile makes it difficult for them to see you in person (politicians and celebrities).

If a patient calls multiple times (more than three times), then the call should be picked up as it indicates an anxious patient. Ask them to message their problem as the doctor is occupied at the moment. Then depending on the problem messaged, one can give an urgent prescription or advice (urticarial, filler complication, and laser burn) and ask the patient to visit the next day **(Table 8.3.1)**.

Another useful method of dealing with odd hours is to have a doctor daily on call who will handle such calls.

However, it is important to identify and treat patients who require after hours consultation. We should not encourage such behavior on a daily basis for casual consultation as with time we shall get

Table 8.3.1: Steps to deal with difficult patients.

	Emergent inquiries (return call immediately)	Urgent inquiries (return call within 1 hour)	Nonurgent inquiries (variable timing listed below)
Complaint/ inquiry	VIP	Fever, chills, general malaise (flu-like symptoms), elevated temperature	Nonurgent patient questions (24 hours)
	Angry patient	Increase in bleeding from procedure site	Nonurgent complaints/ concerns (24 hours)
	Filler complication	New redness and warmth around procedure site	Laboratory orders and nonurgent results (24 hours)
		Increased pain, swelling at procedure site	*Forms:* Return to work and work excuse notes (48 hours)
		Drainage coming from wound/ site of puncture (pus, foul odor)	Prescription refills (48 hours)
		Wound dehiscence (wound coming apart)	
		Urticaria, herpes zoster	
Script to patient	"Thank you very much for your phone call. Based on what you are telling me this is something that we would consider an emergent problem and you should call 112/reach hospital _____ immediately"	"Thank you very much for your phone call. Based on what you are telling me this is something that we would consider an urgent problem. Our goal is to get back to you within 1 hour. If you have not heard from anyone in 1 hour then please call back, my name is… and I will do my best to help you"	"Thank you very much for your phone call. I would be happy to help you with this. Our policy is… If you do not receive your information within this timeframe, please do not hesitate to call back, my name is… and either I or one of my colleagues would be happy to help you"
Clinician action	Return phone call immediately	Return phone call within 1 hour	Complete or sign appropriate paperwork as needed within the time frame listed

occupied or fed up of patients calling/ messaging at odd hours and expecting a reply on the spot.

HOW TO RESPOND TO NEGATIVE PATIENT REVIEWS ONLINE?

- Do not ignore negative patient reviews.
- Ask yourself and your team tough questions—could you have prevented it, was there a miscommunication, is this an isolated case, or is there a pattern; what changes should you make?
- *Try taking it offline*: Respond with a call— answer the review, that their problems will be handled by your team. Many a times, patients put negative reviews to get your attention and may be happy at the end of the call by your explanation and willing to remove the negative review.
- Never divulge any personal information of the patient— even if you are tempted to

answer back on the post. It does not leave a good impression and also violates the doctor-patient confidentiality.
- *Avoid being defensive*: The patient may write mean things in their negative review. Redirect the conversation rather than reply back in the same way. Take control and resolve the patients concern.
- *Do not apologize*: Irrespective of the patient's complaint being minor or major—avoid apologizing. As the patient may use it for a lawsuit.
- *Avoid excuses*: Saying "that is our standard procedure" can only cause more anger in an already angry patient. The patient is looking for a solution and not an excuse. If a mistake was made, acknowledge it. Then focus on the solution.
- *Thank them for their comments:* No matter how bad a review is or even if it is totally unreasonable, it will help you know what went wrong. Thank the reviewer.

TOP TIPS

- Stay calm and professional.
- Try to see the consultation from the patient's perspective.
- Work together with the patient to find a solution and act in their best interests.
- Have a "debrief" with colleagues after a difficult consultation.
- Consider a training session in mastering challenging interactions.

GENERAL CHECKLIST FOR ALL DERMATOLOGICAL PROCEDURES

Dos	Don'ts
• Selection of right candidate for the right procedure	• Never do a procedure in a hurry

Contd...

Contd...

Dos	Don'ts
• Informed written consent	• Never select a patient who has partially made up his mind/unrealistic expectations/psychiatric problems/medical contraindications
• Get necessary investigations	• Never do a procedure just because the patient asks for it
• Practice adequate standards of precautions	• Never lose your temper
• Keep emergency drugs and manpower ready	• Do not charge for a complication
• Documentation—accurate, chronological, complete, and clear	
• Pre- and postprocedure photography is a must	
• Records must be maintained for at least 3 years	

REFERENCES

1. Jackson JL, Kroenke K. Difficult patient encounters in the ambulatory clinic: clinical predictors and outcomes. Arch Intern Med. 1999;159:1069-75.
2. Nguyen TV, Hong J, Prose NS. Compassionate care: enhancing physician-patient communication and education in dermatology part I: patient-centered communication. J Am Acad Dermatol. 2013;68:353.e1-8.
3. Nakamura M, Koo J. Personality disorders and the "difficult" dermatology patient: Maximizing patient satisfaction. Clinics Dermatol. 2017; 35(3):312-18.
4. Armstrong AW. Practice gaps: failure to maximize patient adherence strategies in clinical practice. Arch Dermatol. 2010;146:1430-1.
5. Managing challenging interactions with patients. BMJ. 2013;347.
6. Phillips KA. Pharmacologic treatment of body dysmorphic disorder: review of the evidence and a recommended treatment approach. CNS Spectr. 2002;7(6):453-60, 463.

8.4 Handling Negative Reviews Online and Offline

Anil Ganjoo

INTRODUCTION

Dermatology, like every other stream of medicine, has evolved tremendously in the last few decades. What used to be a simple prescription and OPD-based practice, has now given the way to a highly specialized, procedure-based practice that involves a lot of toil, sincerity, and stress. The introduction of cutaneous surgery and lasers, particularly for cosmetic reasons, has made things all the more demanding.

The patients' expectations in all sorts of cosmetic procedures are very high. Besides, patients who approach the doctor for cosmetic concerns, unlike those who present with medical complaints, belong to a higher socioeconomic strata of the society. They are very well aware of all the developments in the field, especially with google at their fingertips. They do extensive research about not only the procedure but also the doctor they are visiting.

Nobody can escape exposure to social media. Even if you choose to be disconnected from social media, there will be things written about you in numerous fora. In fact, there are no secrets in today's world of social media, and information about your activities can spread like wildfire.

The highly demanding and expectant patients are also hard to satisfy. They come to us with minor aberrations or no defect at all and want only enhancement. So, the level of expectations is very high and the most important part of this kind of practice is to align the patient expectations to more realistic proportions. We hear all the experienced seniors saying "Always promise less and deliver more," and that is the most important mantra of a successful cosmetic practice. If your patient gets more than what he expects, then he will be very happy and thankful. So, never ever promise the patient more than your own assessment of the outcome.

The first and foremost factor required for survival in today's highly competent world of cosmetic practice is having a very clean and impressive clinic with a very efficient and polite staff. Making the patient comfortable even before he or she sees the doctor, goes a long way in creating a positive impression in the patient's mind. During the consultation, the doctor needs to be very polite and open to all sorts of queries. Always try to listen to the patient's complaints very patiently and make him feel that you would be ready to go to any extent to give the best to the patient. The time and effort spent with the patient at the first interaction is the most important aspect of developing a good relation and rapport with the patient. If the patient believes in you and confides in you at the first instance, then it is highly unlikely that he will be negative later, even if things do not go as per his expectation.

Once you have passed this stage and the patient agrees to go ahead with the treatment, try to be as sincere as possible in your work. Give your best to the patient and your sincerity will always keep you safe. Be polite and gentle at all times and make the patient feel that you are really concerned about the patients' well-being. Develop a good rapport with the patient and always try to answer all the queries patiently. Never see the patient or do a procedure in a hurry.

However, inspite of our best efforts, things can go wrong. This situation may arise due to patients not getting what they had expected or due to complications, which are a part and parcel of every cosmetic procedure. Once this happens, the agitated patient can get aggressive and return with the complaints of being dissatisfied with the results. He/she can also go online and write negative things about you and your practice on social media.

In today's world, online reviews have become a part of almost every field and this includes medicine. In fact, a recent survey found that 88% of consumers trust online reviews as much as personal recommendations.[1] This shows that online reviews count, and overall, this is a good thing. Data shows that more reviews translate into significantly more appointments, and this holds true even if some reviews are bad. It is not until a physician's *overall* rating drops to 2.5 stars out of 5 that appointments begin to significantly decline.

Another survey of more than 2,500 patients showed that 82% of participants use online reviews to evaluate doctors, 72% use online reviews to find a new doctor, and 19% use online reviews to validate their provider choices.[2] These numbers underscore the significance of online reviews—both positive and negative—to healthcare organizations' and practitioners' reputations and viability.

For healthcare providers, the need to manage their online reputations is becoming more imperative as review sites increase in popularity. Although negative online reviews can present challenges, providers can implement a number of risk management strategies to address this issue.[3]

HANDLING ONLINE REVIEWS

The following strategy should be followed to deal with the online reviews:[4-6]

- *Respectfully acknowledge the review*: First, acknowledge the review immediately. Be respectful, even if you think the patient is wrong. This person clearly thinks he or she is right, so if you become defensive the whole situation can quickly degenerate. At this stage, it is important to remember that you do not have to commit to a course of action, you just need to commit to showing that you take the complaint seriously and intend to find a solution.
- *Keep it private*: Next, reach out privately. As much as the patient wants you to pay attention, medical information remains a privacy issue and even if the patient shares personal details, it is best not to conduct the discussion openly. You can be sued, this person probably cant be. Avoid confirming or denying publicly that the reviewer is your patient, because this can also contravene patient rights. Offer to help the patient resolve the problem, and when it has been addressed to the individual's satisfaction, ask him or her to be kind enough to revise the review or to confirm publicly that the issue has been resolved.
- *Learn from the feedback:* Now, take a moment to learn from the comments. Often, we do not realize what patients are thinking until they say something, and if it is said in an online review it might be the first time we hear anything about it. Do not discount reviews even when they are inaccurate, because patient perceptions are vitally important to your practice. Learn from the comments so that you can avoid similar situations arising again in future. The one exception, of course,

is when the feedback is fake. Closed-loop sites which only allow reviews from verified patients, are not a cause to worry. But elsewhere online, things are not as above board. Nevertheless, if you have strong evidence that a review is fake, reach out to the site and present your case thoughtfully and reasonably. If they refuse to take it down, make a point of responding online and stating that it is fake. Moving forward, ask patients to review you on closed-loop sites—having a strong set of reviews on a reputable site where users are all verified, offers far more credibility than a smattering of questionable ones across the web. On that note, there is nothing that makes a negative review disappear faster than positive feedback rolling in above it. This works because we all typically look for the most recent information. When patients see negative reviews, they check the date to determine whether things have changed since then. Furthermore, most review sites have limited-length pages, so as soon as there are four or five reviews, a new page is created automatically. Typically, the newer reviews appear first.

- *Strengthen your online presence:* Finally, complement all this with a strong online profile of your own. This may sound like a lot of work, but the more authoritative content you publish online, the less likely your negative reviews are to turn up in Google searches. Develop your personal brand by publishing regular blog posts. Share these via social media accounts and actively encourage patients to post reviews and comments. With this, as with all the above approaches, chances are good that the positive will outweigh the negative.

PRACTITIONERS' VIEWS

In a countrywide survey conducted to get the views of practicing dermatologists on this issue, we could get the following important information as to how these practitioners feel about feel about it:[7]

- Do not take these reviews personally as one can not satisfy 100% of the patients. These patients are unsatisfied in general and not happy with the circumstances they are in.
- When you encounter them, you can make out from their conduct and body language that they can be potential trouble makers.
- In the event of a negative comment being given face to face, take a deep breath, relax, and do not retaliate.
- Just show concern and say that you have taken note of it and would look into the matter on how to get things sorted.
- Entering into verbal arguments with the patient will do no good and will hamper the peace of your mind and also of the clinic.
- Answer all negative reviews gently.
- An apology, *if you feel there has been some complacency*, can really make a huge difference
- Sometimes, the patient just needs some attention and he/she might nag you with a negative comment just to attract attention. The best mantra is to ignore and carry on with good work with a calm mind.

Once the patient has written an online negative review, you can take the following steps:[8]

- Contact the patient and give him a patient listening.
- Answer all reviews gently.
- Quite often, patients just want to talk and once the treating doctor provides sufficient explanation about the condition,

- they take their review back or change them.
- In case of a post-procedure complication, the doctor has to take the responsibility. It is advised to personally make a phone call and follow-up with the patient.
- Listen to their concerns. They need to be assured that the complication is going to be settled down in few days. Request them to visit the clinic and assess the side effects. Offer them a complimentary peel/mask, etc. Stay in touch with the patient till the complication resolves.
- Give a detailed reply to the negative review and explain everything. People who read reviews also read the reply and it also shows that the doctor is serious about his patients' concerns.
- Ask your happy patients to write positive reviews for you. Most of the times, only patients who are unhappy think seriously about writing reviews and the happy ones, who are many more in number, do not care to write.
- Report to Google in case you feel the review is fake or the language used is derogatory. Google removes such reviews at times.
- In case there is a review regarding treatment not being effective, call the patient to explain the scientific reasons behind the inadequate response. Request them to visit the clinic to discuss further treatment options.
- Many times, the reviews raise concerns about the expenses occurred during a visit. In this case, call and mention about the expertise and the expensive equipment involved in the procedures.
- Hire a search engine optimization (SEO) agency to the tackle menace. Such agencies can be of great help in dire situations.

ACKNOWLEDGMENT

Thankful to inputs from Dr Sonali Langar, Dr Rohit Batra, and Dr Anuj Pall.

REFERENCES

1. BrightLocal. Online Surveys. [online] Available from Brightlocal.com. [Last accessed March, 2020].
2. Health S (2018, April 16). How do patients use online provider reviews for care decisions? PatientEngagementHIT.com. Retrieved from https://patientengagementhit.com/news/how-do-patients-use-online-provider-reviews-for-care-decisions
3. Adler EL. (2016). How not to respond to bad patient reviews online. [online] Available from www.physicianspractice.com/marketing/how-not-respond-bad-patient-reviews-online. [Last accessed January, 2020].
4. Chauhan MK. (2016). Managing patient online reviews can make a difference. [online] Available from www.physicianspractice.com/blog/managing-patient-online-reviews-can-make-difference. [Last accessed January, 2020].
5. Cryts A. (2016). Docs, ignore millennials' online reviews at your peril. [online] Available from www.fiercehealthcare.com/practices/docs-ignore-millennials-online-reviews-at-your-peril. [Last accessed January, 2020].
6. Kropf S. (2015). Responding to negative online patient reviews: 7 tips. [online] Available from www.physicianspractice.com/blog/responding-negative-online-patient-reviews-7-tips. [Last accessed January, 2020].
7. Segel R. (2017). Dissed by unhappy patients? Here's what to do. [online] Available from www.medpagetoday.com/Practice Management/Practice Management/62349. [Last accessed January, 2020].
8. Weber S. (2015). How to: Deal with negative online reviews. Physicians Practice. [online] Available from www.physicianspractice.com/marketing/how-to-deal-with-negative-online-reviews. [Last accessed January, 2020].

8.5 Means to Retain Esthetic Patients in Practice

Jyotsna Vinayak Deo

INTRODUCTION

Dermatology is a highly prized medical specialty nowadays. Along with work–life balance was always a given, advances in research and therapeutics have improved patient outcomes. Desire-based dermatology as opposed to disease-based dermatology fueled by emergence of subspecialties of dermatosurgery and esthetics has spawned a new segment of patients—the esthetic patient aka the "client." Traditional clinical dermatologists are no longer mere doctors but "dermatopreneurs," i.e., combination of a dermatologist and an entrepreneur. As the proportion of esthetic dermatology increases in practice, dermatologists have to gear themselves to cope with this new segment by developing the necessary interpersonal and professional skills.

Broadly speaking, there are four levels of cosmetic office practice:

1. *Level 1:* It is essentially a noncosmetic practice. This is the traditional disease-based medical dermatology or skin-cancer surgery practice.
2. *Level 2*: It means that there is a minor focus on cosmetic dermatology; this may be a limited number of procedures on a limited number of days of the week, or clinic hours that are devoted to cosmetic practice. This practice (which we sometimes call the evolving or the transitional practice in cosmetic dermatology) is one that typically will devote resources and collect revenues that show cosmetic dermatology to represent 25% or less of the practice.
3. *Level 3:* It is what we would call a blended or integrated dermatology practice; it is one in which there is a relative balance between the disease and the desire patients, in terms of days per week, number of patients seen, and revenue. The level 3 practice generally is highly evolved in cosmetic practice but still performs a great deal of noncosmetic, disease-based medical, and surgical dermatology.
4. *Level 4:* It is completely and solely a cosmetic dermatology practice. In fact, in this practice they may not even offer any disease-based treatment. These practices may be solely dermatology, in a medi spa setting, or may be integrated with plastic surgery.

Majority of dermatology practices that experience a great deal of success from a practice achievement standpoint are levels 2 and 3. That is, they have some limited focus in cosmetic dermatology, or they have a very integrated blended schedule of patients and procedures that are offered.

The advantage of having an integrated dermatology practice is that clinical dermatology patients are direct feeders to the esthetic practice. Hence, there is less expenditure on advertising. Also, with a variety of services under one roof, there is a greater scope for patients to avail the services multiple times. As the number of interactions increases, so does the trust and the receptivity to procedure suggestions. But all this is possible, only if one learns the art and science of patient retention.

IMPORTANCE OF PATIENT RETENTION

It is always tempting to focus on new patients when developing one's practice, but while doing so, one should not forget about retaining the existing patients. Why? New patient leads could result in consultations, single visit, or a series of visits that can strengthen your bottom line in the short run, but not necessarily in the long haul.

Patient retention, on the other hand, helps to solidify ones esthetic practice on multiple fronts. The key is trust. Once you have established a care cycle for your existing patients and they are happy with their outcomes, this translates into a relationship that is based on trust. If a patient first visits you to have a chemical peel and is happy with her results, the chances are good that she will return for other touch-ups and procedures. If the patient originally came in for one procedure and sees the successful results that other patients are getting from you, she might opt to have one or more of them; or she may ask for your expertise in explaining what procedures she could benefit from. Established patients will likely spend more than a new patient, whose new relationship with you might only be for one issue.

It is five times more expensive to draw in new patients than it is to retain existing ones. Existing patients do not need to be convinced to visit your practice, they already know you and trust you. They act as direct referrals to their family members, friends, and coworkers.

They are, in effect, walking billboards- 24-hour living advertisements and examples of your work and represent free "word-of-mouth" advertising.

Retaining esthetic patients or for that matter a clinical patient in practice is as simple as ABC where A stands for Availability, B for Behavior, and C for Competence, if only one remembers these tenets well.

A is for Availability

A dermatologist should be available when a patient needs one, else the disease would subside on its own. Jokes apart, accessibility of a consultant and ease of taking appointment are of paramount importance. Prominent clinic location with sufficient parking space for vehicles, easy access to public transport, and disabled-friendly access are helpful. The clinic timings should be in accordance with its location, e.g., a clinic in an office district could follow office timings but a clinic in the suburbs where the majority of its clients work in the city could have staggered timings with morning and evening shifts and an afternoon break. In other words, the timings should be convenient for one's target clients.

It is helpful to have a website where patients could book appointments in advance. While booking appointments, enquire if the patient is coming for a consultation or a procedure and allot the slot accordingly. Sending reminder SMS a day prior to the appointment makes the patient feel special and wanted. We also send reminders about follow-ups. In case of cancellation of appointments and unexpected delays (e.g., an unexpected breakdown in the laser machine) too, inform the patients well in advance.

Patients are given a contact number, which they can call in case of a query or an emergency. In case one is out of town, have your staff in the clinic give the reference of your fellow dermatologists, who would be only too glad to reciprocate the favor.

B is for Behavior

A famous surgeon once said, "The patient will never care how much you know, until they know how much you care." Good behavior never harmed anybody but bad behavior is injurious to the health of your practice. It is not just about the patient's experience in your consulting room it involves the entire in-clinic experience.

The staff should greet people warmly while answering the phone and also when they enter the clinic. This politeness should be universal and not just be restricted to patients, but should be extended to every person visiting the clinic. The necessary patient details should be entered in the software.

Waiting area should be uncluttered and peaceful. Handy pamphlets about the esthetic services on offer and educational videos and posters can generate awareness. While waiting for their turn, patients could fill an esthetic interest questionnaire which would help one in gauging their specific desires. Asking patients to fill feedback forms and give suggestions can make them feel you care. The staff should keep the patients informed about delays, because the longer the waiting time, the angrier the patient.

Before the patient enters your consulting room, briefly peruse the questionnaire answered by them as also go through their details which have already been entered at the reception.

In case of a follow-up, go over the previous visit notes.

Always greet patients by name and address them appropriately. Keep your phone on silent mode and give them your undivided attention while listening to their problems. The consultation should be long enough to address the patient's concerns satisfactorily. Give your honest inputs along the way. In case a procedure is recommended, always provide the relevant details, e.g., in a case of melasma, while one can get good results with chemical peels and laser toning, it would be prudent to elaborate on the importance of concomitant sun-protection. Also, it is necessary to emphasize the relapsing nature of the condition and the fact that not all cases respond to therapy. Being realistic in one's appraisal of a patient's problem is always appreciated.

If a patient does not wish to do a procedure, suggest alternative remedies. We live in a country where finances can be a constraint, especially in case of esthetic procedures. Never deride somebody for not having adequate budget. Patients visit us to feel good about themselves, if we cannot make them better, we have no right to make them feel worse. Empathy, sympathy, and compassion always go a long way.

If a patient does go in for a procedure, ensure a good procedure-room experience. Attending staff should not gossip among themselves but rather should always be encouraging to the patient. When an esthetic patient comes for follow-up, they should discreetly compliment them on how good they look. But at no point should the confidentiality of the patient be compromised. It is always good if the consultant and staff are on the same page while interacting with patients. For example, a patient going in for laser hair reduction needs to be explained about the need for touch up and repeat sessions and this should be reiterated at every follow-up. Standards of care and pampering should be maintained at every visit and all the clinic staff should adhere to them.

Medicine is a fickle science and not all patient outcomes are satisfactory. What comes handy at such times is your behavior. Accept your mistake, if you are in the wrong and try to make amends. One of my regular patients, while doing chemical cauterization of her seborrheic keratosis, some of the

Trichloroacetic acid (TCA) spilt over. We apologized profusely and worked sincerely to get the postinflammatory hyperpigmentation under control. Eventually, it did subside. The patient still follows up regularly for other skin-related issues.

Another patient was suffering from a severe case of hormonal acne. As she battled with her polycystic ovarian disease, her acne kept flaring as did her melasma. As she was undergoing infertility treatments, we could only offer topical therapies. But we were trying our best to help her, she could perceive that, so we all persevered together. She still visits us, with her kids.

Good behavior, and honest and effective communication always strengthen a doctor–patient relationship.

C is for Competence

While there is no doubt that competence is imperative for success, without A and B to support it, the practice would find it difficult to attain its full potential.

Competent consultants suggest the best and most cost-effective remedies to their patients. It is not enough to be well-qualified, one needs to be abreast with all the recent advances in ones' field. Reading regularly, attending workshops, acquiring hands-on training, and discussing with one's fellow colleagues helps hone his/her skills. Learning from our experiences and sharing what we know reinforce it further. So try to become the best you can.

This pursuit for excellence should be extended to your staff as well. Train them well. Learn to anticipate problems and troubleshoot in advance.

Lastly, know when to say no, how to say it politely, and know when to refer. It could save your practice.

I hope you find these ABCs of retaining esthetic patients useful.

8.6 Ensuring an Unforgettable Esthetic Experience for a Patient

Sonali Langar

INTRODUCTION

Advances in the practice of esthetic medicine have evolved significantly over the past few decades. Knowledge about esthetics and its acceptance in the society has increased leading the deliverance of more esthetic procedures by the dermatologist. Now seekers of esthetic procedures are well-informed healthcare consumers, who want to participate in their medical care and decision-making process. Doctor–patient relationship has also seen a steady transformation. At one time, providing excellent care was enough to build a successful healthcare practice. Today however, doctors and their staff must also provide high-quality, efficient service to achieve high patient satisfaction and retention. The concept of personalization of medicine has evolved shifting treatment protocols from "disease-centered medicine" to "patient-centered medicine." Thus, conferring good unforgettable experiences to the patient undergoing procedures for esthetic enhancement has become center stage of esthetic practice. Needless to say, good esthetic experiences retain the patients and help in generating good will. A satisfied consumer acts as a brand ambassador by spreading 'word of mouth publicity.' Hence, practicing esthetics in a forthright manner, maintaining quality, and delivering services upfront have been essential. This chapter enumerates various touchpoints that aid in achieving so.

THE CLINIC

The clinic forms the first touchpoint for the patient. Punctuality and starting clinic on time earns respect and reputation of professionalism, and competence for the clinic.

Ambience of the clinic, good lighting, cleanliness, and good housekeeping cast good first impressions. Basic amenities such as provision of drinking water, clean sitting area, clean toilets, and hygienic surroundings should be maintained. Esthetic clinic should have a pantry and a dedicated staff who ensures water, beverage, and snack supplies to the patient waiting for undergoing esthetic procedures. Sometimes for prolonged procedures as full-body lasers, there should be provision of serving wholesome meals.

Clear signage should be allocated to different procedure rooms and the patient should be accompanied by the clinic staff to their specified procedural chamber.

Waiting time for the patient should be as short as possible. Front desk staff should be groomed to keep this in mind. Use of clinic management software can be particularly handy in keeping a track on the time and number of consultations and procedures. Television facility displaying informative or educational channels acts as a good engaging tool for the patient in the waiting area. However, playing self-grandeur depicting videos should best be avoided.

In heavily attended clinics or hospitals, another approach would be call esthetic procedure patients during less busy hours of the day or allocate separate procedural days in a week so as to cut down the waiting time and to impart undivided care.

Majority of esthetic patients demand privacy and secrecy and are not comfortable in disclosing having undergone an esthetic correction. Separate waiting chambers segregating them from general OPD, and allocating individual appointment slots by catering one patient at a time would substantially help.

THE STAFF

The staff are the face value of the center and it need not be stressed upon that they should be pleasant, dignified, and professional in their dealings with the patient. Prompt and disciplined staff helps in generating positive representation of the center. The importance of quality staff cannot be undermined as they support the day-to-day running of the center and provide ongoing care to the patient.

A friendly front-line staff greeting the patient on the phone or on their arrival in the clinic is crucial in building up an initial rapport. Staff should always display a smile on their faces as it helps in establishing an empathic relationship with the patient. It is a nonverbal way of communicating that the patient is valued. This eases out much of the anxiety that the patient may experience walking into a nonfamiliar clinic for the first time.

The other supporting staff should have good communication skills and display quick warm responsiveness to the patient's queries making their experience seamless from the reception to the doctor's chamber. Pantry staff should be allocated the responsibility of offering drinking water, beverages, and light snack to the patients sitting in waiting room from time-to-time.

The staff assisting the doctor/therapist should be well-trained in procedural knowledge and equipment use. They should be provided with industry-specific service training and follow-up renewal training for better handling of the procedure.

Counseling staff should be present in the center to provide supportive service to the patient. Counselors provide information, advice, and assistance in helping patients understand their esthetic procedure. They help patients to amplify their vision and understand the proper potential of the procedure in achieving esthetic enhancement.

It is imperative that the role of each staff must be clearly outlined to them, so as to hold them accountable accordingly for any discrepancies, if they may occur. A sense of sound organization culture in the workplace should be inculcated for a more sustainable level of work culture.

Uniformed staff with their name tags help to build a standardized image of the esthetic center. This also makes the staff feel more valued and inculcates a sense of authority in work place. Patients also consider employees in uniform to be qualified and knowledgeable. They are more satisfied when they seek answers from a uniformed staff. Uniform wear also distinguishes staff from fellow patients facilitating ease of identification and communication.

A feedback policy for the staff should be placed at work place. Feedback clarifies expectations of the patient, and helps the staff to learn from their mistakes and builds confidence. Moreover, the apprehension of a negative feedback encourages courteous behavior and prompt response in response to patients queries.

THE DOCTOR–PATIENT RELATIONSHIP

The doctor–patient relationship (DPR) is the most important defining element in a successful esthetic practice. The importance of DPR can be judged by the fact that a satisfactory encounter with the treating physician can negate all the other lacunas experienced by the patient at the center. The consultation with the doctor should make the patient feel relaxed, understood, and well informed. Some essential key points in maintaining a good DPR are enlisted below:

- *Communication*: Good communication skills are essential in establishing DPR. Effective communication between the physician and patient results in improved medical and emotional condition of the patient, better patient compliance with medical treatment, enhanced satisfaction of the patient toward healthcare services, and lesser risks of the patient's misconduct. Patient's consultation should be elaborate and a two-way communication, with the practitioner listening to and acknowledging the patient's esthetic concerns and existing expectations. The consultation should avidly cover the following points:
  - The patient's reasons for seeking the procedure
  - An explicit, objective description of what the patient is trying to correct
  - The patient's understanding of the procedure and it's financial implications
  - What likely outcome the patient desires and the extent to which this will be fulfilled

- Explanation of the steps of the corrective procedure that will be used, using either accurate diagrams or patient photographs
- The risks factors and complications involved in the procedure
- History of previous cosmetic procedures undertaken and their outcome
- History and nature of body image and appearance concerns, including impacts of body image on psychological and social well-being
- Relevant psychiatric history or signs or symptoms suggestive of body dysmorphic disorder
- Relevant past medical history and ongoing medications
- Advise on change in lifestyle of patient before undergoing procedure as losing weight and quitting smoking.
- Nonpermanency of the effect of procedures should be clearly explained, so that the monetary implications of repeat procedures to maintain results are understood.
- Last but not the least the option of doing nothing should also be discussed as it puts the doctor in a fair upright place.

Sometimes, customising the esthetic procedure for the patient furnish more appreciable and satisfactory results rather than adhering to the patients request for a particular procedure alone. A justifiable approach would be to offer possible treatment options for better results and helping the patient to decide the best option depending upon the patient's age/lifestyle/budget/social and cultural background.

- *Doctor empathy*: Empathy defined as "the ability to understand and share the feelings of another" is vital to ensure a good quality DPR. Being able to feel patient's emotions helps deliver more compassionate care and make the patient feel more comfortable during treatment. Kind words and a little emotional support from a doctor can have a measurable impact on the therapeutic effect, patient's outcomes, and quality of life. Empathy can be delivered in the following ways:
- *Warm introduction*: Introduction serves as the first, integral part of the treatment process. It should be warm and friendly, addressing the patient by name and treating him/her as an individual and not a faceless visitor.
- *Documenting personal details*: Jot down a few personal details of the patient. Document important life updates or significant events and send good wishes from the clinic as on their birthdays and marriage anniversaries. On these occasions, the clinic can offer an discount on pricing of esthetic procedures to generate goodwill. Knowing these personal details about your patients not only convince them you care, but help cultivate feeling of attachment and respect between the two parties.
- *Spending an extra minute*: This might be a tough for physicians operating busy centers. However, adding one minute to each visit and asking how patients are doing generally, not just medically generates a sense of satisfaction in the patient that his/her overall well-being is cared for too.
- *Making eye contact*: If eye contact with the patient is not present, it damages any sense of connection with the doctor. This may be pertinent for centers which use a computer or mobile device in the examination room. Make sure one is not glued to

the screen. Nonverbal body language speaks just as loudly as one's words.
- *Showing support*: If a patient is upset or worried about something, acknowledge their difficult situation. When delivering a diagnosis and treatment protocol, make sure to pleasantly answer all the queries. Additionally, hand over information booklet of esthetic procedures for better understanding. In the event of any untoward side effects arising from an esthetic procedure, display exemplary support to the patient. Say you are there and say it loudly. The author had a patient who developed postinflammatory hyperpigmentation (PIH) to fractional CO_2 laser session. She was rendered full emotional and medical support with subsequent peeling sessions to help resolve PIH. After clearance of her pigmentation, she was offered to stop the treatment and take refund of the payment but she continued to carry on with the sessions saying that "you did not leave me when I needed you, how can I leave your clinic now."
- *Putting yourself in your patients' shoes*: Always treat the patient as you want to be treated yourself.
- *Getting patient feedback*: The best way to gauge your patients' perceptions of physician empathy is asking them a feedback. Design a questionnaire or satisfaction survey on how the patient perceives your services and wants further betterment. If there are lacunas, deal with every complaint, as complaints can be opportunities to build a lifetime of loyalty from a patient. Check the validity, take action to resolve it, and then let the patient know.
- *Sharing articles on empathy with your staff*: Empathy training is as important for the staff as for the doctor, as patients likely spend more time interacting with receptionists, medical assistants, and therapists in the clinic. Thus, a negative interaction with your staff can influence patient satisfaction just as much.
- *Trust*: Trust is a fundamental part of DPR and occurs in a framework of interaction which is influenced by both personalities of the doctor and patient and norms of social systems. Patients will not forget you if they trust you. Trust has also shown to have a positive impact on patient's adherence to medication, patient satisfaction and better follow-up of treatment.
- *Informed consent*: This is based on the moral and legal arguments of the patient's autonomy (independence in decision-making). Physician needs to be honest with the patient and his family in providing genuine assessment of favorable and unfavorable outcome probabilities along with the suggested treatment option.

THE PROCEDURE

- Once the patient enrols, there should be a system of proactive healthcare reminders stating the date and time of the procedure.
- It is important that majority of the procedures should be done by the treating physicians themselves taking assistance from qualified staff. This way the patient feels more safe in being handled by the qualified doctor himself. When prolonged procedures are being performed by the therapist as body lasers, proper introduction of the therapist by the doctor and handing over the patient to the therapist should be in a professional manner. Frequent supervision visits by the

doctor should be made in the treatment chamber to personally monitor the successful deliverance of the procedure. Mid-session coffee/snacking breaks should be offered to the patient undergoing prolonged sessions.
- The procedure should be done under hygienic conditions taking utmost care of asepsis. The modesty of the patient should be upheld by draping the patient and avoiding unnecessary exposure. The patient should be briefed about the steps of the esthetic procedure, so as not to startle patient while doing it. The type of procedure done and the materials used should be communicated and legibly mentioned on the patient's records, thereby maintaining transparency.
- All attempts should be taken to minimize pain during the procedure as much as possible. The liberal use of anesthetic creams, cold compresses, vibrators, and nerve blocks, wherever applicable should be used. Beforehand information of the pain or discomfort that might be experienced during the procedure allays the anxiety and mentally prepares the patient to endure it. Talking to the patient in between the procedure and reassuring that the procedure is being successfully done has a calming effect on the patient. A little amount of pampering makes the patient happy.
- Cosmetic procedures should never be provided without aftercare. All patients should be able to contact the practitioner in the event of any untoward side effect following the procedure. A contact number should be provided to patients in case of emergency and a dedicated staff should be assigned to answer all queries post procedure. In an unfortunate event of the procedure going wrong or developing adverse effect, owning up and taking proactive measures goes a long way in building a concrete physician–patient relationship.

To summarize, unforgettable esthetic experience for the patient streams from better communication with alignment of realistic results, quality and personalized medical attention, transparency in financial dealings along with staff accountability, and sound organizational culture. Combining great service with education and explanation of clinical decisions, you are well on your way to satisfied patients.

TAKE-HOME MASSAGE

- Treat the patient with priority.
- Display warmth and smile while dealing.
- Inculcate sound organization culture at workplace.
- Make staff accountable.
- Align the patient for realistic expectation.
- Give quality and personalized medical attention.
- Maintain transparency in financial dealings.

8.7 Empathy and Ethos of Clinical Practice

Koushik Lahiri, Surajit Gorai

INTRODUCTION

The desire for better patient care leads to the development of many strategies for better service to the patients. When a patient walks into a doctor's chamber, he or she can be compared with a blind person entering to a new house. For that blind man, it will take months together to have a general idea of a room itself. Patients or their relatives are unaware of our medical world. When for the first time you utter the diagnosis, their journey to the uncharted sea of diseases begins. After going home, they will discuss with colleagues, read about it, search on the web, and will have a rough idea about the ailment. This introduction to the new world of disease is not at all a happy experience; it is full of pain, fear, and anxiousness throughout. Any medical term such as "dermatographism" or "mastocytosis" is an alien thing to them. They may correlate it with a "cancer" or "a disease that may kill someone soon" or may take it so easily to ignore it. It all depends upon how they get the information from the doctor. Sympathy and Empathy are two terms that are increasingly getting attached to medical practice. Sympathy is to have the feeling for the patient. Sympathy is also condescending and has the attitude of a favor or charity which patient may not want or even dislike and empathy is to express the feelings accurately to express that doctor is with the patient to help and he understands his suffering.[1] Studies indicate that effective and empathic communication skills may decrease the likelihood of patients filing malpractice claims against their physicians.[2,3] In India also, these claims are alarmingly increasing.[4,5] There are evidences that indicate empathy is an important medical tool that can be acquired and taught in medical school. Clinical empathy is an essential medical skill that can be taught and improved, thereby producing changes in physician's behavior and patient outcomes. The teaching of clinical empathy more widely into clinical practice at all levels of medical school is important. The behavioral aspects of empathy—the empathic response—can be assessed and integrated into medical schools core communication skills training.[6]

SPECIAL CHALLENGES IN DERMATOLOGY PRACTICE

In dermatology, patient care is someWHAT different and is gradually changing from clinical to cosmetic, FROM DISEASE to desire dermatology. Individual patient care with empathy plays a great role. In a clinical setting where diseases such as atopic dermatitis or psoriasis can be controlled, but always there is a chance of recurrence even with the best therapy available, patient satisfaction is challenging.[7] To declare them as an incurable disease is not an easy task. Better to put those diseases in a different way without hurting them emotionally. In the first visit, it can be explained in a bit tricky manner like—in reply to the question "Is it curable?"—Sir/Madam if you take the definition of "cure" as per dictionary, then it means "clearing of lesions" and it is possible in almost all cases like yours. But if you think cure means the disease will not come back again, then it is difficult to say like in all other diseases. But saying so, the doctor should always be very careful about answering the exact question. Like, if patient is asking for a second opinion or in subsequent visits you may be more straightforward. The art of storytelling comes into play in these scenarios as body movements, eye contact, and gestures, all become important. This art somewhat related to experience and can be better with practice. A warm patient–doctor relationship is always necessary and effective communication is the key to it.

PROBLEMS OF CURRENT INDIAN HEALTHCARE

In the recent time, in India, the doctor–patient relationship is gruesome. A lot of factors in Indian healthcare and sociopolitical scenario are responsible for it. On one side, corporate healthcare is on the rise and on the other side, government setup is not well equipped, and is overburdened with patients. Due to advertisement and marketing strategy developed by core marketing people, not guided by doctors, society is getting a message that every disease is curable with the panacea of natural or modern medicine.[8] With cosmetology boom patient expects to get an exceptional beauty with modern technology. Over-the-counter (OTC) sale of topical steroid or triple combination creams are advertised as a fairness cream, lead to some permanent damage to the skin. In India, even with constant and strong action from the Dermatology Society, topical steroid abuse is going on.[9] Assessment of unrealistic expectation is possible with good communication skill and it can be learned.[10]

WAYS OF EFFECTIVE COMMUNICATION

In short duration of dermatology visit, it is a challenge to communicate in a patient-centric way that also fulfills the traditional diagnosis-making approach. Due to a long list of patients waiting outside, eliciting the concerns and ambiguous information provided by the patient makes the communication more difficult. All those things along with a lack of empathetic care lead to the frustrating, dissatisfied patient experience. A few basic principles of patient-centric commutation can be learned.[11]

The relationship between doctor and patient starts when a patient enters the room and ends with an exchange of smile or a concluding remark. The following are a set of practical and evidence-based suggestions to help improve the quality of the doctor–patient relationship in dermatology:

- **When the patient comes in the room:** In work environment, a lot of distraction like cell phones, laptop, books, files on the table, our thoughts and issues unrelated to work may interfere us to make proper eye contact and exchange a smile when a patient is entering the room. Greeting the patient and relatives with respect is very important. We should make a conscious decision to avoid distraction when a patient comes in.[12]
- **How to begin? small talk, guiding statement and pauses**: It has been shown in many studies that small non-medical talks like "how are you today?" increased patient satisfaction.[13] The main difficulty in patient conversation is to extract pieces of information that we need. In another study, it showed that allowing free talk can help to give all necessary informations and it delays the consultation time only by 6 seconds.[14,15] Moreover, when a patient is interrupted once, they never raised their

issues. On average, they were interrupted at 18 seconds. A facilitative statement like "I see," "it's worrisome," and "I can feel your concern," provides more information and increases the bonding.[16] A pause during the interview should not be taken as an opportunity to ask more questions or give a response. Silence allows the patient to think and continue the discussion.

- **When the patient is a storyteller and not stopping:** Most of us fear that open-ended questions allow the patient to talk rubbish for a long duration. In most cases, it is not true but there are some situations when patients are taking a long time we need to shape up the conversation in a proper direction. When it is going to the wrong direction, there are some ways to politely ask them to cut short. We can ask:

"Would it be fine if I interrupt you to ask some specific questions?"

"I need some more detail information on your itching habit. Is it ok to say that?"

"May I ask you some specific questions regarding your sleep habit?"[17]

- **When the patient brings a list of questions?:** In India, it is not that common, at times it is better to concise the conversation with a list of questions as the list itself makes the discussion close-ended and brief. But sometimes silly and unrelated set of questions takes a lot of time and energy. Like the patient comes for psoriasis and also wants to discuss androgenetic alopecia, lack of glowing skin, acne scar, and so on. It is better to humbly request the patient that today we can discuss your most troublesome issue such as psoriasis and we can fix a date after 2 weeks for your hair. As an example, "I can feel that your psoriasis got worse and you want to have a new plan. That is why I need to discuss the scenario with you. Today we have 15 minutes only, so is it ok if I give you an appointment in the next 2 weeks?"[18]

Here in India, the patient may also ask about GI problems, joint problems, and many more from a dermatologist only. In those cases, they should be referred to the concerned professional politely. Keeping the name and number of other doctors handy is useful to refer by name.

- **Reflective listening:** Reflective listening is just to echo the thought that the patient expressed. This technique has an immense impact on the doctor–patient relationship. Like "Ok. Do you mean to say your psoriasis worsen with the application of previous creams? Do not worry I will take care of the issue."[19]

It allows the doctor to verify an issue even if it is silly to a doctor but a big concern for a patient. It also reassures the patient about the fact that the doctor is listening and understanding my issue.

- **Showing empathy:** To identify the feelings and concerns of each patient is important for successful practice. Until unless we can comprehend the actual issue, be the physical symptoms or a psychological one, it is not possible to act on them. Giving a solution according to patient's actual concern is showing empathy. In studies where the patient-doctor interview was filmed and analyzed for empathetic communication, it was found that physicians often allowed the expressions of the patients' emotions to pass without acknowledgment.[20] These missed opportunities to show empathy termed "empathic opportunity terminators,"[21] may hamper rapport building, resulting in poor adherence, low patient satisfaction, and unfavorable clinical outcomes. Often we miss the psychological distress associated with chronic diseases like in a case of psoriasis, they want a discussion on "it's curable or not, not any medicine!"[22] So empathetic discussion revealing the facts related to the disease can break the ice. Personal communication skill training is helpful to address those issues.

Empathy consists of three components: A *cognitive focus* (entering into the patient's perspective), an affective focus (experiencing surrogate feelings), and *an action focus* (explicit acknowledgment of emotions and allowing the patient to modulate the physician's understanding).

An approach to recognizing and addressing emotions is summarized with the acronym NURS.[23]

- *Name:* Make a best effort to name the emotion that the patient seems to be experiencing: You seem upset, or I can see that you are very worried.
- *Understand:* Explicitly legitimize the patient's feelings: Given what you have gone through, I can see why you are feeling this way, or many people feel the same way you are feeling in this situation, it is very understandable.
- *Respect:* Take advantage of opportunities to acknowledge and praise the patient and family for things they are already doing: I can see that you have made a lot of effort to remember to take care of your skin. Congratulations.
- *Support*: Make the patient feel like he or she can trust in the physician and seek help when things go wrong: If your problem gets worse, please be sure to call, or I promise to stick with you until this problem is under control.

What other questions do you have?
At the end of consultation, a simple question "what else can I help you with?" or "what other questions do you have for me today?"[24] provides an opportunity for the dermatologist to conclude, address untouched issues, and calming the patient. In a busy practice with brief office visits, this is a useful way to prevent patients from feeling rushed, while nicely conclude the visit with a smile.[25]

EXAMPLE OF PATIENT-CENTERED COMMUNICATION

Dermatologist: "Hello, Mr Roy. It is very nice to meet you. I see that you are from Durgapur. Durgapur expressway is smooth to drive; I enjoy driving on the road (Small talk)."

Patient: "Yes, it is really good and probably the best highways in Bengal."

Dermatologist: "Tell me why you decided to come to see me today." (Open-ended question)

Patient: "Well, I have few raised bumps over my forearms and legs, sometimes itchy, the main concern is I cannot wear short dresses and everyone asks me about it. So embarrassing! (Brief pause)

(No interruption from the dermatologist)
I have consulted a local doctor; he prescribed me *steroids*. I never knew about them and I came to know only while buying my medicines so I never took them. I took only the allergy medicine and applied a cream called 'Tazret forte' which is not a steroid."

Dermatologist: "I can feel your concern. Being a college student it is tough not to wear a dress of your own choice. Also, you are having fear of taking steroids. (Repeating what you have heard, naming and legitimizing the emotion)

Patient: "Yes, doctor, you seem to understand."

Dermatologist: "I am going to ask our nurse to give you a gown, and after I examine you, we can decide together on a treatment plan. I am sure there is a way we can help you." (Concept of joint decision-making)

Encounter Special Situation

Interpersonal skills are particularly important when we deal with an angry patient, disappointed patient or patient with unrealistic expectations. Besides, computer use during the interview can create a new set of problems for the dermatologist.

Patient Anger

Anger may be a reaction for grief, dissatisfaction, anxiety, or some unrelated event.[26] Like in India doctors are blamed for almost everything in the course of patient care. A big fat bill in a corporate setup, long waiting time, lengthy conversation with the receptionist, and argument with the fellow patient for sitting chair may also be a cause for anger. We usually react to the emotion with similar anger or pour them with additional information or try rationalizing them. Often, a more useful approach is to hear the issue calmly and fix the exact problem if possible. With a patience hearing about the issue, melt them down to a certain degree. The skill mentioned before as "NURS" is particularly useful.[22] Then, if it is due to a known medical fact such as "acne flare-up with isotretinoin" or "retinoid dermatitis" can be explained gradually. If it is not due to the medical part or more of a service giving issue, then politely ask them to seek a solution from the appropriate authority.

Another useful technique is to ask yourself, "what other emotions might be driving a patient's anger?" More frequently than not, the additional emotion is fear.[27] Knowing that a fearful patient is presenting angrily can be helpful in terms of deciding on your response. Responding to the fear component of anger often produces the desired effect of facilitating good communication. So in that case, only reassurance is enough to calm down the patient.

Patient Disappointment

It is very common in dermatology practice. In most of the cases, patient gets disappointed because of a known medical fact, more likely due to side effects of a known topical agent or not having desired response to therapy.[28,29] Like, according to his or her expectation, marks of acne are not going within a month or tinea is not clear after the first visit. To handle the situation, compassionate counseling in the first visit is of utmost importance. The term "I wish things were different" can be used instead of "I am sorry" as an empathic response in situations where patients may be experiencing disappointment.[30] "I wish we had better treatments for your disease," e.g., it creates an alliance with the patient by showing the physician's desire for the patient's well-being. "I am sorry," by contrast, may be regarded with an apology or an expression of pity.[31] Recent studies have focused on the importance of complete transparency, delivering information promptly, providing an apology, and an explanation, and implementing policies to prevent recurrence of the same mistakes.[32] A full discussion of proper responses to medical mistakes and their medicolegal consequences are beyond the scope of this chapter.

Setting Patient Expectations

In one study, dermatologist reported being frustrated in fulfilling psoriasis patient's expectation for an easy solution and inability to understand the disease process.[33] On the contrary, the patient wished to know the etiology of the disease, know all the treatment available, and to get cured at the same time. In general, most patients are hopeful for having a permanent cure for the disease without any future recurrences. They are very reluctant to hear the term "incurable." In this regard, the study highlighted the need for better education of patients about the concept of maintenance therapy for long-term control of psoriasis.

In India, education about health is not only inadequate and misleading but also obtained from nonprofessional sources. In the age of social media to have access to authentic scientific knowledge is difficult and easy to have wrong information from unreliable sources. Moreover here in India, various legally acceptable modes of therapy such as homeopathy, Siddha, Unani, and naturopathic treatment makes the scenario complicated.

It is often advisable to listen first and find out exactly how much patients already know about their diseases, and then fill in the appropriate knowledge gaps. Other helpful strategies include basing the selection of therapies on patient preferences (e.g., does the patient want a cream versus an ointment) and providing written instructions about the treatment plan.[34] Patients might appreciate having an approximate timeline describing when to expect certain therapeutic effects. This is one way to match the patient's expectations with what the physician can provide.

COMPUTER USE DURING THE MEDICAL INTERVIEW

As we are advancing toward e-prescription and e-record keeping, we must be aware of a few facts that may also harm the doctor–patient relationship. A 7-year long study that filmed the physician–patient interaction revealed that the use of computer negatively affected the amount of information provided to the patient.[35] Eye contact and way of conversation were also hampered due to a repeated shifting of gaze from patient to computer screen.

With this in mind, it might be wise to increase physician–patient interactions by engaging patients in relevant parts of the computer screen as much as possible. When turning toward the computer, the physician may wish to name what he or she is doing (e.g., "Excuse me for a moment. I need to type your new prescription into the computer.") Another way to maximize eye contact with the patient is to keep computer entry during the visit to a minimum. This might mean spending a few minutes before the visit to familiarize yourself with the patient's electronic health record and saving computer entry of nonessential information (e.g., laboratory orders, prescription requests, and looking up diagnostic codes) until the end of the visit, after the patient has left the room.[36]

PATIENT EDUCATION AND KNOWLEDGE

Patient education is the process of influencing patient behavior and producing the changes in knowledge, attitudes, and skills necessary to maintain or improve health.[37] Patient education is important for a variety of reasons, including patient satisfaction, knowledge, adherence, and outcomes. Patient satisfaction in dermatology correlates with the quality of explanations and answers to patient questions. Certain aspects of patient education are medicolegal obligations, such as obtaining informed consent for a procedure or discussing potential adverse effects of medications.[38] The Joint Commission currently requires that each hospital "assess the patient's learning needs and use methods of education and instruction that are matched to the patient's level of understanding." A different form of learning aids such as face-to-face interaction, booklets, audiovisuals, and most impotently the internet is the main source of health knowledge nowadays.

The Internet is a growing source of information for patients, with increasing numbers of people searching for health information on the web. The advantages of the Internet include the presence of many types of resources (e.g. written, video, and forums) and patients' ability to gather information at their own pace at home. While the quantity of information available through the Internet is undeniable, the quality of information has been more of a concern. Fortunately, some studies suggest that the Internet is a decent source of information for patients. A study on skin cancer prevention resources found that the preferred sites by experts were also among the most easily found sites.[39]

A systematic review of randomized controlled trials (RCTs) on patient education for atopic dermatitis concluded that "patient education appears to be effective in improving quality of life and in reducing the perceived severity of skin disease."[40]

To provide patient-centered education, the needs and goals of each patient should be elicited. According to the Joint Commission, this includes asking the patient "how he or she prefers to receive information (i.e., reading, hearing, or viewing)." Gathering patient information on language is also highly recommended. One method is to ask the patient directly, "In what language do you prefer to receive your medical care?" or "In what language do you prefer to read health-related materials?"[41]

A patient's health beliefs, if not addressed, may affect compliance and cause unnecessary anxiety. For example, a patient may report that a prescribed corticosteroid cream is not effective, while the actual reason for treatment failure is a lack of application due to fear of thinning the skin. If the dermatologist does not ask, "Is there anything about the medication that concerns you?" then the root cause of the problem will not be discovered. A study on chronic illness patients revealed that medication beliefs were stronger predictors of reported adherence than gender, educational experience, and a number of medications prescribed.[42] Healthcare providers should simplify their educational messages as much as possible.[41]

CONCLUSION

In conclusion, studies have shown that physicians who have been trained to enhance their interpersonal skills receive higher ratings of their overall communication style and are also more likely than control subjects to exhibit specific patient-centered communication behaviors.[43]

This generation all over the world is brought up in a sterile cocoon, in a sanitized bubble. The concept of a joint family rarely exist. It is a nuclear era with only parents and one child. No relatives are encouraged or entertained. They do not communicate nor do they interact among themselves as all are busy. So no relationship gets built up. They get their training in schools where they are mixing with peers from similar background. They never get the chance of getting exposed to the "big bad world" and grow up with a lopsided impression about the world around us. So when they become doctors they are mentally on an elevated platform, an isolated pedestal which makes them (both doctors and patients) even more alienated from each other. This delusion of grandiose and complex of superiority does not help. Induction to the whole society or at least the population served by the hospital is important to serve patients in an empathetic way. In some universities around the globe, liberals arts is being included in medical schools. The students get the knowledge of literature, philosophy, sociology, and history.

Soft skills training are incorporated in the curriculum.

The use of good communication skills has been shown to add minimal time to the visit yet can have a positive influence on subjective and objective measures of health outcomes. It is possible to learn the skills described above and successfully put them into practice, but like other medical skills, excellence in patient communication takes time, practice, and coaching.

REFERENCES

1. Chu CI, Tseng CC. A survey of how patient-perceived empathy affects the relationship between health literacy and the understanding of information by orthopedic patients? BMC Public Health. 2013;13(1):155.
2. Levinson W, Roter D, Mullooly JP, Dull VT, Frankel RM. Physician-patient communication. The relationship with malpractice claims among primary care physicians and surgeons. JAMA. 1997;277(7):553-9.
3. Ambady N, Laplante D, Nguyen T, Rosenthal R, Chaumeton N, Levinson W. Surgeons' tone of voice: a clue to malpractice history. Surgery. 2002;132:5-9.
4. India Medical Times. (2016). 110% rise in number of medical negligence cases in India every year: Study. [online] Available from https://www.indiamedicaltimes.com/2016/11/20/110-rise-in-number-of-medicalnegligence-cases-in-india-every-year-study/. [Last accessed March, 2020].
5. Times of India. (2016). Alarming rise in medical negligence litigation: Study. [online] Available from https://timesofindia.indiatimes.com/city/nagpur/Alarming-rise-in-medical-negligence-litigation-Study/articleshow/55484635.cms. [Last accessed March, 2020].
6. Sessa P, Meconi F. Perceived trustworthiness shapes neural empathic responses toward others' pain. Neuropsychologia. 2015;79:97-105.
7. Renzi C, Abeni D, Picardi A, Agostini E, Melchi CF, Pasquini P, et al. Factors associated with patient satisfaction with care among dermatological outpatients. Br J Dermatol. 2001;145:617-23.
8. Vijaya RM. Medical tourism: revenue generation or international transfer of healthcare problems? Journal of Economic Issues. 2010;44(1):53-70.
9. Lahiri K, Coondoo A. Topical steroid damaged/dependent face (TSDF): An entity of cutaneous pharmacodependence. Indian J Dermatol. 2016;61(3):265-72.
10. Nguyen TV, Hong J, Prose NS. Compassionate care: enhancing physician–patient communication and education in dermatology: Part I: Patient-centered communication. Journal of the American Academy of Dermatology. 2013;68(3):353.e1-8.
11. Makoul G. Essential elements of communication in medical encounters: the Kalamazoo consensus statement. Academic Medicine. 2001;76(4):390-3.
12. Prose NS. Paying attention. JAMA. 2000;283:2763.
13. Eide H, Graugaard P, Holgersen K, Finset A. Physician communication in different phases of a consultation at an oncology outpatient clinic related to patient satisfaction. Patient Education and Counseling. 2003;51(3):259-66.
14. Gross DA, Zyzanski SJ, Borawski EA, Cebul RD, Stange KC. Patient satisfaction with time spent with their physician. J Fam Pract. 1998;47(2):133-8.
15. Beckman HB, Frankel RM. The effect of physician behavior on the collection of data. Ann Intern Med. 1984;101(5):692-6.
16. Lindberg B, Axelsson K, Öhrling K. Experience with videoconferencing between a neonatal unit and the families' home from the perspective of certified paediatric nurses. J Telemed Telecare. 2009;15(6):275-80.
17. Tallman K, Janisse T, Frankel RM, Sung SH, Krupat E, Hsu JT. Communication practices of physicians with high patient-satisfaction ratings. Perm J. 2007;11(1):19-29.
18. Epstein RM, Mauksch L, Carroll J, Jaen CR. Have you really addressed your patient's concerns? Family Practice Management. 2008;15(3):35-40.
19. Coulehan JL, Platt FW, Egener B, Frankel R, Lin CT, Lown B, Salazar WH. "Let me see if I have this right...": words that help build empathy. Ann Intern Med. 2001;135(3):221-7.
20. Suchman AL, Markakis K, Beckman HB, Frankel R. A model of empathic communication in the medical interview. JAMA. 1997;277(8):678-82.
21. Marvel MK, Epstein RM, Flowers K, Beckman HB. Soliciting the patient's agenda: have we improved? JAMA. 1999;281(3):283-7.

22. Richards HL, Fortune DG, Weidmann A, Sweeney SKT, Griffiths CEM. Detection of psychological distress in patients with psoriasis: low consensus between dermatologist and patient. British Journal of Dermatology. 2004;151(6):1227-33.
23. Smith RC. Patient-centered interviewing: an evidence-based method. Lippincott Williams & Wilkins; 2002.
24. Olson KP. 'Oh, by the Way...': Agenda Setting in Office Visits. Family practice management. 2002;9(10):63.
25. Robinson JD. Closing medical encounters: two physician practices and their implications for the expression of patients' unstated concerns. Social Science and Medicine. 2001;53(5):639-56.
26. Breen KJ, Greenberg PB. Difficult physician-patient encounters. Internal medicine journal. 2010;40(10):682-8.
27. Ekman P. Emotions revealed. BMJ. 2004; 328(Suppl S5):0405184.
28. Alzolibani AA. Patient satisfaction and expectations of the quality of service of University affiliated dermatology clinics. Journal of Public Health and Epidemiology. 2011;3(2):61-7.
29. Pichert JW, Miller CS, Hollo AH, Gauld-Jaeger J, Federspiel CF, Hickson GB. What health professionals can do to identify and resolve patient dissatisfaction. The Joint Commission journal on quality improvement. 1998;24(6):303-12.
30. Quill TE, Arnold RM, Platt F. "I wish things were different": expressing wishes in response to loss, futility, and unrealistic hopes. Ann Intern Med. 2001;135(7):551-5.
31. Hassig RA, Balogh L, Bandy M, Doyle JD, Gluck JC, Lindner KL, et al. Standards for hospital libraries 2002 with 2004 revisions. Journal of the Medical Library Association. 2005;93(2):282-3.
32. Lazare A. Apology in medical practice. JAMA 2006;296:1401-4.
33. Mazor KM, Greene SM, Roblin D, Lemay CA, Firneno CL, Calvi J, et al. More than words: patients' views on apology and disclosure when things go wrong in cancer care. Patient Education and Counseling. 2013;90(3):341-6.
34. Uhlenhake EE, Kurkowski D, Feldman SR. Conversations on psoriasis–what patients want and what physicians can provide: a qualitative look at patient and physician expectations. Journal of Dermatological Treatment. 2010; 21(1):6-12.
35. O'Malley AS, Cohen GR, Grossman JM. Electronic medical records and communication with patients and other clinicians: are we talking less? Issue Brief No. 131. Center for Studying Health System Change; 2010.
36. Rao JK, Anderson LA, Inui TS, Frankel RM. Communication interventions make a difference in conversations between physicians and patients: a systematic review of the evidence. Med Care. 2007;45(4):340-9.
37. Qaseem A, Fihn SD, Dallas P, Williams S, Owens DK, Shekelle P. Management of stable ischemic heart disease: summary of a clinical practice guideline from the American College of Physicians/American College of Cardiology Foundation/American Heart Association/ American Association for Thoracic Surgery/ Preventive Cardiovascular Nurses Association/ Society of Thoracic Surgeons. Ann Intern Med. 2012;157(10):735-43.
38. Uhlenhake EE, Kurkowski D, Feldman SR. Conversations on psoriasis–what patients want and what physicians can provide: a qualitative look at patient and physician expectations. Journal of Dermatological Treatment. 2010; 21(1):6-12.
39. Renzi C, Abeni D, Picardi A, Agostini E, Melchi CF, Pasquini P, et al. Factors associated with patient satisfaction with care among dermatological outpatients. British Journal of Dermatology. 2001;145(4):617-23.
40. Leffell DJ, Berwick M, Bolognia J. The effect of pre-education on patient compliance with full-body examination in a public skin cancer screening. The Journal of Dermatologic Surgery and Oncology. 1993;19(7):660-3.
41. Ohya Y, Williams H, Steptoe A, Saito H, Iikura Y, Anderson R, et al. Psychosocial factors and adherence to treatment advice in childhood atopic dermatitis. Journal of Investigative Dermatology. 2001;117(4):852-7.
42. Kaplan SH, Greenfield S, Ware JE Jr. Assessing the effects of physician-patient interactions on the outcomes of chronic disease. Med Care. 1989;27(3 Suppl):S110-27.
43. Roter DL, Hall JA, Kern DE, Barker LR, Cole KA, Roca RP. Improving physicians' interviewing skills and reducing patients' emotional distress: a randomized clinical trial. Archives of Internal Medicine. 1995;155(17):1877-84.

SECTION 9: Managing Special Clinics

9.1 Setting Up and Managing Esthetic Dermatology Clinic

Shehnaz Z Arsiwala

INTRODUCTION

Esthetic dermatology involves consultation and procedure for correction, prevention enhancement, and maintenance of skin conditions which are cosmetically discomforting to the patient. The function of the skin may or may not be affected by these conditions but the psychological implications are stronger and patient seeks to correct them.

Since both general and esthetic dermatology are merged into day-to-day consultations in metropolis cities and even small towns, it is truly difficult and practically impossible to separate the two out, e.g. a psoriasis patients may seek laser hair reduction or an eczema patient may develop acne and progress to acne scars, in such situation, the physician having a practice profile of general as well as esthetic dermatology can handle all concerns of his/her patient from psoriasis control to laser hair reduction.

Addition to a clinic which caters to general dermatology patients can incorporate modifications into a clinic which enables one to set-up and manage an esthetic dermatology clinic.

As is the current trend, the next generation seeks to set-up an esthetic-based clinic at outset, in such a situation the set-up can have esthetic clinic requirements inducted.

A qualified dermatologist is already armed with qualification and knowledge on physiological, anatomical behavior of the skin and is the best to initiate, run, and maintain an esthetic dermatology clinic.

A dermatologist at the helm of esthetic practice has the expertise to select cases for esthetic procedural interventions as he/she is well versed with dermatological medical history of patient, e.g. sound knowledge of markers of cutaneous hyperandrogenism in patients with acne, hair loss, and acanthosis—all of which form the largest figures in consults nowadays.

A few important aspects a dermatologist must keep in mind, while setting up an esthetic dermatologist clinic, can be divided into the "setup-related factors and practice-related factors.

Detailed planning, time, and effort are consumed in setting up a quality care center which must gain reputation of being state-of-the-art and of great scientific setup. This ranges from clinical acumen of the physician, scientific rationale concepts of care, knowledge of equipment and consumables, their applications and maintenance, safety to etiquette and conduct of the ancillary staff, ambience, all at a competitive service price, and all upgraded and updated from time to time.

SPACE (FIGS. 9.1.1 TO 9.1.5)

The clinic space should have a consultation room, a well-ventilated, well-decorated waiting area with services such as washroom and water-drinking facilities for patients, an examination room attached to consulting room, and a single or multiple procedure room depending on the space available. The privacy of patient undergoing examination or procedure should be ensured.

PROCEDURE ROOMS (FIGS. 9.1.1 TO 9.1.4 AND 9.1.6)

Individual procedure rooms should be separated by door/partition/curtains and ensure that laser rooms have no mirrors.

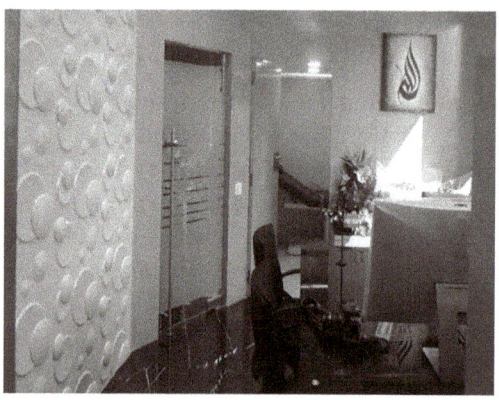

Fig. 9.1.1: Comfortable consulting room.

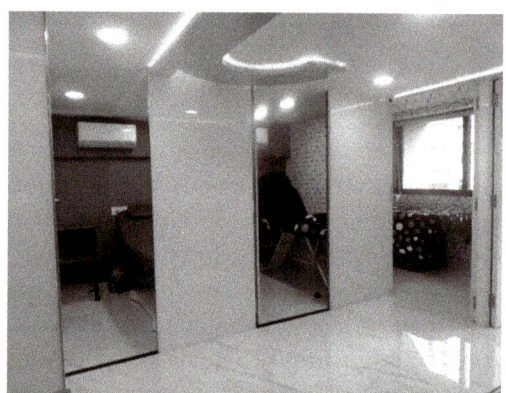

Fig. 9.1.2: Procedure rooms.

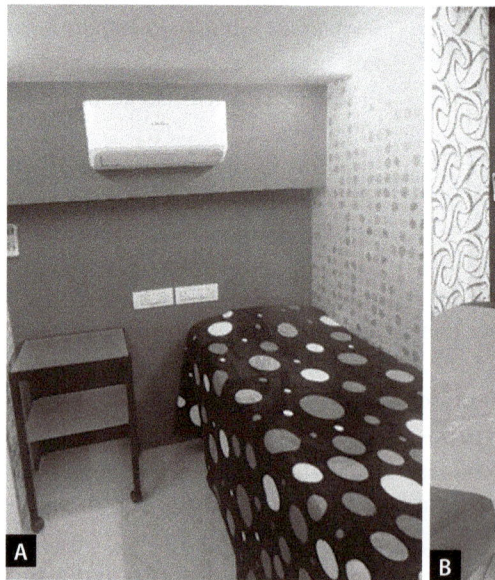

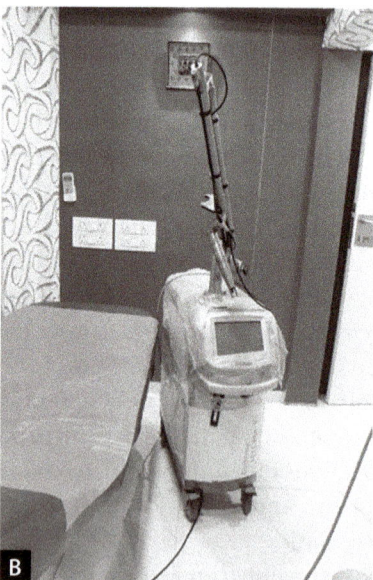

Figs. 9.1.3A and B: (A) Esthetic procedure room; (B) Procedure room for laser.

Section 9: Managing Special Clinics

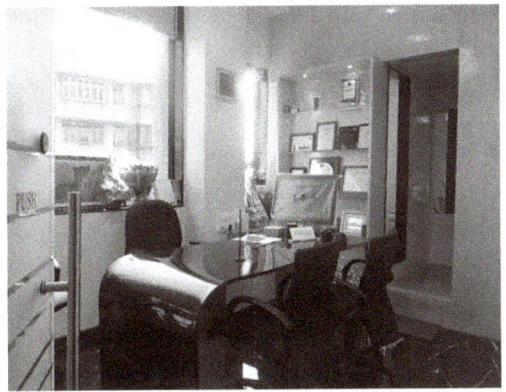

Fig. 9.1.4: Well-lit consulting chamber.

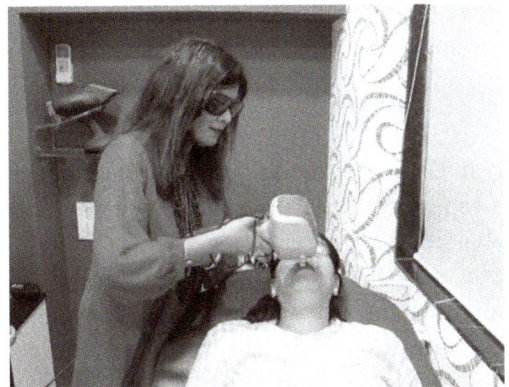

Fig. 9.1.5: Safety protocols during lasers.

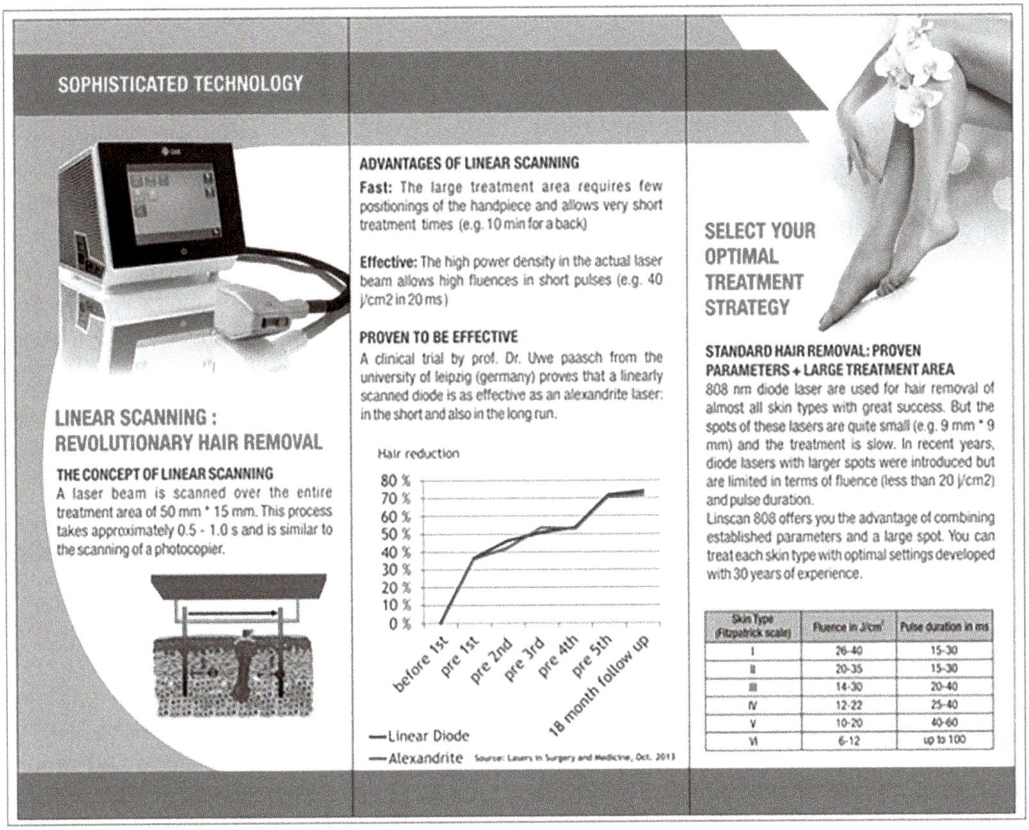

Fig. 9.1.6: Brochure sample highlighting technology for laser hair removal.

A reclining chair or bed for comfortable placement of patients, trolley/shelves for house products, etc., and disposable sheets to prevent cross transmission of infection should be available. Laser rooms should have marked warning signs for irradiation that are visibly displayed. Good lighting and air circulation should be present.

OPERATION THEATER

If an OT is present at premise, it should have a separate entry with a recovery room and all equipment for emergency care should be available. OT should have a comfortable bed, modular and operable by remote or manual change of level/recline. Infection control strategies and daily disinfection protocol and weekly fumigation protocols should be followed.

WASTE MANAGEMENT

Disposable of waste has protocol of segregation of dry and wet and sharp waste disposal according to municipal waste disposal rules should be mandatory. Waste disposal pick up and licenses should be procured.

PHOTOGRAPHY

There should be a separate room for photography documentation with uniform background and adequate lighting. One must invest in a good single-lens reflex camera (DSLR) camera with bounce flash and Wi-Fi facilities available in the camera body. Uniform positioning and standardization of images is very important to compare results in an esthetic set up.

AMBIENCE

Ambience should be pleasant and soothing and relaxing. There should be no clutter in waiting area. Waiting chairs should be comfortable and esthetic, adequate display of services, brochures (**Fig. 9.1.5**) for services, light soft music or a TV in display area with minimal or no sound can keep a waiting patient involved, occupied, and abreast with latest trend.

STAFF

Staff can be in uniforms, but not necessary. They should be decently dressed, if not in uniforms, have a pleasant personality and good communication skills, and should be tolerant and polite in personality. Also, staff should be well trained to handle difficult patients and aggressive demanding personalities, if needed.

ASSISTANT DOCTORS

Assistant doctors should be qualified, well versed with the process of clinic, abreast of latest trends, have good communication skills, and have a general notion on focus and vision of the clinic functions. The assistant doctors serve an addition to the Chief Consultant and also have individual skills and expertise, like peels, injectable lasers, etc. and should work in conjunction with whole team for patient care.

PROFESSIONAL SKILLS

Skill in cosmetic procedures can be acquired through postgraduate observerships, fellowships, workshops, and working with esthetic-oriented clinic.

CONSENT FORMS

Consent forms are extremely crucial for documentation of an informed valid consent in an esthetic dermatology clinic and should be individual to each category of procedures and detailed. Consent should be discussed in patient's own language and signed mandatorily before each procedure. The forms should be stored for at least 5 years and patient is required to sign with complete signature and not initials, for patient's 21 years and above. Consent of parents or guardians in case of minors. If consent is of multiple pages, signature on each page should be obtained. Specification for use of photographs or videos should be added in consent form and patient should have a right to decline. As a general rule, no procedure should be conducted without consent forms.

CONSULTATIONS

Consultations should be detailed with proper history and examination. Mandatory investigations should be conducted. Esthetic goals and desires of the patient should be given priority and procedures should be chosen with safety, efficacy and evidence-based knowledge. Skilled care is premium in improvising procedure outcomes and should be communicated in clear language.

FEEDBACK FORMS

Feedback forms or questionnaire serve to assess the services and updates and improvise on various aspects from quality care to staff, etc. and should be encouraged in patients. Feedback forms also bring out any shortcomings or grievances experienced by the patient and can be addressed amicably.

Accessibility after procedures is vital and every query or concern post-procedure should be addressed. Monitoring or results should be adequate and counseling for post-procedure care should be detailed.

Appointments should be handled by competent receptionists and can be available on phone, Emails or Website online.

INFORMATION

Information brochures serve to educate the patient of latest trends, new updates, and available services and impart the patient with education, also giving the patient an informed choice.

In clinic, information and videos are helpful in educating patient, while waiting for their turn and alleviate any doubts and fears regarding a treatment.

COMPLICATIONS

The center should be well-equipped to handle any complications arising out of in-office procedures, right from vasovagal attack to bleeding or vascular compromise during fillers, etc. A crash cart should be available for same at premises and also access to nearest hospital emergency care for any untoward grave complication should be provided.

SYSTEMS AND MACHINES

Systems and machines should be well maintained, serviced and upgraded and updated from time to time. Technologies catering to hair removal, pigmentation, and rejuvenation should be installed depending on client profile and additional devices for tightening, fat reduction, etc. can be incorporated according to patient profile.

PRECAUTIONS

Safety precautions during procedures, fire precautions, handling of sharps, and waste disposal with standard of care protocol should be adhered with strict vigilance.

Offers, packages, and discounted rates are rolled out by some centers at festival and marriage season, varies according to clientele, and are a personal choice of the clinic management.

Questionnaire regarding esthetic concerns of the patients helps the physician to gauge patient desires.

Confidentiality, which is utmost important, should be maintained.

Acquiring, conducting, and achieving success in an esthetic patient-oriented clinic is a challenge and continuous journey for a physician and his/her team and one must keep abreast of latest scientific trends with safe rationale.

BIBLIOGRAPHY

1. Alcalay J. Dermatology: A medical, surgical and aesthetic profession. Isr Med Assoc J. 2008; 10:404–5.
2. Aurangabadkar SJ, Mysore V, Ahmed ES. Buying a laser: tips and pearls. J Cutan Aesthet Surg. 2014;7(2):124-30.
3. Brennan C. Aesthetic Policy and Procedure Protocols: A "Must Have" for Every Aesthetic Medical Provider. Plast Surg Nurs. 2015;35(3):127-8.

9.2 Trichology Practice

BS Chandrashekar, Preethi B Nayak

INTRODUCTION

In the human body, hair is a major cosmetic display feature. It does not have any vital function in humans, yet it plays a significant role in social as well as sexual interaction. The diagnosis of hair disorder dates back to the ancient Egyptian times. The difficult task in diagnosis of hair disorder is to distinguish between subjective complaints and true disorder, along with establishing the underlying pathogenesis.

Patients usually consult dermatologist with diffuse or focal effluvium, changes in hair structure or color, and scarring or nonscarring alopecia. The key feature in the management of a patient with hair disorder is attributed to the establishment of correct diagnosis. Correct diagnosis of hair disorder is complex and requires detailed evaluation of clinical history and presentation, physical examination, and laboratory tests. Due to the limited therapeutic options in many hair disorders, the practitioner needs to recognize and address this issue.

Who should Practice Trichology?

As trichology is part of the dermatology curriculum in postgraduation, dermatologists are considered true trichologists. In the recent past, hair restoration surgeries have attracted a lot of other specialties, and hence hair transplantation is shared by multiple specialties as a subspecialty.

COMPONENTS OF TRICHOLOGY PRACTICE

- Hair loss
- Unwanted hair growth
- Hair shaft abnormalities
- Inflammatory/noninflammatory hair disorder
- Hair cosmetics/hair grooming/hair care.

SETTING UP TRICHOLOGY UNIT

Trichology being an essential part of dermatology practice, the guidelines and requirements of setting up a trichology unit are similar to setting up clinical dermatology or esthetic dermatology practice **(Fig. 9.2.1)**.

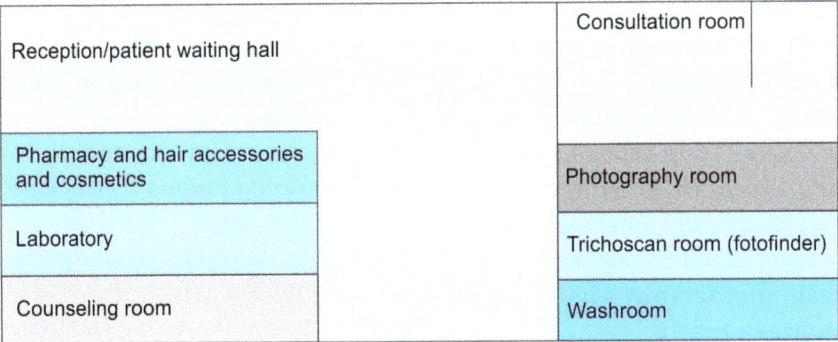

Fig. 9.2.1: Outline of infrastructure of a trichology unit.

The trichology unit may be planned in such a way to accommodate the following:

Common to General Dermatology Practice

- Reception and patient waiting hall
- Consultation room(s) for the physician and the patient
- Examination room
- Photography room
- Laboratory
- Pharmacy and hair accessories and hair cosmetics
- Washrooms
- Laser wing

Specific to Trichology Practice

- Trichoscan room
- Minor OT [procedures such as biopsies, platelet rich plasma (PRP) mesotherapies, dressings, sample collection, suture removal, etc.]
- Major OT (hair transplantation, excision of scalp tumors, flap surgeries, etc.):
  - Preoperative/preparation room, changing room, autoclave room, major OT proper, and dissection/graft-cutting room

Equipment Used by the Treating Trichologist

Diagnostic

Handheld lens, dermoscope/video dermoscope, trichoscan, microscope, Woods lamp.

Therapeutic

Platelet rich plasma centrifuges, radiofrequency unit, cryosurgery unit, major and minor OT instruments, low level laser light therapy (LLLT), and laser for hair removal.

Basic Steps of Approach to the Hair Loss Patient

- Assess the impact of hair loss on psychological well-being
- Evaluation of hair loss
- Differential diagnosis
- Ancillary laboratory evaluation
- Design therapeutic guidelines.

CLINICAL EXAMINATION

Good lighting, a magnifying lens, a dermatoscope, and appropriate positioning of the patient on a chair are prerequirements for clinical examination.

- *Inspection*:
  - Visual assessment of pattern and extent of hair loss
  - Hair behavior (color, shine, texture)
  - Presence of scalp inflammation
- Palpation (pattern, scarring, elasticity, surface changes, and other lesions)
- Examination of other body sites
- Clinical photography—hair density, follow-up assessment
- Hair pull test (a group of approximately 60 hair is held between thumb and forefinger of dominant hand—gentle traction)
- Hair card test
- Hair mount test
- Trichoscopic examination
- Trichogram
- *Other tests*:
  - Daily hair counts
  - Hair wash test
  - Trichometry
  - Trichotillometry

Laboratory Tests

- *Blood tests*:
  - Hormonal evaluation (to rule out androgen excess and PCOS)
  - Thyroid profile
  - Serum ferritin
  - Extended tests (serum vitamin D, vitamin B_{12}, serum insulin, lipid profile, etc.)
- Scalp biopsy (to take 2 punches of 4 mm)
- *Microscopic examination of hair*:
  - Trichogram
  - Photographic trichogram and its modifications
  - Light microscopy (including potassium hydroxide mount)

DERMOSCOPY/TRICHOSCOPY

Hair dermoscopy (Also called trichoscopy, **Fig. 9.2.2A**) usually uses a magnification of 10X and can be combined with still or video images (video-dermoscopy) **(Fig. 9.2.2B)**. Specific changes have been reported on dermoscopy of different conditions affecting the hair. It would also be valuable in evaluating structural abnormalities of hair.

PATIENT RECORDS

It is essential to maintain a database of patient records. It not only becomes easier to remember past details of patients' treatment and procedures, but also helps in building a rapport with the patient. One can use electronic medical records (EMR) to access details of the patients.

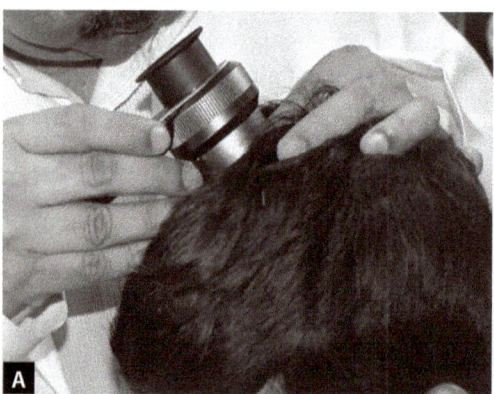
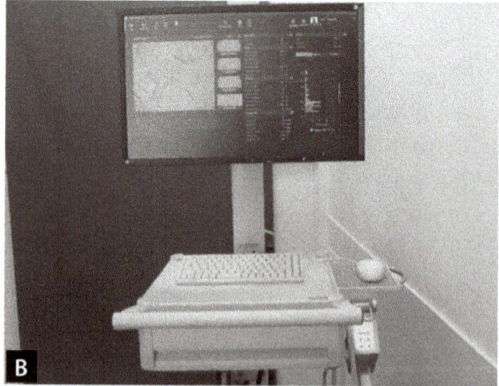

Figs. 9.2.2A and B: Dermatoscopic examination of scalp and Trichoscan (Fotofinder)

PHOTOGRAPHY IN TRICHOLOGY

Clinical photography of hair disorders is an extension of dermatological photography.

Importance of photography in trichology practice:
- Photography plays an important role in documentation of a patient.
- Helpful in counseling, follow-up of patients, and comparing results obtained.
- Useful in the medicolegal cases.
- As patients cannot see the vertex and occipital areas of the scalp, photography helps to visualize these areas and the problems associated with them.
- Helps in counseling patients with body dysmorphic disorders.
- In those patients who are treatment dropouts or have discontinued treatment, photography helps in planning further management.

PATIENT COUNSELING AND LIAISON TREATMENT

In practicing trichology, one encounters several patients for whom the medical approach alone is not enough. For instance, the primary dermatological disease may have secondary psychological impact, such as general anxiety, low mood or social anxiety. Or, some patients may have a comorbid mental illness such as depression. Or, some patients, because of their deficits in stress management, may experience an exacerbation of the symptoms of their skin condition in times of stress, examples being alopecia areata and trichotillomania. These types of patients need psychologically adapted care in dermatology and preferable to work in conjunction with a clinical psychologist for counseling the patients.

DIET AND TRICHOLOGY

Diet is an integral part of dermatology, and is inseparable from trichology practice. A healthy lifestyle is always beneficial to the patient. A trichologist can himself counsel patients regarding hair-rich diet, or he can collaborate with a dietician to do the same, either way, it helps trichologist to develop a stronger bond with the patient and indeed helps in overall improvement of hair and skin condition of the patient.

PHARMACY AND HAIR COSMETICS

Figures 9.2.3A and B show pharmacy and hair cosmetics.

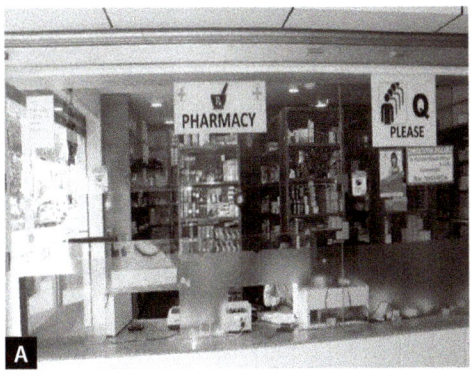 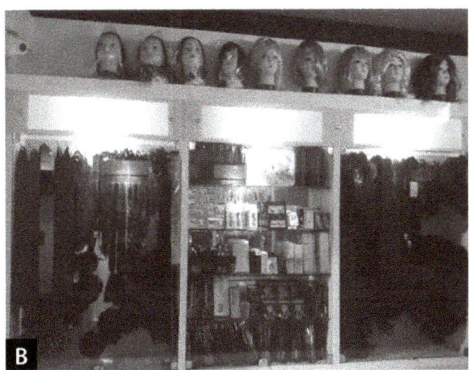

Figs. 9.2.3A and B: Pharmacy and hair accessories and cosmetics.
Source: Obtained permission to reprint from IADVL Textbook of Trichology

DIFFICULTIES IN HAIR PRACTICE

- *Time*: Hair-related disorders are chronic-distressing diseases, which require time and patience of both the treating doctor and patients. Counseling plays a key role. The amount of time the clinician has to spend with each patient is more in hair-related disorder, hence it is difficult to accommodate in busy practice. Trichologist can take help of counselors, dieticians, psychologists, and patient education leaflets, videos, photographs, for patient management, and utilize the short time available more effectively and smartly. Provision of separate trichology clinic is advisable in case if one finds difficulty to provide sufficient time.
- *Finance*: Hair-related products and procedures are relatively expensive. Patient has to be made aware of this from the beginning. Duration of treatment is prolonged especially in androgenetic alopecia, hence, financial commitment has to be realized better.
- *Patient education*: This is crucial in trichology practice. A need to appoint a counselor should be considered. Patient who come for hair-related complaints are usually well informed, a good reasoning and educating the patient helps in long-term management.
- *Internet*: In modern-day practice, Internet is a major hurdle for trichologists. Before consulting a doctor, patients usually go through the internet irrespective of the authenticity and correctness of the content. Patients tend to cross-check the information gained from the trichologist with that available on internet as well. Hence, it becomes difficult to maintain good patient-doctor relationship. It is a better practice to discover from the patients regarding what information they have got from Internet regarding side effects.
- *Infrastructure and instruments*: Dermoscope is dermatologist's stethoscope, but not all dermatologists are well versed and well exposed to it. Video-dermoscope and operation theater facility are available only in higher centers, hence, compromising the trichology practice.
- *Quackery*: Due to low risks and complications, and higher profit, trichology forms a fertile ground for quacks. Quacks are promoting trichology field in a wrong way, and are luring patients with discounted cost, compromising the quality of care. The gap between true trichologist and patients is increasing due to the interference and false propagation by the quacks.

LEGAL ASPECTS

All relevant permissions such as clinic registration with municipal authorities, health authorities, pollution control board, and waste disposal agency are a must. Trichology practice involves both medical risk as well as surgical risk for the practitioner. Cases are likely to be filed in consumer protection court, in case of complication, inadequate care, and patient dissatisfaction.

Professional liability insurance protects the doctor against financial consequences of an error or omission, during the service or professional act, especially during procedures such as hair transplant.

EVOLVING HAIR PRACTICE

From table-chair trichologist to trichologist owning a state-of-the-art operation theater, trichology has evolved through the years. Types of hair complaints, types of patients, patient's knowledge and consciousness about self-beauty, instruments, infrastructure have been changing, so is the trichology practice. Hence, it is trichologist's responsibility to be up-to-date with recent advances in this field and implement it in the practice for the benefit of his patients.

CONCLUSION

To run a successful trichology practice, there are five important components which must be handled well and effectively: (1) Clinical; (2) Procedural; (3) Administrative; (4) Marketing; and (5) Quality control. One should have prior basic knowledge, budget, and plans to reach the determined goal.

As in any practice, the main aim of the trichologist should be to gain patient's confidence, and should always accept that "Patient is always right". Finally, a well-rooted strong knowledge in trichology helps the practitioner to set-up a well-established trichology practice.

ALGORITHM OF APPROACH TO HAIR LOSS PATIENTS

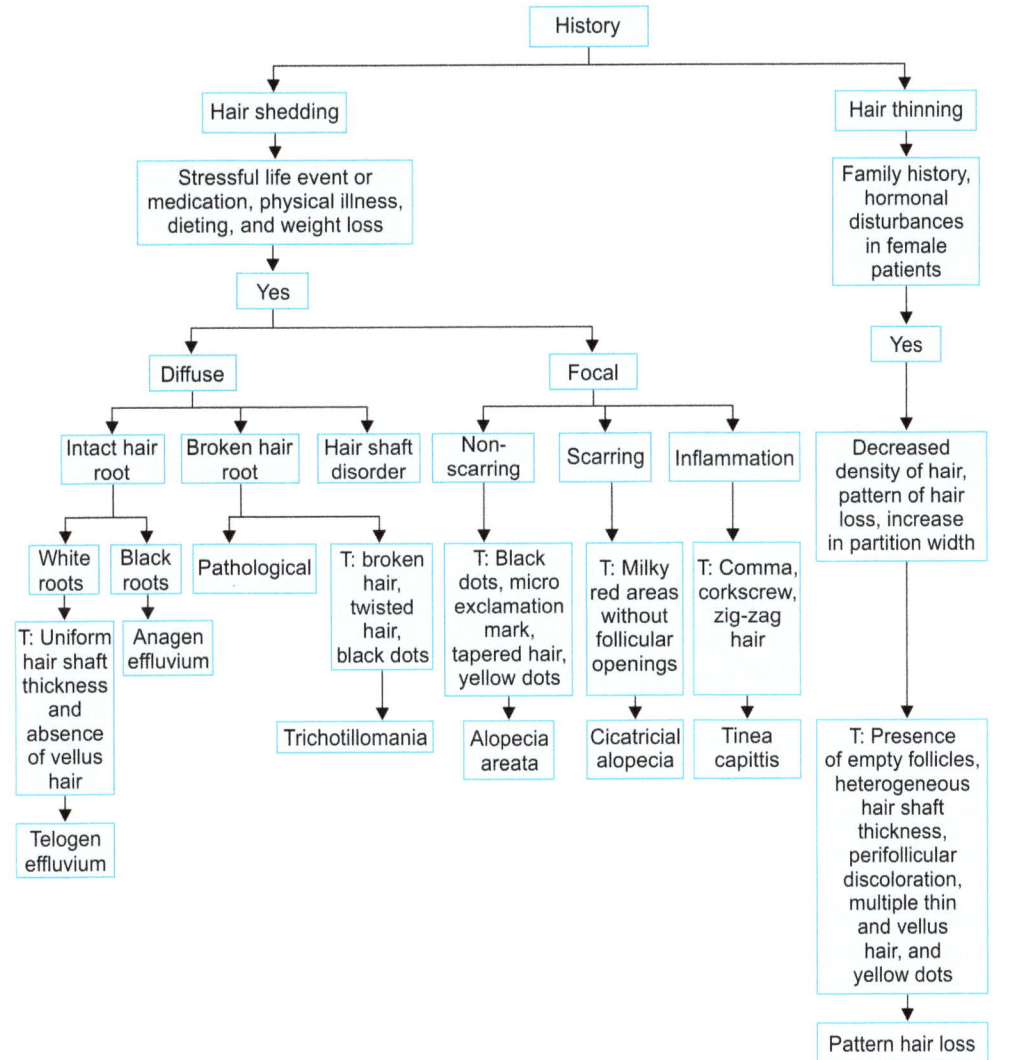

9.3 Setting Up and Managing Allergy Clinic

Kiran Godse, Aditi Jaiswal

INTRODUCTION

The most common allergic disorders in dermatology are atopic dermatitis and urticaria. Urticaria presents with wheals (hives), angioedema, or both, and has a lifetime prevalence of about 9%. The appearance of pruritic, erythematous dermal swellings that blanch with pressure, indicating the presence of vasodilation and superficial dermal edema, is characteristic of wheals. Urticaria cases are classified as either acute or chronic. Chronic urticaria is defined, if daily or almost daily wheals or angioedema are present for >6 weeks. Hence, adversely affecting the quality of life owing to its chronicity. Most of the patients present later after the lesions have subsided, since the lesions are transient, it becomes difficult to understand the disease and its severity. This makes examination also difficult.

Atopic dermatitis, also known as atopic eczema, is a chronic, inflammatory, relapsing skin disorder with generally an early age of onset in infancy and early childhood. It follows a relapsing course with repeated exacerbation and remission, which is characterized by dermatitis with itch. Natural history of atopic dermatitis often involves typical progression including food allergy, allergic rhinitis (hay fever), and asthma. It is accompanied in a majority of patients with a personal or family history of "atopic diathesis". Since the onset is in childhood, most parents are very concerned about the disease activity and the investigations of the same for their child.

Thus taken together, it is imperative that proper specialized services should be provided along with counseling to the patients of urticaria.

INFRASTRUCTURE

- Allergy clinic can be set-up in a clinic, hospital or affiliated with a hospital with inpatient facilities to allow for extended diagnostic work-up and management of exacerbation.
- No specific ideal space required.
- It needs to be able to provide care for atopic dermatitis and urticaria patients of any age, since most acute urticaria patients are children and presenting age for atopic dermatitis is in childhood. Hence would be beneficial, if it is child-friendly.
- Staff needs to be able to communicate adequately with patients in national, local language, and English.
- The dermatologist should exhibit high motivation to help the patients and show understanding that they may be the last resort of patients. Staff needs to convey to patients that they are in good care.
- It is beneficial to display posters depicting about the specific allergy and urticaria in the waiting area of hospital to increase the understanding of patients about their disease.
- Counseling of patients and their families, for example, on triggers of exacerbation, stress, avoidance of non-steroidal anti-inflammatory drugs (NSAIDs), daily-life issues can help to optimize urticaria management.

WORKING

- The hours of working are predominantly decided by the consultant, but sometimes urticaria with angioedema can present as emergency in institutions.
- Structured documentation, recording, and archiving of patient data help in keeping track of patient's progress.
- It is better to keep electronic medical records and an appointment scheduling system to keep patients satisfied.
- Structured history taking by the physicians is essential and a checklist can facilitate this.
- While in the waiting area, patient can be handed a form to fill up in detail about the relevant history, known allergies, and comorbidities. They can also be informed about the do's and dont's for taking care of their child with atopic dermatitis.
- UAS7, UCT scores should be used since these provide for reliable improvement in patient. Same is applicable for atopic dermatitis scoring, i.e. Scoring AD (SCORAD) and eczema area and severity index (EASI).
- Presence of diagnostic measures for urticaria comorbidities and underlying causes such as autologous serum skin test (ASST), basophil activation test (BAT), and skin-prick test would set one apart from the rest.
- Provocation testing and threshold assessment are important in the diagnostic workup of chronic inducible urticaria (CIndU). Standard operating procedures are needed as is the use of appropriate instruments/protocols such as dermographometers.
- Routine allergy testing, even with the Phadiatop or the enzyme-linked immunospot (ELISpot) assays can be used.
- Atopic patch test can be used for atopic dermatitis.
- An inpatient service at a nearby place should be present when one is planning to prescribe biologicals for urticaria and other allergies.
- Patient support groups could be organized in the form of meetings of all the patients suffering from the same disease. This will help them understand the prognosis and improvements seen by other.

NETWORKING

This is an integral part of any practice. The physicians need to know that one can provide treatment beyond the daily medications when not controlled so that they can refer it to an urticaria specialist and an allergy specialist.

- The specialist needs to be able to interact with other specialties for the management of comorbidities, the treatment of patients with differential diagnoses, and to perform extended diagnostics. Hence, it is a two-way communication.
- Patients need to be able to find the clinic via information on the web.
- It is also good to have referral network of physicians.
- Working with patient association at times can be beneficial.
- Collaboration with GALEN centers for UCARE for urticaria and ADCARE for atopic dermatitis will provide an edge over other physicians.
- Making oneself known as an allergy specialist can also be possible by being involved in the academic activities such as publications in the subjects of urticaria and atopic dermatitis.
- Delivering and organizing focused conferences and workshop for practitioners and masterclass for residents would help educate the dermatologists as well as physicians.

SETTING UP AN ALLERGY CLINIC

The following list is needed for setting up and managing an allergy clinic:
- Centrifuge for blood separation for auto-serum therapy
- *Autologous serum skin test*: Tuberculin syringe, saline, lens and measuring scale
- *Emergency kit*: Inj adrenaline, hydrocortisone, avil and oxygen for rare anaphylaxis with omalizumab injection
- Prick test is not useful in skin allergies
- Patch test kit for contact allergy
- Other specialists should be available, such as chest ENT specialists and pediatricians and psychiatrists
- Counselor is needed for most chronic skin diseases
- Support group for urticarial and atopic dermatitis with monthly meeting
- Well-equipped laboratory for doing blood test such as IgE, Immunocap assays.
- Trained nurse to handle skin allergy cases.

9.4 Setting Up and Managing Laser Clinic

Avitus John Raakesh Prasad

INTRODUCTION

Over that past decade, laser dermatology has gained popularity and will continue to do so as more and more dermatologists are getting trained and are looking forward to invest in laser-based procedures. Use of lasers is becoming an integral part of how we treat our patients for various conditions which need intervention where only medical management will not suffice. Setting-up of a laser clinic requires careful pre-planning and execution as they take a part of your working time, income, and definitely need to give return on investment.

HOW TO START?

Locality

a. Starting on a rented space or owned building near a popular place or near a well-known junction, for example, broadway junction, Gandhi circle or a famous road or well-known reference area is ideal. It makes it easier for clients to remember and give reference to other clients.

b. It should be approachable to the clients as many will be coming from long distances. It could be preferably near a main bus stand, railway junction, and metro station. So it will be easier to commute.

c. Do not start in a congested area where parking will be a hassle, the need to start in the center of the city has slowly reduced. A well-known area near the outskirts of the city which can be approached from towns surrounding a major city is also a good idea. Clients nowadays do not like to travel through traffic and many who come for laser treatment will come by their own vehicle which needs parking.

d. Visibility is the key, so starting a laser clinic in a famous area but in a side street and not on the main road might not help a beginner, but for an already established doctor in a smaller town planning to start in a posh area in a big city, it is a different story as they already have patients pool. If it is a commercial complex, starting in the first floor will be better choice provided elevator service is available preferably once side of the clinic is facing the major road.

e. Get information and register your clinic according to the latest rules and guidelines.

Space Requirement

f. A minimum of 500 to 800 sq area is required to start a laser clinic, but having at least 1200 sq ft will give you an option to reallocate space and expand.

g. For beginner who cannot invest in a large space because of lack of funds, you can start in a 300 sq ft area with 150 sq ft for reception and 150 sq ft for consultation and attached minor laser room. Then rent a 500–700 sq feet floor in a side road even a km away which would cost much lesser and calling it your second clinic. Make it your laser clinic and you could refer your clients there with appointments, so you could go there and do you procedures.

h. A typical space allocation is given here:

Room	Minimum space allocation
Reception	150–300 sq ft
Consultation room	75–100 sq ft (can be 150 sq ft, if attached minor procedure bed is in the room)
Main laser room	150–200 sq ft
Minor laser room (×2) (if needed) can be also used for peel, botox and fillers	75–100 sq ft each

Apart from the essential space allocation, there will be a need for additional space requirements, if possible or affordable (**Fig. 9.4.1**).

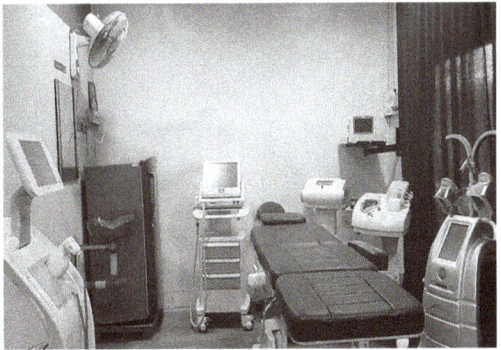

Fig. 9.4.1: 200 sq ft laser room can house multiple devices if there is space constraint to have many laser rooms.

Room	Minimum space allocation
Miscellaneous such as autoclave and laundry room	75–100 sq ft
Phototherapy (full body, hand and foot unit, targeted phototherapy)	150–175 sq ft totally
Washroom	75 sq ft

Interiors

i. Choose a color scheme for your clinic, different color for each room is good idea to break monotony, a clinic is like your second home where you spend most of time awake, make it pleasant for you as well as your clients. Choose a lighter shade like light green or sky blue for your laser room (**Fig. 9.4.2**).

j. Make sure every room, floor, and ceiling is accessible to cleaning as they collect lot of dust over time which is damaging to high-end laser systems. Using designer ceilings is good to look at but definitely difficult to clean. The floor can be covered using vitrified tiles or antistatic materials which are easier to clean. The walls should be painted with antibacterial coat paints which are available now and are washable also.

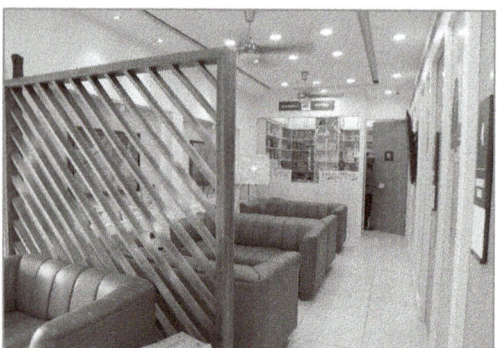

Fig. 9.4.2: Reception.

k. Having sliding door for your laser room is a good idea plus it should have width of 3 feet. By having a sliding door, it helps in saving extra space when you cannot afford to have a larger laser room. Lower depth cupboards or shelves of 1–1.5 feet are ideal to maximize available space **(Fig. 9.4.3)**.
l. Ambient lighting is needed in every room. Laser room lights should be chosen correctly. It should have sufficient central illuminance of 1,000 lux for the laser room and minimum of 40,000 lux in the operating field, good field of light with shadow dilution. It should produce minimum heat.
m. Air conditioning has become a necessity. According to NABH guidelines, at least 20 air changes per hour (ACH) is needed in a laser room of floor area of 10 ft by 15 ft with a height of 8 ft. It come 400 CFM (cubic feet per minute). To simplify, 1 ton AC is required for a 100–150 sq ft area, a 1.5–2 ton AC for a 200–250 sq ft depending on the local temperature of your place. Having a ceiling which is lower around 7.5–8 ft from the floor is ideal to have effective cooling of the room and be able to get 20 ACH. A refrigerator to keep Botox and Fillers and medicines which need cold chain, ice water, and ice cubes for the procedure.

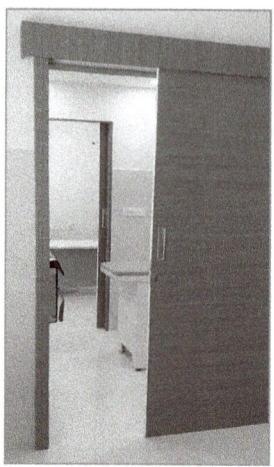

Fig. 9.4.3: Sliding door connecting two laser rooms with the consultation room.

n. Exhaust fan with autoclose flaps is required in Laser room where ablative procedures and laser hair reduction are done, to remove the fumes and smell following the procedure. A good smoke evacuator is also essential.
o. Electrical wiring should have standard wire gauge of 7/20 and if possible three-phase connection for your laser room and phototherapy room. The plug points should have dual 5 and 15 Amp outlet. The plug point should be placed at a foot height from the floor to prevent wires hanging from the walls and hindering mobility for the operator and the equipment. Do not keep the plug point at floor level as it would be difficult while mopping the floor **(Fig. 9.4.4)**.
p. A small adequate wash basin in laser room and preferably a small overhead ceiling tank inside the laser room helps when there is water shortage. Plan to have a washroom in your clinic or at least in your building premises and you need to have it cleaned regularly.
q. Having an uninterrupted power supply in case of power failure is needed. A UPS

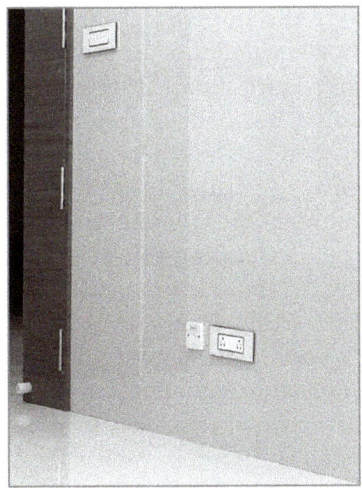

Fig. 9.4.4: Switches position.

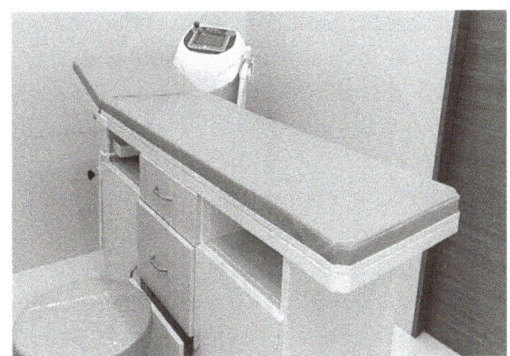

Fig. 9.4.5: Laser bed with drawers to save space.

of minimum 7 KVA is needed in a laser room to power a laser equipment, light stand, and smoke evacuator in case of sudden power shut down. If the power failure happens while the laser is working, it could harm the capacitors and damage the laser equipment. A minimum of 15 minutes back up of 7 KVA UPS is enough, costing between ₹ 75,000–100,000, if you cannot afford a bigger capacity UPS provided you have a generator system in your building or clinic. The capacity of the generator depends on the number and area of room space, number of electrical equipment, AC, and laser required to be running for optimal running of the laser clinic. It is better to invest in a 20–25 KVA generator, if you are planning to put AC in all rooms and upgrading your laser clinic and laser equipment as the newer systems require more power to operate without lag.

r. Making a clinic esthetically appealing, beautiful interior is a must but do not overdo it, as maintenance and cleaning has to be done regularly and it requires staff and time **(Fig. 9.4.5)**.

s. Fire safety, mainly in the laser room, is a requirement by new norms in clinic establishment. Having a sufficient fire extinguisher with regular checking and date stamping will ensure safety. Always keep a record of the last date of service and due date for next service.[1]

Finances

- Investing in a clinic and laser equipment needs careful planning and execution. A basic laser clinic setup requires a minimum of ₹ 30–40 lakhs excluding the rent deposit. Investment in lasers will require a minimum of ₹ 25–40 lakhs. It can even go into a crore. As a beginner, check how much can you earn from procedures after the initial 6 months. Ideally if you take a bank loan for ₹ 30 lakhs for a 5-year period, your repayment with interest, average per day is ₹ 3000, if you can earn ₹ 6000, then you can repay in 2.5 years. Keeping this in mind, if you earn anything above ₹ 6000 per day, that is your profit. If it is ₹ 40 lakhs, then above ₹ 8000 per day should come from your investment to have profit.
- Taking loan from the bank is easier for a doctor, talk with the bank manager

regarding the documents needed. A loan of ₹ 30 lakh can be sanctioned quicker for a doctor. You can take a loan even against fixed deposits which you might have instead of closing them, which will reduce the interest rate.

- The general rule is 20% of your investment in equipment earns 80% of total profit and 80% of investment earns 20% of total profits. Invest in equipment which has multipurpose and faster return on investment. CO_2 fractional, MNRF machine, peels, electrocautery, Microderm and Hydra-facial, intense-pulsed light are few which have a higher return on investment procedures. If there is high-patient pool for hair removal and skin rejuvenation, then a hair removal laser, High-Intensity Focused Ultrasound (HIFU), Q-switched Nd:YAG laser is definitely a good investment.
- Sharing of lasers is good concept, it helps a doctor who is starting practice and cannot invest in lasers on his own due to the cost factor. If three or more dermatologists from the same or nearby place who have a good relationship with each other can invest on few lasers together, it would reduce the financial burden and it will give them options to do various laser procedures rather than working only with one laser which only one can afford. The lasers could be bought and kept in a separate clinic dedicated for laser procedures in an area accessible by group. Patients can be given appointment directing them to that center and each doctor can do for their patients. Ideally, time scheduling will be a problem which should be addressed and sorted out. On the long runs, it will have some pros and cons but if an agreement between the parties is made legally, before investing, stating the norms, it will prevent any misunderstanding in the future.
- Mobile laser clinics is another concept where a full-fledged mini bus can be converted to a laser center. Do not forget to do a power audit to see the possibility of running the equipment. It could also mean transporting the lasers from one clinic to another or between doctors. Transporting lasers should be done with care, as in some equipment the coolant and few attachments such as the articulated arm, have to be removed before transporting. Active Q-switched Nd:YAG lasers is one of the sensitive lasers to transport and in most cases, an equipment technician should accompany the lasers being transported to do a systems check after transport.

Staff

- A minimum of three staffs is required initially for a 25 patients OPD along with 4 to 5 procedures a day. Once the procedure load increases or the number of procedure room increases, you will need one staff extra for each room. When running a full-fledged clinic, remember to keep extra staff, in case someone takes leave. You will need auxiliary staff for cleaning and maintenance.
- Train your laser technicians in the technologies you have or plan to invest. Whether you employ an assistant doctor, nurse, medical esthetician or laser technician, all of your employees will need proper laser training. Laser companies give training to doctors and technicians when buying a laser but the time spent in training is definitely not enough. There are few dermatology centers around the country that offer 20–40 hour training courses. This will help them learn proper maintenance of the machine, taking

safety precaution, and assistance to the laser performing doctor.
- Staff should be trained properly in how to clean the equipment periodically and after a very laser procedure. Cleaning should be done only by a person authorized by you as improper handling can damage the equipment.

Buying Equipment[2]
- Ask guidance from your senior friends or peers about the equipment and company
- Buy from a company which has a larger presence. A company with a service center near your city will be able to help with breakdown and maintenance.
- FDA approved machines are the first choice but not everyone can invest high. If you are planning to buy, be sure of the quality and do not compromise. The cost and quality should be analyzed before buying. Remember, the success of a laser surgeon is in providing results not just having a laser.

Insurance and AMC
- Ask for 1- or 2-year warranty on machine and parts, annual maintenance contract (AMC) should be done immediately after the warranty period is over. Everything should be on paper signed by both parties. Do not agree to verbal guarantee.
- AMC should also include clause for mobility support if possible as lasers are moved from one clinic to another in some cases.
- Get insurance on the machine including fire insurance. Usually an equipment brought through loan from bank automatically gets insured but read and confirm.
- Usual and routine insurance policies do not cover risk of mobility. If the lasers are moved between multiple clinics, then a special tailor-made insurance policy subject to the locations of transport and modes of transport may be designed after discussion with the insurance companies, though this may attract a higher premium rate (also called special contingency insurance).[1]

Other Requirements
- Provision for an emergency crash cart in laser room, oxygen cylinder, real-time pulse-oximeter, and blood pressure monitor.
- An external cooling or cryogen-spray equipment is needed while operating few lasers such as hair removal lasers or fractional lasers to reduce pain for the patient and increasing comfort during the procedure.
- Eye protection for both the patient and the operator is essential. An opaque or specific-laser protection goggles are used for the patient. When laser is done near the eye or eyebrow, then use of an eye shield (COX II eye shield) is definitely needed to prevent any damage to the eye. For the operator, the green goggles filters the light from 190 nm to 1,800 nm which is ideal for most lasers except ablative lasers such as erbium or CO_2 which require higher wavelengths cut-off but the orange goggles filters only between 190 nm and 540 nm and from 900 nm to 1,700 nm which is not suitable for using Ruby or Alexandrite lasers since it does not filter 694–755 nm. Please make a note of the wavelengths filtered by particular goggles which are printed on the goggles before using it.
- Pest control, mainly cockroaches and rats, as they can damage the wiring and circuits inside your equipment.

- Protocols charts for cleaning, preparing for procedure, emergency management, and complication management.

CONCLUSION

Esthetic and laser dermatology is a growing field of dermatology. Many technologies are available to choose from. Choose in which you are confident and what your patient condition needs. A good esthetic clinic set-up is essential for success and return on investment. A careful planning and adequate investment is the first step.

REFERENCES

1. Dhepe N. Minimum standard guidelines of care on requirements for setting up a laser theatre. Indian J Dermatol Venereol Leprol. 2009;75:101-10.
2. Aurangabadkar SJ, Mysore V, Ahmed ES. Buying a laser: Tips and pearls. Journal of Cutaneous and Aesthetic Surgery. 2014;7(2):124-30.

9.5 Setting Up and Managing a Pediatric Dermatology Clinic

Ravi Hiremagalore

INTRODUCTION

Pediatric dermatology deals with skin problems in children. These problems can be unique to the age group or could be the same issues seen in adults but have to be managed differently. A child is not a miniature adult. The surface area for absorption of a child's skin is much more than an adult. Hence, topical agents used for treatment have to be appropriate and judiciously prescribed. Also, a child has an inherent fear of strangers. This makes examination also difficult in a child and even various procedures as simple as even a skin biopsy. In the current day scenario of a nuclear family, parental anxiety is immense and at most care needs to be taken to deal with this. In such a case, some of the conditions would be over treated, which could have otherwise been managed conservatively. There are some conditions such as Gianotti Crosti syndrome (GCS), atypical viral exanthems, staphylococcal scalded syndrome, linear IgA disease of childhood, birthmarks, and genodermatosis that are typically seen only in children. Awareness of some common benign skin lesions of newborn is necessary to reassure anxious parents and avoid unnecessary treatments. Conditions such as vitiligo, alopecia areata, and lichen planus have to be managed differently in children and can vary in the various age groups. To illustrate an example, care should be taken to prescribe immunosuppressive agents in toddlers and younger since they would need live vaccines given as part of the immunization schedule. Steroids in the prepubertal age for some of these autoimmune conditions may not be preferred since it might hinder the growth spurt. Surgical management of vitiligo may not be a suitable option in children since stability is very difficult to achieve in such cases. Taken together, it is imperative that we need training and specialized services for pediatric dermatology.

TRAINING IN PEDIATRIC DERMATOLOGY

Currently in India, Fellowship-Training Programs in Pediatric Dermatology are available in Bangalore Medical College and Research Institute, Indira Gandhi Institute of Child Health, and CUTIS Academy of Dermatological Sciences, all of them in Bengaluru and JIPMER, Puducherry. The duration of fellowship training is 12–18 months. Minimum qualifications include MD or Diploma training recognized by the Medical Council of India (now National Medical Commission). The first three centers are affiliated to and awarded by Rajiv Gandhi University of Medical Sciences (RGUHS), Karnataka. Also, one-month observerships are awarded by the Indian Academy of Dermatologists, Venereologists and Leprologists at Christian Medical College, Vellore, Tamil Nadu, India.

INFRASTRUCTURE

Pediatric dermatology practice can be in an individual clinic or institutionalized. There is no ideal space requirement for practice. However, it should be spacious enough to accommodate a large waiting area for kids to move around. It should include a designated play area **(Fig. 9.5.1)** with child-friendly equipment particularly to cater for toddlers. Older children would need access to simple activities such as coloring and drawing and children of all ages should have appropriate reading books to keep them engaged while waiting. This would certainly reduce anxiety of parents while they wait. The waiting area should be as safe as possible since the patients are primarily children who are prone to accidents. There should also be a designated area for nursing mothers to feed the baby **(Fig. 9.5.2)** and diaper changing stations so that cleanliness and waste management can be done as per requirements.

WORKING

The hours of operation are predominantly decided by the clinic or hospital. However, it is not mandatory to work into late evening hours since dermatology is not an emergency. The outpatient in a hospital

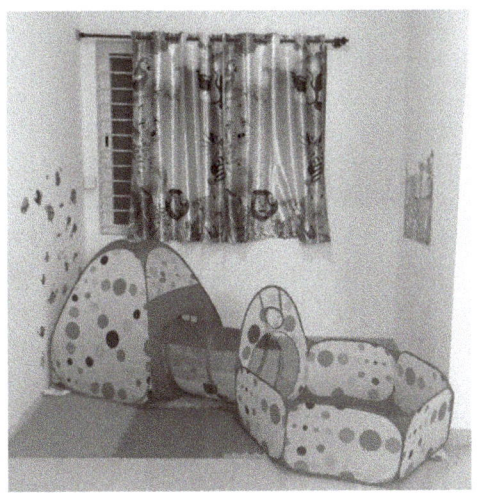

Fig. 9.5.1: Designated play area for kids.

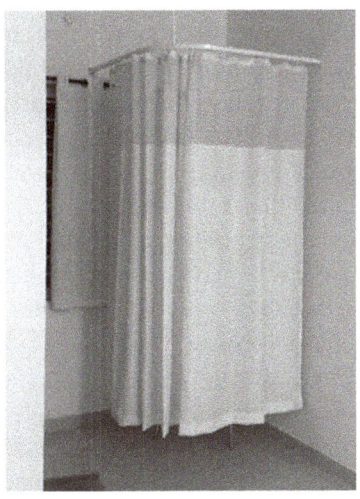

Fig. 9.5.2: Baby-feeding area for nursing mothers.

setting has to be in a pediatric facility and not the general or dermatology facility. This has the advantage of the infrastructure being child friendly and enables interaction with pediatricians and pediatric subspecialists. The latter is very important for a successful pediatric dermatology practice. As in other dermatology practices, it would be good to have an electronic medical record and an appointment scheduling system. This avoids prolonged waiting time, which is very pertinent in children.

Moreover facilities such as NBUVB, patch-testing, and KOH examination need to extend beyond the regular working hours since most school-going children are free only after 3 pm in the afternoon. There are instances that need special attention since the age group is pediatric. Firstly, the pediatric dermatologist should be aware of some of the common pediatric cartoons and characters so that he/she can make the child's anxiety less while examination or during a procedure. Some examples of scenarios specific to be considered are phototherapy units and procedures. Since whole body narrow band is a closed chamber, it would be appropriate to allow one parent inside and to have some stickers or child friendly cartoons displayed inside if possible. Alternatively, parents can be encouraged to read something the child likes from outside so that the child feels safe. Similarly, it would be preferable to encourage parents to show some cartoon program their child likes while doing procedures. This can sometimes avoid procedural sedation. Some of the aspects in pediatric dermatology have to be institutionalized since it involves care in an emergency setting. The classical example is treatment procedure requiring sedation. This is done in a pediatric emergency setting by the pediatrician. The classical indication would be extensive molluscum contagiosum and particularly near the eyes that warrants therapy. Access to pediatric emergency would certainly help complete a pediatric dermatology practice. Procedural sedation should never be done in a clinic setting. It would be nice to give the child a reward, like a chocolate or sticker for his cooperation during the clinic or procedure.

NETWORKING

This is an integral part of any practice in particular pediatric dermatology since it is predominantly a referral practice. Pediatricians are the main referring physicians. Moreover there are certain scenarios when a constant dialogue is necessary between the dermatologist and pediatrician. Hence, it is important and imperative to have a network with pediatricians. One of the simplest ways is to send a feedback note on the child referred. This can be done informally on a smartphone or can be structured through an email or a letter. This has to be integrated into the pediatric dermatology practice so that a dedicated time can be spent for this purpose.

PITFALLS AND CHALLENGES

- As with any subspecialty practice, one of the major challenges in starting a pediatric dermatology practice is referral. This primarily comes from pediatricians since they are the first point of contact for kids. Occasional referrals come from dermatologists mostly for management of severe atopic dermatitis that has not responded or for the treatment of warts and molluscum contagiosum that are progressive despite topical therapy. This problem can be addressed through proper networking and teaching.

- Treatment protocols for pediatric age group are not readily available for most conditions. This limits the development of a standard uniform practice in pediatric dermatology.
- Another important challenge is nonavailability of certain medications used in dermatology in pediatric suspensions such as dapsone, griseofulvin, and acitretin. This can be overcome by having a pharmacy that has appropriate licenses to compound these drugs as suspensions.
- Financial sustainability is an important issue in pediatric dermatology practice.

Hence, it is more appropriate to have it established as a part of an institution. Additionally, research can be a good complement to a pediatric dermatology practice.

CONCLUSION

Pediatric dermatology practice is very different from general or cosmetic dermatology. It is not just prescribing creams. It involves a lot of counseling and viewing in the eyes of a child. This requires sound up-to-date knowledge of the various conditions combined with passion.

9.6 Establishing Hair Restoration Surgery Practice

Venkataram Mysore, Sajin Alexander

INTRODUCTION

Hair loss is a cause of concern for people worldwide. Androgenetic alopecia is the most common cause of hair loss in males and over the past few decades, hair restoration procedures such as hair transplantation have ushered in a new era in clinical practice.

From the patient's perspective, it is a life saver from the never-ending agony of hair loss where there is no other treatment option available while for the doctors or clinicians it has become a golden goose that is considered to be risk-free, easy, comfortable and a steady revenue provider to be exploited by the clinics. It has been such a success that an establishment can survive merely by providing this one technique.

Everyone, from urologists, nephrologists, pathologists, anesthetists to ayurvedic doctors and even quacks, without prior formal education, is trying to stick their hands into this honey pot.

However in reality, it is a difficult practice to establish due to certain facts that cannot be left unaddressed like:
- It is a time-consuming surgery therefore not easy to fit into a routine practice
- Requires a team
- Requires infrastructure

REQUIREMENTS FOR HAIR TRANSPLANTATION PRACTICE

Before setting up a practice in hair transplantation, every doctor needs to fulfill certain basic requirements as no one can ease into any field without them. They can be broadly categorized into the following six subheadings:
1. Training
2. Skill

3. Manpower
4. Instruments
5. Infrastructure
6. Marketing

Even with the above basics mastered, without proper time management, no dermatologist can become proficient in this field as it is often detrimental to practice of general dermatology/surgery and becomes difficult to integrate into an existing busy dermatology practice unlike esthetics and lasers.

TRAINING

Training in the procedure is the most important step. Knowledge of the different layers of the skin and structure of the hair alone without the scientific know-how of the technique is insufficient for a dermatologist to start a practice in hair restoration.

Training is difficult to obtain and only a very few authentic centers offer reliable training.

Once this training is achieved, it becomes important to train the support staff as well for smooth functioning of the clinic.

A beginner also needs to learn:
- Infiltration, nerve blocks
- Tumescent anesthesia
- Basic and advanced life support skills
- Ability to handle emergency situations

SKILL

Hair transplantation is a skill and labor-oriented technique which requires:
- Hand to eye coordination—which is an important requirement to avoid transection.
- Surgical skill is required which is greater than that acquired during usual dermatosurgery training.
- Surgical expertise in dissection, hemostasis, suturing, and wound care.
- Organizational skills to arrange a team and to direct and lead them.
- Counseling skill is another important tool in the dermatologist's armament which is needed for the following categories of patients:
  - Patients with unrealistic expectations
  - Young immature patients
  - Patients who scout around different doctors
  - Patient who ask for quotations
  - Patients who refuse to take drugs.

MANPOWER

Manpower is an important requirement and is needed at different levels.

A team of 4-6-8-10 assistants is needed which take part in various steps of hair transplantation. It takes about 3–4 months for training of assistants and requires repeated practice and persistence. The dermatologist/surgeon should guide their training by keeping the following points in mind:
- Supervision of dissection by staff is crucial
- The awareness that many do not acquire the skill
- Giving emphasis to patience, motivation, and dedication
- Adequate remuneration to keep the staff.

The skill of both the dermatologist and his/her team also depends on the number of cases he/she performs, the more the daily cases, the more expertise one gets, and the more expertise one garners, the more cases he/she receives.

Viewing videos of other successful dermatologists/surgeons and by practicing on banana leaves or beetle leaves for dissection and on putty/clay for insertion helps to a great extent.

INSTRUMENTS

- Dissection needs self-illuminated binocular stereomicroscope with magnification of 5–20 which enables better visualization of the follicular units as well as special knives or scalpels with blades (no. 11 or 15) to dissect the grafts.
- Manual punches (sharp or blunt) ranging from 0.7 mm to 1.2 mm or motorized versions (Maximum 10,000 rotations per minute) may be used for extraction in follicular unit extraction (FUE).
- Single- or double-bladed scalpel with blade no. 21–23, skin hook, and scissors are required for extraction in follicular unit extraction.
- Chiller tray and holding solutions such as unbuffered saline, plasma-lyte A, and ringer lactate solution are also required to keep the graft from drying.

INFRASTRUCTURE

None of the above-mentioned processes would be fruitful without adequate space or room for the procedure. This involves not merely a room but a logistical infrastructure as it is not profitable to do the procedure in a nursing home.

- *Waiting room*: A comfortable, preferably, separate room is required for the patient. The room should be well lit with posters, brochures, and facilities for viewing computer presentations and websites as the need for consultation is long for each patient. Presence of a receptionist at the front desk to guide them is also necessary. A counselor/junior doctor is essential to do the initial consultation and counseling.
- *Operation theater*: A proper theater is indispensable for hair transplantation procedures. Ideally, the theater of dimensions 12 × 14 size is required, equipped with pulse-oximeter monitor, emergency trolley, resuscitation equipment, and a defibrillator. Always keep a standby anesthetist.
- *Dissection room*: The next most important step after harvesting the punch grafts is the dissection which requires utmost concentration and patience. Therefore, a room with dimensions 12–14 ft with specific dissection tables, comfortable chairs, adequate lighting, and microscopes with 4x magnification are basic necessities.

MARKETING

Perhaps one of the most overlooked step in the establishment of a practice in hair restoration is marketing. With modern society becoming more and more tech savvy, it becomes prudent that young doctors use media to his/her advantage.

CHALLENGES

Being a newcomer to the world of hair restoration practice, one would face many challenges. A few of the challenges are:

- *Unrealistic expectations because of Internet and Media hype*: In 2002, 1,000 grafts were considered as a mega session while now 2,500 grafts are considered a mega session. Giga sessions over 4,000 grafts are also being performed. So, there is more pressure on a newcomer.
- *Disinformation from alternative medicine practitioners*: 'A little knowledge is a dangerous thing', would aptly sum up this issue and there are many clinical

practitioners of other disciplines who spread disinformation that finasteride causes impotence and infertility and that minoxidil causes blood pressure changes. Explaining the actual facts to a patient exposed to such an information can be an uphill battle.
- *Trichotherapists*: Blind faith in quackery and other agencies could pose a problem at convincing and counseling some patients.
- *Need for validation*: Demanding patients who need guaranteed results can pose a problem in counseling before and convincing after hair restoration.
- *Patients who are internet savvy*: These patients believe anything they read off the internet and have an unshakable belief that transcends even the opinion of the specialist in that field.

Tips for Newcomers Planning to Start a Hair Restoration Surgery Practice
- Be realistic
- Be honest and transparent
- Underpromise and over deliver
- Do not sell transplants
- Do not underemphasize importance of drugs—unless drugs are taken, they will continue to lose existing hair.

CONCLUSION

Starting a hair restoration surgery practice may seem as a very tempting prospect to many budding young dermatologists/surgeons today but as easy as it may sound, in reality, it involves a lot of labor and patience. A successful practice involves multiple factors that should be tailored to the needs of the patient, keeping in mind what is best for them.

SECTION 10
How I did it?

10.1 Journey from Lotions to Lasers

Ganesh S Pai

When I joined postgraduation in 1977, dermatology was one of the last choices for postgraduation. Unknown to many then, it was an emerging field and its full impact would be known only two decades later. Rook was a two volume textbook, HIV was yet to be discovered as a disease, and leprosy and sexually transmitted diseases (STDs) were an important segment in practice!

Dermatology was practiced with lotions and creams. In government hospitals, patients were asked to bring their own bottles which would be filled with benzyl benzoate for scabies, calamine lotion to soothe the skin, liquid paraffin, and various tinctures such as gentian violet, Castellani's paint, and coal tar lotion. In addition to these, treatment options included other messy ointments with petroleum jelly base such as salicylic acid ointment, sulfur ointment, and coal tar ointment.

In the years to come, a variety of cosmetically elegant steroids creams, antibiotic creams, moisturizers, and whitening creams were marketed by several companies. Subsequently, a range of cosmeceuticals, sunscreens, and immunologicals hit the market.

Opportunity which enhances medical care arrives all the time. Unfortunately, nobody can predict the timing because they depend on invention and scientific advancement. In the mid-eighties, phototherapy and cautery machines became very popular in institutions and clinics and dermatosurgery, such as grafting in Vitiligo, became common practice. These machines were, however, not expensive to own and were affordable to doctors. Patients were billed reasonable charges.

As the years passed by, after virtually close to two decades of practice, violently disruptive technology arrived in the form of lasers in India. Around this time, similar disruption took place in a variety of specialties such as high technology scanning machines in radiology, C-arm in orthopedics, and intraocular lens in ophthalmology. Embracing laser was akin to reinventing our practice. It required developing fresh skills, educating patients, and diverting savings, and financial resources to the purchase of these lasers.

At the stage when doctors earn a substantial income, they have a choice of either reinvesting in their clinic by planning expansion and purchase of lasers or resorting to purchase of illiquid properties, farm houses, and unrelated business.

The dawn of the cosmetology era had just broken out and there were great opportunities to upgrade my practice. There was no road to follow and I had to make my own road. It took a large investment to setup a new clinic with 3,000 sq ft of space and all my savings of two decades were used up in this venture in 1997. One by one, lasers were added, starting with the erbium laser and then followed by hair removal laser, carbon dioxide and QSW laser.

The first 10 years till 2008 were used to buy this bunch of devices. With progress of time, nonablative devices, such as radiofrequency devices, gained prominence for tightening skin, stretch marks, pores, and wrinkles and these were installed between 2012 and 2014. Upgrades of the earlier generation of lasers were done every 5 years with a buyback option by the companies. Cryolipolysis and Pico QSW lasers were the last investments in 2017 and 2018.

After 7 years of establishing my laser and cosmetology practice, in the year 2006, I found it difficult to divide my time between half a day of teaching in the morning and half a day of practice in the evening. This was never a problem during the period between 1979 and 1999 as I had only a consultation practice and I enjoyed postgraduate teaching very much. After all the heavy investments in laser machines and manpower, I found that the time spent in teaching crippled my return on investments. At this point, I had left lotions completely and moved on to lasers.

The loans can be difficult to repay especially if the demand for cosmetic services does not rise exponentially. Financial planning is therefore important and instead of buying a clutch of machines, I bought them sequentially.

The challenge I faced 20 years into my practice was whether or not to take a plunge into cosmetology and ramp up practice in a field which was uncharted territory. I could not afford failure as I had put in all my savings into a large cosmetology center with laser devices humming in many rooms. In a small city, it is difficult to establish purely cosmetology practice. I had to convert dermatology clientele into cosmetology patients. The flow of acne, acne scar, accident and burn scars, moles, hirsutism, and hyper pigmentation are prime targets for conversion to cosmetic practice in a dermatology clinic amidst another group of patients with psoriasis, eczema, fungus infection, and hair loss. In retrospect, right time to invest in lasers is when we have outpatients of thirty cases a day. Any laser practice commenced prematurely would lead to financial disaster.

There are certain other ideas which must be incorporated into a successful cosmetology practice to sustain its longevity. In the initial few years, it is easy to manage issues of growth through leadership, direction, and creativity. In the second decade of cosmetology practice, the volume load of patients in a successful clinic would have grown exponentially in geometric rather than arithmetic progression. To sustain this, growth will only come through delegation of responsibility to an assistant or senior staff in the center. Collaboration with other dermatologists and hospitals which do not offer such facilities is important to sustain flow of new patients.

Cutting down of red tape requires quick decision-making abilities and means staying nimble footed to eliminate wasteful expenditure. Finally, the most important for middle-aged or older dermatologists is a crisis of health which we so often take for granted. We doctors generally have a poor health profile compared to other people in society. We are more prone to obesity, diabetes, and cancers primarily because we under exercise and overeat, that too at odd times of the day.

The entire edifice of a carefully nurtured, heavily invested, and technologically sound cosmetology clinic can come apart if this were to occur.

What of the future? Into the seventh decade of my life, the challenge is to stay healthy, motivated, and invested for the practice of cosmetology is like riding a tiger. The ride is great but it is perilous to dismount for the tiger will eat you up. The heavy investments in a cosmetology practice are similar to a ride on the tiger.

10.2 Single Clinic to Multiple Clinics

— CP Thajuddin, Jyothi Kannangath

INTRODUCTION (MENTION WHY IS THIS NECESSARY, WHEN IT BECOMES NECESSARY)

When you run one clinic, your time and energy will be spent on that particular clinic. Since it is a solo clinic show, there is a limitation of growth. When you become more popular, and people come to know your expertise in your specialty, they will start coming to your clinic from distant places also, if you can train and delegate your work to some ethical and loyal doctors with trained nonmedical assistant, you will be making more revenue in multiple clinics than a single practice. Moreover, each center will promote or compliment the other. There may be seasonal fluctuations in different locations, so multiple clinics will balance the cash flow.

Transforming single clinic to multiple clinics is not difficult but needs certain skills and planning.

Before starting: You should have a clear vision. From where you want to start and where do you want to reach?

May be you can just do a 5WH and 1H session

- *Why?* Why am I going for multiple clinics? Do I have a strong reason for that?
- *What?* What is that I am going to gain out of that? More revenue? Better reach and popularity? Providing employment to many?
- *When?* When am I going to do this? Is the time apt? When should I have the 1st branch in place? When am I further expanding?
- *Where?* Where am I going to start my next clinic? Is there enough potential there? How are the competition placed in that area? Is the infrastructure cost (rent/lease) right in that area? Do the customers have the right approach to the location?
- *Who?* Whom I am going to have there to run the clinic? Are they having the right attitude and experience? Are they having the positive thinking and ability to manage?
- *How?* How am I going to get the right building? How am I going to invest? Where are the resources coming from? How can I manage my consultation timings?

Once you have the honest answers for the above questions, you are ready for the next step.

Think and plan. It is not a good idea to start multiple clinics in the beginning of your practice without a strong foundation and an extraordinary qualified team.

FIND YOUR SPECIALTY

No matter how narrow it is. From cosmetodermatology to cosmetosurgery with or without out lasers, etc., communicate convincingly. If you believe in yourself, show it. Do not start multiple clinics just because someone else is doing well.

Some would like to go for a solo practice or work in a well-established clinic or would like to attach them to a multispecialty hospital. Few more ambitious doctors would plan for multiclinic or franchise. It all depends on how big your dream is.

WAYS AND MEANS

Nurture your first clinic to near perfect position, and replicate. Think about your visits, you cannot visit all the clinics all the time. You can travel fast till your physician asks you to slow down. Aim should be that the multiple clinics should run in your absence too.

When you move on to multiple clinics, the first thing is to brand your clinic and implement centralized administration and accounts and follow the prepared processes and procedures. Initially you will have very busy schedule including managing, and promotional training activities, etc. Do not forget the legal aspects of running a clinic.

HOW TO SUPERVISE AND MONITOR ACCOUNTS?

- Find the right people and place.
- Do not just dream about the goal. Work toward the goal. Consistency is the key.
- Run away from negativity. Try to remove the negativity from inside your mind too,
- Stay away from people with lots of "good ideas." There will be many "well wishers" to give you free advices.
- We live in a world of copycats. It is okay, to copy. We will always get some ideas from already established clinics.
- Like a Satan, make yourself happy first. Happy mind makes sound as music. If you are happy; you automatically make the people around you and the organization happy.
- You should be mentally and physically and spiritually healthy. Healthy enough to accept the success and failures.
- Do SWOT (strengths, weaknesses, opportunities, and threats) analysis.
- Find your strength, weaknesses, opportunities, and threats.

Here are the 9 Ps to keep in mind for your multiple clinics to be successful.

1. *Passion*: Passion is worth billions. It attracts patients. Even more clearly, it helps to keep those patients—for life when you have passion you never work or struggle. It is a joyful flow of experience. Work hard, but work smart.
2. *Planning*:
   - Plan your future:
     - *Short term*: 1–3 years
     - *Medium term*: 3–5 years
     - *Long term*: 5+ years
   - Begin with the end in mind. Keep your vision, mission, and targets clear. Where do you want to be and how do we get there. Find a good financial source. You can find medical or nonmedical partners or get a loan. Bankers are the best partners since they won't interfere with your work and dream. Give a designation to yourself like chief doctor or chief clinical officer or chief executive officer.
   - *Plan your visits*: Select your days and time for visiting the other clinics.

Know the culture and pulse of the people in that area. In south India itself, practicing time of doctors maybe little different in each states/area.
- Keep good ethical doctors as assistants and train them well, let them know your dreams and make them to participate in your programs.
- You cannot do all the work yourself. Delegate your management job to someone whom you can rely on and concentrate on your practice more.
- This is little tricky initially, you may lose concentration on your service.
- The aim should be that your 1 hour work should equal 10 hours of pay.
- X to 10X *(If you have multiple centers, you are delegating your works to others and the income will multiply, still you will be working less. Remember! Your time cannot be multiplied).*

3. *Product*:
- Whenever you are self-employed, you are in business. We all are entrepreneurs by default. Albeit, we do not get marketing training from our medical colleges.
- You are the product and need to sell yourself. Package yourself just like what you look into a product while making a purchase. Give attractive package with esthetics, good functionality, interesting features, and offer durability.
- Your package is your service. Give after treatment follow-ups and support.
- Try to get the best equipment. For example, get lasers which are USFDA approved.
- Build trust. Build consistency in everything you do.
- Keep ethical thinking! Keep integrity and that is the fundamentals of all the success especially while running multiple clinics.

4. *Place*: Locality is important. People should have easy accessibility to your clinic, with good parking area.

5. *People*:
- Business is about people.
  - Make a good team. If you are thinking big, choose the right ones. Better to hire somebody near to your location or give them accommodation nearby.
  - Communicate to everyone in the organization. Security guard of your organization too has a message to the patients.
  - Conduct regular meetings. Know your staff well. Listen to their problems.
- No harm in doing little micro management, if necessary. Nothing wrong with it.
- Make your team feel important, listen to your inner voice. Happy people make free marketing tools, because they are the key assets. It is their manners, tone, knowledge, body language, ability and profound effect, even though as doctors we provide the treatment but its them who provided the service.
- Imagine like a cycle chain. You have to oil it regularly for a smooth ride. If any link is broken, repair it or change it. If any of your team is slowing down your journey, find a solution or replace.
- Listen to your patients. You are not always right.
- Now all quality certifications worldwide are moving from patient satisfaction to patient delight.
- Provide the patients more than they expected.

6. *Process and procedures*:
    - It is advisable to have a QMS (quality management system) preferably ISO 9001, ISO 14000 certified by an external accreditation body to give an appeal and credibility.
    - This will provide your organization with quality manual where each and every process procedure are explained, monitored, measured, and recorded.
    - This needs to cover from the parking lot to the patient satisfaction index.
    - Need to take good care of appointments, token/ID card training, written physical evidence.
    - Ambience and cleanliness is very important.
    - Keep visual communication aids such as displays, posters, and banners to continuously communicate the vision and the policies to your staff. Images speak volumes but only if you let them.
7. *Pricing*:
    - The more it costs, the better it seems in esthetic practice.
    - Build choices into your pricing for your services too. Think about it keeping GST in mind.
    - Do not charge less. Give better services.
    - The low price position kills.
    - The perception of quality to price is directly proportional, in other words higher the price better the quality.
    - Price creates perceptions, and then creates satisfaction.
    - Push price moderately higher, not very high though. Higher prices just do not talk, they tempt.
8. *Promotion and branding*:
    - Need to advertising promotions, improve public relations, do direct and indirect marketing, personal selling, etc.
    - Perception of the service rather than reality.
    - It is a good idea to have people recall your brand. For that purpose, you can have uniform color code, logos, staff uniforms, print materials, etc.
9. *Problems*:
    - Perception of the service rather than reality. Sometimes services are 'unsought'. All patients won't articulate much, may be frustrated.
    - Our service can't be tested before treatment...So there is a little risk. Good counseling before the service will help. Take time for counseling. When you become more and more busy, let others who are well-trained do the counseling part.
    - Keep P/PC balance (Stephen R Covey). P = Production; PC = Production capacity. It holds true for the equipment and the staffs.
    - Maintain the people's equipment's, and clinic's facilities in proper way. If the people are tired or the machines are worn out, the result will be disappointing.

KNOW YOUR PATIENT'S EXPERIENCE/SATISFACTION

- You must have a well-defined mechanism to monitor and measure the feelings of the customer in all the clinics. There are various methods to do that like customer feedback form, touch screen smiles at billing counter or at any place where they can see easily, etc.

- Have a customer satisfaction index monitoring mechanism with specified targets.
- Also another very important thing is to monitor the employee satisfaction index too. A happy employee always drives happy patients.
- Let problematic patients handled by proper hands.
- Try to get more promoters and fewer detractors.
- Introduce procedures to the existing patients and make new patients.
- Introduce existing patients with new procedures.
- Give new procedures for new patients.

CONTINUOUS IMPROVEMENT

- What is the role of the manager? He is not working with his hands or doing any procedures.
- He must be the person who works on continuous improvements.
- It should be a 360-degree approach and with measurable results:
  - Better experience and satisfaction for the patients
  - Better work environment for the employees
  - Better housekeeping and hygiene
  - Easy to understand and due process and procedures

PHARMACY AND LABORATORY

- It is better to have a pharmacy license and if possible laboratory facility in all the clinics.
- For running multiple clinics in an ongoing process, one needs to have patience.
- If you are looking at new geographic area, get updated with the latest technology and new methods in our dermatological procedures, need to outsource IT, legal advices, etc.
- You can change the organization from proprietorship to partnership, or to limited liability partnership or private limited company.
- All work is meant to achieve financial gain so as to be able to eat and live comfortably. This is the most naked way of putting across the truth. No commercial activity is for charity, not even healthcare.
- Accept that no one is for everyone, and find the best fits.
- If you do not like the result, change the approach.

FAST DECISION MAKING

- This is very important in today's dynamic economic environment.
- If any center is not doing well, check the problems, try to find a solution, wait for maximum one year to improve, and still if the center does not run well without your presence, close down. Do not want more headaches than little revenue.
- Smart work with passion and consistency can do wonders. If you miss these be informed that you would soon lose your time and money.

How did you start and expand?
We started with a small clinic in a small town in 1999 and then realized the potential of laser treatments. Since not many people were doing lasers in India, patients used to come from all over India for treatment to our small town, at that period of time. Accessibility to my clinic was less, so I started thinking to move to bigger cities.

What problems you faced?
The most common challenge one would faced is attrition from both medical and non-medical employees, with added problem of pilferage.
During the initial days of our practice, we used to transport machines from one clinic to

another, which lead to some damages to the machines.

How did you overcome them?
- We reduced attrition rates, making involvement of medical staffs, gave regular training on new equipment, and freedom with adequate pay. We encouraged attending training courses, workshops, and conferences and also provided incentives and shares revenue of our established centers.
- For nonmedical staffs, we conducted regular "free" camps in all out centers to motivate them and arranged regular get together or picnic to make them feel like family.
- Regular monitoring and CCTV cameras helped in controlling pilferage. Our chief accountant does visit all the centers on a regular basis.
- Now we have almost stopped transporting the machines. Machine breakdown and long down time was another issue. We need to buy instruments from experienced and reputed distributors. Buying from new distributors is a little risk; now there are plenty to choose. Annual maintenance contract is important.
- Yoga and regular workouts helped in keeping a better health. Balancing family life and practice was another challenge. Spending quality time with the family and friends who like your company will be helpful.

Have you later cut down on some centers?
We had to shut down one clinic due to multiple factors.

If so why?
Some of the reasons were mismanagement, our sudden withdrawal of visits to that particular clinic, poor building, greedy building owner, attrition, spoiled employees and pilferage.

10.3 Dermatology to Dermatopathology to Hair Transplantation, the Journey

Venkataram Mysore

Disclaimer:
Some parts of this text are autobiographical- an attempt to narrate my journey ending as a hair transplant surgeon. The same should not be interpreted as pompous and indulgent.

The story began with my entry into dermatology in 1983. My friends remarked: My God, you joined dermatology!!! why???

1983: Dermatology was known for the stink, stain, sting of the creams; there were lots of diseases, but few drugs. There were diseases with long names, long discussions on them, but treatment was in one line. There were a handful of drugs, but with lots of indications such as Dapsone, Griseofulvin, Clofazimine, Chloroquine, and Tetracycline.

There was little opportunity for further training, nor enough challenge intellectually. And then there was an immunology explosion which expanded our knowledge of diseases: Pemphigus, psoriasis, dermatitis-Langerhans cell, SALT concept and immunofluorescence. Thus, dermatopathology was one subspecialty which was challenging intellectually.

With in this desert, there was one beacon of hope for training: Dr PN Behl, Father of vitiligo surgery, who had started the skin institute in Delhi. He was the only one to teach surgey, radiotherapy, lasers and dermabrasion.

So the interests in pathology and surgery were kindled simultaneously.

1993: The Royal College of Pathology, London announced diplomat examination in dermatopathology and I decided to take it. It was a natural choice; dermatology and dermatopathology are visually-oriented specialties–keen observation is everything. Clinical dermatology after all is macroscopic pathology. The examination not just lead me in to becoming a dermatopathologist, but also helped me authoring a book on the subject.

Then came a decade of rapidly changing trends in society and in dermatology:
- Increased longevity
- Changing tastes and attitudes
- Media hype
- Increased awareness
- Increased affordability
- Newer treatments
- Demand for simple and safe treatments; weekend/lunch time treatments.

The disease dermatology that I had learnt changed into desire dermatology, with invasion of lasers, surgery, and esthetics. This also meant that patient became a client, with the client being the king. Commerce set its foot into practice, where marketplace was the laboratory, with a quick transition of drugs and devices from laboratory to clinic. Internet invaded our lives.

Procedural dermatology brought respect and reputation to the dermatologist and also challenges.

One field which made startling progress was hair transplantation (HT). In 2000, my relative who was balding asked my opinion about HT. I knew little and, hence, had to read. The reading left me fascinated. Follicular unit transplant (FUT) and mega sessions had just been reported. And I decided to learn HT and landed with Jung Chul Kim in Korea.

WHY HAIR TRANSPLANTATION?

- Dermatology and dermatopathology are visually-oriented disciplines and hence require brain-eye coordination. Hair transplantation is a skill that, in addition requires hand-eye coordination. Having already mastered the first, acquiring the second skill was not after all very difficult.
- Dermatology often requires repetitive treatments while, hair transplantation consists of repetitive steps within a single treatment.
- So in many ways, it was a natural progression into hair transplantation.

Great things are done by a series of small things brought together   —**Vincent Von Gough**

Thus, the further steps of progress: FUT, FUE and BHT were smooth.

What is the message of the above?
- Change is inevitable
- The only thing that is constant is change
- Learning is continuous.

What is needed is the mindset; mindset to change, mindset to adapt.
- Carol Dweck, Professor of Psychology, Stanford stated that there are two types of mindset:
  - Fixed mindset which regards that intelligence is a fixed trait—capabilities are like shoe size or height, they can not grow
  - Growth mindset which states that intelligence can be trained; the brain is a "growth organ". Capabilities are like muscles which can be developed by working out.

The questions to be asked are:
- Do medical colleges and medical practice encourage fixed mindset?

- Or do they limit students to certain yardsticks—the beaten track?
- *Albert Einstein stated*: Education is what is left behind after you have forgotten what you learnt in college.
- It is therefore important that we need to have the growth mindset which means college is only the start of a life-long learning. Medical practice is a weapon to achieve.

Medical practice has changed now:
- It is more and more about doing what is needed and what is wanted. What is needed can be different from what is taught. Doing well is examples of prominent personalities in doing good.

There are several examples of prominent personalities in dermatological history who have left a mark by their ability to acquire capabilities: Marion Sulzberger, Jeffrey Klein, William Rassman, and others.

What did these men have? They had:
- Ability to try again and again
- Ability to learn again and again.

The questions to be asked therefore:
- Does today's dermatology education stimulates lifelong learning?
- Does it create possibilities and capabilities for future learning?
- Does it prepare our young dermatologist for the field?

Getting ahead in school is about smartness and hardwork. Getting ahead in life is about learning skills and working with other people. Learning through relationships is therefore vital. Life is a combination of team sport and long distance running and a chain of dependence-independence-interdependence. Dermatology and hair transplantation are great examples of this adage.

10.4 Small Town, Big Success: How I did it?

Manjot Marwah

INTRODUCTION

I, Dr Manjot Marwah, completed my residency from Mumbai and moved to Hamirpur in Himachal Pradesh in 2013, that is nearly 6 years back. Not many doctors have taken this leap of moving to a small town, but I have no regrets or looking back after I made this decision. I have practiced in Mumbai for a while and had a very successful run as we are a family of dermatologists. Maybe that is the reason for me to move easily since I knew that in my absence my brother will be looking after our Mumbai clinic along with my uncle. I shifted to Himachal after my marriage and started clinical practice within 1 month of marriage.

Currently, I have a clinic in the center of Hamirpur with all dermatosurgery, laser, and hair transplant facilities. Hamirpur is a small town with no railway connection and the nearest functional airport being 4 hours away. The total town population is 17,060 and its total area is just 5.2 km. Most of the population here are farmers or government employees. This was quite a change from our routine clinical practice in the metropolitan city. But I made it big, and this is my journey.

SETTING UP A CLINIC

When I shifted in 2013 and decided to start a practice here, the rental prices were very reasonable. I took a moderately sized space in the building where a senior pediatrician was practicing. My clinic has one consultation room, a shared reception and two procedure rooms. The infrastructure of my clinic was very basic but well maintained. I got basic stationary printed for the clinic, made a self-made website online and started off with basic dermatology setup. The only machine I purchased was an electrocautery initially. The bus transport system slows down after 5 PM, hence I started practicing from 9 AM to 5 PM only.

CONSULTATION FEE AND EXPENSES

Since the average income in the town is 8,000-10,000 per month and the average doctor fee was ₹ 100-150, I kept my fee at minimum in par with other physicians at ₹ 100. The local civil hospital in town also has an MD Dermatologist, where consultation charges are ₹ 10. Hence raising the fee has always been a difficult option in a small town till date.

However, other expenses are minimal in small towns. Since electricity is available at a subsidy in the entire state, the average electricity bill along with three lasers and air conditioners running every day comes about ₹ 6,000 only. This was such a surprise when I got the first electricity bill after shifting from Mumbai, this bill seemed like a joke. Any dermatologist living in a metropolitan city will agree with me.

FINDING STAFF

Finding trained staff is another hurdle in a small town and the most difficult part is retaining them. Most of the young population looks forward to shifting to a bigger city. Hence it is important to always have extra staff and pay them as per the standards in the big cities, not as per the small town standards. Only when the staff is well paid do they stick to working at the same place. I started with one staff and currently have a team of seven staff members in my clinic.

DERMATOLOGY PRACTICE

As I had joined a running clinic, my initial few months I would receive one to two patients which were referral from the other doctors in the clinic. I conducted and visited medical camps organized by NGOs, but realized that none of the camp patients actually turned up in the clinic. The only benefit of the camps was the press and media coverage, this helped in people finding out that I was practicing in the clinic. Another thing that indirectly helped was attending social functions, getting to meet people and being seen more often. Over 3 months, the few patients that had visited me had spread word and I had a regular flow of patients, up to 10-12 per day. Slowly the word started spreading and currently I see patients from four neighboring districts on a regular basis, with a patient inflow of 65 per day as an average. I concluded that the best way of marketing was by word of mouth, so focused on increasing my facilities and introduced chemical peels, minor cosmetic treatments like micro-needling for scars and microdermabrasion for rejuvenation.

DERMATOSURGERY PRACTICE

I started doing free vitiligo surgeries for all females with stable vitiligo and limited patches in my initial years. This helped in spreading the word that I was treating vitiligo around the neighboring villages. Normally in small towns it is a taboo to discuss about vitiligo or reveal that one has vitiligo. So when the surgeries started happening, it encouraged referral and there was a good flow of vitiligo patients too.

A few other procedures and surgeries that I am regularly doing at minimal costs are ear lobe repair, microblading, blepharoplasty, hymenoplasty, and recently autologous fat grafting. It is easier to start the dermatosurgery practice in a small town. People do not like to travel far for minor surgeries, they prefer if it can be done in the same town. A patient for blepharoplasty came to me in my initial days when I was not confident. I counseled him that I will do it, but we may need a corrective surgery to correct the asymmetry if it occurs. Once the patient consented, I was more confident in doing the surgery and mastering it in the following few patients. This is how I have been able to learn different dermatosurgeries, by revising the literature and putting it in practice.

LASER SETUP

Within the first 6 months, with a lot of anticipation I invested in my first laser. A diode for laser hair reduction. This was a low budget reassembled machine that suited my budget at that time. This was also one of the biggest hurdles, since people in small towns have not heard of lasers. They fear this word and link it to hazardous rays. Introducing lasers required a lot of patient education, newspaper articles and pamphlet distribution, but once the results started coming, the response was very good. Not only did the laser patients increase but my dermatology patients started increasing too. Within the first 8 months itself, the laser investment was recovered. My charges for laser were extremely minimal since I wanted the population to first accept it. Being the pioneer, involves a lot of effort in awareness and marketing. The response was very good. After the first 2 years I invested in a high end Q-switched Nd-YAG. I realized that there is a lot of demand for tattoo removal in my state since one boy in every family is asked to join the defence forces, and tattoos are prohibited in the army.

Hence, understanding the sociocultural practices helps in deciding the demand and the type of patients one will encounter. This helps in deciding which equipment one must invest on. For example, every town has its own characteristics just because my colleague purchased a CO_2 laser and is benefitting from it, does not imply that it will be favorable to me too. Hence before investing in any laser, it is worthwhile to start dermatology practice and understand your local demands and patient mentality.

HAIR TRANSPLANT SETUP

I had not expected a good response for hair transplantation when I started practicing in my small town. However, since I was trained in hair transplant, I had put up a few before after pictures in my clinic. Through the visiting patients, I started getting queries. I kept a counseling book with pictures. Similar to lasers, hair transplant was also unheard of and needed patient education. I did my first hair transplant 6 months after starting my practice. I started advertising and writing educative articles in the local newspapers, the response and queries grew. I made training modules and trained my inhouse staff for implantation of grafts. Initially only one of them was able to do it and I used implanters and implanted myself. Then slowly and steadily my staff became more confident and increased their speed. Currently I do two to three surgeries a week in my clinic. I even receive patients from metropolitan cities who drive down because of good references.

MY CAREER GROWTH

In 2018, I decided to take a leap and open up a second center in a neighboring city, Jalandhar (Punjab). Jalandhar is 3 hours away from Hamirpur but has much denser population and a higher per capital income. I started realizing that I wanted to work on esthetic dermatology and there was not much scope in my small town. Hence took the decision of opening a second center. This is a 2,500 sq ft center in the middle of the market in Jalandhar. For the first one year, I had to struggle a lot with the travelling and getting the infrastructure ready. Then the hurdle of buying lasers and paying off the loans. But it had not been for my steady practice in Hamirpur, I would never have been able to expand to another town. Currently I work 3 days of the week in Jalandhar and do only esthetic procedures and surgeries and I have assistant dermatologists to help me. The other 3 days I practice in Hamirpur.

MY HURDLES

Starting in a small town, there are not many hurdles. Since there are fewer dermatologists in these areas, it does not take very long to make a name. A very common issue in small towns is that everyone knows each other and people expect free treatment. This used to bother me a lot initially when I had fewer patients. As the patient load increased, this did not affect me. Everyone who comes to the clinic can see there is a long waiting line, and respects my time. Seeing five to six patients free of charge is normal on any average day for me. I also faced few issues with the language, especially if the patient did not know Hindi. My clinic staff helped me out during such times.

Initially faced few issues when I started doing hair transplants. Many patients refused to believe that a female will be doing it. They believed that a male doctor was more capable to do it. To overcome this, my husband who is also a doctor, would help me out. He would counsel the patient, explain the procedure, and get him comfortable with the idea of the surgery and me doing it. In some cases, he would visit and observe in between the surgery, wherein the patient felt reassured that a "male doctor" was around. This was required only in the initial days. As the number of surgeries increased, patients come asking for me directly.

SUMMARY

Practicing in a small town is a personal choice and comes with its benefits and drawbacks. Family life and personal time is always more when practicing in a small town and even clinic expenses are low. However, it is difficult to introduce newer procedures and facilities to such population. Every new treatment or dermatosurgery introduced requires a lot of time and dedication in patient education in the initial days. Acceptance for newer treatments is slower. After a few years of practice, you may feel that your career has reached a standstill and growth becomes difficult. They only way to overcome this is by continuously updating your skills or starting up another center, like I chose to do.

I am glad that I moved to a small town in my initial years of practice and have never regretted this decision. It has helped me to become a better doctor and a more selfless human being. Even if I have a successful practice in my new clinic, I would never leave my small town practice for the job satisfaction it offers.

KEY MESSAGE

1. Start small. Understand the response and then invest in machines and devices.

2. Do not overcharge, focus on actually helping the patients. That is what gives you a good reference. After all, word of mouth is the best publicity you can get.
3. Bring in novel techniques. Initially the hurdle of patient education will be there, but it will pay off heaps and bounds.
4. Use the local media as an educative medium rather than for advertising. Paid articles will always respond better than paid advertisements.
5. Train your staff well and pay them well.
6. Join the local IMA (Indian Medical Association), this helps in networking with fellow doctors.
7. Keep updating your knowledge. My patients many a times feel very satisfied when they know I have gone to attend a conference. They ask me on their follow-up if there is any new treatment to treat their condition.
8. Have a pleasant personality. Since it is all about interpersonal relationship in a small town.

10.5 How I did: Establish a Large Dermatology Center

BS Chandrashekar

INTRODUCTION

In the changing scenario of medical practice, the way in which patients choose their physician is changing, dermatologists need to change the way they grow their practice. Dermatologists have their own brand and business which is unique to our speciality, which helps in growth of practice. The common ways to grow one's practice are:
- Patients should get the best experience, as in today's world of digitalization experiencing is believing
- Adding services what your patients need and requests
- Using electronic medical record (EMR) tools and practicing photography from the day go as dermatology is a visual speciality
- Adopt the latest changes in treatment options
- Take into the account why patients are leaving your practice
- Extend your relationship and build your personal brand
- Physicians referrals
- Involve your staff in strategies, goals and action plans.

In the context of establishing a large center, let us look into the model which I established; CUTIS Academy of Cutaneous Sciences (CACS). It is an institute where education and research, service to community, and more importantly patient care are given highest priority, with utmost professionalism and utter discipline.

THE DAWN

"The beginning is always the hardest" is true!

Back in 1997, we started as a make shift clinic in a small space of 365 sq ft, with 10–20 patients a month. Now, the institute is spread over 35,000 sq ft, with 5 floors, 12 consultation rooms, procedure floor with 20 rooms for lasers, peel, botox and filler state of art operation theatre facility, minor operation theatre, phototherapy room, waiting lounge, photography room, video dermoscopy room, recreation club and fitness center for staff, cafeteria, pharmacy, catering to the needs of around 400 patients per day.

It started with one doctor and has turned into reality with a total of 80 staff, including 22 dermatologists. It started with table-chair dermatology, and has grown to evolve into super specialty dermatology center. It started with no prefixed goal or aspiration to achieve what it is today, an institution.

EVOLUTION

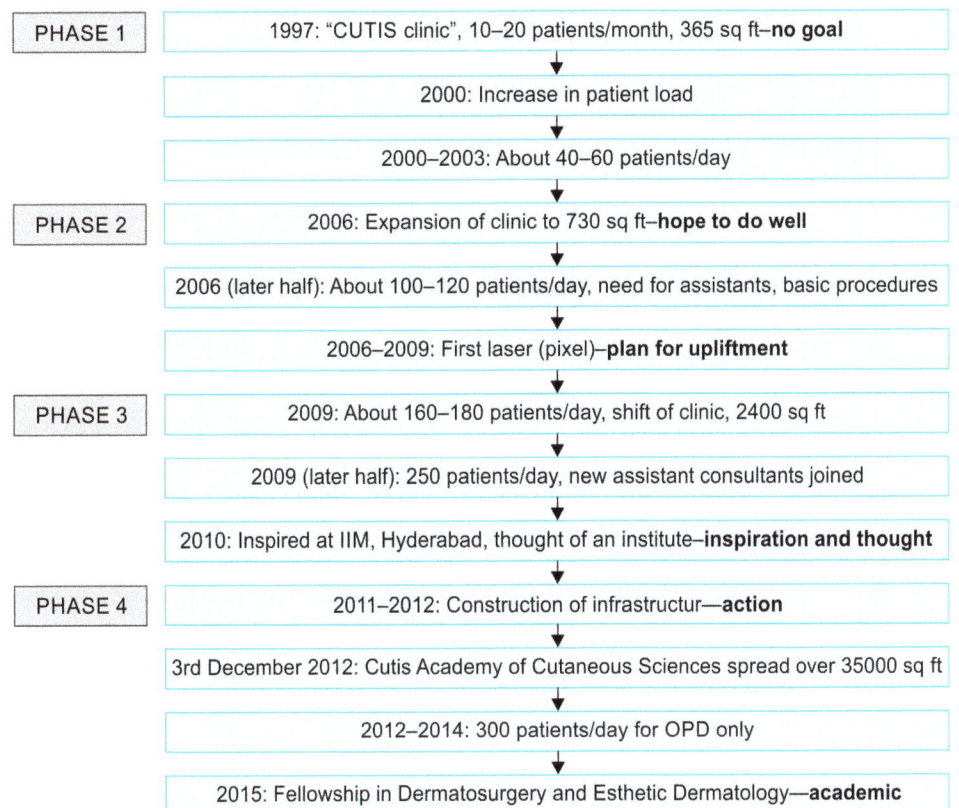

WHY OPEN YOUR OWN PRACTICE?

The first and the most important question is why start your own dermatology practice.

Opening your own practice is an exciting way to take the practice of dermatology into your own hands. Unfortunately, it is also complicated and challenging. To ensure success, it is critical to have a clear and detailed plan at the outset that can help keep things moving on schedule.

The inherent risk, upfront expenses and difficulty of opening one's own practice may explain why the fresh pass outs look for opportunities in health industry

There is no universal formula for starting a medical practice. It might be worth your while to consult a professional colleague who has started dermatology practice before and is aware of the potential pitfalls. An established dermatologist will understand the variables and help you plan accordingly. New practices might need to hire contractors to outfit their new offices. Overall, many common items must be on your checklist when building your practice from the scratch.

My beginning: I had clear cut intention of starting my private practice from the day I passed my MD. As everyone else, I was looking for economic stability first hence joined a medical college to work as I was interested in academics as well. During those times, I did not interact with any of the established dermatologist in the city. Even today I repent for not consulting seniors. If i would have done it, the incubation period of my practice would have reduced. I would not have struggled for 5 long years to see the light of good beginning. Now the times have changed, guidance is available in and around in the form of internet, practice promoting workshops and open-minded professional colleagues who guide and show the right path.

THE FOUNDATION

At the heart of your growth plan is the successful medical practice you built. This is the foundation for everything moving forward. By matching your service excellence with your medical skill and intuition to a growth plan that fits your needs, you will be in a position to look into your patients' changing needs.

Maintaining your current patient base is crucial to business success, as is continuing to grow your base with new patients. As a dermatologist, you know how important an individual's image is, and that same mentality should be applicable to your practice.

Growth has its risks, but the right strategy can deliver stability, security, and long-term profits. Once you have assessed the current strength, weakness, opportunities, and threats to your practice and how well you are equipped to handle them, you can move on to the next stage—building a strategy for growth.

My foundation: When I started it was hard to build a base, all the strategies to promote practice were under taken. Meeting family physicians, general practitioners, pediatricians, physicians, and gynecologist for referrals. Newspaper articles on various skin ailments were published, and addressed few dermatology-related topics in some meetings of family physicians. Although it did not fetch much what I desired, but definitely brought an awareness among public and peer groups that a dermatologist is available in this particular area. At the same time, I had to leave the medical college because of unforeseen circumstances. Then, I had to look out for filling the 9 AM to 4 PM gap, hence, I started roaming around 60–80 km/day in search of patients in many polyclinics and hospitals. Finally, after putting so much of effort I realized that best PRO for any practice is one's own satisfied patients. To improve satisfaction level of current patients I introduced small procedures such as acne extraction, chemical peels, etc. This not only fetched new patients and extra revenue but also changed my image to a cosmetologist and dermatosurgeon alongside clinical dermatologist.

HOW TO GROW YOUR DERMATOLOGY PRACTICE TO ESTABLISH THAT DREAM BIG CENTER

The professional life of most dermatologists, pose a difficult path. We go through immense amounts of prolonged studying, and then work for years—if not decades—to acquire the technical acumen and artistic skill. And then, after dedicating this massive amount of time and effort, at least few of us take the entrepreneurial route, choosing to start our own private practice. It is entirely a new journey, with a whole new set of skills, this time, in business. But where along the way did we learn how to become business owners? Where were we taught, how to grow our practice and take it to the next level? For many of us it is the biggest (or only) gap in our education.

Where to Begin?

Even if you are happy with your current performance, it is important to keep looking for ways to develop. If you do not, you risk allowing your competitors the room to grow and take practice share from you, which could seriously weaken your position. Going for growth may therefore begin with consolidation of your current practice. To devise a successful growth strategy, you need to know exactly what shape your practice is in. This will help you to ensure your practice is properly structured and grow in right direction.

Consolidate your Existing Performance

While you may be spending more time and resources on developing the practice, you need to be sure that the core of your practice is still performing well. It is vital not to neglect your existing patient base as this remains fundamental to your growth and provide the regular money flow you will need during this phase.

Timing is critical to the success of any growth strategy. Answers to the following key questions will help you judge if the time is right:

- Has your practice come to a stage of expansion, or is it working at full capacity?
- Do you have the resources and system in place to carry on your existing practice while targeting expansion? Do you want to sit in the same place or anywhere else?
- If new initiatives are likely to disrupt existing practice, how will you ensure your patients do not lose out?

You may have to consider including additional staffing, refining clinical processes, and equipment, or outsourcing certain area such as laboratory, pharmacy, etc. in order to give you the flexibility to pursue a growth strategy.

My consolidation: Eight years in to the practice what I looked at is to consolidate by several measures, like expanding clinic space, modernizing interiors, regularizing appointments, standardization of procedures, employing more staff and assistants to ease out work, and to improve time given to the patients. One of the important steps taken by me is towards investment. I followed the path of self-finance to add technologies, to start pharmacy and laboratory which gave extra income to further consolidate my finance. I started to re-invest 30% of the revenue generated out of the practice by depositing it in a separate dedicated account which was utilized only for investing in clinic upliftment. By this time there was substantial increase in number of patients, assistants and revenue too.

DREAMING BIG…IT'S IN YOU, ONLY IN YOU

Shift Your Psychology

The first thing you have to realize is that the chokehold on the growth of any business is always the owner. And while 20% of that chokehold may come down to mechanics of running a practice, a staggering 80% has to do with one's mindset and thinking—that is, one's own fears, limits, and stories about why one's practice is not where one want it to be.

Most people think that they need to redirect their focus toward new strategies to make real change. But while strategy is absolutely important, it is the wrong sequence to start with. What is the strategy for being fit and healthy? It is not that complex, yet 70% of Indians are technically considered incapable, because it is not a strategy problem; it is a mindset problem.

Take a moment and think about your perceived limitations. (It might help to think of them as "reasons" you cannot achieve something). For most of us, here are some of the common ones we are preoccupied with:
- It is so hard to find a reliable long-term receptionist or a manager or a technician. They either leave after a few months or a year, or I have to fire them. The cost of that kind of turnover is killing my bottom line.
- I have to stay in urban areas to keep volume of patients up, but then the overhead I am paying rent which cuts deeply into my profits.
- Patients get so frustrated from dealing with their improvement status that they cannot ever be fully satisfied customers from start to finish. They subconsciously blame us for their poor compliance.

It is easy to throw your hands up and say, "I have tried everything." But if you keep saying that, then you will undoubtedly convince yourself that your growth is limited. The reality is, the only limits that exist are the ones that you create for yourself, and it is those that prevent you from reaching your achievement goals. Once you come to understand what your limiting beliefs are, you can begin to shed those constraints.

It is time to decide that you are no longer going to tolerate the way you are running your practice until now. It is time to decide that you deserve more. Your staff deserves more, too, and they deserve to see that there is a different way. Step out of the state of learned helplessness and resolve that you are going to arm yourself with the tools and strategies necessary to make real, lasting change in your practice towards becoming an entrepreneur.

FALL IN LOVE WITH YOUR PATIENTS

Your practice has a purpose and direction. And that purpose has nothing to do with you, it is about your patient. Do not fall in love with your practice; fall in love with your patients or even your ideal clients.

Understand who your patients are: What do they want? What do they fear? What do they desire and how do you meet those needs for them? How can you give them the experience that they want?. *Remember whatever said, shown, read, or done, experiencing is believing.*

Answering these questions will allow you to create a culture where every single employee in your practice will know what is your purpose, and you will collectively is able to add more value than anyone else. Forget about having satisfied customers. Satisfied customers will go away when a better offer comes along. What you want is a raving fan. You have to over-deliver in a way that makes you irreplaceable to them. When you can do this, you will be able to make your way towards dominating practice scenario.

My dream: Academics was always my priority. It was still a big lacunae in my profession. After leaving medical college I was missing teaching which was my passion. I happened to attend a workshop on medical leadership at IIM, Hyderabad which began a thought process in my mind of establishing a center not only for Professional growth but also to integrate teaching, training and research. This was a big challenge which required strong mind set. Capacity to take risk and a clear vision. This time I had to take a huge bank loan to establish the center.

FACTORS WHICH PROMOTED THE GROWTH OF CACS

- Clinical skills
- Communications skills
- Inception of photography and computerization from the beginning
- Upgrading technologies and infrastructure at regular intervals
- Seeing dissatisfied patients on priority
- Not too strict about fee structure
- Providing medicinal samples liberally at right time for a right cause
- Cordial with colleagues and fellow professionals
- Healthy and commendable relationship with industry
- Attitude of love everyone hate none
- Involving colleagues and staff in decision making
- Work like a family supporting each other at times of distress and enjoying each one's success.

CHALLENGES FACED!

Few of the constraints faced and fought in the due course of the growth are; Finance especially during the initial days, manpower, choosing technology, and gap between therapeutic promise and response. Few of the strategies not followed; no marketing by any means, no website till 2012 and no referral fee.

THE CLOSING REMARK

Dermatology specialty has grown as a tree with many branches, and we have nurtured each and every branch with care, perseverance and commitment, so as to improvise and provide superlative treatment to its patients, and have created a platform to research, create novel treatment alternatives in dermatotherapeutics and to ignite young minds.

What do you really want? You have to decide what is most important to you and what are you doing all this for. If you are just doing it for the money, you are eventually going to burn out. Because no matter how much money you make, if you are not fulfilled, then you will never be happy. Remember, *success without fulfillment is the ultimate failure.*

10.6 Adopting/Incorporating New Techniques in Practice

Maya Vedamurthy, Deepak Vedamurthy

INTRODUCTION

A technique is the purposive application of skills or knowledge or both by a healthcare provider to a patient. A procedure is a combination, often quite complex, of provider skills or abilities with drugs, devices, or both.

Medicine is a continually evolving discipline, and if physicians fail to adopt new techniques in practice, they will find themselves left very much behind their competitors. We were no exception to this rule. Fortunately, our physicians-motivation-adaptation (PMA) scale was good enough to run the race.

This quote always propelled us.

"Do not wait; the time will never be 'just right,' start where you stand, and work with whatever tools you may have at your command, and better tools will be found as you go along."

—**George Hebert**

At the same time, this often-repeated quote by our professor, Prof. Patrick Yesudian, would caution our enthusiasm.

"Be not the first by whom the new are tried nor yet the last to lay the old aside."

—**Alexander Pope**

The above two quotes always influenced our decisions in incorporating/adopting new techniques in our practice.

As a practitioner of clinical and esthetic dermatology, it was inevitable for us to introduce new techniques in practice, which had its pitfalls, in addition to its benefits. Ensuring the safety of a new technique has its challenges.

PITFALLS OF NEW TECHNIQUES

- Not regulated in the same way as drugs
- Insufficient data to ascertain the truth
- Fear of peer reviews
- Resistance to acceptance by patients and colleagues
- Lack of guidelines
- Risk of liability
- Cost often high

Our implementation would eventually depend on the sum of factors that influence acceptance and resistance to the new technique. We make sure we incorporate only procedures that are postmarketed and not on research or clinical trials. It was always difficult to strike a balance as adopting new techniques remained the prerogative of esthetic dermatology. We would carefully consider the safety and efficacy before dissemination into clinical practice. The learning curve for technical competence is critical for a complete understanding of the benefits, harm, and optimal application of a new intervention. We would explore a wide range of alternative therapies/techniques to validate our acceptance.

Hence we laid my criteria to help us decide to adopt the new technique and position it in our practice.

Factors that influenced our decision making in introducing a new technique—3Es
1. Evidence
2. Experience
3. Exploratory design/exploration

Evidence

To us, the priority is medical evidence. We were aware that we are not a scientists to innovate or to do research. But we would go through medical literature or other resources to gain knowledge about the proposed new technique or we would talk to experts in the same field or even experts in another field who use similar technique, e.g., we discussed the handling of laser with my ophthalmology friends as they started using laser much earlier than us.

'Primum non-nocere' (again often repeated by Prof. Patrick Yesudian) was our motto.

We always intended that medical evidence should include efficacy and safety. We understand that introducing a novel technology into clinical practice is like introducing a new scalpel in the operating theater. We always keep in mind that new medical technologies, unlike others, emerge from a process that is far less systematic and certainly less linear.

We would also speak to colleagues with similar interest or attend workshops, e.g., we have heard and read about chemical peels in the early days of my career and was looking for an opportunity to learn more about it, as it was not available in India at that time. We suddenly came across a workshop on chemical peels organized by the national skin center at Singapore in 1995. We just decided to go and explore. We were convinced of the procedure as we found it fairly simple, easy to perform, safe, and effective, and so we returned home with a handful of chemical peels. But the courage to start on my dark skin dampened our spirit. We waited to have a Caucasian patient to gain that first experience and confidence to move forward.

Pitfalls I Encountered in Evidence-based Esthetic Medicine

We realized that every product or procedure introduced in the market should be viewed with skepticism until proved otherwise. We should not go overboard in the early stages of introduction, e.g., when dermal fillers were first marketed we had two permanent fillers introduced to dermatologists, e.g., polyalkylimide and polyacrylamide. One of them was widely promoted and extensively used by a large chain of skin clinics. With this evidence, we ventured to use it in our practice until we realized they were no longer recommended due to lack of safety. We then realized that today's evidence is often in tomorrow's dustbin.

We had many more similar lessons to learn as well as undo our mistakes, e.g., using artificial hair fiber implants in alopecia, use of conventional TCA chemical peels in dark skin, etc. On the contrary, evidence-based aesthetic medicine had its benefits too. We realized that aesthetic practice is a service industry based on our patients' needs. One such practice we found rewarding was the use of dermal fillers in hand rejuvenation, which we initially thought would be difficult to incorporate in our practice. Use of dermal fillers for hand rejuvenation as an antiaging procedure was promoted extensively in the Western world, but surprisingly it was well-received by our patients too.

Experience

Experience as a health provider and as the patient undergoing the new technique was helpful to decide the adoption of the same in clinical practice. The learning curve for technical competence is critical for a complete understanding of the benefits, side effects, and optimal usage of a new technique. So we would choose our staff, friend, relative, or at least a patient who trusts us over the years for medical competence. Once we gain confidence in the procedure, we would proceed to disseminate it into clinical practice.

To gain experience as a patient, we would opt to be a volunteer or try the technique on ourselves to obtain insight and to completely understand the benefits for optimal application of a new intervention, e.g., before launching Botox in the country, there was a pre-launch workshop organized by Allergan where an international trainer was brought in to demonstrate injection techniques. As we were keen on seeing the results on ourselves we volunteered to have our crow's feet injected, and this boosted our acceptance to start it in our practice. Similarly, we have tried most of the techniques in our practice on us personally to ensure optimization for a better outcome.

Exploration

Before adopting a new technique, we explore a wide range of alternative therapies/techniques to validate our acceptance. We would also consider financial criteria such as return on investment and manufacturer/suppliers support system. While we weigh the patient's benefits for adopting new technology, we also weigh the risks associated with these to a physician's practice. We do not get excited about introducing new tools aggressively, but we integrate it into our practice slowly and judiciously.

We explore the cost-benefit analysis, the cost being the patient's expenses, and the benefits being their clinical outcome.

How we decide to buy expensive laser machines in our practice—Real-world scenario.

Our motivation here is to get the best available treatment for our patients. We do understand that there are no gains without pains. We usually depend on our database and study the market response before buying an expensive laser/machine. We do not jump on to every machine that hits the market. We have a basic principle that the laser should give us professional credibility, and we do not buy machines that are sold to beauty parlors, salons, spas, etc.

We usually buy them through bank loans, and we make sure we will be able to survive the monthly EMIs. We prefer to compete on quality than price, so we prefer to achieve a break-even policy in the beginning and concentrate on profit later. When we are confident of this equation, we venture to acquire the new laser/machine and to accept the new technique in our practice.

The next major step after accepting the new technique is the implementation in practice, which we needed to execute carefully.

We follow Ps similar to that of marketing practice

The Ps include:
1. Product selection involving the new technique.
2. Patients selection
3. Promotion

Product Selection

Choosing the right product for the technique is very important. We prefer to use high-quality products from a reputable manufacturer. We compare the products on the market and choose the one which we would be ready to use on us. We do not compromise on cost if it assures safety and efficacy. We prefer to choose products which have labels like FDA approved as it offers at least safety to our patients and our practice.

Patient Selection

Patient selection is equally as important as product selection. We choose the right patient to have a satisfying result. Having chosen the patient, we do confess that we are using a new technique that is added recently to our practice and the reason for which we choose to do it. We also allow them to choose conventional techniques if they are wary of the new technique. It is banal to say that the field of aesthetic procedures (from both user and provider perspectives) is complex as it involves the patient's consent and desire to choose the technique. We are compelled to scrutinize the social, economic, psychological status of the individual before adopting a new technique. We take written informed consent for the new technique which includes a list of alternative treatment options available that can be carried out and a list of risk and expected complications that may arise with the new technique. We clearly explain the advantages of the newer technique and the purpose for which we have chosen it. We believe collaborative decision making and written informed consent are fundamental components of safe clinical practice when adopting new techniques (ensuring the safety of new techniques has its challenges).

Promotion

Promoting new techniques should be timed carefully and early enough as the late introduction of a new technique may deprive the patients of adequate or "state of the art care." We understand that at this time, we do not have guidelines from professional bodies, so we go slow on promoting or adopting the new technique.

First, we educate our associates and staff on the new technique, and they, in turn, are expected to inform patients and help them make decisions that fit their beliefs, values, and choices. As a principle, we do not use social media to promote any of our products and do not rely on them for marketing purposes.

We train and credential our staff to do the new technique before dissemination into practice, which helps them to balance responsibilities to patients and clinical practice. We make sure that they also track the outcome of new techniques.

Pricing also influences the dissemination of the new technique. We make sure that the technique always represents good value for money. We take suggestions and surveys from manufactures and market to make sure our patients feel they are paying the right price for a new technique.

CONCLUSION

We always have trepidations while introducing new technologies. Finally, we redirect our thoughts and focus on our motto to "we can do it" also called "Rosie the Riveter" after the iconic figure of a strong female war production worker. This American World War II Wartime poster has inspired us to adopt and disseminate new techniques in our practice safely, effectively and judiciously.

10.7 Managing Association Work with Practice: Striking a Balance

Umashankar Nagaraju, Priyanka Agarwal

INTRODUCTION

Striking a balance is the key to life. When your work and personal life go out of balance the stress level is likely to soar, hence a harmony between the two is a must.

The situation becomes further challenging when your work includes managing association work as well as your private practice. Association in any organization is for the welfare of its members and society on the whole. It is managed by a group of members chosen to do so, which includes mainly a president, secretary, and executive committee. Secretary is the driving force in any association. Association activities are implemented by the secretary with the help

of his/her executive members. To restore harmony between association work and practice a few practical strategies that we need to put into practice are:
- Time management
- Share
- Schedule
- Efficient and trained staff
- Make up for the lost time
- Being honest
- Unplug
- Healthy lifestyle
- Learn to say "NO".

TIME MANAGEMENT

We need to define our priorities and based on that our time. Divide your time accordingly, e.g. how I do that is by fixing the time from morning 9-11 AM for association work and 12-6 PM for my practice and remaining for my family.

As the saying goes "There is never enough time to do everything, but there is always enough time to do the most important thing".

SHARE

"Share if you care"

Be open to those closest to you about your work life be it to your spouse or young children at home, so that they have a better appreciation of your efforts, of what drives you or keeps you away from them. Sharing of information is very important as pertains the association.

For example, being a secretary I am entitled to share all the association activities with the president and the other executive members for which meetings are carried out and also on the other hand keep the members informed about the minutes of meeting which I do is by means of emails. Conferences are planned so as to keep the members informed and updated about the latest developments. Conferences are also an important platform for social interaction and sharing of knowledge and experiences between its members.

SCHEDULE

It is always better to plan things ahead so as to avoid conflicts as much as possible. Not to forget that the life we have chosen as doctor, by its very nature means that there is no such thing as schedule. However, as far as possible we should try sticking to a plan per day that would make life a lot easier and organized.

As pertains the association work a calendar of events is planned for the year and subsequently implemented. Meetings have to be planned well ahead of time so that the resources can be economically utilized. Conferences too have to be planned in advance so that it involves a good participation from its members. How I cope up with it is by proper scheduling of the events.

EFFICIENT AND TRAINED STAFF

As the quote goes "*Too many cooks spoil the broth But Many hands make light work.*"

So the staff involved at the place of association work as well as at your practice place should be efficient and trained. The staff should be well versed with the use of latest technology whether be it computers, I pad or mobile especially in the present era where everything is technology dependent. Continuous training is a must so as to keep them updated. They must be well versed with their job profiles.

At my practice work place I entrust my clinic staff with photography, setup of procedure room, positioning and preparation of patient. I have also efficiently trained them with postprocedural care, guidance and counseling of the patients which saves me some time.

Whereas at my association work place my work is to supervise and give instructions on how the activities are supposed to be carried out.

MAKE UP FOR THE LOST TIME

Post of secretary in an association involves a lot of traveling as meetings are held in different parts of India and abroad. Frequent traveling (around 4-7 days per month) to the head quarter is essential for the smooth functioning of association to continuously monitor and motivate the staff such as manager, assistant manager, accountant, office assistant and class 4 employees.

So when I am traveling my practice is managed by my assistant doctors and I make up for it by devoting some extra hours for practice once I am back which is impossible without my family's cooperation.

BEING HONEST

"Honesty is the best policy"

Be true to yourself. We can rationalize anything and everything, e.g. I can easily justify myself for a missed family dinner or a gathering by telling myself I am working to give my family a better future but the fact persist I could not make it for the occasion because I was more passionate about something else.

It is the passion which is the driving force. In very simple terms it means we are more involved or more focused in a particular thing because we enjoy it, we thrive on it, not because its forced on to us.

So being equally passionate about everything is important. We cannot ignore practice for association work or family for practice striking a balance between the three is equally important.

UNPLUG

In the present era, technology being so advanced it enables us to work anytime anywhere be it on a moving train or waiting for a cab or at home. However, working on a moving train or waiting for a cab may buy us some grace time to reply emails or other things but working at home may not be justified.

Today work is like to invade our personal space until we know how to recreate boundaries. Leave work at work.

Keep computers and laptops turned off at home. Avoid the use of mobile phones as well. Time is our most valuable asset we can give your families so better to go unplugged when with family.

HEALTHY LIFESTYLE

"Health is wealth"

Staying healthy is the key to everything so to adopt a healthy lifestyle is a must. Which includes a good diet as well as some exercise. Some studies suggest that exercise helps relieves stress by releasing feel good hormones called endorphins.

For example, since I do not get a lot of free time to exercise I prefer to use stairs instead of elevators and escalators that adds to a few extra miles I walk per day.

LEARN TO SAY "NO"

Last but not the least learn to say no be it to a patient who lands up to your clinic after the closing hours without prior appointment with no serious illness or a coworker at association asking you to super head an extra projects or activity.

Epilogue

(Great) Grandfatherly Advice for Young(er) Dermatologists and Dermatologic Surgeons

Lawrence M Field

Philosophical counseling from their elders is generally not sought by "young dermatologists". A listing of the "Golden Rules" of practicing successful dermatologic surgery has never been proffered. Many younger physicians try to expand their practices by expensive marketing to accomplish successful practices, seemingly unaware of the already existing, prudent, and proper ways adopted by their seniors. In building and maintaining your practices, expensive advertising budgets will never equal the tried and tested basic truths, which may be perhaps slower, but infinitely more sound. This great grandfather seeks to enumerate a few of those time-tested tips for his younger colleagues through this letter:

1. Integrity, honesty, and ethics are the cornerstones of success. Financial security follows closely and is critically interrelated.
2. Charge fairly and appropriately. Be charitable towards people, and extend yourself to do charity work.
3. Office esthetics, waiting room appearance, cleanliness, neatness, washroom area care all impact on your patients and their families as much as your own skills.
4. Be generous with your time and effort in providing patients and their families with the information they need to make intelligent and informed decisions. You will thus, seem not arrogant. "Customer service" is critical.
5. Know how many times your telephone rings before it is answered, and how many are put on hold for extended periods of time—these can identify potential problems.
6. Be prompt with your schedule. To be late does not increase your importance in the patient's eyes, but may well be interpreted as rudeness and arrogance. If late, apologize, and mean it!
7. Be charitable towards your colleagues. Teach and share with them whenever possible. You will share their good fortune and happiness, and earn their respect and gratitude.
8. Criticize not, that you not be criticized. Professional enemies last forever!
9. Protect the referring doctor from patient criticisms when possible. It will be most deeply appreciated, for most adverse statements return to that same doctor who was being criticized via that same patient or the family.

10. When referred a patient, only do that which was requested of you. Never violate this rule, or be prepared to lose all future referrals by that individual and his/her friends. Emphasize to the patient requesting you to do more, that it is unprofessional to do more than that for which the patient was referred to you.
11. Establish and insist on good, warm, professional, and ethical relationships between your office staff and the staff of your referring physicians.
12. Know what your referred patients and those referring physicians need, and exceed those needs and expectations. Excessive charge complaints are disasters for you.
13. Learn from anyone and everyone who has knowledge, which may benefit your patients. Cross "specialty lines" and professional lines are necessary to accomplish this.
14. Read, study, discuss, practice.
15. Keep formal records of your surgical training and document your learning experiences, in addition to standard CME credits. Photographs and operative reports help.
16. Learn techniques to minimize patient discomfort, both physical and emotional. Extend these considerations to their families.
17. Establish a network of consultants friendly to you, and then do not hesitate to seek consultation when in doubt.
18. Your presentations and publications become your specialty's means of giving you earned honors and accolades. Be meticulously honest in both. Your intraprofessional reputation depends on it.
19. Get an academic appointment and find the time to teach. You will be rewarded in many ways, as respect from others and from one's self increase as time passes. Patients love their own physicians to be teachers and givers.
20. Stay alert to the failings of your colleagues. Become an interventionist only via proper professional channels and medical societies. Avoid lay lawyers and media when they seek an opinion on your colleague.
21. Be quick to send your records in response to requests from other physicians. Offer to help in any way you can in the future care of the patient.
22. Express unhappiness with professional nepotism and program control by any self-appointed "chosen few". Fight it openly and aggressively.
23. Engage in a continuing study of all appropriate journals, going back as far as it is possible to do. Browse your medical center library monthly if possible, or whenever the opportunity presents itself.
24. Attend appropriate meetings to expand your dermatological surgical knowledge and skills, especially meetings of your local association, the American Society for Dermatologic Surgery, the International Society for Dermatologic Surgery, the American Academy of Cosmetic Surgery, the American Society of Liposuction Surgery, and your local and state dermatologic surgery societies, and, when possible, cross-fertilize with plastic, eye, ear, anesthesia, etc.
25. Always use/obtain the highest possible quality sutures, staples, equipment, instrumentation, etc. The finest work requires the finest materials.
26. Surgical personalities are generally impatient personalities. Be patient and know yourself by taking the time to obtain and chart histories and/or blood

work regarding possible hepatitis, HIV, bleeding dyscrasias, etc., whenever applicable.
27. Answer phone calls from physicians as quickly as possible, and from patients and their families the same day. You should never be too busy for these courtesies. But, in so doing, remember your patient's rights to privacy when talking to the family!
28. Look and act like a surgeon if you are representing yourself as a dermatologic surgeon. This includes gloves, mask, surgical cap, surgical top, sterile milieu prn, etc. Your surgery room(s) should represent the state-of-the-art in surgical suites, and be reserved for appropriate procedures.
29. Your "comfort level" may, at times, be in competition with or at variance with your "competence level". At such times, as and when you feel uncomfortable with what you are performing (or about to perform), stop. Wait, get consultation, or refer.
30. Turn down patients whose families are against you doing a particular procedure. That family may never be happy, and can easily set an initially happy patient against you with all the undesirable sequelae.
31. Observe many. Watch, listen, filter. If you must disagree with that which you are observing, politely do so outside the patient's presence. You should not criticize, and remember, "There are many roads to Rome", i.e., many ways to do things. Experiences and results vary.
32. The more you know, the more you learn-always.
33. Remember who taught you-praise and thank them openly. It will humble you, and remind you of the long path you have taken to knowledge.
34. Forget you have not had complications—it means nothing to the one case in which you do. Approach each as that case.
35. Always err on the side of conservatism, most especially with cosmetic procedures. Law suits last a miserable 3–5 years, or more.
36. Models and body builders seek perfection—even if they deny the same to you. Caution is the word.
37. Ethnic, cultural, religious differences and sensitivities exist between people. Learn, observe, and practice.
38. Never hire a new employee without the acceptance of your previous employees. Jealousy, rancor, dissatisfaction lurk, and office performance suffers.
39. Always remember it is a privilege to practice medicine-practice it both as a science and as an art.
40. Work diligently for respect-both from yourself and from others. Both are hard-earned, and worth every possible effort to achieve!
41. Extend this list by adding your own rules.

These are here for your consideration. And the author hopes and believes that these are as relevant, important, and vital to his younger colleagues as they have been to him.

Reproduced with permission: J Cut Aesth Surgery Year. 2008;1(2):104-5.

Part 2
Plastic Surgery

- Section 11   Starting Off
- Section 12   Marketing
- Section 13   Growth
- Section 14   Essentials

SECTION 11

Starting Off

11.1 An Introduction to Plastic Surgery Practice

Sanjay Parashar, Aniketh Venkataram

Medical practice has seen a paradigm shift in the last decade or so. The field is moving away from one of necessity to one of demand. Nowhere is this more true than in the field of cosmetic or esthetic surgery. Esthetic surgery practice is constantly evolving with improving technologies, better understanding and advancing infrastructure.

During training, the emphasis is on acquiring surgical skills. After residency also, plastic surgeons have multiple learning opportunities to hone their skills, and technologies to aid in learning process. But what after that—is a question faced by many young plastic surgeons. This is compounded by the fact that many life skills are not learnt during the hectic grind of residency such as administration, leadership, marketing, communications and finance, etc.

Due to this lacuna in training, many surgeons take missteps early on in practice. Most surgeons want to start their own practice. They have their own funds or they take loans—in both situations there is pressure to generate revenue to meet the expenses and earn profit. Many start spending on marketing erratically, using misleading information to gain public attention. And when a client steps into the office, whole attention is to "convert" them to patients. Oftentimes the patient is brought to the operating room and a surgery is performed—only to realize the patient is unhappy and has gone through unpleasant experiences. Some may get exploited by corporates.

Due to our lack of knowledge, we look to other professionals for help. And again we can be misled or overcharged. Another issue is that nonmedical professionals are not aware of the nature of business (practice) we are in and the unique challenges we face. A marketing person looks at you as a commodity and patients as a consumer. A financier will critically analyze your books and look for "bottom-line" failing to account the "Goodwill" that helps to keep the wheel rolling in medical practice.

The goal should be to build a long-term sustainable practice with sound fundamentals that has sustainability and scalability. The reputation of a plastic surgeon depends upon first and foremost their visibility (so do not retreat in your comfort zone, go out and let others know who you are!), integrity, and honesty. This is assuming they have the basic skills to perform surgeries and are committed to good postoperative care. A medical degree, training and skills do not guarantee success in practice, because remember everybody has that. So your success depends upon how different you are, how you promote yourself and how you manage people and your practice.

It is important to be critical about ourselves and identify our own strengths and weaknesses, through a "SWOT analysis". It simply means your Strength, Weaknesses, Opportunities you have and Threats that can affect your practice and business.

So, the aim of this book is to fill these gaps in training, to produce well rounded medical professionals. In this book the chapters cover most aspects of business management from acquiring skills (clinical and nonclinical), creating infrastructure, communicating with people, establishing a referral base, to grooming yourself and leading a team of experts to run a successful practice.

There are many challenges from acquiring clients, performing safe surgeries, dealing with complications, patient dissatisfaction, litigation, dealing with competition, rising costs, demanding employees, rapid technological advancement and so on and so forth. Relax, take a deep breath, where there is will there is a way! And remember "What goes around comes around". Be good, do good and you will earn all the goodness. This book is just a start to help you deal with the turbulence you may face setting up your practice.

The contributors in this book have gone through a learning curve, not only clinically but also in practice management. They have put together their years of experience and learning in this book to help guide the new generation. This book is for new Plastic surgeons getting into practice, surgical residents and for existing practitioners to improve the quality of practice.

11.2 Acquiring Skills and Mastering the Art of Plastic Surgery

Karishma Kagodu

INTRODUCTION

As a plastic surgeon we are programmed to think that knowing every surgical technique is of utmost importance and that the operating room (OR) is where plastic surgeons belong. I have grown to now believe that there are many other crucial skills involved in mastering *"The Art of Plastic Surgery".* Expanding the horizons of knowledge in class and polishing the skills in the OR is just the beginning....

Our entire residency training program is aimed to educate and train us in basic plastic surgery knowledge, technical expertise, surgical skills and getting accustomed to working long grueling hours. Way back as a general surgery resident, my inspiration to become a plastic surgeon grew working under a dedicated cleft and reconstructive surgeon. For me plastic surgery became exciting, diverse, with a tremendous variety of conditions to treat—a true *"The Head-to-toe Profession".*

On joining the training program, one must be ready to take up this broad and challenging subject, yet at the same time not be content with the stipulated 3 years of rigorous training.

One of the most deeply ingrained memories from my typical residency days involved—anatomy flap dissection, early morning seminars, being grilled by "The Boss" during rounds, followed by hectic surgeries and OPD. Looking back, we always waited to run back into the OR, but now I feel otherwise.

The following were the important lessons that I have learned over the years and would like to share with you…

LESSON 1

"Experience the outpatient consultations" besides just attending surgeries. Remember, trauma/burns/reconstructive surgery patients are totally different from cosmetic surgery patients. The counseling for each of them is different. *"Communicative skills"* are rarely thought of as important during residency, but become essential in the future private practice. Being attentive, using the right words, learning to decipher the patient's mind, making direct eye contact, while planning the procedure in the back of your head takes years of experience. Meeting and working with as many plastic surgeons as possible in the initial years can give you the much needed heads up in the right direction.

After the completion of the stipulated 3 years we tend to feel like the *"King of the World"*. Hold your horses as it is only the beginning.

A plastic surgeon is now in a dilemma on which path to follow *"Private Practitioner or Academician"*. In the past, most surgeons joined Medical Colleges and Hospitals and climbed up the ladder till they were the heads of departments and great teachers. I too thought of the same during my residency. I believed I needed to do reconstructive surgery for years and then eventually switch to cosmetic surgery.

LESSON 2

Reconstructive surgery definitely lays the foundation for a good cosmetic surgeon, but cosmetic surgery also has an equally long learning curve extending beyond those stipulated 3 years.

I believe a *"Private practitioner can also be a good teacher"*. This will involve fellowships, traveling to attend CMEs and hands-on workshops. These are critical requirements, in the initial years post residency, if one wants to pursue a successful career in trauma/burns/onco-reconstruction/cosmetic surgery.

How do you Know where and when to Begin?

My career actually took off when I realized my passion, which was cosmetic surgery.

I followed and recommend the following guidelines:
- No matter which subspecialty, it is essential to realize what you really want.
- Do not get influenced by anyone, you just need to follow your heart and it is never too late to make a start, either post residency or even years later.
- Plastic surgery is an ever-changing, complex field, where innovations in surgical procedures and techniques are continuously happening the world over. Choose the subject and the surgeon, visit and learn from them.
- One of the greatest attributes of our profession is the vast diversity of subspecialties to choose from and I believe one can really be *"The Master"* if one focuses for years on that subspecialty. Most great surgeons worldwide that I have

known, have done just that. Although some exceptional few have mastered multiple subspecialties.

LESSON 3
Know what you Want…Follow your Dream…The Pursuit for Knowledge is Endless…

When I was first exposed to the cosmetic surgery world, I was totally fascinated and in complete awe. I decided to follow my passion for the subject and started hunting for fellowships, and started mailing every surgeon in the world who I felt I could visit and learn from, taking into account logistics, funding and time away from home, as some or all of these factors come into play. Some of us have family commitments, few are newly married, and funding could also be an issue for some. I worked day in and day out to save up and then decided where I could travel, how long I could stay and yet not compromise on my learning.

After 2 long and fruitful years I had completed my initial learning journey starting with esthetic body contouring, breast and face procedures, with renowned plastic surgeon, Dr Sanjay Parashar at the Cocoona Esthetic and Day Care Centre, Dubai. Followed by specialized training with the biggest name in Rhinoplasty Dr Nazim Cerkes, at Istanbul, in Turkey. I then trained in microsurgical onco-breast reconstruction and esthetic breast-related procedures with Dr Venkat Ramakrishnan at St Andrew's Centre of Plastic Surgery in Chelmsford, UK. Finished my Facial Esthetic Fellowship—DAFPRS, Italy with Dr Giovanni Botti and last but not the least, I decided to visit our very own pioneer Dr Srirang Pandit in Pune. I have revisited Dr Nazim Cerkes twice more to refresh my rhinoplasty learnings. I still call Drs Pandit, Nazim, Botti and many of my seniors for advice on complicated cases.

"Fellowships are Essential for Acquiring Skills required in our Profession."

LESSON 4
Culminating the Dream: All of this Struggle—"What is the Goal?"

For me the *"Goal"*, was to open my own cosmetic center, complete with world-class equipment, and high standards of safety and professionalism. Besides numerous cosmetic and plastic surgical techniques, I had also learnt practice-enhancing and marketing strategies which are something that is not touched upon in our residency days. There is an art of convincing the patient to undergo the correct procedure after identifying the patient personality.

Why all this?

By the time the patient reaches the point of direct interaction with the doctor, they must be partially convinced and at ease about the clinic and the doctor with just the ambience, positivity, non-intrusive nature of the staff and most importantly the short waiting period. The rest lies in your hands and in your skills as a doctor.

One cannot emphasize enough the importance of *"right planning and execution"* which is where your hard earned *"technical and work experience"* will come into play.

A well-planned or with the best equipment will always be your unique selling proposition (USP). Photographic documentation, appropriate medicolegally safe consent forms with meticulous patient records are essential in making your clinic a wholesome place.

Patient privacy and confidentiality as well as not allowing patients to cross paths during and in between treatments will make the client feel secure and are also of paramount importance. These are important aspects you observe during fellowships and they cannot be taught as such.

Finally, finding a good marketing team, having a plan in mind and organically growing on social media is important. Marketing strategies are plenty, choosing the right one for yourself is essential.

TIPS AND PEARLS ON PURSUING FELLOWSHIPS

- Research the field of plastic and cosmetic surgery and which centers around the globe have provisions for pursuing a fellowship.
- Once you know your areas of interest, apply to individual universities or surgical centers.
- Make sure you are well informed about the surgeon's practicing in those centers, the kind of work they pursue and if that fits into what you want to pursue.
- Whether fellowship or observership—choose the right surgeon, with the experience that you feel will help you in the future.
- Some surgeons are amazing teachers—these qualities one sees in their presentations during conferences. Hence attend CMEs/conferences/live surgical workshops—to identify your mentors.
- Plan a visit to Europe/UK/USA (having a vast number of plastic surgeons)—visit as many surgeons in a short period as possible. Even if it is just for 10–15 days—you will pick up some crucial pointers from each of them. I did this on my Europe trip of 3 months. During my Italy DAFPRS Fellowship with Dr Giovanni Botti, I also visited Dr Gino Rigotti (Fat Grafting), Dr Enrico Robotti (Rhinoplasty). I also clubbed in Botti's Best Face Conference—got to assist Dr Nuri Celik, Dr Ruth Graf, Dr Mario Pele and went to Istanbul for the first ENT-Plastic Surgery combined rhinoplasty symposium.
- Stay updated—attend national/international meets in your field of interest live workshops are always better according to me.
- Stay in tune with the latest technology and instrumentation—incorporate them in your practice.
- Update surgical skills by revisiting your mentors or meeting new colleagues.

SUMMARY

- Acquiring surgical skills and academic knowledge is very important, but the ability to convince a patient to believe and trust in you is the key to a successful practice.
- Mastering the art may take forever, but your passion and honesty must not dwindle. The constant desire to acquire new skills must not end.
- We all are artists in our own right, on a mission of paving a successful path for ourselves in our chosen field.

11.3 Golden Rule of Success: Mastering Personality Development

Sanjay Parashar

"In the history of the universe, there has been nobody like you and to the infinity of time to come, there will be no one like you. You are original. You are rare. You are unique. Celebrate your Uniqueness."

—*Gurudev Sri Sri Ravi Shankar*

I agree with gurudev: Our uniqueness defines us. It is what helps us define our lives. And working on ourselves in order to produce a diamond from a stone is a continuous process.

INTRODUCTION

According to the definition, personality development is the relatively enduring pattern of the thoughts, feelings, and behaviors that distinguish individuals from one another.[1] Although, it is development, in the field of esthetic plastic surgery it needs to be adapted to the best of its form. We are in the business of making people look better, and it has to start by being better.

In medical schools and colleges, doctors are taught to be professional, humble and passionate with patients. But how many take that advice seriously? Most successful doctors are known for their arrogance and attitude. We seem to have forgotten the gift of medicine is to be imparted along with great courtesy and etiquette.

In general medicine and surgery patients do not care much about the personality of the doctor as long as they are successfully treated and cured. Most of them come as they do not have a choice, they are chasing an illness and looking for a cure. However, in elective surgery, particularly in esthetic practice the patient has a choice. Choice changes everything.

Before we go on to personality development let's look at what makes a patient select a plastic surgeon? A plastic surgeon will go through two checklists.

- *Checklist one*
  - Qualified
  - Experienced
  - Skillful
- *Checklist two*: Those that make it through the first checklist, will have to then live up to the expectations on the second one.
  - Vibes
  - Personality
  - Grooming
  - Integrity

It is the "vibes", surgeon's personality, grooming, the way they talk manner of speaking, how comforting are they, how assuring are they, and how they make the patient comfortable. It is the right mixture of all these characteristics that gives an edge to a surgeon.

I believe, if you are running an esthetic practice it is important that you satisfy these five senses of the patient.

1. *Sight:* Clients/patients are very observant. They look around and they look at you. For them everything needs to look good. The clinic interior, décor, staff grooming, surgeon's appearance, paper work, tidiness, etc. After all, they expect you to make them look perfect. So you need to be perfect too.

2. *Smell:* The place and people need to smell good. Most clinics smell of hospital odors. Humans are scared of the hospital because of the smell of alcohol, antiseptic blood or other such strong smells. This makes them anxious. A pleasant odor reduces their anxiety and helps to calm them down.
It is important that your practice does not smell like this. Imagine you are going to a spa and you smell stale mop, sweat or any other unpleasant odor. How would one respond? One would clinch their nose. The clinch sends a strong signal of dislike to the brain; there are a lot of points lost. It is tough to recover from this.
3. *Sound:* Sound is important for comfort. It starts with the tone of the receptionist and other staff they interact with, the music playing and the sounds that the equipment used in your clinic makes. As long as one keeps these sounds in check, the patient will also keep their behaviors in check. The principle at play here is— What you give is what you get!
Gentle music, soft-spoken conversations, soundproof rooms with loud equipment are the way to go.
4. *Taste:* Yes, the water, coffee you serve at your proactive is equally important. Make sure the water is clean and served at the right temperature given the temperature outside. Imagine serving warm water in the summer or cold in the winter. At my practice here in Dubai, we have ensured we have good coffee and with multiple choices, I do have many patients and visitors, who say—doctor I come here for the coffee. I love it.
With these five senses, we are going beyond the two checklists I talk about. I am telling you to connect to them on a level they are not even aware of but we all know it is important.

5. *Touch*: This one is my favorite. Be gentle with your patient, the way you examine and treat will help them trust you more. As this is what you the doctor controls directly and cannot pass on the blame to anyone else.
I often see the doctor, during the treatment or examination moving the patient face, head, etc., without consent. This leaves the patient feeling roughed up a little. I suggest developing a habit of talking through to these steps,—I would like you to move your head to the right and look at the...Rough handling and abrupt movement scares patients and makes them more anxious.

And the last sense—the 6th sense. I always tell my team the 6th sense is the most important of all. I call it "love at first sight", where the patient feels an instant connection with the doctor, staff and the clinic as soon as they lay eyes on them. Mastering the 6th sense is a knack that one can acquire, when they master *the 5*.

All these senses are important to one's personality. Your personality consists of:
- Grooming and dressing
- Personal hygiene
- Attitude
- Behavior
- Communication skills

GROOMING OF THE DOCTOR AND STAFF

A recent study demonstrated that a doctor's appearance is an important requirement and these include wearing a clear name-tag (77%), neat grooming (65%) and professional dress (59%).[2]

Professional attire is associated with honesty, knowledge, discipline and better care. I believe a clean white dress in the form of the doctor's coat or a plain white full sleeve shirt with a tie gives a commanding position to the surgeon and patients tend to take them more seriously. A clean unstained surgical attire, which has a name, and designation clearly mentioned is also impressive to the patients.

A colored checkered shirt, half sleeves and tees give a casual look and patient does not take them to be very professional.

Likewise, proper footwear is a mandatory wear. A flip-flop, unpolished shoe, or worn out shoes may not be seemed very impressive.

Similarly women can wear an apron or a formal office dress or traditional dress with plain and light colors.

Hair grooming is equally important, in men well-groomed hair and in women nicely tied hair appears more professional and above all it is hygienic.

Patients do pay attention to your hair, skin, body and dress. A patient who is asking for hair transplant will pay attention to your hair, a patient with skin pigmentation, wrinkles or acne will look at your skin and patient coming for liposuction will certainly take notice of your tummy. It is up to us how to represent ourself if we have to be the role model of our patients.

Looking after your skin, hair and body are important elements of grooming.

PERSONAL HYGIENE

Surgeons, estheticians, technicians often come in close contact with patients, while performing procedures or assisting procedures. Bad odor is single most deterrent to patients and that carries a bad impression and may even refrain the patient from coming back. Foul oral smell and poor dental hygiene is also not accepted well.

As a leader you need to lead by example and you need to train your staff so they understand the importance of personal hygiene.

Ensuring your staff brushes after each meal they have in the office and applying body deodorant frequently is a good idea.

I always keep extra pair of scrubs and office clothes in my clinic and change if I feel I have sweated a lot. This often happens with surgeons who are running around all the time.

ATTITUDE

A positive attitude is necessary to spread positive vibes in your clinic among the colleagues, staff and patients. Being passionate for what you do is extremely important to impart confidence to the patients. Patients see your dedication and devotion to your job and it assures them you will do the job well.

Being compassionate is also very important; to understand the patient's emotion and pain gives them the comfort they are looking for and reduces their apprehension. Listening more than speaking is an age-old therapy to treat human psyche. I spend about 70% of my consultation time listening.

BEHAVIOR

No matter what, we are being judged all the time by our patients, staff, colleagues and vendors. They make a certain impression about us and that affects their decision. And not only do they carry that with them, but also they spread it around.

Like your clinic or hospital, is a brand, you are a brand too. Your behavior is an important part of brand building. Building a positive image is crucial to your success. Image travels like wildfire, I believe in "What goes around comes around".

Control on language and temperament reduces the anxiety of the patient, staff and yourself as a surgeon. Do not let your emotions take control of situations, but learn to control your emotions. This will help you stay focused and calm during challenging situations.

"When pride comes, then comes disgrace, but with humility comes wisdom". Often knowledge and experience makes one believe invincible, but in our profession, we know very well that not everything is in our hands. No matter how much we know and how best we can perform, there may be below par results and we may not be able to satisfy all our patients. Having humility does not mean embracing mediocrity or being incompetent, it just means understanding your limitations and accepting mistakes if there are any.[3]

Having a sense of humor improves rapport with patients. Being friendly and making them laugh reduces their anxiety and makes them feel more approachable. However, it has to be in good taste and noninsulting. When you see a lot of patients in a day you may go through a lot of different emotions and face challenges from angry, upset and dissatisfied patients. Resetting your mood before you see the next patient is a real talent one must possess for a successful practice.

COMMUNICATION SKILLS

The most important part of communication skills is "listening". A "patient" listening helps you clearly understand the needs of the patient and gives confidence to the patient. If we are distracted (telephone calls, texting, computer surfing) patients may feel unworthy of our attention and if we are too rushed they may feel undeserving of our time.

There are certain basics of practicing good communication. Patient and empathetic listening with both "ears and eyes" is necessary to focus on what patients are saying and this is so important to give them a satisfying result. Just listening while you are performing other tasks such as looking at a computer screen or phone does not give confidence to the patient. They feel neglected.

The increasing dissatisfaction and lawsuits against doctors have a common denominator that "you were not paying attention to what the patient wanted". There is enough evidence in the literature to suggest poor communication between doctors and patients is an important attributing factor.[4] The hour of the need today is to have a formal training in communication skills in the medical curriculum and training of practicing plastic surgeons.

All the above five elements are necessary not only for the plastic surgeon, but also for the whole team. These habits need to be inculcated in your team as your staff are the one that are the gateway to your practice and also they hold the hands of the patient and provide them postoperative support.

We all know surgeons are hardworking, practical, organized, obsessive and maybe perfectionist, but surgeons are also perceived as arrogant, hostile, impersonal and egocentric. Have you realized dermatologists and estheticians see more patients than plastic surgeons in esthetic practice? The reason is patients/clients feel less intimidated and they feel they may have a more patient listening from them then a surgeon. And, that they may have a less painful and scary solution to their problem.

You need to define, practice, demonstrate and preach the professional standards that are necessary to keep the image not only for you, your center but also to the whole esthetic plastic surgery industry. You need to define and display integrity and commitment.

Personality development is a key skill that will help you stand out. Be aware that flamboyance, overconfidence, is counterproductive.

REFERENCES

1. Caspi A, Roberts BW. Personality development across the life course: the argument for change and continuity. Psychological Inquiry. 2001; 12(2):49–66.
2. Au S, Khandwala F, Stelfox HT. Physician Attire in the Intensive Care Unit and Patient Family Perceptions of Physician Professional Characteristics. JAMA Intern Med. 2013;173(6): 465-7.
3. Chochinov HM. Humility and the practice of medicine: tasting humble pie. CMAJ. 2010; 182(11):1217–8.
4. Virshup BB, Oppenberg AA, Coleman MM. Strategic risk management: reducing malpractice claims through more effective patient-doctor communication. Am J Med Qual. 1999;14(4):153-9.

11.4 Setting-up Documentations in your Practice

Milind S Wagh

OVERVIEW

A very experienced and respected plastic surgeon colleague would often relate anecdotally about hundreds of patients he had operated and treated over 20 years of his practice, doing a particular procedure with remarkably consistent good results. Based on the same, he was invited to give a prestigious oration on this subject at a meeting of his peers. This necessitated that he goes back to his records and archives to find documentary and photographic evidence to back his claims. To his chagrin, he found that his clinical records were woefully poor, incomplete and in some cases completely absent. He simply could not find evidence of enough cases to present to bolster his oft-repeated anecdotal claims of success and had to shamefacedly acknowledge the same.

A colleague performed a face-lift on a patient under general anesthesia with due informed consent taken preoperatively for the procedure. Intraoperatively, he found that he also needed to perform a lower eyelid blepharoplasty on the said patient to ensure a comprehensive rejuvenation. Consent had not been taken for the same in advance but the surgeon was clear in his mind that this needed to be done in the patient's best interests and went ahead with the procedure. Postoperatively, the same was explained to the patient as soon as she recovered from anesthesia. The patient was upset that this was done without her prior informed consent and even with the final result being quite pleasing the surgeon was sued. The law was quite clear on the matter...that in an elective procedure with no life or death consequences, any additional procedure without the patient's express specific prior informed consent was beyond the clear brief given to the surgeon and should not have been done. The surgeon had to pay a six-figure compensation to the patient in this case.

Another colleague had a torrid time operating and managing a particularly fussy VIP patient who, postoperatively would not follow his instructions and often simply not show up for regular follow-ups as planned. After a while, she was completely lost to follow-up and would not answer calls or reply to text messages. Six months later, the surgeon received a legal notice that the patient was highly unsatisfied with the result and was filing a suit against him in the Consumer Court. The surgeon had photographic evidence of the operated area preoperative and postoperative with dates, had maintained meticulous records of his consultation notes, his operation notes, detailed write-ups of his postoperative and follow-up instructions as well as text messages and phone calls with screenshots recording that the patient had received and read the messages but had not responded. This diligent record keeping on part of the surgeon ensured that the court dismissed the frivolous suit.

A lady underwent breast augmentation surgery with implants 12 years before, with a plastic surgeon in another city. Her implants had settled well and were not giving her any trouble. The patient however wanted them replaced because she had read on Google that implants should ideally be changed after a certain number of years. She visited a different plastic surgeon in the city of her present residence and insisted that she wanted the implants changed. She had not preserved any records related to the previous procedure, so the current specialist had no information about the volume and type of implants and the plane in which they had been placed. Clinical examination yielded only partial and imprecise information. The patient was reluctant to undergo imaging studies to ascertain this information. A quick call to the colleague who had done the previous procedure and a request to check his records helped—all the information that was necessary was still available and helped immensely to plan the patient's implant exchange surgery.

The four diverse examples or case studies mentioned above exemplify the vital importance of documentation of various kinds in clinical practice across specialties but more specifically in our field of plastic surgery. We tend to think that maintenance of documentation and records is important only in cases of litigation. Yes, its importance in medicolegal evidence, for insurance claims and for labor compensation cannot be overemphasized. However, even without the Damocles' sword of litigation hanging over us, it is in our own interests to have a detailed documentation and record of every patient because it is equally if not more crucial for:
- Medical education
- Epidemiological research
- Presentations in conferences and publications in peer review journals
- Readily available information related to treatment, past, present and future
- Medical audits and statistics

All of us who completed our medical courses and training programs look back upon those days with varying degrees of nostalgia. While the fun times as well as the tribulations and struggles of those days are often recounted and discussed, we also remember those days because our responsibilities were limited to following instructions and learning under the protective umbrella of a senior colleague and/or a teacher. When we emerge Chrysalis-like from our training programs with a freshly minted degree or diploma in the specialty of our choice and plunge into the uncertain world of clinical practice, that protective umbrella is suddenly no more and we find that we are directly and personally responsible and independently legally liable for our actions vis-à-vis any and all patients that we see and examine, consult with, treat and manage surgically or otherwise. We are firmly within the ambit of not only the medicolegal implications of every decision and move of ours but also within the purview of the Consumer Protection Act, which the law of our country, in its "wisdom", has included our profession in.

PERMISSIONS, REGISTRATIONS AND INSURANCE

The first documentation that is mandatory when one starts practice in any state of our country where one wishes to practice is *registration with the corresponding State Medical Council* **(Fig. 11.4.1)**. This includes basic registration for the MBBS degree and then add-on registrations for postgraduate degrees/diplomas and super specialty degree/diploma. This is also of critical importance in securing attachments to hospitals, as they will ask for all the requisite registrations with the concerned state medical council before even scrutinizing your documents. Practicing and doing surgery in another/second state now mandates that a separate registration be done with that state council before practice is officially allowed in the said state.

If one starts a clinic of his/her own, then the surgeon also needs to be registered under the *Shops and Establishment Act*. In the event of starting a day care center or nursing home/ lying hospital with overnight patient stay, requisite *permissions from the local Municipal Bodies* and registration of the facility with them is mandatory. This often also involves acquiring a *change of user certificate* if a residential property is converted to a commercial property, which is the category that a clinic or nursing home/hospital falls under. It also requires *fire safety clearance* from the local fire department. Since any clinical surgical establishment is likely to have change of wound dressings, injections, even minor procedures under local anesthesia, the generation of biological waste, blood and bodily fluids and use of disposable syringes, needles, etc., requires a *Memorandum of Understanding (MOU)/ Annual Maintenance Contract (AMC) with a local biomedical waste disposal agency*.

Those who practice cosmetic surgery from which the total income per year from all sources is likely to exceed ₹ 10 lakhs also require to be *registered for Goods Service Tax (GST)* **(Fig. 11.4.2)**, so that the same can be paid regularly on income and input tax credit availed from vendors when GST is paid by the surgeon on what he/she buys to use in his/her practice. It is absolutely vital that

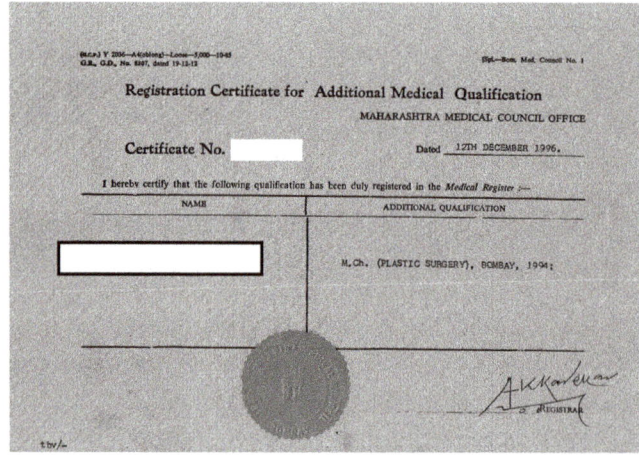

Fig. 11.4.1: Registration certificate for additional medical qualification.

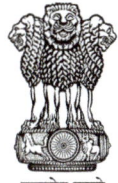

Government of India
Form GST REG-06
[See Rule 10(1)]

Registration Number:

1.	Legal Name				
2.	Trade Name, if any				
3.	Constitution of Business	Proprietorship			
4.	Address of Principal Place of Business				
5.	Date of Liability				
6.	Period of Validity	From		To	NA
7.	Type of Registration	Regular			
8.	Particulars of Approving Authority				
Maharashtra Goods and Services Tax Act, 2017					
Signature					
Name					
Designation					
Jurisdictional Office					
9. Date of Issue of Certificate					
Note: The registration certificate is required to be prominently displayed at all places of business in the State.					

This is a system generated digitally signed Registration Certificate issued based on the approval of the application by the jurisdictional tax authority

Fig. 11.4.2: Registration certificate.

the esthetic surgeon be registered for GST. The service tax officials have a very stringent scrutiny policy and make income tax officials look like angels.

Another important component, which must be paid attention to, right from the beginning of practice, is *Medical Indemnity Insurance*. As a plastic surgeon, this may cover all aspects of plastic surgery, except cosmetic surgery. There are a few insurance companies, which now also cover cosmetic surgery for an additional or larger premium. A minimum annual cover of ₹ 50 lakhs is advisable, whereas it should preferably be at least ₹ 1 crore for those who regularly do cosmetic surgery. Medical indemnity insurance is the mandatory lifeboat for any surgeon doing esthetic surgery. There are occasions galore in our country where the surgeon has been saved by his indemnity policy when accosted with consumer court lawsuits, however frivolous or false they may be.

Many states mandate that the doctor's qualifications and degree certificates be on display in his clinic or be available to the patient to examine if requested. It is always a good idea to also display currently applicable membership certificates of any professional associations, national and international, for the benefit of patients.

A few years ago, the Maharashtra Medical Council had even sent out circulars to all registered medical practitioners in the state "requesting" them to even display their fees structure for consultations and follow-up visits in their clinics.

OUTPATIENT DOCUMENTATION AND MEDICAL RECORDS

Registration and EMR Entry

Each new patient who visits the clinic and is seen by the surgeon must be registered in his medical records. These may be done in the traditional way by maintaining a book register with entries detailing the patient's name, age/sex, address, contact number and date of visit at the very least. It is now more and more convenient to maintain these records electronically feeding the same information into the computer using electronic medical records (EMR) software, a plethora of which is available at a wide range of one-time buying costs and recurrent costs for updates. Our clinic records each patient in the time-honored way of noting the relevant information on paper every day. The receptionist then translates this to the electronic form on the weekend when she has more time on her hands. An audit of the same is undertaken with me at the end of every month to ensure that all the information has been properly entered and saved.

Patient Questionnaire

Every new patient should be given a common patient questionnaire **(Fig. 11.4.3)** to fill while in the waiting area, with all the details related to his/her personal history, current and past medical, surgical and obstetric history, history of current and past medications, allergies, comorbid conditions, addictions and vices. It should also mention the reason why the patient wishes to see the surgeon and should state that all the information provided is genuine and correct to the best of the patient's knowledge. It should be signed by the patient with the date and time clearly written in the patient's own handwriting as far as possible. At the beginning of the consultation, the doctor must read the same and run through all the information provided, both positive and negative, with the patient, add his own notations and sign with time and date. This questionnaire is an important part of the clinic records. This questionnaire is maintained in the paper form and a scanned digital form in my clinic, for ready reference whenever the patient revisits. It saves a lot of time and lets the patient know that the information she has provided is available with us in case there is any discrepancy, duplicity or temptation to hide or falsify information in the future.

Consultation and Follow-up Visit Notes

A detailed history-taking and clinical examination is invariably part of our consultations. However, it is not enough to only do that, the same must be penned down, any significant issues underlined or

Patient Information

Name			Surname		
Date of Birth	Age	Gender	Height		Weight
Address			Contact No.		
Reason for Visit/Procedure Desired					

Medical and Surgical History

	Yes	No	Details		Yes	No	Details
Diabetes				Thyroid			
Hypertension				Bleeding tendency			
Stroke				Varicose Veins			
Heart Attack				Jaundice			
Asthma				Kidney Disorder			
Chest Pain				Acidity			
Pneumonia				Urine Infection			
Anemia				Eye Problems			
Blood Transfusion				Ear Problems			
Tuberculosis				Seizures			
Recent weight Loss/Gain				Syncope/Fainting			
Constipation				Mental Illness			
Smoking				Alcohol			
Any other Medical History:							
Other Medications				Allergies			
Previous Surgeries				Anesthesia-related Problems			

Gynecological History

Pregnancies	LMP	Could you be Pregnant Now? Yes or No

I certify that I have disclosed my medical history truthfully to the best of my knowledge

Patient Signature   Date

Fig. 11.4.3: Patient questionnaire.

highlighted and the clinical impression and possibly the treatment plan as discussed with the patient and their relatives must be noted on paper and signed with date and time. Any tests/investigations suggested should also be clearly written with instructions on when and where they should be done. Photocopies or digital scans of these consultation notes must be immediately taken by the doctor's receptionist/staff and the same retained in the clinic. If an EMR is being maintained, the same must be uploaded there with dates and times.

The same holds true for any and all follow-up visits of the patient, irrespective of whether he/she has been operated or not. In the case of follow-up visits, special notation must be made on the date on which the patient has been instructed to return for reassessment. It is also important to record any missed or lapsed visit dates with notes made about how and when the patient was reached out to and reminded. This can form part of the EMR.

I personally believe that the time has come for audiovisual recording of consultations with the patient's consent. This of course cannot include the patient's clinical examination, especially if it is of areas that the patient is uncomfortable revealing or even the patient's face if consent is not given for the same.

Investigations Done

Photocopies and/or digital scans of all investigation reports asked for and done by the patient must be taken and stored for the doctor's records. This is important not only for reference at any time in the future but also in case the patient either accidentally misplaces the same or maliciously suppresses them in the event of litigation. In the case of X-rays, CT scans; MRIs and other imaging studies, photographs or digital copies of the same should ideally be retained.

Clinical Photographs

Ours is a field where clinical photography and documentation is an integral part. Documentation of our results by preoperative, intraoperative and postoperative photographs in different standard views with standard lighting and background forms the mainstay of our treatment timeline for our own records as well as to share with the patient. Ideally the patient's written consent must be taken for all photographs. In fact, refusal of consent should also be documented with the patient's signature. Any photographs used on the surgeon's website or for digital marketing need express written consent from the patient. Any objection to the same at any time in the future, even after previous consent, has to be respected and the particular photographs deleted as per the patient's wish.

Preoperative Instruction Sheet

A comprehensive preoperative instruction sheet with pertinent points related to specific surgeries being ticked or crossed should be available to give to each patient on his/her preoperative visit **(Fig. 11.4.4)**. This should include instructions for fasting prior to surgery, any medications to be taken prior to surgery with names, strength, number of doses and the time/date to be taken. Any instructions related to stopping smoking or alcohol intake as well as stopping any other medications are to be included. The surgeon must run through the same, point by point, with the patient and confirm that it has been noted and understood by the patient and any accompanying kin. I make sure that I call on the patient and a relative 1–2 days prior to surgery in most cases and take the time to sit down with them to go over the preoperative instructions and clarify that they have understood the same. There have been occasions when I have postponed elective surgery on the morning of the procedure if the patient has, for example, not stopped smoking, has not been fasting adequately or has not taken his/her medication if deemed important enough. It is simply not worth

Name: Date:

2 Weeks Before Surgery

STOP Smoking—smoking decreases blood supply to skin and complicates healing

STOP: Aspirin, Warfarin, Ticlopidine, Clopidogrel, Heparin, Ibuprofen, Vitamin E (high doses), Ginseng, Ginkgo biloba, garlic and green tea

Arrange for accompanying person

2 Days Before Surgery

Confirm that all preoperative investigations are complete

Measurements for PRESSURE GARMENT (whenever required)

1 Day Before Surgery

WASH operative area with Betadine cleansing solution/chlorhexidine solution

Remove hair from operative area/arm pits/private parts

Tab PAN (40) at _____ PM

Keep hospital bag ready—reports/GARMENT/change of clothes/medicines/ID card/toiletries

NIL BY MOUTH—No food or water after _____ PM

On the Day of Surgery

Shower normal; wash operative area with Betadine cleansing solution/Chlorhexidine solution

Brush teeth normal—avoid swallowing excess water

NO tea/coffee/breakfast

Tab PAN (40) at _____ with 2 sips of water

Tab Disperzyme at _____ with 2 sips of water

DO NOT take diabetes medication

Take blood pressure/thyroid, etc. medications (as advised by doctor)

Wear loose fitting clothes (e.g. pants with elastic bands/top with front closing zipper or buttons)

Please remove all metallic objects (rings, ear-rings, bracelet, anklet, necklace, etc.) off your body, at home

Please carry all reports/GARMENT to the hospital

Please report at _____ Hospital at _____ AM

Any Other Instructions

Fig. 11.4.4: Presurgery instructions.

it to lament later and ascribe a sequela or complication to the patient not obeying your instructions adequately. The onus lies not only with the patient but also squarely with you.

OPD Procedure Consent Forms

Often minor procedures are carried on an OPD basis under local anesthesia in the surgeon's office. A separate consent form for the same must be available for the patient

Patient name:_____ Date of birth:
Diagnosis:_____ Contact no.:
Procedure:_____ Anesthesia:

I, the undersigned, acknowledge that I have understood the above procedure (operation) that I am to undergo, under_____ anesthesia

Further, I have been explained the following in the language that I understand.
1. the nature and effects of the above mentioned procedure/operation.
2. the nature and effects of the anesthetic medicines and procedures.
3. that, any further alternative operative measures may be necessary during the course of the operation I hereby permit Dr _____ to do so.
4. that, Plastic and Cosmetic surgery is a mixture of science and art and one cannot guarantee a specific result in any individual.
5. the postoperative recovery and all the potential complications associated with the procedure.
6. that an assistant surgeon/s and/or nurses will be required, which I acknowledge.

I have had an opportunity to clarify all my queries regarding my procedure (operation) and I have been explained the preoperative precautions, procedure details, postoperative recovery care, possible risks and potential complications of my procedure (operation) and anesthesia to my satisfaction.

I agree to have clinical images/clinical photographs/video recording taken for the purpose of operative planning, postoperative comparison and research work.

I undertake to follow all the instructions regarding the preoperative advice, procedure (operation), post-operative care and visits that Dr _____ will give me both prior to and after the procedure (operation).

I acknowledge that it is my choice to undergo the above procedure (operation) and I give consent for the performance of the above procedure (operation) on me.

Patient's signature:_____ Date:

I confirm that I have explained the nature, expected benefits, potential risks and complications of the procedure to the above mentioned patient and/or parties responsible for the patient.

Name of doctor: DR.
Signature:
Date:

Fig. 11.4.5: Procedure consent form.

to read, understand and sign. A possible standard format is shown **(Fig. 11.4.5)**.

Receipts

All patients must be given printed receipts for fees received for consultations, and follow-up visits signed by the staff and preferably countersigned by the surgeon. The receipt must mention the patient's name, date of payment and mode of payment (cash, credit/debit card). In the case of card payment, a duplicate receipt must form part of the clinic records. Any deposits made by the patient in lieu of partial payment of surgical charges, etc., must also be acknowledged with a receipt (with duplicate or carbon copy), which in addition to the basic information mentioned earlier must also note the reason for payment. Any money refunded or returned to the patient or owed by the patient must also be recorded with the same details. All this information should ideally be uploaded into the EMR.

Certificates Issued

We often issue certificates of current treatment, leave of absence from work and fitness to resume work to patients who are under our care and operated by us. A meticulous record of the same must be maintained. All certificates should ideally be addressed to a specific person or organization. A generalized "To whosoever it may concern" certificate can often be misused by the patient without the doctor being aware of it. All certificates should be related to a specific issue such as planned date of surgery, estimated hospitalization time, time period of rest recommended, restrictions on physical activity, date from which work can be resumed and a final fitness certificate to resume all activities. Care should be taken to stick to genuine specific facts in the certificate without resorting to falsehoods under pressure from the patient. All certificates must be clearly dated in the present, it is unwise to provide a certificate with a retrospective date and a doctor does so only as his/her own peril. Ideally time duration of not more than 2 weeks should be attested to in any certificate. Subsequent ones given at regular intervals if necessary can prolong the period as required. All certificates must be signed personally, stamped with the surgeon's rubber stamp or seal and the registration number/state medical council added. All certificates should be countersigned by the patient or have his/her left thumb print. Interim certificates given to a relative without examining the patient are to be discouraged. We would do well to remember that such a certificate from a surgeon is a legal document that is taken cognizance in the court of law and must stand scrutiny for our own well being.

INPATIENT DOCUMENTATION AND MEDICAL RECORDS

Admission to a hospital necessitates a whole bunch of different types of documentations to follow the hospital protocol and often based on guidelines from quality control and accreditation organizations such as the ISO and National Accreditation Board for Hospitals and Healthcare Providers (NABH). Listing or detailing all those documentations that a hospital keeps records of is well beyond the scope of this chapter. However, it is also necessary for the individual visiting surgeon to maintain some records and documentation related to his management of his patient while admitted in hospital. It is wise to remember, "what is there in the records never happened in the eyes of the law". The highest court in the land has ruled that patients are entitled to have complete access to their indoor papers and treatment records and must be provided a copy if requested. It is therefore in the hospital and doctor's interests that the documentation of each patient's treatment is precise, meticulous, comprehensive and contemporaneous.

Numbering and Labeling

Each page of the patient's indoor paper must have the printed label with the patient's details on it and numbered chronologically. This makes sure that no loose pages are missing and also prevents deletions and additions in case of litigation.

Visit Notes

Every clinical visit made by the surgeon to the patient for assessing his/her progress needs to be documented meticulously. Beginning with the date and time of seeing the patient during each visit, the notes in legible handwriting should detail the patient's clinical progress since the previous visit and highlight any issue that is specific and important with regard to the treatment being given or the surgical procedure carried out. It should clearly mention any change in medications since the previous visit, both additions and deletions, and countersigned. It should also mention any fresh tests asked for or done, with the latest values of the same. Any restrictions or allowances with regard the patient's ambulation/positioning, etc., should be clearly noted. As far as possible, no erasures, overwriting or inking out should be done.... any alterations must be with a single cross through, which is countersigned and then rewritten. *Abbreviations are too avoided consciously.*

Doctor References

Any references made to other specialists and the reason for doing so should be mentioned on paper, with date and time. Follow-ups on the same, after the reference has been seen, should be notated.

Inpatient Investigations

Copies of all investigation reports carried out on the inpatient must be retained by the hospital since the originals need to be handed over to the patient.

Discharge Card/Notes

In most hospitals, it is the resident medical officer who writes the discharge note which is given to the patient at the time of leaving the hospital. While it is supposed to be a detailed summary of the important aspects of the patient's treatment in hospital, it is often hurried, sketchy and woefully incomplete. Ideally, the entire discharge note, which is evidence of the entire inpatient treatment, should be dictated and personally checked by the primary consultant under whom the patient is admitted, before it is printed and handed over to the patient. A complete copy must be retained by the hospital and attached to the indoor paper when it is moved to the medical records department. I make it a point to read the patient's discharge summary myself before it is printed, make the necessary changes, additions and deletions, knowing fully well that this is not only just the instructions to the patient but also an important medicolegal document.

DOCUMENTATION FOR OPERATED PATIENTS

Consent Forms and Site Marking

A detailed informed consent form for each procedure is preferable, rather than a general consent form for all. It must clearly mention that the risks and benefits of the procedure and any common complications related to the procedure have been explained to the patient in a language he/she understands. The patient and a relative must both sign the consent with date and a witness and the surgeon should countersign with the time and date as well **(Fig. 11.4.6)**.

A similar but separate consent form for anesthesia with necessary details, signed by the patient and relative and countersigned by the anesthesiologist for the case, must be part of the inpatient records.

An additional safeguard is a site marking form. The marking of the site of surgery in a printed illustration, as shown in **Figure 11.4.7**, must be carried out and signed by the surgeon and countersigned by the patient and relative, with date and time. Any refusal to allow site marking must also be noted.

Operation Notes

Detailed step by step operation notes mentioning anesthesia, position of the patient, any infiltration of fluids and salient steps of the surgery performed, intraoperative findings, suture material used in different planes, any

UHID No. _____ Patient Name: _____ IP/OP No. _____ Age. _____

Sex: _____ Bed No: _____ Ward _____

I hereby authorise the performance on me/my patient_____(son/daughter/wife/husband of) _____ the following surgery/procedure _____ to be performed by or under the direction of [Name of the Doctor]_____together with associates or assistants who may be employed by the clinician for my Medical Condition.

The procedure has been advised by Dr_____ and Dr_____has discussed with me in detail, and I understand and acknowledge the following has been explained to me in the language known and understood by me:.
1) The nature and purpose of the proposed surgery/procedure(s)
2) The following risks involved in the proposed surgery/procedure(s)
   a)
   b)
   c)
3) All possible alternative treatment choices available to me
   a)
   b)
   c)
4) The possible benefit of the proposed surgery/procedure(s)
   a)
   b)
   c)
5) It may be necessary to administer section and/or anesthesia (local, nerve block, regional) for this surgery/procedure.
6) Tissues or blood may be removed and used for diagnosis and treatment of my condition, and these may be disposed off sensitively and appropriately by the hospital and its staff.
7) That no assurance/guarantee has been given by any one as to the results that may be obtained.
8) Postsurgery/procedure follow-ups.
9) I have read and fully understood this entire form. I have asked the Clinician all the queries I had and they have been answered to my utmost satisfaction. I hereby accord my consent for the above mentioned surgery/procedure.

PERSON	NAME	SIGNATURE	DATE	TIME
Patient or Next of Kin (NOX)				
Witness				
Surgeon				
Interpreter, if required				

(The consent is valid for the current admission or current visit for the above mentioned procedure)

Fig. 11.4.6: Surgery/procedure consent form.

implants, meshes and drains placed are a crucial aspect of surgical documentation. Their importance cannot be emphasized enough. The notes must be dictated or personally written in legible handwriting as soon as possible after the procedure is completed, preferably immediately while details are fresh in the surgeon's memory. If dictated, the transcription must be checked and any corrections made at the earliest.

UHID No._____Patient Name:_____IP/OP No:_____Age:___
Sex:_____Bed No:_____Ward:_____

Use diagram below for marking the correct surgical site in the following situations:
If the patient refuses to be marked.
If the surgical site involves genitalia or other site with a left/right distinction that cannot be marked.

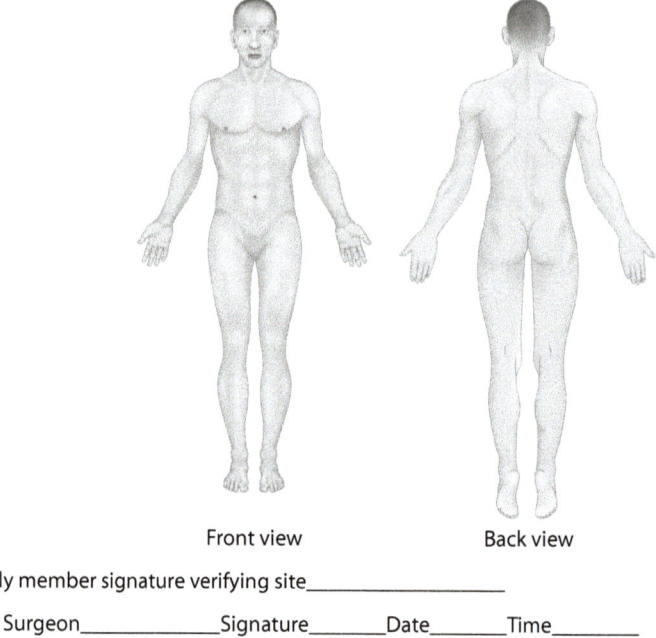

Front view   Back view

Patient/family member signature verifying site_____
Name of the Surgeon_____Signature_____Date_____Time_____
This form is to be placed in the top of the chart for reference during the surgical procedure.

Fig. 11.4.7: Site marking.

They must be signed and dated by the surgeon. I make it a point to write as detailed an operative note as I can, mentioning each step of the surgery, any relevant findings including those which were not clinically detected or were a surprise during surgery, any maneuver out of the normal which was necessary to circumvent or avoid any problems, any difficult dissection due to scarring, the area in which the same was detected. I also elaborate on the all volumes infiltrated injected, aspirated, details of all implants (with their labels) placed, sutures taken, their types, and the kind of suturing done. Detail is never wasted.

Postoperative Orders

Just as crucial are the postoperative orders detailing the patient's treatment immediately after surgery. The medications to be given to the patient, the dosage, the route of administration and the daily regimen must be written by the surgeon or assistant and checked at every visit. The surgeon must ideally countersign any alterations or stoppage of the medication.

In summary, as seen above, there are a lot of essential documentations that we require to maintain in our day-to-day practice. They are not difficult to adhere to, once a protocol is established and followed assiduously. Ignoring them with the lofty view that we are surgeons and not accountants or record-keepers is not only to be like an ostrich with its head in the sand; in today's day and age, it is indeed foolhardy and irresponsible. How critical, proper, timely and meticulous documentation, is in clinical practice today cannot be overemphasized, especially in a litigious field such as plastic and cosmetic surgery.

TIPS AND PEARLS

- India is an increasingly litigious society. Doctors also seem to have become a favorite of the lay public for censure and even physical assault. In such a scenario, meticulous documentation and maintenance of clinical records must become a matter of habit and normal routine.
- Documentation is important not only in cases of potential litigation and police inquiry but also for the purpose of medical education, epidemiology, medical audits and statistics, readily available information related to treatment, past, present and future and for presentations in conferences and publications in peer review journals.
- We must always remember that we are directly responsible and independently legally liable for our actions vis-à-vis any and all patients that we see and examine, consult with, treat and manage surgically or otherwise, irrespective to our affiliations to corporate hospitals and other clinical institutions that we do not own ourselves.
- We are firmly within the ambit and purview of the Consumer Protection Act which the law of our country has included our profession in. As such, we are essentially service providers who are directly answerable to the law for all our deeds and actions. What is not there in the documented records does not exist in the eyes of the law.
- Though we are probably the most law-abiding of all professionals, we appear to be targeted for harassment more than other profession, for reasons only known to the government. Hence, it is critical that we make sure we have registration with the requisite state medical council in the state/s that we practice in, registrations for GST in case of esthetic surgery with prompt and transparent payment of GST on a monthly basis, adequate Professional Medical Indemnity Insurance to cover for any potential litigation and permissions with the local administrative bodies for our clinical establishments. We must also make sure to keep them current at all times.
- In this digital era, rather than relying on paper documentation which is perishable, it is wise to digitalize and backup all records and documentation as soft copies and upload to the cloud so that it is both preserved as well as readily accessible in the present and the future. Investment in a good EMR software as well as adequate secure cloud storage is never wasted.
- Protecting our own interests in our clinical practice, while being competent ethical professionals should be the guiding force and mantra for all of us.

11.5 Patient versus Client

Lokesh Kumar

INTRODUCTION

Medical practice since ancient times is considered a noble profession. During the practice of medicine a bond and relationship develops between seeker and giver. Seeker being patient puts tremendous amount of faith in giver who in turn is the medical professional. He/she is bound and governed by strict code of medical ethics to provide selfless adequate care to the seeker. Personal gains to the physician take a back seat and may not be the prime incentive to provide compassionate and competent care to the seeker.

This sort of sacred relationship has suffered a setback in modern times, for the reasons beyond control of both seeker and giver. This relationship needs a relook and has to be redefined in the changing scenario of modern time. The patient—age old term used for seeker in medical practice is being slowly replaced with client in the modern practice of medicine.

PATIENT VERSUS CLIENT

However, there is a fundamental difference between a patient and client. If we understand this difference, both seeker and giver can benefit in maintaining their relationship with each other while safeguarding themselves against the perils of both.

A patient is a person seeking advice from a physician for a medical condition, and expects his physician to use his medical knowledge to find a right diagnosis and suggest appropriate treatment for his problem (illness in the present context). The patient has very little knowledge of his condition and has to largely trust his physician to give right advice and treatment. The physician on the other hand is under obligation to respect this trust and provide best possible solution to his patient's problems. A doctor-patient relationship thus develops in which the former is kept on a slightly higher pedestal and later plays a more passive role.

A client on the other hand has some amount of knowledge of his condition, can self-diagnose and seek treatment even for a condition which may not be necessarily a disease but treating it may be desirable for enhancement of normal body function and appearance. There is a financial aspect of this relationship too, which plays significant role in this as client is seen and factually is necessary source of revenue generation for the practice. This relationship is more business-like in which both parties are at equal playing field. This kind of client-based relationship has come in forefront with emergence of medical esthetic business.

Most people visiting a medical esthetic facility behave and expect to be treated like clients. The 'good old doctor' may unwittingly be forced into the shoes of a medical business professional, with no experience of this field.

So to summarize the patient is literally a sufferer whereas client is more like a customer. The patient is helped with an obligation while to a customer, we provide a service and he/she pays for it. Even though in modern medical practice, most patients also pay for treatment, but the fundamental difference remains.

Now the basic question remains: Is there any need to define and segregate both these groups?

In modern healthcare when more and more patients are paying directly for their care, the thin line differentiating patient from a client is fast fading. The patient, who is aware of his rights and paying for the services, is behaving more like a client. In this changing scenario it is important for all medical professionals to understand the needs of a client and deal with them adequately in order to be successful.

Taking a big leap from being a pure doctor to a medical business professional

In view of lack of training in the business aspect of medicine in medical education, it is important to learn these skills before jumping into practice and to keep mastering and refining the skills of dealing with clients.

I would like to give here ten commandments to help in making a smooth transition.

1. Once upon a time there were patients and patients only. Other professionals such as lawyers, accountants, prostitutes, etc., now doctors too have clients. The sooner we absorb this fact the better.
2. For some it is difficult to imagine treating patient as a client, but it is better to give up this hierarchal relationship and make way for a more collaborative relationship.
3. Turn yourselves into a patient listener as a client is not merely a passive seeker, but is knowledgeable about his needs.
4. Be ready for your patients (sorry clients) to be armed with fresh internet knowledge. Work your way around this to suggest the best possible solution for their needs.
5. Convert your facility to be more client-friendly rather than patient-friendly and learn to appreciate the different needs of both these groups.
6. It is never too late to learn the business aspect of medicine as money is as important to you as much as your clients. If it is tough for you then hire some dependable staff to deal with this aspect on your behalf.
7. Appreciate the fact that a client may have a friendlike attitude toward you and expect the same from you. There is no harm in this as long as he does not take undue advantage of this. You can still have a professional attitude and maintain a distance without jeopardizing the relationship with your clients. If need be hire someone with oratory, listening and convincing skills to do the job on your behalf.
8. Learn to read alarming signs in your client's behavior and avoid those client who can be potentially harmful to you and your practice even at the cost of monetary loss.
9. Every client however friendly—is a potential litigant so there are no short cuts with record-keeping while dealing with clients.
10. Medicolegal issues are part and parcel of client-based relationship and sooner we understand this better it is. Be prepared to deal with the situation as and when it is thrown at you.

DILEMMA OF DEALING WITH UNREASONABLE CLIENTS

Unreasonable clients are a reality in today's client-based practice and at times it is difficult to deal with them despite of your best practice attitude and experience. Unreasonable clients are of two kinds. Some people are unreasonable in their behavior while others are unreasonable in pushing their unreasonable demands. It is important to identify these two groups of clients. The former group may be easy to deal with as they are mostly attention seeking individuals and your trained staff can easily deal with them with a little bit of pampering. It is the latter group of people who are difficult to deal with because of their unreasonable demands. Unfortunately, there is no absolute formula to deal with them and the decision on how to deal with them may depend on case-to-case. If the demand pertains to deficiency in service which can be corrected, it is easy, but if the demand relates to asking for a particular type of treatment which you do not think will benefit him/her, or rather may be harmful, you are well within your right to say no to such clients.

This brings us to another question—how to say no and whether you have absolute freedom to say no? In a client-based practice where the most treatments offered are for elective problems it is easy to say no and you are well within your rights to say no. How to convey this is a different matter altogether and depends on your personality, the amount of unreasonableness your client depicts and whether you want this client to return in your practice or not.

DEALING WITH DISSATISFIED CLIENTS FROM OTHER PRACTICE

Every now and then you will encounter clients who had unpleasant experience in the hands of others. These clients are a test of your tactfulness of extracting information without alarming them and without expressing anything against a colleague even with subtle hints in your behavior. It is important to differentiate between dissatisfaction arising out of a client's own personality disorder and actual unfortunate setback in someone's hands. Your ability to judge the situation correctly can save you lots of embarrassing situations otherwise you can be almost sure that you will be added to the list of previous doctors your client has visited.

11.6 Three Pillars to Success: Quality, Service and Safety

Medha Bhave, Amiti Shah, Neha Chauhan

WHAT IS QUALITY?

"Quality is never an accident. It is always the result of high intention, sincere effort, intelligent direction and skillfull execution.

Uncontrolled variation is enemy of quality."

—**William Foster**

Parameters of Quality of a Cosmetic Practice

The Facility

- Reception of a patient
  - *Appointment system:* An easy appointment system, preferably

online is need of the hour. Ensure you keep enough time for patient.
- *Courteous receptionist/patient coordinator:* Receptionist should be well knowledgeable of the services, facilities, approximate costs and postsurgery recovery. She/he should have confidence in the services that you provide, to be able to convince the patient and satisfy all their queries. They often turn to her/him for an independent testimony of the doctor's work. An efficient receptionist can facilitate follow-ups and treatment of the patient. She/he can be crucial in earliest detection of a discontent and angry patient. Timely information to the doctor can save potential litigations.
- *Respect patients time:* Reschedule appointment well in advance in case of emergency.

▪ Ambience
- Ensure a clean, comfortable, and soothing ambience with provisions for drinking water and clean toilet.
- Display your qualifications and registration.
- Display rates of common procedures, consultation and follow-up charges.
- Display patient information material for services, procedures and new treatments to a reasonable extent with local language options.

▪ *Professional interactions:* Privacy is the most important factor in plastic and cosmetic consultations. The patient should be able to open up to the doctor in order to bring about all the relevant details in clinical as well as medicolegal points of view. It is a good idea to have checklists for the common problems that the doctor treats as well as procedures. This avoids overlooking key steps or documents. Create a small book in the form of clinic or hospital manual that uses flowcharts for quick reference to the sequence, patient undergoes after coming to the clinic or for any surgical or nonsurgical procedure. For example, a typical laser hair removal patient coming to OPD continues as shown in **Table 11.6.1**.

▪ *The staff:* In addition to hospitality training, the staff needs to understand the therapy and their side effects. Training and certification of staff is the sole responsibility of the clinician in charge.

The Clinician

▪ *Clinical/surgical skills and competence:* Essential attributes in skills of a doctor includes–
- Working within limits of specialty (referred as surgical privileges of a surgeon defined by international accreditation committees).
- *Timely reference:* Patients may have associated clinical problems that require timely referrals.
- *Detailed history*: Requesting the patient to fill a medical history form enlisting medical illnesses, e.g., diabetes, medications such as blood thinners and previous surgeries. A patient undergoing cyst removal or ear lobe repair may have undergone a cardiac bypass and consuming blood thinners such as aspirin, clopidogrel. It is imperative to stop these medications at least 4–5 days prior to the surgery.
- *Undergoing adequate training prior to performing any procedure:* Associating with a senior mentor will help discussion about problematic cases and surgical supervision.

Table 11.6.1: Clinical record of laser hair removal (LHR) patient.

- Name
- Age
- LMP (Last menstrual period)
- Are periods regular?
- Examination
    - Height
    - Weight
    - BMI
    - Acne
    - Areas of hirsutism
        - Side burns
        - Cheeks
        - Upper lip
        - Chin
        - Submandibular area
        - Others
            + Chest/Abdomen/back
- Investigations
    - Pelvis USG to rule out PCOS
    - Endocrinology reference if needed
- Explain the LHR
    - Procedure in detail
    - Side effects
    - Expected outcome
    - Number of sessions with margin
    - Cost involved and mode of payment
- Schedule a Laser hair removal appointment. Explain to the patient that no depilation creams or waxing should be done 2–3 weeks prior to LHR. Clipping the hair or shaving can be undertaken
- Receptionist to remind patient 1–2 days before the scheduled date.
- Procedure
    - Consent
    - Clinical photograph
    - Shaving
    - Cleaning the part with sterilium
    - Check the machine
    - Patient to be seated on the chair
    - Protecting goggles to the patient
    - Apply cold jelly with prior warning
    - Explain the procedure in short, warn about machine noise and feeling of warmth
    - Record parameters used after verifying previous records and noting history of burns, etc. in the past
    - Carry out LHR
    - Apply cold compresses
    - New prescription of sunscreen and twice a day application of hair growth inhibitor
    - Remind extrusion of dead hair postlaser
    - Schedule next appointment and reminder
- Enter details of parameters used and complications if any in a record sheet

Being a part of plastic surgery associations including Whatsapp group may be helpful for case discussions and advice. However, be careful before sharing confidential patient information as this may have medicolegal implications. Careful concealment of patient's identity is imperative.

- Honesty and transparency in discussion about options, with open mind to economical and cultural background of the patient.
- Monetary gain should always be the last priority. For example, syringe liposuction of 50–100 mL daily is practiced by many nonqualified doctors as remedy for inch loss. A qualified plastic surgeon should never fall for such half-hearted measures doomed for failure just for earning profits. Thus, a doctor's fiduciary responsibility must always be upheld.
  Many clinicians perform small surgical procedures in their clinics instead of hospitals. In an unequipped clinic, it is hard to deal with allergic reactions, vasovagal shock and other emergencies. The post-hair transplant deaths in India shed light on inadequacies in management of daycare cases in clinics. It is important to detect incipient complications at earliest and treat properly. In case of any doubt about outcome, strive to get best opinions, admit the patient and observe instead of postponing such precautionary measures.
- *Regular updates in knowledge:* Register relevant degree with medical council/ attend specialized hands—on courses and get certification.
  - Get accustomed to local law and remember your medical ethics.
  - Follow guidelines by relevant bodies and authorities.
  - Participate in continuing medical education and keep evaluating your own work.
- *Experience:* Maintaining records, trying to get long-term follow-ups and honest, critical evaluation of mistakes and results contributes to rich experience that grows by sharing with colleagues and juniors. "One cannot make ALL the mistakes in life" as Dr Ralph Millard, the cleft surgery doyen quoted.

Equipment and Disposables

Buying The Food and Drug Administration (FDA)-approved equipment is very expensive but legally safe. It is legally binding to have annual maintenance contract of equipment. Complications such as burns with lasers are known complications but clinician is protected in the court only if proper maintenance of the machines can be proven in the court of law. The disposables should never be reused to prevent transmission of diseases. This is particularly important in case of filler syringes and botox vials which are partially used. Always use fresh needle to draw neurotoxin if it is going to be stored for use in another patient later.

Outcome Audits, Reviews, Feedbacks

"Quality in a service or product is not what you put into it. It is what customer gets out of it."

—**Peter Drucker**

Regular audit of outcomes and various aspects of service such as infection control, complication rates is not far from being imposed under clinical establishment act. Various patient satisfaction scores and outcome scores are available for many types of surgeries. These should be regularly used to objectively measure success of surgery and procedures. Detailed description of clinical quality measures requires detailed, coded maintenance of records pertaining to following aspects:[1]
- Patient demographics
- Details of admission and operative procedure
- Details of anesthetist and anesthetic

- Details of surgeon
- Clinical outcome indicators

One should remember the dynamic nature of surgical procedures and constant improvements needed. Going beyond patient satisfaction to find faults and improve oneself is key to not only quality but also innovations. One may, thus, redefine norms of quality of given procedure.

Need for presence on social media, patient appointment apps and digital marketing has already made way for likes, comments and reviews on various platforms. These should be looked upon positively as a way to improve quality of care. Occasionally some adamant, misinformed patient can create undue trouble on digital platforms. One dissatisfied patient managing to go viral can spoil the rating on social media. We should try to use only those platforms that give us opportunity to file our reply and clarification.

Regular presentations at clinical meets to validate own results is useful but not available to most of the colleagues as usually select established speakers are invited for meetings. The local associations can play useful role by conducting sessions to allow local clinicians to present their work, even if it is a me too work. A panel of local experts can moderate it.

Health Insurance Portability and Accountability Act (HIPAA) compliant registry can be maintained about surgeries and complications. Thus, self-regulation to limit rates of complications and standardize the outcomes within the small local community of plastic surgeons can be undertaken. This can tip the balance in favor of a surgeon in medicolegal cases.

COSMETIC SURGERY: A SERVICE INDUSTRY

The cosmetic surgery industry is a service-oriented practice, which relies heavily on patient satisfaction. We do not nurse the ill or provide emergency care. We are treating healthy individuals who consciously decide to have enhancement procedures performed on certain parts of their body for overall mental and physical wellbeing. They are not patients in true sense of the word. But the fact, contrary to patient's expectations, is that they develop symptoms more severe than their original problem in the postoperative period, albeit temporarily. They develop pain and swelling where there was none. The result takes long time to be fully visible. The patients are simply not ready for these unless preempted and counseled.

The rampant growth of shortcut yet ineffective beauty clinics by nonqualified individuals, with huge marketing budgets has changed the mindset of our potential patients. They want painless, quick-fix solutions lasting forever, without any suffering or side effects; at the rates available at such clinics! As cosmetic surgeons, we face challenge to be honest on one hand while not be intimidating to frighten off a patient and deprive him/her of advances in the treatment. The key to this balance lies in a well-curated service to the patient.

The Core of Service: Personalization, Trust Building and Branding

The personal touch is incredibly important in guaranteeing higher patient satisfaction in cosmetic surgery. Any procedure requires commitment from the doctor and trust from the patient. The personal touch at each contact point—the surgeon, nurses or other staff—is crucial for a positive patient experience in terms of safety, security and best outcome. We work hard to offer our full attention to our patients from the initial consultation all the way to the recovery period and beyond. This aftercare service concept helps build our patient base as well.

"People do not buy goods and services. They buy relations, stories and magic."
—**Seth Godin**

The pillars of trust building in cosmetic surgery practice are knowledge, skill, expertise and their application in an honest, transparent and well-communicated, consistent way.

A well personalized service goes long way and gets recognition as a brand. Branding will help expand our practice to touch new horizons.

Information in the Digital Age

Today, as everything goes digital, the way in which the patients' access and consumer information has revolutionized. They have all kinds of information at their fingertips for any purchase decision. Thus, the consumer habit, naturally is that even the cosmetic surgery patients want to know about the surgeon, the procedure and reviews before a face-to-face consultation. In fact, it is in the interest of our work that patients should know about qualifications, so that they approach the right doctor and not fall for freebies and discounts offered by quacks.

For decades, advertising in the medical industry has been frowned upon and according to code of ethics—unethical and illegal. However, with the onset of digital media, digital marketing is important in order to make sure our patients are consuming truthful information to make the right choice in cosmetic surgery. Ethical advertising is the best way forward. This means clarifying board certification, offering a genuine biodata, stating risks upfront and sharing real patient results and reviews (with their consent).

In the context of the Internet, "information sharing" is a more accurate term than advertising. Honest and open information sharing with the public can help create awareness, build trust and empower patients.

The patient should have clear instructions about perioperative procedural details **(Table 11.6.2)**.

Cost of Service

One of the most common issue is the cost of service. The cosmetic procedures are not covered by insurance plans. So, the patient needs to bear the full cost. It can be a great dissuasion to patients. For example, a lipoma removed with a combination of liposuction and extraction through a small incision is unlikely to be compensated unless the doctor makes special effort in communication. Cashless payments are not available at all. Offering payment options to spread cost burden over a few months or working at hospitals with more affordable service can be appreciated by patients. Nevertheless, the doctor needs to ensure recovery, be ready to handle problems if the outcome is compromised.

Cosmetic procedures are never only for the rich. More and more middle-class patients are opting for cosmetic surgery due to increased demand socially and for jobs in hospitality and showbiz. However, we continue to raise awareness around fraudulent doctors who claim to offer same procedures for a very low price but compromise on quality hygiene, care as well as products. The patients should be educated about quality of implants, neurotoxins and fillers that make the service look costly. It may be useful to let them participate in buying process wherever possible, for example implants. If they can get invoice in their name and pay directly, they may be convinced better. Thus, transparent services certainly can be unique selling proposition (USP) of your brand. In long run, compromise in cost will pull down the quality of service. Another important factor adding

Table 11.6.2: Perioperative checklist.

- Name
- Age
- Name of procedure
- Schedule
    - Date of admission
    - Date of surgery
    - Tentative date of discharge
- Hospital address to report to
- Contact number
- Contact person
- Instructions
    - Nil by mouth from ----- AM/PM
    - Take water till--------AM
    - Medicines to be omitted----------------------- for ------------- days
    - Medicines to be taken in the morning of surgery with a sip of water -------------
    - Remove all ornaments
    - Get all reports
    - One adult must accompany the patient
    - Carry a photo ID (This may soon become essential, though it is not so at present)
- On admission
    - Indoor case paper formalities
    - Plan of surgery by admitting doctor
    - Informed consent with surgeon and anesthetist as well as patient and Kin's signatures
    - Shift to OT at-------------------AM/PM
    - Operation records
    - Detailed operation notes
    - Postoperative orders
- On discharge
    - Detailed discharge summary with status on discharge
    - List of medicines with duration
    - TO DO and NOT TO DO lists
    - To report if--- list
    - Contact person and number in case of emergency
    - First follow up
    - Tentative suture removal
- On last follow up
    - Schedule of follow up for next year
    - Special precautions to be followed
    - Monitoring and maintenance

to cost is payment for good staff. Suffice it to say that if you throw peanuts, only monkeys will come.

Legally Bound Service

As patients seek service from us, we need to uphold their rights while covering ourselves with professional indemnity as accidents do happen despite most meticulous, continuously updated and even audited service. Though audits have not been common in Indian practice, one should be prepared for outcome audits in near future.

SAFETY IN COSMETIC SURGERY

"Primum non nocere", a principle enunciated by Hippocrates is one of the most important principles in Medicine. Modern patient safety improvement movement began in 1999, when a report titled "To Err Is Human: Building a Safer Health System" was published by The Institute of Medicine, USA.[2] Surprisingly, very little data is available from India on patient safety except for a few papers on needle-stick injuries, reuse of syringes and biomedical waste management.[3] Since cosmetic surgery involves operating upon otherwise "healthy" patients who desire to have a more desirable appearance, safety assumes all the more importance.[4] There is minimal or no margin of error here and any untoward event such as complications and mortality are more vehemently highlighted by media as compared to those occurring with other surgeries which are done for curing a patient.

The authors outline the following steps for improving safety of cosmetic surgery patients:

- *Clinics/institute for conducting the surgeries:* Must conform to "The Clinical Establishments (Registration and Regulation) Act", 2010 and provide a safe environment to conduct the surgeries.
- *Education and licensing of the surgeon:* Board certified plastic/cosmetic surgeons to maintain the basic standards of outcome should conduct surgeries. There should be periodic licensing and re-examination of the cosmetic surgery practitioners to evaluate their competency and knowledge of safe practices. Action must be taken against unsafe providers to warn/deter them from conducting the same. Organizing continuing medical education (CME) that also provide earn credit points to retain certification may also be a step to ensure that the cosmetic surgeons keep up-to-date with the latest protocols that improves patient safety. Besides the surgeon, the entire support team of anesthesiologists, technicians and nurses must be well trained to ensure highest standards of safety.
- The surgery:
  - *Assessing suitability for cosmetic surgery:* Understanding the motives of the patients behind seeking cosmetic surgery, their expectations and desires from the surgery; is as important as acquiring the technical skills of performing cosmetic surgeries. Patients who are clear about the condition, have realistic expectations, understand the possibility of complications and are ready for follow-ups are ideal candidates for cosmetic surgery. Patients who are confused must be offered further consultations to evaluate their suitability for cosmetic surgery. Patients with body dysmorphic disorders may need counseling by psychiatrists.
  - *Evaluation of the deformity and execution of surgery:* Detailed history taking and examination, proper planning and conducting surgery in a relaxed, unhurried environment[5] are important for patient safety. Special attention must be given to conditions such as age, diabetes, obesity, smoking habits, systemic diseases, nutritional status, radiation history and immunosuppressive conditions; all of which can have serious bearing on the final outcome of the surgery.
  - *Special groups:* Cosmetic surgeries in adolescents should be carefully evaluated. This group is undergoing body and emotional changes and may not be able to make correct decisions that may lead to regret/depression or even suicidal tendencies later. It has been shown in studies that most adolescents who were dissatisfied

with their body image at the onset of teenage were satisfied with their body appearance at 18 years of age.[6] Hence, it requires an extremely guarded approach while dealing with this group of patients seeking cosmetic surgery.

- *Use of implants/foreign materials:* Only the implants/fillers/neurotoxins/peels approved by the regulating bodies should be used.
- *Approved machines with regular annual maintenance with documentation thereof:* This includes lasers, diathermy, anesthesia machine and other gadgets we use. Regular review and elimination of expired medicines is important. Even in a clinic a stalk of emergency medicines, intubation set, pulse oximeter, glucometer should be maintained.

- *Miscellaneous:* Conducting mock drills at regular intervals to simulate crisis situations during surgery and managing them can improve the efficacy of the team in responding to any unforeseen emergency that may occur in future during a real surgery.[5] *Tie-up with a tertiary care center*—for any unforeseen emergency.

Despite the best efforts and following the latest protocols, the surgeons may sometimes face difficult situations that may land them in courts. The authors suggest the following to ensure safety of the surgeons:

- *Saying "No":* As prevention is better than cure, the following category of patients are deemed unsuitable and must be politely refused for surgery as they are bound to be less than satisfied with the surgical outcomes:
  - Those seeking surgery in attempts to please spouse/partner or in hope of promotions.
  - Body dysmorphic disorder—those who perceive their deformity in excess.
  - Patients with unrealistic expectations.
  - Overtly critical, suspicious, aggressive and ill-behaved patients
  - Emotionally unstable patients as their ability to cope with surgery is diminished.
  - Any patient not liked by the surgeon or the staff.
- *Take help/give help:* Second opinions, specialist references for evaluation and investigations, talking to a colleague whose dissatisfied patient approaches you instead of jousting, training in nonclinical arts, e.g., communication skills and how to deliver bad news in case of untoward events are few factors that avoid litigation.
- *Professional indemnity:* Last but not the least having a professional indemnity is must for all practitioners of cosmetic surgeries considering the high incidences of litigation lawsuits in cosmetic surgeries.[7,8] Also being member of local governing bodies of cosmetic surgery may help in case one encounters a difficult patient.
- *Association and peer groups:* It is high time for associations to have proper legal cell with panel of lawyers and experts to help a member in problem.

BIBLIOGRAPHY

1. Royal College of Surgeons. (2016). Professional Standards for Cosmetic Surgery. [online] Available from https://www.rcseng.ac.uk/standards-and-research/standards-and-guidance/service-standards/cosmetic-surgery/professional-standards-for-cosmetic-surgery/. [Last accessed January, 2020].

REFERENCES

1. The Royal College of Surgeons of England. Outcome Measures for Cosmetic Surgery: Clinical Quality Indicators.

2. Institute of Medicine. To Err is Human: Building a Safer Health System. Washington DC; National Academy of Sciences; 1999.
3. Lahariya NC, Choure A, Singh B. Patient safety in maternal healthcare at secondary and tertiary level facilities in Delhi, India. J Family Med Prim Care. 2015;4(4):529-34.
4. Dean N, Foley K, Ward P. Defining cosmetic surgery. Aust J Plast Surg. 2018;1(1):95-103.
5. Taylor JR. Patient Safety in Plastic Surgery. Can J Plast Surg. 2004;12:3.
6. Rauste-von Wright M. Body image satisfaction in adolescent girls and boys: a longitudinal study. J Youth Adolesc. 1989;18:78-81.
7. Marchesi A, Marchesi M, Fasulo FC, Morini O, Vaienti L. Mammaplasties and medicolegal issues: 50 cases of litigation in aesthetic surgery of the breast. Aesth Plast Surg . 2012;36:122-7.
8. da Silva DB, Nahas FX, Bussolaro RA, de Brito MJ, Ferreira LM. The increasing growth of plastic surgery lawsuits in Brazil. Aesth Plast Surg. 2010;34:541-2.

11.7 Setting-up a Day Care Esthetic Surgery Clinic

Rajat Gupta, Tejaswani Diwakar

INTRODUCTION

Day care surgery is well established in developed countries for its medical and economic advantages and is fast catching up in developing countries. The concept of day care surgery is well acceptable to the surgeon and the patient alike. The pros of day care surgery are:
- Shorter waiting period for the patient
- Better rationalization of cost of surgical procedures
- Less pain and rapid recovery due to advancements in anesthesia and surgical techniques
- Early mobilization of patient
- Early return of patient to their homes resulting in reduced risk of nosocomial infection
- Less loss of pay due to early return to work

In patients of ASA grade I, except for tummy tuck, a gamut of esthetic surgeries is performed as day care procedures in our clinic. Liposuction of less than 4 L, gynecomastia surgery, breast lift, breast augmentation with fat filling or implants, breast reduction, rhinoplasty, Brazilian butt lift, vaginal rejuvenation, hair transplant, face-lift surgery, dimple creation, face slimming with buccal fat pad removal, upper and/or lower lid blepharoplasty, lip reduction, bull-horn lip lift, chin augmentation, fat grafting of the face or hand are just to name a few.

Our patients are advised to be fasting from 12.00 AM and get admitted in the clinic by 7.00 AM. They are operated in the morning and all except patients of tummy tuck surgery or patients with comorbidities are discharged by 7.00 PM. The concept of day care surgery is very appealing to the patient and surgeon and with the right set-up and skills every cosmetic surgeon can conduct the majority of his/her surgeries as day care procedures.

Before a surgeon decides to start his/her esthetic day care clinic, they should ask themselves three questions.
1. Where do you intend to set up the clinic?
2. What are your skills?
3. How much capital can you invest?

The location to set up the clinic is an important factor as the land value or rent varies from region to region. This can take up a considerable amount of the budget. Various factors need to be considered while zeroing in on the location of the clinic. The location should be prominent, well connected to major cities and have ample options for boarding and lodging making it convenient for outstation and international patients to visit and stay. The neighborhood of the clinic should be safe and preferably sophisticated. It would be beneficial to have the clinic close to the main road making it easily accessible.

The surgeon should be aware of his skills and should be clear regarding what procedures will be performed by him/her in the clinic. The surgeon also needs to consider if he/she will appoint another consultant to perform procedures, in which he/she is not well-acquainted with. This will dictate the instruments and machinery to be purchased or rented and also the manpower to be employed. One need to be reminded that investing in expensive and niche technique does not always guarantee that the investment will pay off.

Finally, the most important factor is the capital that the surgeon can invest. The amount needs to be budgeted in terms of the land value, décor of the clinic, machinery and human resource. While deciding on the capital investment, the surgeon also needs to keep at the back of his/her mind the monthly expenditure after starting the venture which includes EMI on bank loans, remuneration of staff, servicing and maintenance of equipment, electricity and water bills, and various taxes besides personal expenditure.

Having answered the above three questions, planning can be made in three phases:
1. Premises
2. Human resource
3. Tools

PREMISES

The first impression may not always be the last impression, but it does have a lasting impression. The client is subconsciously assessing the surgeon even before the one-on-one personal interaction. Therefore the premises of the clinic should be appealing.

The name and logo of the clinic should be self-explanatory or at least indicative of the treatment modalities offered and the clients that the clinic caters to. The clinic's name and logo should be artistically presented outside the clinic and there should be sign boards which facilitate the client to reach the clinic without any hassle. The clinic should be easily accessible to everyone, including the disabled, if not situated on the ground floor.

The entrance to the clinic should be neat and have information regarding all the doctors providing consultation in the clinic as well as their field of expertise.

The interiors of the clinic should exude subtle elegance. The clinic should be spacious or created in a way to appear spacious. Neutral shades should be used on the floor and walls. Lighter shades are soothing and make the space open and bigger while darker colors make the space appear smaller. Also, some dark shades are known to aggravate moods and emotions. The clinic should be well illuminated preferably with LED lights rather than fluorescent lights. Capitalize on the natural light. The ceiling should be white for good and uniform illumination of the clinic. The luminaire should be classy and not too loud. Use mirrors, indoor plants, paintings and statuary judiciously. The clinic can be air-conditioned, with Wi-Fi connection and under CCTV surveillance.

The clinic space can be segregated into the following areas:
- Reception desk
- Visitors lounge
- Patient coordinator or counselor's chamber
- Doctors consultation chamber
- Examination and photography room

- Procedure room
- Surgical area
- Storage
- Pharmacy
- Restroom
- Kitchenette

The reception desk is a focal area and there should be enough space for the staff to work comfortably. It can double up as the billing counter also. Being the busiest area in the clinic, it will be equipped with telephone, computer with or without a printer, card swipe machine and stationary. However, efforts should be made to keep the clutter out of sight.

The visitors lounge or waiting area should be designed thoughtfully. There should be enough furniture—chairs, couch and sofas available for people of all sizes. Few cushions make the seating area more comfortable. Coffee tables with bottled drinking water and latest reading materials should be placed close to the seats. There can be racks with pamphlets and brochures with information regarding the various technologies available and the procedures performed in the clinic. Also, there can be an audio-visual display in the form of TV screens placed strategically which educate clients and their relatives on common conditions that are managed in the clinic—the symptoms and signs, pathophysiology of the disease, preventive measures, investigations required, various treatment modalities available, side effects or complications of treatment, before and after images of patients treated in the clinic and testimonials by satisfied clients. There can be "Wall of Fame" in the waiting room which has framed degree certificates, awards and certificate of appreciation as well as wall-mounted photographs of the surgeon clicked with his mentors or celebrity clients which will further strengthen the patients' faith in the surgeons' abilities. There may be a prayer area in the visitors lounge. Having a coat hanger, umbrella rack or a mobile charging point is optional. There should be a clean restroom close to the waiting room.

The patient coordinator or counselor's chamber should have provisions to measure the patient's height, weight and blood pressure. Having already interacted over the phone or mail before the formal consultation in the clinic, the client will be at ease to meet a familiar person first. The coordinator can then lead the client to the doctor's chamber and introduce the client to the surgeon.

Doctor's consultation chamber should be designed keeping in mind the sanctity of the doctor-patient relationship with utmost importance paid to maintain confidentiality and privacy. The conversation between the client and the surgeon should not be overheard by people in the visitors lounge. Light background music may be played, but should not interfere with the conversation. The room should be spacious with a desk and chairs across for the surgeon and the client. There should be additional furniture for the accompanying person. The room can have shelves with books pertaining to the subject. The awards and mementos received by the surgeon may be displayed. The surgeon can have graphics in print to explain the pathology and procedure to the client. The room should be well lit with a full length mirror and hand mirrors. These aid in discussing problem areas and ensure that the surgeon, the client and accompanying persons are on the same page while discussing treatment planning. There should be a comb and a trichoscope in case the surgeon specializes in hair transplant.

There may be a separate examination room or a section of the doctor's chamber may be separated by screens for the purpose of examination. The examination should be done in complete privacy. The area should be well-illuminated and have a full length mirror, hand mirrors, measuring tapes and other device required for assessing problem areas. A DSLR (Digital Single Lens Reflex) camera and a black or green screen as a backdrop are extremely useful for clicking standardized photographs and maintaining a record in the laptop.

In every esthetic clinic there is generally a procedure room to conduct nonsurgical procedures such as fillers, botox injections, silhouette thread lifts, chemical peels, platelet-rich plasma (PRP) treatments and medical facials. The room is equipped with procedure tables, overhead lights, centrifuge machine, packaged products, local anesthetic agents, sterile gloves, needles, syringes, gauze and waste bins as per BMW regulations. Suture removal may also be done in this room.

The surgical area comprises:
- Changing room
- Scrubbing area
- Operation theater
- Recovery room
- Sterilization room
- Laundry

The changing area should have OT gowns with color coding for surgeons and staff, caps, masks, plastic aprons and OT footwear. The gowns may have the clinic name and logo embroidered on it.

The scrubbing area may have one, two or three station scrub sinks and may be manually operated or hands free. It may have knee operated soap dispenser, digital timer or infrared sensor water control.

The operating room should have:
- Surgical table with electronic table movements, providing Trendelenburg/reverse Trendelenburg, kidney bridge, lateral tilts and head, leg, back section.
- Surgical table accessories such as arm support, leg support, body support, etc.
- Operating stool and chair
- LED surgical lights with or without HD cameras
- Anesthesia machine
- Defibrillator
- Oxygen and Nitrous oxide cylinders
- Electrosurgical unit for monopolar and bipolar cautery including accessories such as patient electrodes, hand-pieces and foot pedals.
- Surgical instrument set including lighted retractors, breast tourniquet and funnel for breast implant insertion
- Suction machine for anesthetic purpose and for liposuction
- Centrifugation machine
- Surgical light source and monitors for endoscopic surgeries
- Energy-based devices such as power-assisted liposuction (PAL), Vaser™, CO_2 laser, minimally-invasive radio frequency ablation machine
- Back table with lights and microscope for hair transplant
- Deep vein thrombosis (DVT) pumps
- Weighing scale
- Medical cabinets and casework with anesthetic and surgical consumables
- IV stand, instrument trolley
- Waste disposal as per BMW regulation
- Patient shifting trolley

The postoperative recovery room should be comfortable and close to the nursing station. It should consist of remote controlled bed for patient, couch for the attendant, monitors to assess patients' vital parameters, IV stand and a bell system to call the nurse. The recovery room should have attached wash room. It can have a locker for storage of patient's valuables.

Sterilization room should consist of autoclave and ethylene oxide sterilization (ETO) machine. The OT staff should be specifically trained to dismantle and sterilize the parts of energy-based devices and other expensive equipment. Preferably the graphics from the instruction manual may be pasted on the wall of the sterilization room for quick reference.

A laundry area is required for washing reusable gowns, drapes, etc., or this service may be out-sourced.

The storage room is essential for storage of drugs, IV fluids and other consumables, e.g., cannulas, catheters, endotracheal (ET) tubes, etc. A refrigerator may be required to preserve medications that need to be stored at lower temperatures.

Some clinics also dispense scar modulation, skin and hair care products. A pharmacy counter can be set up near the billing area for this purpose.

Any center performing day care surgeries should have a kitchenette with a microwave, refrigerator, burner hob, wash basin and utensils to provide beverages and food for the staff and in-patients.

HUMAN RESOURCE

Human resource generally comprises:
- Front office staff
- Patient coordinator/counselor
- Laser technician
- Hair transplant technician
- Nursing staff
- OT technician
- Housekeeping staff
- Surgeon's assistant
- Anesthetist

The front office staff must be well-groomed, courteous, fluent in English as well as vernacular languages and should have a working knowledge of the various procedures performed in the clinic. The front office staff could be wearing a uniform with the logo of the clinic embroidered on it.

Patient coordinators are important members of the team. They are the first person that the client interacts with either by email or call. They should be well-trained to question the patient regarding their concerns, obtain information/images, answer the patient's queries, inform the approximate estimate of the treatment, to fix an appointment with the surgeon in the clinic or through video chat, schedule the procedure as per the convenience of the surgeon and the patient and finally to maintain telephonic follow-up of operated patients. As they play a bridge between the patient and the surgeon, a patient coordinator should possess good communication skills and should preferably be someone with a medical or paramedical background.

It would be beneficial to employ a technician who has been trained in certificate courses to assist the surgeon in hair transplant and laser procedures.

The presence of an experienced senior nurse in the team is invaluable during the preoperative, intraoperative and postoperative management of the patient. She should be knowledgeable about patient positioning, painting and draping, sequence of surgical techniques, functioning of the various instruments and energy-based devices and also regarding sterilization of the equipment.

The OT technician should be well-versed with commonly used anesthetic and surgical machinery. He should also receive training in handling and maintenance of the newer power-assisted plastic surgical equipment.

Cleanliness in the clinic should be of top priority. Housekeeping staff should frequently inspect and clean the waiting area floor and tables, sanitize the washroom, return the magazines or brochures to the stands and replenish water bottles.

If a plastic surgeon can afford to appoint a junior doctor to assist him/her in the surgeries, it will prove to be a major advantage as the on-table decision making and assistance skills of a trained doctor is unmatchable.

Working with a single anesthetist/constant team of anesthetist has the advantage that he/she is well-acquainted with the OT machinery and consumables. We have left the protocols and buying of anesthesia equipment on our anesthetist team only. Since they are the experts in their field, it is our belief that we should not interfere in their work. I believe one should not compromise on anesthesia machine, medicine/drugs and other equipment. A good rapport between the anesthetist, OT staff and the surgeon ensures smooth functioning of the OT set-up avoiding miscommunication and unnecessary delays. At the same time, it is recommended that one should have a tie up with a nearby superspeciality hospital. This helps in shifting the patient to the hospital set up in case of any eventuality.

TOOLS

The surgeon must judiciously invest in technology for medical as well as nonmedical purposes. As mentioned earlier expensive technology does not guarantee that the investment will pay off, however some are worth considering.

Liposuction is the most commonly performed day care surgery and it is also a component of tummy tuck, breast reduction, face slimming, neck lift and fat grafting procedures. In our clinic, we use power-assisted liposuction (PAL) device such as Microaire and ultrasound-assisted liposuction (UAL) device, e.g., VASER. From our experience power-assisted infiltration and aspiration reduces operating time and surgeon fatigue to a large extent. VASER helps in emulsification of fibrofatty tissue and helps in better skin redraping giving superior results in contouring surgeries than conventional liposuction methods. Therefore, investing in energy-based liposuction device may prove to be immensely fruitful in the long run. We also have minimally invasive radiofrequency ablation devices, e.g., Thermi which can be used in conjunction with liposuction or as a single modality to tighten lax skin in face, neck, arm and thighs. ThermiTight can also be used for nerve ablation to reduce pain after tummy tuck procedures. ThermiVa is used as an adjunct in vaginal rejuvenation procedures. Use of Piezotome has revolutionized our rhinoplasty technique leading to more pleasing results.

We sometimes use cosmetic surgery simulation software to educate patients and accompanying persons about the results of surgeries such as rhinoplasty, breast lift/augmentation, chin augmentation, liposculpture, etc.

In a time of increased litigation against doctors, one cannot be too casual regarding record-keeping. In our clinic, we use technology like Doxper to instantly digitize case sheets, prescriptions and inpatient records using smart digital pen and encoded paper which is linked to the surgeon's iPad or mobile phone through an application. The data gets saved on the devices in real time and can be retrieved as and when required. It would be wise to invest in a technology which stores data without involving extra time or effort by the surgeon.

Starting an independent esthetic surgery clinic may be a long-awaited dream-come-true for some surgeons. Doctors would have invested their entire lives savings into the project. Some would have taken large amounts of loans from the bank. It would only be wise to get a good insurance cover for the clinic and review the terms and conditions regularly.

11.8 Setting-up Inpatient Clinic with Operation Theater

Lakshyajit D Dhami

INTRODUCTION

Health care is one of the most important industries in India, of which the esthetic surgery and cosmetic procedures are one of the fastest growing in recent times.

A rising population, longevity, health awareness and increase in affluence are the driving force behind this growth. Though there is a very strong network of public, private and corporate hospitals in most of the cities and towns, there still exists a gross lacuna in adequate inpatient and outpatient facilities. The major hospitals are mainly focussed on providing tertiary and intensive care facilities and lack specialized and focused esthetic—surgical and nonsurgical facilities.

Small surgical inpatient clinics with operating room facility, also commonly known in India as surgical nursing home, provides primary and secondary health care mainly in nonintensive areas of specialty care, not just in small or big towns spread across India, but also in major metropolitan cities such as Mumbai, Chennai, Bengaluru or Delhi.

These clinics are an ideal small business model, with minimal investment required in infrastructure and/or equipment. They are also being run either by an individual or a group of doctors or a family of doctors with similar, diverse or complimentary surgical facilities being provided under one roof.

Esthetic plastic surgery, hair transplantation and other cosmetic procedures are unique superspecialties, which do not require either a large floor space area or expensive tertiary care equipment or any specialized expensive technology to be provided in-house under one roof. These inpatient clinics can be setup with minimum basic infrastructure as a small single specialty nursing home. However, there may be an individual need for specialized esthetic surgery-related equipment.

Setting-up such a clinic by an individual doctor could pose a challenge to the novice consultant, who has no formal training of either planning, starting or running a small business model of a well-functioning and profitable nursing home.

There are a few basic guidelines that the entrepreneur consultant must follow to execute a successful model of inpatient clinic that he/she is venturing into:

DEVELOPING A BUSINESS PLAN

The first question that may arise "is owning and running a nursing home feasible and profitable?"

Yes it is.

So what are the advantages?

Typically, esthetic surgery patients are all self-paid. The mediclaim insurances does not cover the cost of these procedures and, hence, an individual patient/client desirous of cosmetic surgery is very conscious about price and would like to save every single rupee without jeopardizing the outcome of the surgery.

An esthetic procedure easily costing upward of 2-3 lakhs in a corporate hospital would only cost 10–1.5 lakhs (approximately 50–60% less) in a single-specialty surgical nursing home. A consultant performing these procedures in a corporate setup would on an average earn just about 20% of the total bill, while he could easily earn upward of 50% of the total bill in his own center. This will make him earn an overall 25–50% more. He also is, his own boss and can plan his schedule most suitable to his style of working.

A personalized quality, ethical and patient-focused health care is easily delivered at these small focused nursing homes with not only remarkably reduced cost to the patients, but also significantly increased earnings and profit for the doctor. The clinic helps to create a niche expertise in specialized esthetic procedures and excels in providing care linked to the expertise of the owner consultant.

If the owner doctor desires to service the vast healthcare needs of his/her target communities, then he/she needs to be able to get visiting consultant on board from other complimentary specialties. Alternatively, collaborating with other nursing homes in the vicinity, with focus on noncompeting specialties can help him/her develop mutually benefitting referral pathways, and optimize on each other's strengths.

GETTING FINANCES

Start with creating the financial project for the inpatient healthcare unit with operating room facility. Start the process in reverse. Make a list of premises and all the equipment that is needed in the nursing home.

- *Calculate the cost of premises:* Ideal carpet area requirement is minimum 1000 sq ft to preferably 3000 sq ft, depending on whether it is a single doctor owner or multispecialist owner practice. Also add stamp duty, change of user fees and transfer fees to the purchase price.
- Add the cost of interiors, furniture, air conditioners and desired decoration.
- Add the cost of medical and surgical equipment as per the list described below for in-house facility.
- Once all these costs are totaled, add routine day-to-day running costs including maintenance charges, electricity charges, salary of the staff and marketing costs for each month of the first year of the launch.

There are numerous avenues available to finance this project. The funds can either be self-provided or from family members or friends or it could be partly from any bank or nonbanking financial institute. Loans to a consultant are easy to obtain and are available at attractive interest rates (It is easier to obtain a loan after couple of prosperous years of clinical practice and against the mortgage of premises to be purchased).

A sound and promising projected income report will have to be prepared with the help of a chartered accountant as a prerequisite to be submitted to either a bank or nonbanking financial company (NBFC).

IN-HOUSE FACILITY PLANS AND EQUIPMENT

- Indoor rooms for major liposuction, abdominoplasty, breast reduction surgery, facelift surgery that would mostly require an overnight stay facility. Body lift surgery, arms/thigh plasty, gluteal augmentation may require more than 2–3 days stay.

Patients' beds with overnight stay facility preferably 2–3 rooms with 1–2 beds in each room, attendant bed/sofa cum bed, bedside lockers/tables, etc. Minimum

required 50-100 sq ft per bed, with one washroom/toilet per two beds.
- Consulting rooms with patient examination table—minimum 100 sq. ft.
- Operation theater (OT)—minimum space 200/250 sq ft with OT table, OT lights, anesthesia Boyle's apparatus with continuous oxygen and nitrous oxide supply together with isoflurane and sevoflurane vaporizer, CO_2 level sensor monitoring, continuous monitor with SPO_2+ECG+BP (with printer for recording preferable), basic anesthesia equipment including laryngoscope, endotracheal tubes, regular north pole and south pole, laryngeal mask, emergency tracheostomy set, defibrillator, spinal and epidural anesthesia set, suction machine, electrocautery unipolar and bipolar, radiocautery, mayo trolley, patient transport trolley, general instruments with drum and autoclavable boxes, specialized instruments for specific esthetic procedures.

  Any special equipment cost can be added as per the specific need and expertise of the specialist concerned.
- Store room with facility to store O_2 and N_2O cylinders (60-80 sq ft).
- Autoclave room (with ETO sterilizer if desired) (100 sq ft).
- Minor OT dressing room (100-150 sq ft).
- Laser/ancillary device procedure rooms (minimum 100 sq ft each).
- Pantry—50-100 sq ft
- Nurse room/staff changing—room (100 sq ft).
- Waiting area—100-200 sq ft with one toilet for OPD patients.
- Photography room (100 sq. ft.), the consulting room can double up as one in case of space constraint.

PICK A LOCATION

The place can be either an independent unit or a part of a commercial establishment with adequate facility to register under the Clinical Establishment Act. The location is very important from the viewpoint of easy approach and accessibility to the target client base desirous of various cosmetic procedures/surgeries. It is advisable to have 2-3 parking spaces available for visiting doctors and patients.

BUILDING PLAN AND INFRASTRUCTURE

The structure of building should have adequate height (minimum 9 ft), round the clock water supply, 24 hours electricity with sufficient (4-6 hours) backup and efficient sewage system. In the clinic, patients' rooms should have adequate ventilation (openable windows for quick evacuation of patients and staff, in case of fire), should be well-illuminated with access to daylight. The corridor and the staircase should be wide and obstruction free for easy movement and quick evacuation in an emergency. There should be access to wide elevator of minimum size 6 × 3 feet, which can easily accommodate patient stretcher. The inpatient room's doors and passage should be wide for free and easy movement of stretcher and wheelchair.

STAFFING THE NURSING HOME

A small inpatient clinic with operation room (OR) would require at least one nurse and one ayah bai on duty 24 × 7. It would require a minimum of four nurses and four ayah bai to be employed taking into consideration 8 hourly shift duties and one weekly off. For the OR, there is a need to employ a trained scrub nurse and a ward boy to help during surgeries.

The front desk would require 2–3 receptionists to handle the phone calls and OPD. A part-time/full time accountant is recommended to relieve the surgeon of admin and accounting work. For some specialized practices, there may be a need to hire a marketing person to handle and oversee different marketing mediums and communications.

LICENSES AND INSURANCE

Acquiring a No Objection Certificate (NOC) from the builder and housing society beforehand is a must as there have been many instances of doctors who suffered major financial losses, litigation and mental agony due to noncompliant society members. Registration with local authority is an absolute prerequisite and all their norms should be known and adhered to.

"I started my nursing home in Mumbai almost 30 years back. I could establish my nursing home on the second floor of a housing society without a separate staircase/lift as the norms at that time were relaxed. Later about 10 years back, when BMC changed the rules under the high court's ruling, we were faced with the dire situation of having to shut down our nursing home. With the help of the Local Medical Association, we could somehow get a Change of User for our premises as a Nursing Home as we had preexisting Registration with BMC for many years and there was no specific objection from the society members. However, we did end up paying a huge penalty to the tune of ₹ 12,50,000/- at that time."

Registration with the Pollution Control Board and tie-up with an agency for medical waste disposal is also essential to avoid huge penalties. Besides the doctors and staff, the establishment also requires a separate errors and omissions insurance cover.

MARKETING AND EVALUATING THE PRACTICE

Display of well-worded and attractive signboards outside and inside the premises are an excellent marketing tool. How the practice is marketed depends on the demographics of the target patient population. One must consider how the peer group physicians and nursing homes attract patients and apply appropriate strategies and tactics.

It is extremely essential for the surgeon to keep a sharp eye on the balance sheet of their nursing home on a regular basis to ensure that it is a profitable venture at all times.

Last but not the least, in the initial period of setting up the nursing home, the surgeon may have to tighten his belt in order to service the loan he may have taken for the premises and equipment. However, once the loan is repaid, and he is debt free, his earnings will increase substantially. Also when he decides to retire, the setup can prove to be his cash cow, if rented to another young surgeon of the same specialty who in turn would benefit from the established practice. It can even prove to be his retirement fund if he decides to sell it off at an increased market value of the property.

SECTION 12
Marketing

12.1 Developing your Brand

Karthik Ram

WHAT IS A BRAND?

Different people have defined it differently but billionaire entrepreneur Kevin Plank nailed the essence of the word when he said— "Brand is not a product; it is not one item. It is an idea, it is a theory, it is a meaning, and it is how you carry yourself."

WHY IS A BRAND IMPORTANT?

For doctors, their reputation or image is their brand. Branding is important because it makes an impression on your clientele and helps them know what to expect from the practice. What sets you apart from other doctors is your brand. So, a lot of thought has to go into brand development.

HOW TO DEVELOP THE BRAND?

Begin with the end in mind. Each person has a different end in mind. In this context, the end could be the ultimate image that the doctor wants to project. Visualizing this image is the starting point.

- *Set your mission, vision, and values:* This is a vital first step as it defines the brand's goal for its customers, employees, and owners. Chart out the short- and long-term goals. Where do you see yourself or what do you plan to achieve in the next 2 years, 5 years, 10 years and so on? Once the ultimate goal is set, work hard toward it.
- *Selecting the brand name:* Your brand name should be simple and practical. It should indicate your core area. Do not go blindly with the advice of marketing "experts" who suggest exotic sounding words which do nothing to communicate the strength of your brand. If your key area is surgery, opt for a name that points to this. If Chennai Plastic Surgery had been christened *Elysium* or *Rendezvous*, it would have taken us ages to convince people about what we do. The brand name must convey what the practice plans to do.
- *Choosing the logo:* Much like the brand name, the logo should also convey the message. It could be as simple as the first letter of your brand name in a creative font; it could be a complicated doodle of any part of the anatomy. Irrespective of what it is, a logo should be easy to recall as images are powerful and help people make the association with the brand.
- *Taking care of taglines:* Taglines have to speak about your services and must not be generic. You might argue that some of the most popular taglines are generic. Iconic

ones like *Just Do It, I'm Lovin' It, Think Different*, etc., come to mind. Remember, however, that these multibillion-dollar companies have been around for years and have poured a huge fortune into building their brands and hammering the taglines into our minds through aggressive advertising and marketing.

Creating a tagline need not be tricky. List out your core areas. Do not worry if it is a long sentence. Keep editing and trimming the sentence until you are able to express your key area in the shortest possible number of words.

- *Reinforcing the name, logo and tagline:* The actual work begins after finalizing the above aspects because these have to be reinforced. How do you do this? The ideal way would be to organize a grand launch event to let existing customers from your earlier individual practice know that you are now moving to a branded practice. Ensure that existing marketing channels and materials are updated to reflect the changes.

  If finances permit, then it is ideal to appoint a brand manager or hire an experienced branding agency to work out a brand strategy that ties these aspects into a cohesive whole and lends a much-needed focus to the business.

- *Staying visible and active*: Visibility builds positive brand perception. The more the visibility, the better the recall rate for the brand. Ensure that the brand is displayed in places where the public spends the maximum time.
  - *In clinics:* In all prominent areas like waiting areas, on the walls of consultation suites and treatment rooms, on coffee-table magazines, etc.
  - *In public places:* In areas where the public is likely to see the brand repetitively and frequently. For example, on the back panel of buses, on hoardings next to busy junctions, highways, etc.
  - *On social media:* Most people, especially the youngsters, are on social media, so it could act as a powerful medium for brand promotion. Whatsapp, Facebook, Instagram, etc., could help reach out to a large number of potential clients. Remember that there is no panacea. Different mediums work for different places. Find out the best approach through trial and error and customize accordingly.

- *Integrating the brand into your marketing:* As mentioned, visibility increases brand appeal. Integrate the brand wherever possible.
  - Staff uniforms should carry the brand logo. Objects such as towels, tissue papers, bedspreads, etc., can have logos imprinted on them at a nominal cost.
  - The logo should appear on almost all giveaways to clients: prescription pads, product takeaway bags, pens, coffee mugs, etc.
  - The logo and the tagline must appear on all brochures (printed and electronic), follow-up e-mailers, newsletters, etc.

- Innovative ideas to make your brand memorable—innovation is key to brand promotion.
  - *Feedback:* Asking for feedback and acting promptly on it with consistency gradually makes a brand memorable and likeable. Pay special attention to negative feedback. Reach out to the clients and ask them the reason for their feedback. You will soon learn to

differentiate between idle complaints and constructive criticism. Ignore the former with a smile; act on the latter with urgency.
- *Advertisement:* Ensure that the advertisements carrying the logo are subtle and esthetic, with a human touch and at times, a sense of humor. The ads do not have to be about the direct promotion of a service.
- *Blogging:* Blog on topics that offer solutions to frequently asked client questions and concerns. Ensure that the blog contains the latest and updated information, so that it makes the clients curious enough to keep revisiting the page, thus indirectly creating a connect.

- *Expanding the reach of the brand:* In the initial days of your practice, project yourself. Ensure that people correlate the surgeon and the brand. Once you achieve it and the volume picks up, you can detach yourself and solely promote the brand as it slowly incorporates a team of surgeons, to enable smooth functioning even in your absence. Most brands are initially associated with a single surgeon; however, later you have to bring in other members and form a team, if your aim is to expand.
- *Other marketing mantras:* Your marketing activities should be a set of tools to aid you in expanding your brand and reaching your goals. Keep the following points in mind:
  - *Target clientele*: What is your target clientele? Understand its needs. Observe the trend—what are the procedures they commonly opt for? Structure your marketing agenda based on the clientele.
  - *Have patience:* Patience is the keyword while establishing a brand. Take advice, seek suggestions, but ultimately chart a plan that works best for you. Initial marketing costs will always be on the higher side. It might be a couple of years before you finally find your niche.
  - *International reach:* Once you establish yourself nationally, gradually start promoting your brand internationally. With time and experience, you will have a fair idea about how to respond to the international queries you receive. Understand their behavior and needs. Do not overpromise and underdeliver. Be truthful. Remember, there is no better marketing tool than positive client feedback. Before starting the practice, understand government rules and regulations like Foreign Regional Registration Office (FRRO) and Forex. Good legal compliance speaks well of the brand and increases credibility among international patients.
  - *Trademark and copyright:* This is a necessary step if you are planning to spend a lot on branding.
  - *Consistency:* People identify a brand with its stability. Once you have finalized the important aspects of a brand, stick with it at least for a few years so that the brand gets rooted in public memory. This includes keeping the practice location or the registered office unchanged.

Congratulations from the bottom of my heart on your new venture!

TIPS AND PEARLS

- Branding when it comes to cosmetic practice is more about how you make

- people feel. The best advertising is done by satisfied customers.
- Social media marketing has forever altered the face of esthetic marketing and will continue to do so for many more years to come. You either have to learn how to use it or get left behind.
- Innovation remains the key to stay ahead of competition in esthetic practice. Make sure that you build a team that supports this culture and consistently evolves.

12.2 Websites and Search Engine Optimization

Aniketh Venkataram

INTRODUCTION

There was a time not too long ago when having a website was considered a luxury. In today's mobile world however, it is essential. Doctors are traditionally not very tech savvy and often have difficulty figuring out the online world. This chapter aims to provide some basic information on how to have a good performing website.

WHY DO I NEED A WEBSITE?

This question is similar to asking why do I need a clinic? Your clinic is a location where people can find, meet, and interact with you. A website accomplishes the same thing in the virtual world. It is your identity, your brand, and your persona on the internet. With the advent of smartphones, the amount of time an individual spends on the internet has skyrocketed. Nowadays, people are becoming habituated to looking up any place or product online before physically going there. If you do not have a good website, you might not have people coming through your door.

Building a website has been extensively covered in the dermatology section, so here we will be focusing on search engine optimization.

WHAT ARE SEARCH ENGINES?

Because there are so many websites, it became essential to have a tool to navigate and find what you are looking for. This led to the birth of search engines. Search engines go through all available websites on the internet and build a catalog of them, so that when you search for something, it provides you with what it thinks are the best options for what you are looking.

WHAT IS SEARCH ENGINE OPTIMIZATION?

In simple terms, it is the process of trying to get your website to rank as highly as possible on a search engine. Because there are so many websites for any given topic, if you want your website to be seen, it is important you rank highly, preferably on the first page of a search engine. Studies have shown that most users do not go past the first page of Google. The higher you rank on a search engine, the more visitors you get. The more visitors to your site, the more they interact with you.[1]

It is important to distinguish search engine optimization (SEO) from search engine marketing (SEM). Search engine optimization refers to improving the ranking of UNPAID results, i.e., you do not pay any money to the search engine to increase your site's visibility. Search engine marketing refers to the process of placing ads with search engines for them to be visible easily.

HOW DO SEARCH ENGINES WORK?

Search engines are programmed to analyze a website's content and understand what that site is about. It does this by using programs called spiders which scan and analyze websites. These spiders pick-up keywords and catalogs the website under that keyword.

A keyword is any word or phrase that the search engine considers relevant. A single website can be ranked under more than one keyword. The more relevant a website is considered for a particular keyword, the higher it ranks.

All of this information is fed into the search engines algorithm. This algorithm is a complex formula (that is proprietary and unique to each search engine). The algorithm then decides what ranking to assign to each website for that keyword.

While keywords are important, they are not the end-all to your website's ranking. Earlier search engines relied on them exclusively, which meant that they could be manipulated. Modern search engine algorithms employ a much more holistic approach to calculating your ranking.[2]

WHY IS GOOGLE THE BIGGEST SEARCH ENGINE AND HOW DOES IT WORK?

Initially there were many competing search engines. Google however, quickly overtook all of them. This is because it built a huge index of websites and was much faster than others. It gave incredibly relevant results and used the most advanced technology.[3]

No one can claim to know exactly how the Google algorithm works. One key change that Google made was to introduce personalized results for searches. This means that Google keeps a record of your prior internet activity and searches. It then tailors the results of a particular search for you. In essence, if two different people perform the same search, they can get two different lists of website with different rankings.

WHAT ARE THE FUNDAMENTALS OF SEARCH ENGINE OPTIMIZATION?

The Google algorithm is constantly being updated and modified. What this means is that there is no "hack" or quick way to rank highly on Google. Your website should be built on strong fundamentals to provide the best user experience and Google will reward you accordingly. The principles to be kept in mind are discussed next.

Relevance

The most important thing to remember while building your website is to make it relevant. Your website should be focused on plastic surgery and aim to provide as much useful information on the topic as possible. Search engines keep a track of how much time a person spends on a website. If someone reaches your website for a particular search but then leaves your site quickly, Google downgrades your ranking for the search the next time in favor of a website that keeps the user engaged for a longer time.

Consistency

Your website should be easy to understand both for a user and for a search engine. Having a common theme and scheme across your website makes for a more pleasant user experience. To achieve this, keep your website well organized and consistent, both in terms of design and content.

Build for the Long-term

As mentioned before, you should look at building a strong website for the long-term. Beware of anyone who promises to get you on the first page of Google within one month. They might achieve this by using black hat tactics. That might work initially, but the Google engineers will almost always eventually close these loopholes and might even downgrade your website for using them. Try to avoid hacks which might work in the short term, but which would ultimately be punished by Google.

Remember your Aim

The aim of your website is to get the most conversions. There is no point in having a high ranking and high traffic of people visiting your website, if they do not like what they see and call you.

HOW TO BUILD YOUR WEBSITE FOR SEARCH ENGINE OPTIMIZATION?

The most important thing to keep in mind while building your website is to keep it user-oriented. That should be your first and last concern.

Organization

Keep your website organized. If you have a lot of pages on a lot of topics, organize them into groups (or silos), and have a separate landing page for each silo. This makes it easier for a user to navigate your site and also for a search engine to index your site. Try to make it as intuitive as possible.

Design

While your design should be eye-catching, it should not slow down your website or make it difficult to use. Google values loading time very highly. Choose a simple functional design that works for you, and make it consistent across the website.

Content

Search engines love variety of content. Apart from text, use pictures, videos to your advantage. Remember that images can come up separately in Google's image search. Videos can drive traffic from YouTube. Having different types of content caters to different audiences. It is important to create your unique content and not copy from other sites. Google punishes plagiarism.[4]

Mobile Friendly

It is *imperative* that your website be mobile friendly. Two-thirds of all internet use today is done on mobile devices. Mobiles overtook desktops in 2015.[5] This is a fact that can be missed as the website is usually made on a desktop. Do not forget to see how your website reads and performs on a mobile phone.

Updates

Once your website is up and running, the work does not end there. It is important to keep updating your website with news and information. Search engines give a higher preference to websites that keep adding new information, rather than remaining static.

HOW DO I USE KEYWORDS EFFECTIVELY?

You might have surmised by now that keywords are very important toward your website's, SEO. In order to use keywords effectively, you must first decide which ones to use. Do some research to decide which keywords you want to use for which pages on your website. Choose the most relevant keywords. As mentioned before, there is no point using keywords which drive a lot of traffic to your site if that does not lead to conversions. Apart from basic general keywords, do not ignore more specific ones. While these might not lead to as much traffic as more general ones, the traffic they do generate is more likely to convert.[6]

Once you have decided your keywords, distribute them effectively in your website. Some places you can use them include headings, image titles, captions, and judiciously in the body of your matter. Be careful to avoid stuffing them in your site. This can be downranked by Google as it will deem it to be spam.[7]

CONCLUSION

There are many more advanced techniques to website building and SEO. The aim of this chapter is to provide a basic understanding and fundamentals for you to start with. It is important to understand that SEO is not a one-time job and there is no shortcut to it. Search engine algorithms are constantly being changed. Rather than trying to understand the algorithm and manipulate it, the best course to use basic principles to provide a relevant, useful website that adequately represents you and your practice.

TIPS AND PEARLS

- Having a website is essential in modern practice.
- Understanding how search engines work, helps optimize your website.
- Build a website for the long term, do not look for hacks.
- Relevance and user experience is key in building a good website.

REFERENCES

1. Ortiz-Cordova A, Jansen BJ. Classifying web search queries in order to identify high revenue generating customers. J Am Soc Inf Sci Tec. 2012;63(7): 1426-41.
2. Demers J (January 20, 2016). "Is Keyword Density Still Important for SEO". Forbes. Retrieved August 15, 2016.
3. Jarboe G (February 22, 2007). "Stats Show Google Dominates the International Search Landscape". Search Engine Watch. Retrieved May 15, 2007.
4. "Google Search Quality Updates". Google Blog.
5. "Inside AdWords: Building for the next moment" Google Inside Adwords May 15, 2015.
6. "The Most Important SEO Strategy". clickz.com. ClickZ. Retrieved April 18, 2010.
7. Kesmodel D (September 22, 2005). "Sites Get Dropped by Search Engines After Trying to 'Optimize' Rankings". Wall Street Journal. Retrieved July 30, 2008.

12.3 Traditional Marketing (Offline)

Sandeep Sattur

"Soliciting of patients directly or indirectly, by a physician, by a group of physicians or by institutions or organizations is unethical"
—**MCI, Code of Ethics Regulations, 2002**[1]

INTRODUCTION

The permeant dispersion of the media with cosmetic treatment promotions has amplified the demand for the same.[2] The situation is

Table 12.3.1: Comparison between internal and external marketing.

Internal marketing	External marketing
Marketing orientation within the organization itself	External marketing is where your message is directed to prospective new patients who do not know you
Having a clear practice identity Telling patients about your services Friendly and warm manner towards patients	Collateral Materials Yellow pages Advertising Patient and community programs Web strategies
There is little or no cost Small target audience (only people who enter the clinic)	Higher cost attached But reaches a much larger audience
It takes time and often requires an active effort from the doctor and staff	Mostly passive, no active participation from doctor
Results are seen as a "slow burn"—it builds (with consistency), but slowly	Can be explosive if planned well

skewed for the doctors—on one side the Medical Council of India (MCI)[1] prohibits advertising by doctors and on the other side the Consumer Protection Act (CPA)[3] equates them with business or service providers making them accountable. Speaking logically, as the CPA treats the doctors as service providers or traders, they should be ethically allowed to promote their services or trade[4] but that is not so.

The irony of the situation is such that since doctors cannot advertise, they remain at a disadvantage compared to the rapidly mushrooming hair and skin beauty clinics. The debate about whether a doctor can market himself/herself or not will continue but a plastic surgeon or a dermatologist will have to walk a tight rope while promoting cosmetic surgery services all the time remaining true to the ethical guidelines prescribed by the MCI.[5]

MARKETING

The word marketing immediately conjures an image of advertisements in most people's minds. But actually marketing is everything a doctor is and does, his ethics, culture, clinical skills, etc. These are the foundations upon which all other aspects of marketing are built. *The first step to successful marketing is to have right ethics and honesty, if these are missing, then no amount of marketing will be able to rectify the damage.*[6]

TRADITIONAL MARKETING (OFFLINE, NONDIGITAL)

Traditional marketing is much more than only use of nondigital media such as print, television, radio, etc., for promotion. Traditional marketing involves integrating all aspects of a doctor's practice from setting it up to the promotional activities. Traditional methods could be internal (whether the marketing is within the clinic itself) or external (direct approach to the prospective patients) **(Table 12.3.1)**.

Step 1: Master Technical Aspects

Before starting practice, it is important that the doctor be reasonably accomplished in a broad set of clinical skills. It is important to ensure adequate training and competence before performing any procedure on the patient.[7] Keeping abreast with the latest in the field through continued education is another important factor.

It is a big advantage if one can identify and focus on his/her strengths early in his/her career. Understanding your niche helps to define your practice, which in turn helps you to identify the specific patient population who would need your services.

Step 2: Clinic, Equipment, and Staffing

Patients today research the doctor, and factors, which help the patient choose between different doctors, are the "*determining attributes.*" These attributes could be years of medical experience, clinical skills, latest technology and equipment, atmosphere in the doctor's office or ease of getting an appointment, cost of treatment, recommendation of doctor, closeness to home, doctor's visibility in the media, etc.[8]

Many factors impact the patient's thinking even before meeting the doctor. This begins with the entry of the patient into the clinic:

- *Ambience in the clinic:* It should be tasteful and subtle but not opulent. It should convey the doctor's esthetic sensibilities. Very expensive or loud furniture and carpets and other accessories can have a negative impact on the patient. Privacy and confidentiality are crucial to esthetic practices and so, it is ideal to design the reception in such a way that other patients in the waiting room cannot hear the conversation between the patient and the receptionist.[9,10]
- *Equipment:* Apart from providing efficacy for the treatments, having the latest and updated equipment for the clinic helps to boost the image of the clinic. Choose the equipment in a gradual or stepwise manner.
- *Staffing:* The initial encounter of a patient with the receptionist over the telephone is important. The person who answers the clinic's phone can either be the clinic's best first impression or be the worst marketing call.[6] This encounter will decide whether or not the patient will make an appointment for a consultation or not. Similarly, the staff manning the reception is crucial to the success of the esthetic clinic. Not only they are required to have good administrative skills, but also possess people skills and help to convey a feeling that the clinic cares about them personally. More importantly, they should be well-versed with the products and procedures available at the clinic.[9] The importance of the staff behavior with the patients is conveyed very well in a survey conducted for hospital magazine that showed that 87% of the consumers considered courtesy of the staff as an important factor in considering their choice of hospital.[8]
- *Price/cost:* Pricing is one of the key components of marketing. When starting out, most doctors struggle to find the right price for their services, which will be higher than their working cost. Classic economic models postulate that supply and demand are interrelated and that both contribute to the pricing of goods.[19] However, studies have not shown this to be true to esthetic surgery practices. Procedure pricing is driven by a combination of local economic factors, consumer demand, and surgeon supply. The results suggest that local economic factors such as cost of living, real estate values, and population size are particularly influential in price setting.[20]

Step 3: Location

Location (place) is one of the 'P's of the four 'P's of marketing. Location matters a lot to an esthetic practice and aids the marketing. A right location can offset flaws in business promotion but the wrong location can kill the best marketing idea.[6] Location is not just about a physical address but also about convenience. Location should be determined based on accessibility by all modes of transport, demography of the patient population, existing hospital, esthetic clinics around, availability of parking and surrounding area (cleanliness, slums, etc.). All these factors can play a big role in prospective patients' perception of a clinic and its staff.[11]

Step 4: Market Research

Market research is often the most time-consuming step, but it is the key to optimizing your marketing efforts and budget. Firstly, before you finalize a location it is important to study any esthetic clinics in the vicinity.[11] Get details about their practice and how do they advertise. The best way to find out is to look up their websites, Internet ads, brochures, etc. Identify if there are any lacunae in their range of services. Including these services in your practice would help fulfill the needs of patients from that geographic location.

Step 5: The Marketing Plan

Adopt best international practices in marketing but modify them to suit local, legal, and cultural context. But always stay within the ethical guidelines. Marketing is something that is not taught in medical school and where marketing is concerned, doctors should not be a "do-it-yourselfer". It is best to hire the right market talent.

Choosing a marketing agency and setting goals:

- Check if the marketing agency has previous experience in healthcare or medical marketing.
- What is the plan—is the agency offering you a comprehensive strategy rather than standalone tactics?
- ROI (return on investment) and budgeting—it is prudent to have everything in black and white with the agency regarding rates, fees, retainers, and any potential "extra" charges before starting the marketing campaign. You must ensure that your investments are correctly and accurately tracked and are yielding measurable returns.
- Creativity and style quotient—creativity is an important tool for success of a marketing strategy, whether online or offline. A look at the agency's creatives would give an idea of how innovative they are with respect to creativity.

Step 6: Creating an Identity

Creating a brand identity helps to create schema that help consumers decide whether to initiate or continue use to a product or service. Branding constitutes the very beginning of the marketing communications process.

What do you stand for—it is important to establish the core value that you offer or the identity you want to convey. This is integral to the marketing strategy. First of all, make sure you are clear on how you want to be perceived by the community/peers and patients. Identify what sets your practice apart and gives you a competitive edge, or focus on strength of your practice that answers a community need.[13]

This identity should clearly reflect your mission and ethics and should be consistent in all of your marketing messages.[11] After you have defined your practice identity, develop a logo, which will represent you and the clinic. The logo and the name will be a part of the branding exercise and will be used in all the stationery and your website. A consistent theme (colors, fonts, etc.) should be replicated not only in the stationery, but also in the decor of the clinic and the staff uniforms. This helps the recall value. It will be even better if you get a tagline/slogan for your practice. A memorable tagline or catchphrase that perfectly sums up what your business is all about and also works as a perfect partner for your logo. These are small things that add up finally in a well-planned marketing campaign and brand building exercise.[11]

Step 7: Preconsultation Promotional Activities

Collateral Materials

As mentioned earlier, content creation to aid patient education is an important aspect of marketing for doctors. The collateral materials (brochures, credentials, achievements, accreditations) could help not only in informing the patient about the scope of services, but also create a positive impression in the mind of the patient before the patient even meets the doctor.

Brochures/literature kit: Patient education on each type of service that the practice provides is a part of content creation exercise. Brochures should be tastefully designed and must be informative.

A television or an LCD screen in the reception area can run audiovisuals pertaining to various procedures priming the patient to these services that the doctor has to offer and can be an important marketing tool. This helps to alleviate the irritability that some patients have due to the waiting period.

It is helpful if the information material is printed not only in English, but also in Hindi and the local language.

Display of Credentials and Achievements

The curiosity that most patients have in knowing about the doctor's background can be satiated by tastefully and esthetically displaying credentials such as degrees, diplomas, awards, etc. If the doctor has been quoted in some newspapers or if there are written testimonials or thank you cards from patients, these should be displayed properly. Pictures depicting participation at conferences or making presentations at meetings or certificates of attendance at national and international meetings help to convey the fact that the doctor has good standing in the field and is academically oriented. If the doctor has any publications or has authored books or contributed to textbooks, these should be prominently displayed. These small efforts help to create a positive impression about the doctor even before meeting him.

Doctor's Attire and Conduct

It is imperative that the doctor is dressed appropriately, as most patients critically evaluate the doctor. It is best to be dressed formally or in surgical scrubs. Wearing very expensive accessories or loud clothes can have a negative impact.

Accreditation of the Doctor and Clinic

Accreditation conveys formal recognition by an independent authority in terms of complying with the industry standards of practice and patient care. We do not have special accreditation authorities for outpatient surgery, but in our country getting the clinic accredited to National Accreditation Board for Hospitals and Healthcare Providers (NABH) or International Organization for Standardization (ISO) helps to put the clinic in better light and shows that most norms are being followed where standard of care is concerned.

Being a member of professional associations indicates your standing amongst your peers and this also validates your credentials and quality of your services. For example, a plastic surgeon can be a member of Association of Plastic Surgeons of India (APSI), Indian Association of Aesthetic Plastic Surgeons (IAAPS), International Society of Aesthetic Plastic Surgery (ISAPS), Association of Hair Restoration Surgeons of India (AHRS), and International Society of Hair Restoration Surgery (ISHRS) and the dermatologist can be a member of Indian Association of Dermatologists, Venereologists and Leprologists (IADVL), American Academy of Dermatology (AAD), AHRS, ISHRS, etc. Patients look upon these associations as endorsement of your clinical capabilities and you being listed as a member can help to improve your visibility when the patients are looking for doctors providing specific esthetic services.

Step 8: External Marketing—Media

Media coverage helps to give third party endorsement to the doctor or clinic like no other factor.

Print Media

As of now formal advertisements in newspapers are considered unethical by the MCI except to make a formal announcement in press regarding the following: (1) On starting practice, (2) On change of type of practice, (3) On changing address, (4) On temporary absence from duty, (5) On resumption of another practice, (6) On succeeding to another practice, and (7) Public declaration of charges.

This being a onetime allowance one cannot plan marketing with advertisement in the print media. However, there are other ways that doctors have used newspaper coverage to their advantage. The use of editorials (sponsored advertorials) can be a way of promoting oneself in the print media. Strict adherence to ethical guidelines is necessary and the following points amongst others must be followed:

- All information must be accurate and must not create false or unjustified expectations.[12]
- Do not use deceptive or misleading images.
- Avoid self-aggrandizement by using terms such as "world-famous," best in the country" or even "pioneer," as they are not factually substantiated and specifically prohibited by the code of ethics.
- By leaving out the downsides of the procedures or not putting disclaimers will amount to omission of information and technically make the editorial misleading.
- Quoting testimonials is also considered misleading as only the good reviews get quoted.
- Fee structures and costs may be advertized as long as the information contains enough information that the prospective patients are neither misled nor unduly induced to seek services at that clinic. Also mentioning free consultations is tantamount to luring patients to more expensive treatments or tests.
- Most importantly the advertorial must be basically educative and not be selling any procedure or treatment.

State medical councils have pulled up doctors on the grounds that they did not adhere to the ethical guidelines. Actions by the medical councils have ranged from reprimanding to actual suspension. Hence, one must keep the above points in mind before indulging in any promotional activity.[15,16]

Another important factor regarding print advertising is the cost. Usually the marketing avenues for esthetic practice in the print media are expensive and most of the times do not justify the ROI.

Due to a plethora of local languages, it is important to consider the language of communication to be used in all forms of print communications. It is always helpful to have the print marketing in English, Hindi, and the local language.

Yellow Pages

Of course, things have changed since the time that every household, which had a telephone, had a yellow pages directory. The physical yellow pages have been replaced by the numerous digital yellow pages, which are accessible on the smart phones.

Radio

Talk shows and interviews on the radio, as long as they are educative and fall within the guidelines could be considered. These help in improving credibility of the doctor but may not translate into actual increase in number of patients coming for consultation.

Television

Similarly, television chat shows also help but as it is an audiovisual medium and has a higher viewership, the benefits accrued from a television talks how would be higher. Depending on the channel on which it is aired, the viewership will decide the reach of the show. During the talk show proclamation as to the status of the ranks of competence of the doctor or quality of the services should be avoided.

The commonality between advertorials or radio and TV talk shows or persons looking through the newspapers is the unspoken question in the mind audience members. If through these media one can have a message to answer those questions, the promotional activity would definitely succeed.

Budgeting for media marketing has to be done carefully as this has considerable expense attached to it.

An audit done every quarterly will help crystallize the marketing plan based on the returns achieved by that particular activity.

Step 9: External Marketing— Exposure to Peers and Public

Being invited to speak at social meetings like those conducted by the service clubs or local medical associations can elevate your status to a celebrity expert and not just another doctor. Most people are not very comfortable to speak in public but one has to overcome these fears if one wants to promote oneself in the field. Public presentations and speeches are very good marketing tools (even though the target audience is limited) that help doctors to stand out. It is a good platform to educate the public and even your own fraternity. When speaking at doctors, meeting, you can showcase your academic and professional skills and create an impression amongst your peers.

Step 10: Word of Mouth

A doctor's work/results will speak more than any advertisement. Oral or written recommendation by your patients about your services to prospective patients accounts for a strongest marketing tool. It is a slow process but the success is guaranteed. Studies have suggested that in the health field, like consumers in other fields, patients are very concerned about the quality of service.[17] Better service of doctors leads to a positive word of mouth and this helps patients in making a choice of the doctor/clinic.[18] A satisfied patient will never hesitate to refer another patient. At all times, doctors should strive at providing quality services and this is the most important factor that will promote footfalls in the clinic through word of mouth.

Creating new footfalls would be an important aspect of marketing an esthetic practice but showing common courtesies to existing patients like making follow-up calls to check on them or wishing them on their birthdays, etc., goes a long way in establishing long-term relationships with the patients.

RETURN ON INVESTMENT FOR MARKETING SPEND

In relation to medical practice, return on investment basically refers to the increased patient footfalls in the clinic as compared to the money spent on a particular activity. Return on investment describes the fact that value has resulted from an investment of time, energy, or money. In finance, ROI is depicted in the formula:

ROI = (Investment proceeds–cost)/ (investment),
or

ROI = (campaign net return)/(campaign invested cost).[21]

In online marketing, it is easier to track the ROI as the sources can be traced. Where traditional marketing (offline-internal as well as external) is concerned, determining the ROI is difficult as money invested today may have an unpredictable impact today but show some results in the future. One of the ways is track the source of your patients. Every patient who calls the clinic, sends an e-mail or comes in for consultation should be tracked and it is important to ask the patient "How did you come to know about me/the clinic." Doctors are not trained for devising or planning a marketing campaign and if a significant budget is available, it is best to involve specialists like an agency for the same. If a marketing agency were involved then the regular (monthly, quarterly) marketing audit report would help to decide which of the activities are fruitful and which are not.

POINTS TO REMEMBER

- Never lose the objective of the marketing—creating an identity for yourself, improving visibility, and most importantly educating the patient.
- Ethical marketing will take time but the long-term results will be more sustainable.
- Marketing should never be misleading.

SUMMARY

The ethics and culture one cultivates within one's practice form the most important foundation on which all other aspects of marketing will build. A doctor's ability to strengthen human relationships through marketing will determine the success of the practice. At all times, being ethically responsible in all aspects of marketing will hold good in the long run.

REFERENCES

1. Indian Medical Council. (Professional Conduct, Etiquette and Ethics) Regulations, 2002. [online] Available from https://www.mciindia.org/documents/rulesAndRegulations/Ethics%20Regulations-2002.pdf [Last accessed January, 2020].
2. Lorenzo PD, Casella C, Capasso E, et al. The Central Importance of Information in Cosmetic Surgery and Treatments. Open Med (Wars). 2018;13:153-7.
3. http://ncdrc.nic.in/bare_acts/Consumer%20Protection%20Act-1986.html and https://indiacode.nic.in/bitstream/123456789/1868/3/A1986-68.pdf#search=[Last accessed January, 2020].
4. Nagpal N. Should Advertising by Aesthetic Surgeons be Permitted? J Cutan Aesthet Surg. 2017;10(1):45-7.

5. https://ijme.in/articles/from-the-medical-council/?galley=print [Last accessed January, 2020].
6. Norman J. What no one ever tells you about marketing your own business: real life advice from 101 successful entrepreneurs. USA: Dearborn Trade Publishing; 1999.
7. Sacchidanand SA, Bhat S. Safe practice of cosmetic dermatology: avoiding legal tangles. J Cutan Aesthet Surg. 2012;5(3):170-5.
8. Strauch L. Hospital advertising in the beginning: marketplace dynamics and the lifting of the ban. J Econ Bus Hist Soc. 2004;22:229-40.
9. Bhangoo KS. The art of consultation. Indian J Plast Surg. 2014;47(2):167-74.
10. Sachdev M, Britto GR. Essential Requirements to Setting up an Aesthetic Practice. J Cutan Aesthet Surg. 2014;7(3):167-9.
11. Use Strategic Marketing to Maintain a Healthy Practice. J Oncol Pract. 2009;5(6):305-8.
12. Ethical ways for physicians to market a practice. Committee Opinion No. 510. American College of Obstetricians and Gynecologists. Obstet Gynecol 2011;118:1195-7.
13. Williams J. The Basics of Branding. Available from https://www.entrepreneur.com/article/77408 [Last accessed January, 2020].
14. Rudden D. Can You Hear Me Now? Marketing Essentials for Audiologists in a Noisy Health Care World. Semin Hear. 2016;37(4):325-39.
15. https://www.apnnews.com/medical-council-of-india-to-investigate-advertisements-by-doctors-in-violation-of-the-code-of-medical-ethics/
16. http://www.gmcgujarat.org/pdf/advisory-regarding-advertising-in-medical-practice.pdf [Last accessed January, 2020].
17. Lu N, Wu H. Exploring the impact of word-of-mouth about Physicians' service quality on patient choice based on online health communities. BMC Med Inform Decis Mak. 2016;16(1):151.
18. Lin SH, Lin TMY. Demand for online platforms for medical word-of-mouth. J Int Med Res. 2018;46(5):1910-18.
19. Krieger LM, Shaw WW. Aesthetic surgery economics: lessons from corporate boardrooms to plastic surgery practices. Plast Reconstr Surg. 2000;105(3):1205-10. Available from https://www.ncbi.nlm.nih.gov/pubmed/10724282 [Last accessed June, 2020].
20. Richardson C, Mattison G, Workman A, Gupta S. Pricing of common cosmetic surgery procedures: local economic factors trump supply and demand. Aesthet Surg J. 2015;35(2):218-24.
21. Gould DJ, Nazarian S. Social Media Return on Investment: How Much is it Worth to My Practice? Aesthet Surg J. 2018;38(5):565-74.

12.4 Online and Social Media Marketing

Amit Gupta

DIGITAL MARKETING

It is the new mantra for all plastic surgeons. Increasing competition from qualified and unqualified doctors and our limited knowledge of marketing only increase our challenges in this field.

- There is no paucity of patients looking for plastic surgery services, however, how many of them reach your practice?
- How many people in the world know you exist?
- How many of your own patients know all your services?
- How many new patients can your practice handle?
- Do you have an infrastructure to handle the increased flow of leads once you start digital marketing?

- Do you know that leads are never a problem, it is the conversion that is the bottleneck?

It is essential that you create the necessary infrastructure, workforce, systems and workflow to handle incoming leads. I will elaborate in question and answer format, to make it easy-to-understand.

What is Digital Marketing?

Creating an online presence, via visibility in the electronic space, is digital marketing. If today you are not online, you are invisible. It will be difficult to prosper and grow at a healthy percentage on a quarterly basis leading to stagnation and eventually your practice may be wiped out. On the other hand, an expanding business will outgrow others. So let's seriously focus on online presence and the various modalities.

- Website
- Search engine optimization (SEO)
- Pay-per-click (PPC) and google AdWords
- WhatsApp marketing
- Facebook
- Instagram
- Others

Online or digital marketing is the visibility created via the internet, while the conventional marketing works offline that is without the dependency of internet. Every business needs to be online. A start up needs to be online to gather more customers, and grow. A well-established business too needs to be online to maintain its growth. Even global brands as Kodak or NOKIA, can get wiped out if they fail to innovate and grow.

Why Digital Marketing and not Offline Marketing?

Online marketing is always on. A potential patient can see it any time, all the time. Offline marketing, like magazines, newspapers, TV ads, banners, posters, billboards are limited by:

- *Cost:* Offline marketing is much more expensive.
- *Need repeated insertions*: Public recall is very low, and many repeated insertions are required for brand recall.
- *Limited visibility*: Offline modalities are available to only some people at some times.
- Today no brand can survive on offline marketing alone. Rarely a brand like Maggi can survive only on name and brand recall. Despite that Maggi markets continuously.

Why is Digital Marketing Important for Plastic Surgeons?

Doctors have not been trained in any form of marketing, let alone digital marketing. Plastic surgeons lack skills of patient interaction, patient retention, cross selling, and we look down upon marketing as a crime. We have never been taught basic marketing, because medicine is considered a service to humanity, and doctors have maintained a holier than thou attitude, where the patient has to come to a doctor, and not vice versa. Times have changed. With the availability of unlimited information at the click of a button, patients today have choices, and we as professionals need to tell them that we are doing good work.

I will give a brief statistic that might interest you. The first 2 charts **(Figs. 12.4.1A and B)** are search volumes of hair transplant in India and in USA. Average number of searches are 5 lakhs a month in India and 7 lakhs a month in the USA. Imagine that is the search volume in just 2 countries for just one key word. There are a large number of equally

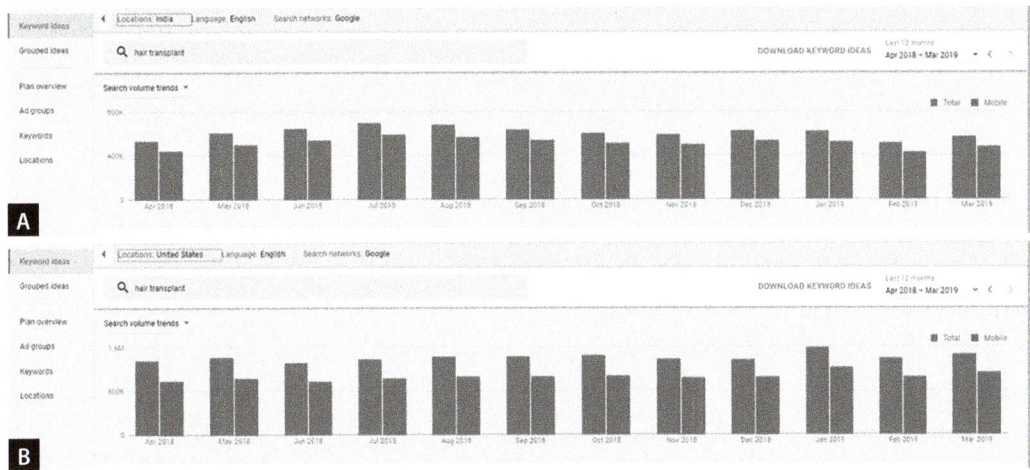

Figs. 12.4.1A and B: Search volumes of hair transplant in India and in USA.

significant key words in hair transplant. This tells about the market size of hair transplant in the world today:

The next few charts **(Figs. 12.4.2A to C)** are also interesting. I have put the search volumes of breast implant as a key word in India. Watch the trends month-wise, city-wise, and platform (device)-wise.

- 83.7% of searches are made on mobile devices. Largest numbers of searches are from Bengaluru followed by Delhi and then Mumbai.
- 2.25 lakhs searches per month and 40% are for hair transplant. So you can imagine the demand for each of these procedures.

What is Google Drive and how is it Useful for Plastic Surgeons?

Google drive is a feature of Google mail or Gmail. You log onto your mail and click the triangle **(Fig. 12.4.3)**.

The triangle is the drive. The drive is the storage for all things that are important, data, pictures, excel sheets, videos, word documents, PowerPoint presentations, etc.

The advantage of drive is that saving is real time, and it can be accessed at any place on earth, via laptop or mobile. The complete clinic software can be run real time on Google drive. Basic clinic enterprise resource planning (ERP) solutions can be created on Google drive in the form of flowchart management (FMS), which can be used to not only store data, but also create schedulers, reminders, follow-ups, etc.

Let's talk in terms of revenues and profits—every clinic needs to have clear appreciation of its numbers. What is gross profit, net profit, fixed expense, variable expense, receivables, and net profit?

An appreciation of numbers leads one to plan what they want to create as a future of the center. Once the numbers start emerging, it will become clear that to double your profits, you need to double your revenue, which means you need to double your efforts to get leads. Playing with numbers is one of the simplest ways to actually make profits.

What are the Digital Marketing Tools Available (Figs. 12.4.4A to C)?

- Website
- Landing page
- Social media

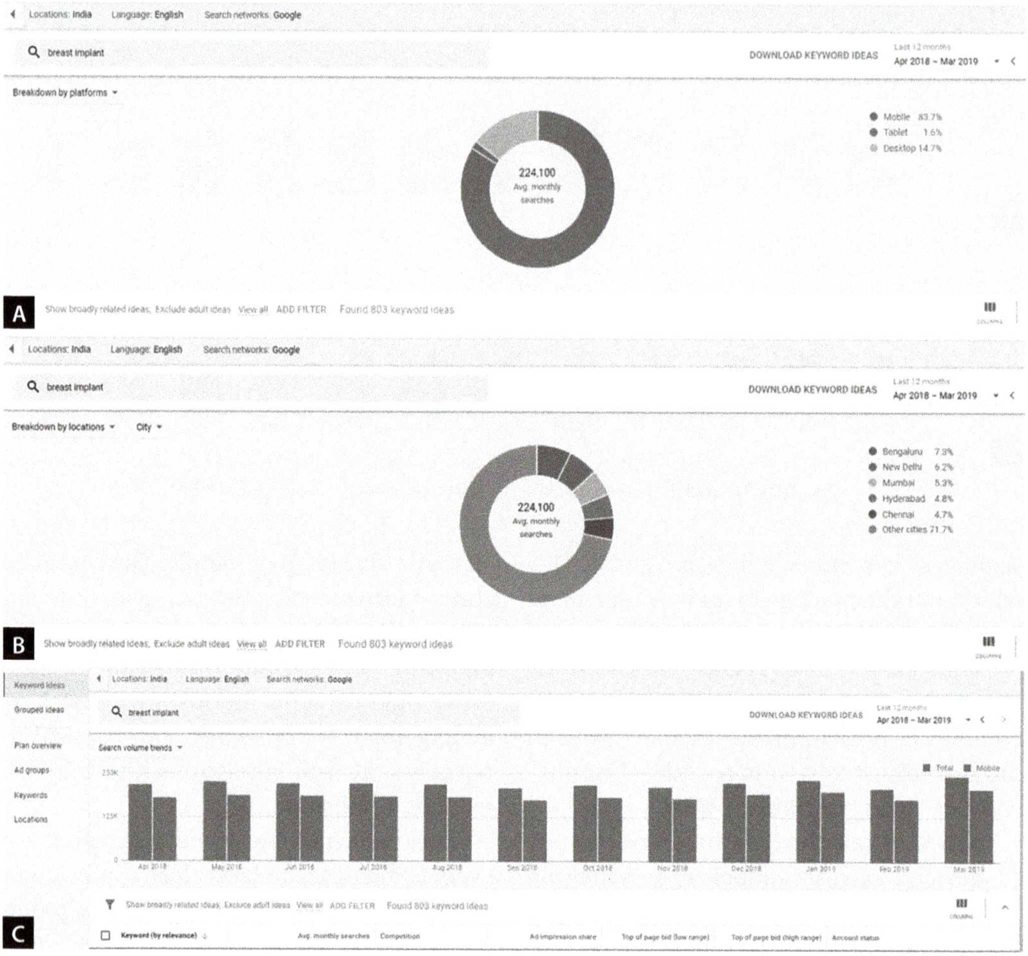

Figs. 12.4.2A to C: Search volumes of breast implant as a keyword in India.

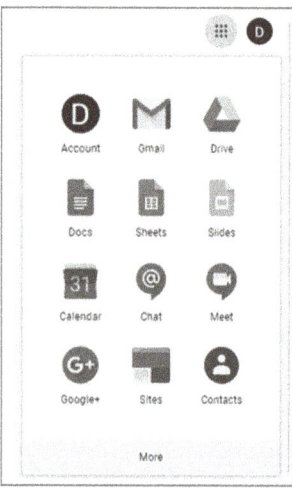

Fig. 12.4.3: Google Drive.

What is Website and Landing Page?

A website has multiple pages and it gives the viewer all the details about your practice, team and services. The viewer may or may not be interested in all the details, but has to select his service from the bouquet of services presented, via home, back buttons, etc.

Landing page: It is more specific to a product or service, and does not confuse the customer with unnecessary information, e.g., a customer may be looking for hair transplant, while the website also displays information on liposuction, Botox, breast, etc., which is not of great interest to him, leading to loss

Section 12: Marketing

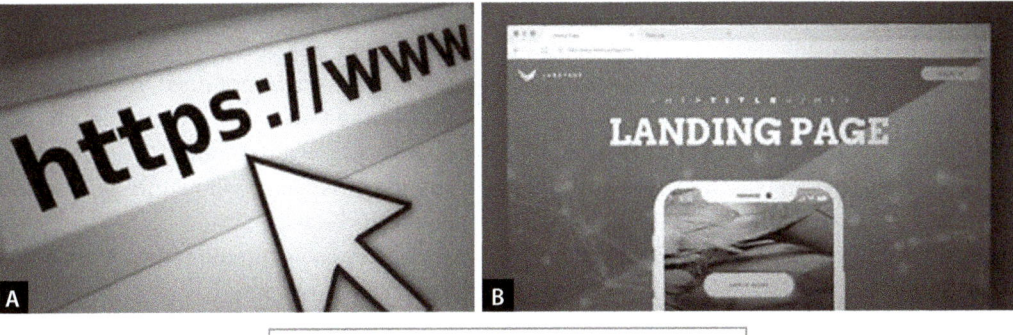

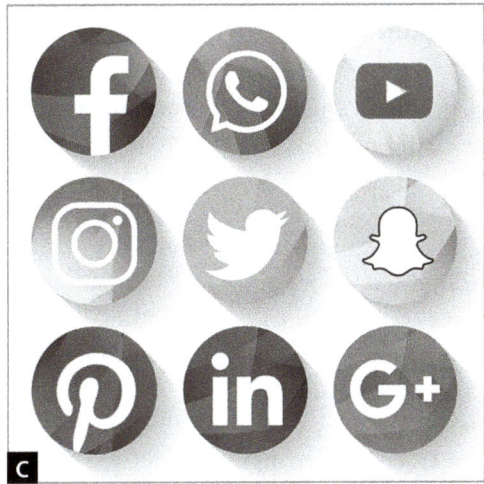

Figs. 12.4.4A to C: Digital marketing tools: (A) Website; (B) Landing page; (C) Social media.

of interest and skipping over the website. Whereas a landing page will be specific and not allow the customer to divert, while focusing on call to actions (CTAs) such as call now, look for more, book now. It is typically more action oriented with a lot of information in small space, direct, nonconfusing to the customer, cheaper to make and maintain, at the same time being more profitable.

Google AdWords work better with landing pages, since the information is specific, with a direct call to action information. Landing pages can be thought of as a mini website.

SOCIAL MEDIA CHANNELS

Live channels include Instagram, Facebook, Snapchat, and YouTube that offers live streaming.

Basics of live streaming:
- It is really important to be clear with the objective.
- Social media can backfire. Any wrong statement, surgical step can mess up the video.
- Go live with a clear script; create a Q&A session for best results.
- The video should be 2–7 minutes.
- Viewership will be higher only if the content is clear, crisp, has education and not marketing, and shows that you care.

Why is Live Media Important?

- Gets the audience a chance to see you in reality
- Creates a chance for direct interaction between you and the audience

- You can get instant clients by being clever, witty, and informative
- Putting live stories on the channels allows your channel to be prominently displayed on your subscribers screen. Every time they log on, they will see your channel first. This creates a chance for the audience to see how artistic, creative, and busy you are.

How to Create Good Content for Videos?

- *Title:* Always create a title that attracts attention. General titles will not work at all. They should be short, attractive, and focused to the video.
- *Duration*: 2–7 minutes.
- *Set up*: It is not mandatory to have a professional camera set up and microphone. But the script should be ready beforehand. A good mobile phone is adequate to get a good video.
- Watch competitor videos to get an idea of the content.

How to Set up Campaigns on Facebook, Google, and Instagram?

- Most important is to decide the target audience:
  - Age
  - Sex
  - Lifestyles
  - Hobbies
  - Regions—regional, national, and international
- Decide your key words
- Plan your budgets and daily spends
- Monitor your spends based on leads generation. Always be ready to cancel any campaign if you get bad quality leads, or are not getting any leads. Keep strict checking of your budgets at all times.
- Google AdWords, Facebook ads, and Instagram ads can easily be started on your own; you do not need a professional to manage the ads. Agencies charge anything between 10 and 15% of the total spends. It is easy. Follow the rules stated above and start.

To master social media today. A few rules for the social media are:

- A clear understanding of your target audience
- A clear understanding of the scope of each media
- Understand what are ground rules of each media—like a breast implant surgery might be banned on insta but it is ok on YouTube
- Create content which engages
- Create content which respects the time limits of each media—some media have 10 second limits, some have 1 minute. Some media have a limit on the size of the video
- Monitor your campaigns— this medium can burn money like it is not funny at all
- Select regions, audience, tastes for each medium carefully, especially important for pay per click (PPC)—these are money vanishing tools if they are not monitored.

SUMMARY—80:20 RULE

Everything will not work for everyone. Over the course you will realize that some of these are more useful than the rest but beyond financial viability. On the other hand, some of these are cheap, but not worth the efforts (time and manual effort). Therefore, once some methods have been tried and tested, start categorizing according to 80:20 rule. This rule states that of all the activities, 20% of activities will bring you 80% revenue, and vice versa.

TIPS AND TRICKS

- *Define your budget*: Social media can burn money, be clear in your objectives. Do you have clear finances? Do you want to pitch for the most expensive key word?
- *Do you have the team to handle leads*: 93–94% of leads generated from social media are either useless or fake. But the center needs to have good resource management to handle these.
- *Define your audience*: What strata of society are you catering? Do you want to cater to low budget or high budget patients? The marketing campaigns need to be tailored accordingly.
- *Focus on free marketing channels first*: Instagram, YouTube, WhatsApp.
- *Put limits on your PPC spending*: It can leak like crazy.
- *Identify negative SEO*: Competitors may pull down your campaigns unethically by doing negative SEO on your PPC.
- Maintain a good customer relations team.
- Be real with the concept of ROI.
- *Create a sales funnel:* Lead generation is easy, work on conversions.

12.5 In the Box Thinking, Salesmanship

Sanjay Parashar

DEFINITION

I was asked to write about "Out of the Box" thinking to develop our practice. I believe the secret is getting the basics right, as most of us forget the basics and start venturing out which may eventually be counterproductive. So, lets begin with In the box thinking!

Salesmanship in a medical practice sounds unorthodox. We surgeons are supposed to serve the patients who need our service. But how do we overcome two challenges every business faces?

1. How do the patients findout what you do?
2. And why should one choose you over others?
   Now you must be thinking.

These two challenges are also your main objectives to be able to maintain a healthy practice.

There is enough written material and books available to tell you about how to be better at salesmanship. I will not be telling you that I will share what worked for me, how I differentiated and established my practice. Also, do not misunderstand me—I will not be telling you how to lure patients with lower prices, outstanding/unrealistic results or false advertising. Rather, I will insist on how important it is to be ethical and a fair salesman. Out of the box thinking is not the answer to marketing a clinic. Getting what is in the box already right is the answer.

Through the ages, a doctor and his practice flourished through word of mouth and referrals. The patient would come to a plastic surgeon only when referred by a physician and the surgeon then provides all information to the patient and the patient would undergo surgery. Similarly, in the past if people needed to buy any product, they will go to a store where a salesman would explain all details and the purchaser then buys it. The power was in the hands of the salesman. Now, things have changed. It is the other way around. The power is in the hands of the consumers. They have all information readily available to them and they have the power to compare, select, choose, and bargain to the best of their advantage. Similarly, in plastic surgery, the power is in the hands of consumers. Patients want to have all the information they need in advance, they research online before coming in for a consultation and if you are not out there on the Internet, they will not find you. So, having a good website and social media presence is an absolute must. I am sure you knew that already, as this is nothing new. So, if you do not have a good Internet presence, get that right immediately. That is the key for them to find you.

So how do you find your edge? Why will they choose you?
Let me tell you the secret that I learned very early on—it is identifying a service-gap. I started my practice in Dubai where there were senior, internationally known plastic surgeons, well established and already doing what I wanted to offer. So, I studied the market and trend and I found a niche…Honesty! It was surprising that something that we all take an oath for was missing. I realized people wanted an honest plastic surgeon who would give them the right information and help patients make the correct decision keeping patients' interest first in mind. I counseled to make them feel confident about themselves first, like themselves first, and recommend a cosmetic procedure only if it truly would help them be a better of themselves. I was starting in a new city, I needed all the money I could get, but I did not let the fear of bills give-out wrong advices. It was a slow start, but laid a strong foundation, these patients became my "ambassadors". I gained respect, popularity, and a following. Until today, I am known for my honest opinion and people come to me for a second opinion. And I help them make their choice, even if I am not the operating surgeon for them. Likewise, you need to find your edge by identifying the service-gap in your market and fill it. In some places, it could be lack of technology, in some it could be the quality of service or protocols, the list is endless. So, identify this gap, and work toward filling it.

Go beyond the basics.
A good plastic surgeon has the skills needed to get the surgery done. But is that good enough?

What matters is…
- How good are you at your consultation?
- How differently you perform the procedure?
- What else are you focusing at that others may not?

Doctors are popular for not listening and always being pressed for time. We hardly give adequate time to patients and answer all their queries. It is because we do this day and night and its repetitive and mundane for us. But for the patient, it is the first time. He or she is more likely to go with the doctor who listens. So, work on your consultation skills.

While protocols are extremely important, but having one's own technique and style is important. So when you meet patients, educate them on how you will do the procedure differently. How your technique is devised with experience and delivers better results and safety.

The final shot in your armor—Beating the Competition.

You can only do that by focusing and laying emphasis on things that your competitors are not focusing on. Most plastic surgeons these days are busy finding the best ways to market and attract patients, I want you to focus on three basic things 99% of places forget to implement.

1. *Providing the ideal environment for the patient:* We all take pride in our setups, but do patients feel the same? Think from the patients' perspective and make the changes needed. What is good for you may not be considered good by patients who help us pay the bills. So, ensuring comfort is a priority at your practice.
2. *Safety:* What can you do to prevent complications, how can you minimise pain, how can you provide great outcome that is sustainable or at least reproducible?
3. *Create great experiences:* A patient who experiences a lot of pain, discomfort or bad outcome or generally has a bad experience will always talk negatively about your practice and the procedure, e.g., liposuction, abdominoplasty. This creates a negative image of the procedure and the discipline by large. Your responsibility is to create a successful image of the procedure you are performing so the plastic surgery discipline gains its credit.

A patient who undergoes a successful liposuction with minimal discomfort, swelling, and bruising and achieves significant result is the best form of marketing for you. An abdominoplasty patient if recovers smoothly without complications and a nicely placed scar will be happy to talk positively about it.

So in the beginning, focus on doing the right thing in the right way. A point will come when you have created enough positive experiences and you are confident and will feel the need to increase your work. Then, and only then, is the right time to promote you. Because you are then telling the truth and not making up and misguiding the patients.

"Salesmanship" does not imply hard sales like a car salesman. We are in the medical business; a smart-sell might get us from Point A to B. But to sustain at Point B, one needs to get the basics right. Become a salesman with integrity, dept, and best in your field.

The Civil Law considers esthetic surgeon, healthcare provider, and patients as "consumers". And consumers expect 100% satisfaction and if anything goes wrong immediately after or even up to 24 months of your treatment, they can sue you for monetary compensation. So, whether you like it or not, you are selling your service, so better do it the perfect way.

UNDERSTAND PATIENT PSYCHOLOGY

Once you have mastered the above basics, you can then look at mastering patient psychology. It will help you gain advantage on the negotiation table and tailor your strategy and grow your business beyond expectations.

When the patient has come to you for a consultation, apart from clinical and medical history you need to understand the patient psychology. I am not talking about Narcissism and Body Dysmorphophobia, I am talking about patient psychology that allows him or her to choose you for their surgery.

There are broadly five kinds of personality in patients seeking surgery:

1. *Nervous patient:* He or she wants to improve looks, but is afraid of complications and side effects. They are looking for safety, assurance, and credibility of the surgeon. They will be nervously sitting in your waiting room and looking around to see for assurances. They are observant of the quality and meticulousness you are offering. They may not be worried about the cost; they want quality and safety. This is where you have to assure how safe your procedure is and give them enough proof of it.

2. *Ignorant patient:* They have body issues they want to address but are ignorant about options and are basically seeking information. These patients need education and may require coming back later. Many of these will drop out once they realize the journey they have to go through. You have to be very patient to answer all their questions proactively without showing signs of impatience or irritability. Once you establish trust, sooner or later they will either bring their business back to you or refer you patients.
3. *Perfectionist:* These patients have quite good knowledge about what they want and the procedure in details. They would have consulted many doctors and are looking for the "Best" who could help meet their expectations. You have to be careful to decide if you want to accept this patient. If you are confident and are perfectionist yourself, you may give them satisfaction, or else stay away from them. In these patients, you need to under promise and over deliver, if at all you operate on them.
4. *Bargainers:* These patients are aware of the procedures and are aware that they have many options to go to. They are looking for best deals. If you do not provide them, they will go to the next door. I think we should not encourage them because to cut down on cost means to compromise on quality or to reduce your time and effort. Both are detrimental to the outcome. To get the best result in a safe way you need to provide your expertise, postoperative care, and vigilance and use best quality products. If you show disinterest in their bargains, they may come back to you.
5. *Plastic surgery addicts:* There are two kinds of plastic surgery addicts:
   (a) One who had surgery and is not satisfied and may be a perfectionist. They keep doing surgeries hoping to get the perfect result. You need to be cautious of them. They are a lawsuit waiting to happen.
   (b) Some who had already experienced the benefits of plastic surgery procedures. These patients are quite positive and do not require extensive counseling. But it is your responsibility to stop them if they are going overboard. Because when they go overboard and their looks show it, it is your work that gets blamed, not their addiction.

"Out of the Box" thinking...
My mantra is " Innovate before its duplicated." I believe in constant innovation, as ideas are open to all for implementation.
Let me share some of the things that will help you get more ideas. Ideas crop up when you think what patients want, understanding their psychology is a skill that needs to be developed.

- *Offer them insurance policy:* One of the fears patients have is what if things go wrong. Nobody likes complications; the worst is the fear of death or lethal complications or even problems that may lead to additional treatment, surgery, and cost. Offer your patients some security, it could be getting medical insurance for complications or offer some insurance within your capabilities to alleviate their apprehension. Our priority for any treatment is to have "NO COMPLICATIONS", we have worked hard to make it true. First

5 years we had literally less than 0.05% complications without any major or lethal problems. The clinical audit in 2018 showed 0.08% complications. We are now confident to provide our patients our own insurance policy to cover most immediate and early complications.

- *Patient education:* Identify ways to educate people and in their own language. You need to understand your target audience be it local, regional or international and speak in their language. Get translation services, in-house translators, and learn few dialect yourself that help to break the barrier to communicate further. Keep looking for different medium to reach them, follow the trend, look for newer ways, and keep learning. There are a lot of resources available to learn business stuff, it is time to read them.

- *Circle of network:* There are many sources of referral; they come from media communications, patients, doctors, etc. You need to be more enterprising so you develop a wider network. Your vendors and suppliers can help a lot in spreading the word around. There are lots of businesses and professional networking groups you can participate. Remember, you need to be subtle in what you ask for; the primary goal is to let them know who you are and what you do. The hospitals you work in, the staff there, nurses are your entire referral source if not directly, indirectly. What goes around comes around!

In a nutshell, apart from your education and skills, you need to gather these skills to give confidence to your patients and get your practice going.

SECTION 13

Growth

13.1 Setting-up Goals

James Roy Kanjoor

INTRODUCTION

Though medical practice is considered as a business model, there is an element of pain, healing and outcome or results of the patient—the "customer" in the business scenario. These health issues make medical practice different from regular businesses in the sense that it is more closer to heart and health. Our specialty skin and plastic surgery, especially esthetic surgery is even more different because our clients are not patients and do not have any pain before we start our management.

It is important to set goals that address the best interests of our patients. "A happy, satisfied patient is our ultimate goal." This mission statement is the foundation for an optimal medical practice.

Medical practice cannot be successful if there are no walk-in patients.

Goals should target the following areas:
- To increase the number of patients—*marketing goals*
- Setting a goal in quality of care—*practice goals. In business world, it is referred as operations*
  - Provide complete patient care in a timely manner
  - Complete transparency and honesty in clinical and administrative management
- To set high standard of clinical care—*surgical goals*

Setting a goal in an individual procedure for patient safety and surgical outcome. For example, when liposuction is planned for a patient, the goal should be an elastic skin quality capable of redraping to an esthetic shape in a calculated period of time.

When a cosmetic breast surgery is planned the goal should be an esthetic breast with an acceptable scar.

The initial goal should also take into consideration finance, facility and finesse. If your goal is to have a total esthetic care under one roof and due to many reasons, it may not be possible to start altogether in one go. You can stage it. When my center "Roys" was conceived, due to financial and technical reasons (to identify the right product suppliers) I started the outpatient section initially followed 1 year later by full fledged operating room (OR) complex in the first floor.

If you have an existing center for many years, you just need to improvise and the latent period may be short. On the other hand, if it is a project conceived from the seed stage, you need to have good reserve for 2 years to meet the day-to-day expenses and run the establishment according to your expected goals. I mortgaged my house to get a loan to build and run the center for 2–3 years. Gold loans and shares also helped us stay afloat.

Over the years you must be smart enough to study your goals, review them, *modify them to grow* with the changing trends, lest we miss the boat.

It is natural to slow down over the years with age and even more so if you are all by yourself. How to overcome this phase? Involve young minds—young, energetic plastic surgeons who are filled with more energy and positivity in your practice. What I am trying to focus on now is teamwork. For example, when we plan a lipoabdominoplasty for a patient, I propose a team of two to do the initial liposuction followed by a team of two for flap elevation, repair and dermolipectomy and the last team to do the meticulous suturing. In case of additional problems such as incisional hernia or intra-abdominal adhesions, I involve another team of general surgeons to handle it. With evolving healthcare system in India, group practice in a full-fledged facility with surgical intensive care is going to be the norm and for us the surgeons, peace of mind at the end of the procedure. *So our goal should be to form a team of like-minded and passionate colleagues to share and support.*

We should also have a proper referral system to clinical nutritionist, bariatric surgeon, dermatologist, etc., for a comprehensive management of the patient.

MARKETING GOALS

A fully satisfied patient will refer another. This is a typical word of mouth referral and it takes time. Rational marketing is crucial to success of the business.

Investing in marketing services can be expensive but is inevitable. Visibility and presence in the Internet and digital media help visibility in the search engines. Honest feedback is a stepping-stone in the progress of the center. Digital marketing as well as the display boards has limitations in displaying the product, as our product is—the before/after results of procedures. It should be modestly displayed that is acceptable to the public and within the legal framework. Exposure of body parts and revealing patient's identity have legal and moral implications. It is always better to show your own patient's postprocedural results while concealing their identity rather than an unrealistic result available on the Internet.

Informal meetings in social clubs, ladies clubs, etc., will help spread the message and allow you to display your personality and build relationship with people.

The expanding patient referral system is the key to a successful practice and there are many ways of doing it, e.g., asking patients to give testimonials and directly requesting them to spread awareness.

A monthly or quarterly review of the system of marketing should be in place to assess the efficacy.

PRACTICE GOALS

Quality care includes efficient team for coordinated work, efficient communication with the patient, well-synchronized patient flow, efficient protocols and administrative management.

Once the patient reaches the center, the workflow efficiency should get the patient to the doctor as early as possible. Efficient front office personal should be able to coordinate with the doctor and patients to prevent unnecessary delays and reduce pressure on doctors.

Effective communication is the prime step in establishing the trust between doctor and patient. Patient listening, spending adequate time in explaining the procedure, outcomes, possible complications and the inevitable scars should be very clearly explained preferably with visuals.

Well-tuned protocols for each step in the management entail a foolproof smooth completion of the procedure. For example, in cosmetic surgery when the decision is made for a procedure on a particular date and time, the sequence of laboratory investigations, anesthesia assessment and arranging the anesthesiologist, preparing the room and OR, consent preparation—all these steps should progress smoothly and sequentially without any undue delay.

SURGICAL GOALS

Surgical goals include safe and successful outcome of the patient not only on short term but also long term. This is an era of lifestyle modification targeting a good quality of life, both in health as well as in style—body figure helps to achieve long-term sustainable outcome.

There should be protocols in place for preoperative assessment, intraoperative period and postoperative period to ensure safe and successful outcome.

GOALS THAT WILL HELP TO PROGRESS

A periodic review of our work, finances, manpower and targets for a specified period is an essential step to evaluate ones performance. Once the system is in place and work is progressing, this process will help us think in the lines of expansion either within the center or outside.

There is going to be maintenance and upgrading of the civil, mechanical, electrical and technical gadgets. About 25% of the profit should be reinvested to maintain the center. The goal should be to expand gradually rather than impulsively. For example, if it is an exclusive surgical facility, try to add nonsurgical technologies that do not require you to work hands on.

Expanding to other cities has its own challenges and it requires extensive homework, extra hours of work and huge investment. On the other hand, if your partner with like-minded plastic surgeons who can invest, partner and associate with you it helps overcome many challenges.

Yet another model is franchising, but that may be too much for a beginner and may not work out as expected due to its own sets of problems.

It is good to have goals prioritized. The first priority goal is always making the first center a successful model.

SETTING GOALS IN TRAINING

Establishing a successful system requires ongoing training and learning for all nurses, doctors and rest of the management team. Whenever a new idea is conceived, have clear protocols to follow, and that should become part of the teaching modules in the future. Each protocol needs evaluation and updating on a regular basis. Involve senior doctors and staff who have seen and established good protocols so that there is a regular teaching system in your center. This training program is very important for the specialty to grow at the same time helps the center to have good recognition in the society.

13.2 Expanding your Practice

Manoj Khanna

INTRODUCTION

The career of a doctor has limitations with regard to time. In spite of your busiest efforts, it is not possible to work more than 10–12 hours a day consistently for more than 5–6 days in a week and may be 250–300 days in a year. When one's expertise and goodwill exceeds this time limitation, it may be necessary to plan growth in both the vertical and horizontal directions.

It is at this juncture in the career of a doctor that he/she has to think of introducing the concept of corporate culture into his/her practice. But this is not an easy procedure and has many pros and cons which have to be evaluated before taking the bold step.

While vertical growth is more controllable and under one's direct control and supervision, horizontal expansion needs provision of corporate culture with proper manpower and management to achieve properly encoded standard operating procedures (SOPs) to achieve proper success.

VERTICAL EXPANSION

As mentioned earlier, it is the easier of the two components of growth as it is directly under your control and supervision. Additional facilities can be added to your practice and competent surgeons added to your faculty to improve the output of the center where you are working. Although it is not humanly possible to do every surgical step of every procedure, you can train your personnel, including consultants registrars and paramedics to execute some steps which are routine that can be achieved by practice and supervision.

But this process of vertical expansion needs supervision and guidance over the entire unit to be able to replicate the same results which have given you your stature and goodwill. This is a time-consuming affair and needs a proper check at each and every step. It is only then you can leave certain steps of the procedure to your subordinates in order to be able to churn out more volume of work in the same possible maximum available time and thereby create growth. Of course, certain critical and vital steps of every procedure must be carried out by you to be able to avoid flaws in the results. This is even more challenging when procedures are done under local anesthesia where the patient is awake and on the lookout for your presence. Procedures such as hair transplant, injection of Botox and fillers, laser hair removal, peels and other cosmetic procedures, e.g., scar revisions necessitate your presence in the surgical room almost all the time if demanded by the patient. Many patients demand that you do the entire procedure which can also be a speed breaker in your daily routine and a hurdle to your time management.

Additionally, you must have well-trained staff for postoperative care. Although the steps are routine for every patient and can be done by your staff, it may be necessary to give your personal time, however little, to each of these postoperative cases for their satisfaction. Proper time management is of utmost importance. Space permitting, it is better to have two or more rooms that allow you to speed up the consultations and follow-ups without wasting time in bringing the patient in and out of the consultation room. I remember late Dr Gus Colon in New Orleans using six different rooms for consultation and postoperative visits where he would move fluently from one station to the next and thereby saving a lot of time in executing his services. Similarly, well-trained staff with affixed protocol can save a lot of time between procedures on a busy operative day. It was amazing to see Dr Constantino Mendieta in Miami finished a procedure and started the next one in the same OR within 9 minutes. Extubation of the patient, shifting to the trolley, evacuation of the patient from the OR, cleaning the OR, bringing in the next patient, antiseptic dressing and draping followed by intubation—all were done within in the stipulated 9 minutes. This needed a lot of practice and coordination, but can be achieved with proper time sense and responsibility by different members of the staff.

Vertical expansion can also be done by adding consultants to your practice. Of course, all of these should be well qualified and have enough surgical expertise to maintain the reputation of your clinic and practice. There can be different areas of expertise of various consultants and their experience and efficiency could be an attractive feature for your clinic or hospital. But this also needs careful screening while appointing these consultants and also needs a vigilant eye at least during the initial period to ensure that your standard and reputation is maintained. You also need a good back office to maintain all records, treatments done, pictures before and after, and all other clinical material required for future records and also medicolegal records. Moreover, you also need a strong billing system to avoid any loss of revenue or misappropriation of funds which is possible in a big setup.

Doing all of these may sound easy, but there are many practical problems. You might encounter consultants and staff eating into your practice and taking your patients away or find leakage of funds at various points in the system. Your reputation could be at stake for any errors committed by your consultants or juniors that will directly tarnish your reputation.

HORIZONTAL EXPANSION

Unfortunately, a doctor cannot be a businessman while he is running a full time practice. Either the doctor becomes a businessman by curtailing his medical practice or appoints others to take care of the business while you can still pursue your medical practice. This is the biggest challenge for any medical practitioner looking at horizontal expansion.

Horizontal expansion begins with the opening of new clinics which can be in your own city or elsewhere, depending on the demand of the specialty.

Horizontal management needs much more business acumen and management skills. It needs to include a corporate culture in your practice and it is essential to have a corporate office with proper staff to look into different centers in different cities.

- A CEO (chief executive officer) with an assistant if the chain is big
- A CFO (chief financial officer) with his team to take care of finance
- HR (human resources) with their team to recruit people in different specialties and centers
- CRM (customer relationship management) to take care of relationship with patients and their management

- Marketing head with the team to look into to all purchases and expenditure along with advertising and promotions.

This setup itself incurs a significant expenditure and has to be maintained from the income of all the clinics in different locations. Also, you need to appoint personnel at different positions with proper scrutiny and meticulousness as "a single bad fish can rot the pond."

Expansion has to be planned with proper setup and locations must be identified properly before venturing into new clinics. In any new location, one must study the geographical needs of the area and the venue to where you want to open a new clinic. Good interior work in alignment with the quality of all the other clinics must be supervised and proper equipment and the correct staff must be recruited. It is essential to have someone responsible for a particular clinic which usually is a clinic manager with the team of people. Having obtained the appropriate machinery required for the clinic it is now essential to employ well-trained doctors who can look after the facilities to be provided at that center and also generate revenue to sustain it. It is important to remember that any new clinic needs at least 6 months to be able to break even and one must have patience during this period to be able to reap good dividends. There must be a reporting system where the head office is informed about the daily activities of the clinic and its revenue as the chances of leakage are very high in the sites which are away from your direct supervision. You must install CCTV in all clinics, especially those away from your city which can be monitored by you regularly. This is also important to remember that registration in different states in India has to be done individually and all licenses and permissions must be procured before beginning such centers. It is important to display clear signs that the facility is under CCTV security and avoid cameras in places of examination which can affect the privacy of the patient as it is deemed illegal.

The challenges of the horizontal chain of the clinic include maintenance of identical standards, retention of staff, prevention of pilferage and revenue losses and continue effort to advertise and promote to attract clients to sustain the clinic. All this needs a lot of business skill and has to be left to others, including your CEO to look after and manage. It is important to maintain patience while you trying to break even as some centers may take up to 1 year to be profitable. Many a time expenses such as depreciation and other hidden costs are overlooked, leading to a much lower income than what you see in the balance sheet.

Once your clinic has started generating positive revenue you also have to build a corpus for that particular clinic for further expansion and new equipment being able to sustain itself with changes to compete in the market. All these need a lot of business acumen.

CONCLUSION

I think it is best for doctors to acquire some business skills by reading, or getting some qualification before venturing into this field which can be a burden on your time, taxes a lot of your intellect and may provide revenue but has the risk of giving you a lot of stress and strain. Probably it is best done by someone who enjoys a challenge of opening a chain and running it successfully rather than looking at its financial returns.

It is difficult for one to be a successful doctor and a successful businessman at the same time and one aspect will suffer for the other whenever given more preference. It is of utmost importance to find the right people in every department to have vertical or horizontal expansions. You must have enough finances when you begin the expansion, there will be setbacks and situations where not all centers or even sections will throwback money and you will have to compensate that loss by profit in other sectors.

TIPS AND PEARLS

- Vertical expansion is easier and more under direct control than horizontal expansion.
- Ensure quality staff at all the levels to provide results equivalent to your standards and the patient's expectations. Personal intermittent supervision is essential to maintain the reputation of your brand.
- Horizontal expansion, especially beyond your station of work needs corporate management, and an administrative team is essential.
- Business acumen and knowledge is vital for horizontal expansion and be willing to be a businessman, although it is very difficult to be a good doctor and a good businessman.
- Know your limits and do not take more in your plate than you can eat.

13.3 Facial Esthetic Plastic Surgery: A Business Perspective

Ashish Davalbhakta

INTRODUCTION

Facial esthetic surgery is a subspecialty by itself. It has grown by leaps and bounds in the last two decades due to the technological advances and its innovative application to the problems people face.

Your facial esthetic practice should no longer be restricted to surgery and should encompass nonsurgical treatments as well. Surgical and nonsurgical treatments go hand in hand and are not absolute alternatives but are complementary to each other. Often, surgical therapy starts when nonsurgical ends. If the whole spectrum of treatment for a particular problem are not offered in the same clinic, there is a bias toward selling what you can offer and having disgruntled patients when the offered treatment does not show satisfactory results.

Another important service vertical is the wellness section. The wellness services include services, which maintain the health of the skin and prevent deterioration. Thus, a modern esthetic facial unit should have a facial esthetic surgery, facial nonsurgical cosmetology and wellness components.

SPECTRUM OF SERVICES

It is important at the start to prepare a comprehensive list of services and display the same in your clinic. It could be digital (as in the website) or running it on a TV screen or print (brochure). In the nonsurgical facial esthetic section, the list of services could include hair loss treatments, under eye dark circle reduction, skin pigmentation correction, antiaging treatments, sagging correction, acne and acne scars treatments, permanent LASER hair reduction services, skin glow treatments, etc. Facial esthetic surgery procedures can extend from hair transplant for baldness, eyelid tucks, facelifts, brow lifts, neck lift (platysmaplasty), rhinoplasty, ear setback, cheek and chin augmentation, dermabrasion, acne scar surgical treatments, fat grafting, double chin reduction, dimple creation, etc.

Facial rejuvenation service classically extends across the nonsurgical to surgical spectrum. The young need maintenance and preventive care—mostly facials, skin creams, regular exfoliation, hydration, and sun protection. A time comes when wrinkles become evident and needs Botulinum to reduce the wrinkles and prevent skin from thinning where it buckles the most. Hollowing or deflation happens with advancing age and needs filling. Once skin laxity sets in, nothing short of blepharoplasty, brow lift, facelift or neck lift works.

Cosmetic dentistry could become part of a facial esthetic service. A good set of teeth and a smile are part and parcel of facial esthetics. Investment in a dental chair and a tie-up with a dentist interested in cosmetic dentistry would be complementary to your practice.

As evident from above, there are many conditions that may be treatable with nonsurgical and surgical treatments. A patient of active acne may seek treatment for acne scars after his active acne has subsided. A patient being treated with Botulinum or fillers, may reach a stage where nonsurgical is no longer effective in delivering the desired result, and may be willing to consider blepharoplasty or facelift. Hence, it is essential to have the whole spectrum offered in your clinic. Referring a patient to somewhere else does not work. Patients who are bonded to you, or trust you, want to have all treatments under your care, even if you do not treat them yourself.

ESTHETIC PRACTICE VERSUS MEDICAL PRACTICE

Once you start your practice, the first issue would be awareness of your facial esthetic practice. For the esthetic practice, news about the clinic does not spread by word of mouth as easily it does for medical practice. People are hesitant to speak about their esthetic treatments, unlike any other medical services. To hope that your happy patient will help grow your practice exponentially may be disappointing in esthetic practice. Hence, there is a need to market and be visible to people.

FACIAL ESTHETIC PATIENTS AND HOW THEY DIFFER FROM OTHERS

A facial esthetic patient is one who looks at himself in the mirror a lot, or is in the habit of having his or her pictures taken. She has observed changes in the face or noticed something which he or she feels needs to be rectified. He or she may be obsessed and if they are, they will be hard to please. Their expectations could be high and their expectations will have to be met to satisfy them. At the consultation before surgery, these traits will have to be recognized and their expectations should be rationalized.

Most facial esthetic patients want improvements with minimum downtime. They are unwilling to accept any scars, bruises or swelling from the procedure. They have to be explained in clear terms what to expect, so they can plan their post-treatment activities. Often, they do not realize this and have an important appointment, or engagement to go to, and can get upset if they bruise or swell.

A facial esthetic patient may come with a request to look good but not be sure what exactly they want or will make them look good. They often say, "you are the doctor, you tell what I need". This is a trap to avoid. It shows the patient is not clear and if you tell them what would help them look better, there is a probability that they may still not like the change and blame you for it.

I have often had requests from some youngsters to change their look completely so that they are unrecognizable. On close questioning, they reveal that they want this so that their partners' family does not recognize them. I try to dissuade such patients. Their expectations are unrealistic. Be wary of any patient who has a request that you feel is unrealistic to meet. Often, I see patients who have a particularly minor issue, that is hard to see on examination. I do give them time, take photographs and load them up on the computer, analyze to see if there is something not esthetically right in terms of ratios and proportions and if I find nothing wrong, I will dissuade the patient from having anything done.

Facial esthetic patients will also not want their identity revealed. So, they are hesitant to allow their pictures to be taken or used for promotional activities. I make it absolutely compulsory to have pre- and post-photos taken for each and every patient, however they are kept for records only. A consent form is filled in and often most patients will not mind if their photos are used for medical and educational purposes. For those you are offering discounts, it could be on a precondition to allow use of their photos for marketing. Often patients may be willing to sign a consent form for marketing use of their pictures, in lieu of a discount.

LEADS AND CONVERSION OF LEADS

Due to this difference in esthetic practice and medical practice, a facial esthetic physician should implement modern marketing and sales principles in his practice, especially if he or she wants to have a busy facial esthetic practice. An inquiry becomes a random lead. If you feel you can help that person, it becomes a potential lead. Getting that lead to your clinic and a consultation takes consistent, sustained effort and interaction. After a consultation and after you have explained a treatment plan, that lead becomes a prospect. The sales team has to now chip in and handhold the prospect till he signs up for treatment. Only after the patient pays for treatment can he be labeled as conversion. In esthetic practice, this process is long drawn out and it is worthwhile in setting up a system to handle this. It has to be automated and will ensure a steady stream of conversions in your clinic.

HOW TO INCREASE CONVERSIONS IN CLINIC

Converting a facial esthetic prospect is an art. There are various techniques to do that and are covered elsewhere in this book. However, from a clinician's standpoint, a proper thorough consultation is the first step. To come across as genuine, honest, knowledgeable and willing to give time to understand what the patient really wants is the key. Giving ample time for consultation, answering all their queries goes a long way in building a lasting impression.

A morphing software of some sort, either 2D or 3D helps in communicating with the patient better and helps them understand what change is possible. It helps them understand what to expect and reduces the fear of the unknown. If they like what they see, they will most likely sign up quickly. I use it for rhinoplasty or nose reshaping the most. Often, facial restructuring such as chin augmentation, cheek augmentation can be morphed fairly well. Even the change possible with fillers can be communicated well.

Having a database of pre- and post-operated patient's photos to show to prospects helps them see the results you are likely to deliver. It will improve their confidence. Hence, it is important for a facial esthetic physician to learn the art of documenting all patients with good photographs.

A past patient chatting with the prospect and explaining how smooth or easy the process was in the postconsultation phase is also very useful.

It is a natural tendency of patients to opt for nonsurgical treatments. I believe if properly counseled at the consultation, they can be guided to the most appropriate treatment for themselves. The facial esthetic surgeon should not look like he has a bias for surgical over another nonsurgical, but be able to point out the pros and cons of surgical over nonsurgical properly. Often when explained the limited duration of the improvement with nonsurgical treatments, patients tend to go for surgical treatments which have long-lasting improvements. Showing them photographs of patients who have undergone nonsurgical and surgical treatments can also point out the subtle improvement with nonsurgical and significant improvement that can be achieved by surgical. This helps them choose surgical if they do want a significant improvement.

STRUCTURE OF A FACIAL ESTHETIC SURGERY PRACTICE

As mentioned earlier, the facial esthetic practice is different from a medical practice. Although we as doctors run it, they cannot be perceived as medical units. People, who come to a facial esthetic unit, although we might call them patients, are not ill. They are fit people like you and I and feel vain when they see seriously ill patients seeking your advice and care. It would be wise to segregate these two receptions or practices completely. As a corollary, a soothing, peaceful ambience, pleasant, friendly and caring staff works well to make esthetic patients feel welcome.

Having a day surgical unit/or an operating suite incorporated in the facial esthetic practice is a huge advantage. A lot of facial esthetic procedures can be done as a day surgical procedure. Blepharoplasties, scar revisions, mole excisions, under chin or cheek fat liposuctions, hair transplants, even rhinoplasties, chin and cheek augmentations, in ASA type I patients can be done as a day surgery. The revenue model of the day surgery unit is far better than a simple clinic.

It would be better if the front desk/customer care executive are from the hospitality background. It takes customer service to the next level. They understand what customer service means as it is ingrained in their basic training.

Although you might have ANM/GNM nurses to help in the surgical patients care, therapist in the cosmetology section, should be preferably Cidesco trained or from parlor background. Laser hair reduction service, electroporation, assisting in peels, cryotherapy application, facials, assisting in mesotherapy are some of the services which they can do very well. Their skills in preparing the room for a treatment, or facial massage skills come handy and give a nice touch to a facial esthetic practice.

A patient coordinator will be a very important part of your practice. A one-point contact for all your patients. It would be nice if this coordinator receives the lead on the first visit and escorts the lead from the reception through every step of consultation, then stays in touch with the prospect, through the sales process and finally after conversion. A friendly face, who will handhold the patient through his or her treatment. You will find these patients, who have taken treatment years ago, first contacting this coordinator when they wish to come back for further treatments.

A marketing and sales manager is important as these two elements are a 24 × 7 pursuit. Such positions in the health industry are hard to come by. Hence, they have to be recruited from the industry, and then trained.

A practice manager with good administrative skills, HR skills and some accounting skills should be able to look after the rest. As the practice grows, it might be possible to look for a specialist in each of these fields.

EQUIPMENT OR TOOLS IN A FACIAL ESTHETIC CLINIC

An examination/facial couch which can double up for injection of Botulinum or fillers good overhead spotlight is a must in each and every therapy room.

Photographic equipment is mandatory. Facial analytic software, 2D/3D morphing software studio lighting are optional but useful.

Laser for hair reduction, whether diode, long pulse ND Yag or IPL and Q switch Nd Yag for pigmentation treatment are helpful adjuncts. Finally, either a CO_2, or Erbium Yag/Erbium Glass ablative laser for skin and scar resurfacing can add value too.

Electroporation or sonoporation devices to help driving mesotherapy cocktails, or vitamin C into the dermis. Microdermabrasion, or hydrotherapy devices that help in polishing the skin can be added based on patient demand. Skin tightening devices such as radiofrequency or high-intensity focused ultrasound are useful for sagging facial skin.

WELLNESS

Wellness is defined as the state of being in good health, especially as an actively pursued goal. Wellness is an active process of becoming aware of and making choices toward a healthy and fulfilling life. This active process to keep facial skin and structure healthy needs to be emphasized in your clinic. Patients/clients need to be educated that they should actively/consciously work toward maintaining their facial skin health. Regular use of exfoliants, moisturizers, sunscreens, intermittent peels, nutritional supplements are necessary for maintaining the skin health. Radiofrequency skin tightening or platelet-rich plasma (PRP) facials to remodulate healthy elastic collagen and boosting the skin from time to time, adds to the preventive maintenance program of the skin's health. Adding this perspective to your clinic makes your facial esthetic service complete.

SUMMARY

The modern facial esthetic practice has changed considerably. There is a need to incorporate best business practices with best clinical skills. Just relying on one without the other does not work. A concerted effort is needed to develop and maintain a facial esthetic practice. A lot of emphasis has to be given to lead capturing, conversion, patient satisfaction and overall customer service. Your constant endeavor has to be to make every patient an evangelist, who will voluntarily talk and praise your services to others.

13.4 Building a Rhinoplasty Practice

Kapil S Agrawal

INTRODUCTION

Although rhinoplasty is a common plastic surgery procedure performed worldwide, it is considered a challenging one. Rhinoplasty is not so difficult for a qualified plastic surgeon to perform, but it is extremely difficult to produce consistently good results.

HOW TO GET RHINOPLASTY TRAINING AND DEVELOP SKILLS?

During the residency program, rhinoplasty exposure is limited and to be proficient in it requires a lot of ongoing learning and experience.

- *Learning the basics (training):* After acquiring the board certification in plastic surgery one must concentrate on one's field of interest and try to gain knowledge of the subject by:
  - Thorough reading of rhinoplasty texts and updates
  - Understanding the anatomy and functional physiology of nose
  - Actively assisting or observing a master rhinoplasty surgeon
- *Develop rhinoplasty skills by:*
  - Watching edited videos
  - Attending video or live operative workshops
  - Hands on cadaveric dissection to get acquainted with the original anatomy, planes and feel of tissue as well as practice of opening the nose, performing the crucial steps and then closure to the perfection
  - Keep analyzing the nose of people around, find the problems, make a plan and do mock surgeries in mind.

Before starting your practice, attend fellowship programs and spend some time with rhinoplasty surgeons to learn the intricacies.

HOW TO CHOOSE YOUR PRACTICE?

If you have economic support or an existing family run clinic or hospital, it is an easier path. Those who do not, need to know their options.

Types of Practice

- Institutional
  - Public hospital
  - Private hospital
- Own practice
  - Solo (nursing home/day care center)
  - Partnership (medium size plastic surgery or multispecialty hospital)
- Freelancing.

If your primary interest is academics, you may choose a medical college or public hospital to start your career. Others may choose to do private practice.

The options are multiple but you have to choose according to your area (locality) of practice and economic support. In my opinion, freelancing is a better option to begin with, it allows you to provide your services to multiple centers/hospitals, reduces financial burden and stress of managing a center in the beginning of the career. Once you have more exposure and experience, you can then choose to start your own center or hospital or you may seek partnership.

When you begin your practice, choose simple cases to avoid complications. On the other hand, you may not have any control on the type of cases you get and may not be able to refuse difficult cases. The caveat is attempting difficult cases and having failures will negatively affect your practice. The solution is to find an experienced rhinoplasty mentor who can help manage these cases.

There are two ways to accomplish this:
1. Either mentor operates in your facility with you assisting or
2. Elect to operate in your mentor's OR.

Few questions you may have at this point:

1. What are the simple cases to start with?
For a beginner, correction of minor irregularities of dorsum, be it depression or bony hump, are the best cases to start with.

2. Open versus closed—is it necessary to learn both techniques?
One must be a master of one of the two approaches and should be well acquainted with the other too. Acquaintance with other approach while pursuing one gives you an opportunity to treat patients on its merit. Sometimes a difficult case which you start with closed approach may need to be converted into open and on the other hand, one of the patients may demand a closed approach while you feel comfortable using open approach. For a beginner, open rhinoplasty is the best to start with as it gives a chance to understand the anatomy and intricacies of all deformities and an opportunity to correct it precisely.

3. When to say no? How to recognize an unsuitable patient?
- Patient with unrealistic expectations is always a bad candidate
- Patients with very thick and sebaceous skin demanding a very slim nose with sharp tip
- Patients showing photos of any model or film star and demanding a nose similar to him or her
- Patients having esthetic and functional problems for which open approach is necessary but asking no change either in shape of the tip or dorsum, which is not possible while using open approach
- Anything that you believe is beyond your capacity should better be denied.

4. Secondary rhinoplasty—at what stage of practice to attempt?
Once you feel comfortable doing different types of primary deformities and getting consistently good results that is the time you can attempt simple secondary deformities such as mild depression or irregularity of dorsum or tip.

A big question is—is it possible to balance rhinoplasty with all other cosmetic procedures, or eventually will you be a rhinoplasty surgeon alone?

Answer is yes; it is possible to balance different cosmetic procedures along with rhinoplasty.

However, if the surgeon has developed an efficient team, and is giving consistently good results satisfying oneself and the patients and, even the colleagues have developed faith, so much that they refer lots of rhinoplasty cases then it is better to concentrate only in rhinoplasty.

HOW TO PROJECT YOURSELF AS A SPECIALIST RHINOPLASTY SURGEON?

There are many ways to promote yourself as a rhinoplasty surgeon:
- Brochures/photo album/banners/display TV screen with before and after results in

the waiting room educate patient in the waiting room. However, ensure you have permission/consent by the patient to allow display of his/her pictures.
- Distribute the brochures and related information to colleagues and general practitioners in the city.
- Social media presence is a must these days
  - Website
  - Facebook page, Twitter, blog writing
  - You tube videos
- Print and electronic media—articles regarding public awareness.

STAFF RECRUITMENT AND TEAM BUILDING

In private clinic, you must have a well-groomed receptionist-cum-clinic manager who is trained to manage the clinic, counsel the patients and answer all enquiries on web and phone. An additional technical staff is required for documentation, record maintenance and managing clinical photographs and videos. You have to build an operating team with the good assistant surgeon, qualified operation theater (OT) nurses and competent anesthetists. In a hospital setup, you need resident doctors, ward nurses and other support staff to manage the patient in wards.

OTHER ESSENTIALS

Your qualifications, fellowship and membership certifications mentioning your interest and training in rhinoplasty must be displayed in your office for your prospective patients.

Having fixed surgical packages for certain types of deformities attracts patients and alleviates their worry of being overcharged. It is important to have a proper indemnity cover for yourself and an insurance cover for the clinic/hospital. Hire a chartered accountant to know your taxes and liabilities. It is wise to invest your profit prudently.

INSTRUMENTS AND EQUIPMENT

Irrespective of type of practice, you must have a complete personalized set of rhinoplasty instruments. Rhinoplasty usually does not need complex equipment except a rhinoscope for the surgeons who are trained in doing rhinoscopy and septal modifications using scopes. Apart from instruments, you must have a 2X or 2.5X loupes and fiberoptic headlight.

WHAT SHOULD BE THE PROTOCOL WHEN YOU START RHINOPLASTY PRACTICE?

One must follow a standard protocol before taking the patient to OT:
- *Proper consultation with the patient:* Minimum two consultations or if possible, three consultations are needed to understand the psyche of the patient. It gives the same opportunity to the patient to understand you and your plans. Write down desires of the patient and analytical points obtained by you on clinical examination.
- *Preoperative photo analysis (homework):* This step is the most important of all. With the advent of digital photography, the things have become very easy. All standard views must be taken.

Frontal, lateral, oblique, basal, "Text-neck view" and smiling view. The best analysis of the nose is done with the help of these preoperative photographs. Photographic analysis is the best way to train one's eyes to analyze clinical deformities. Photographic documentation also helps during surgery and later as medicolegal evidence.

- *Operative plan:* Writing out a step-by-step operative plan against the analyzed and documented clinical deformities is mandatory and helps for future references.
- *Execution:* Operative plan and preoperative photos must always be put in the OT for reference during surgery. Intraoperative photos and videography of crucial steps must be done. Before final closure, photographs must be taken in lateral, basal and cephalic views to assess the nasolabial, nasofrontal and nasofacial angles, dorsum, dorsal esthetic lines, symmetry of nostrils, projection of tip and to ensure all deformities are corrected.
- *Follow-up:* Regular follow-up in postoperative period not only takes care of the patient but also gives an opportunity to learn from our mistakes. The process improves our experience. Observing the healing pattern of the patient allows us to counsel them regarding the swelling and changes in the nose shape over time.
- *Revisions:* Residual deformities or a poor result may need revision surgery. These failures are a great teacher. We must take this opportunity as a learning experience.

KEY MESSAGES

- The willingness to always learn, work hard, be honest toward profession as well as patients and a commitment to excellence are critical in the evolution of a rhinoplasty surgeon.
- Much more can be written on this topic but due to space constraints the author has penned his experiences in brief and hopes that upcoming surgeons would find it useful in the process of building their rhinoplasty practice.

BIBLIOGRAPHY

1. Agrawal K, Raghav S. Management of complications of Medpor® implants in rhinoplasty. Plast Aesthet Res. 2017;4:54-6.
2. Agrawal KS, Pabari M, Shrotriya R. A refined technique for management of nasal flaring: the quest for the holy grail of alar base modification. Arch Plast Surg. 2016;43(6):604-7.
3. Agrawal KS, Sandeep S, Shrotriya R. Text-neck view: a new photographic tool for assessment of nasal dorsum in crooked noses. Plast Reconstr Surg. 2016;138(1):165e-167e.
4. Agrawal KS, Shrotriya R. Ossified costal cartilage during rhinoplasty: a surgical dilemma. Indian J Plast Surg. 2015;48:327-8.
5. Daniel RK. Mastering Rhinoplasty. New York: Springer; 2004.
6. Tardy ME Jr. Rhinoplasty: The art and the science. Philadelphia, Pennsylvania: WB Saunders Company; 1997.

13.5 Body Contouring Practice

Milan Doshi, Aditya N Patil

INTRODUCTION

The pursuit of "ideal" body shape is not new to mankind. From the temples of Khajuraho to the paintings and sculptures of Michelangelo and Leonardo da Vinci, the aspiration for body shape is evident throughout history. What has changed, however, is the concept of "ideal". In the past, a voluptuous female was considered desirable whereas being thin and lean is the thing of today.

Multiple factors such as the advent of social media, an improving economy and an increase in popularity and acceptance of bariatric surgeries among the public have led to an increase in awareness regarding body contouring in developing countries such as India.

In the past, apart from sporadic reports, there were very few standardized techniques, which could be reproduced reliably. During the later part of the 20th century, many significant events took place in the field of body contouring. Of note were the standard abdominoplasty as described by Pitanguy and (dry) liposuction that was described by Illouz. Modifications in techniques (wet, superwet and tumescent infiltration) and devices (power, laser and ultrasound-assisted devices) were described in the years to come. The advent of laparoscopic surgery has added a new lot of patients for body contouring after massive weight loss in the recent years.

Research is on a furious pace in this field and almost every other day, more and more medications and nonsurgical methods of body contouring are being described. These advances create confusion and apprehension between both the doctor and the patient. At the same time, it has also become inevitable for the modern-day cosmetic surgeon to be equipped and well versed with these procedures. A detailed discussion on different techniques is beyond the scope of this chapter. It is also important to know the intricate details of setting up a cosmetic center, which have been dealt with elsewhere. This chapter attempts to talk about developing a practice in body contouring while touching upon the newer aspects of the trade.

BODY CONTOURING SCENARIO

Understanding the need of people is the most important step in setting up your practice. Every person desires to have a healthy life and a perfect figure. The first approach is through diet and exercise. If the desired result is not achieved, one wishes for a quick fix by visiting a specialist. These specialists may also include unqualified practitioners. Most of the people tend to choose a nonsurgical approach to begin with and only a few of these patients move up the "ladder" to consent for surgical intervention, which thus represents only the tip of the iceberg as far as demand for body contouring is concerned. People tend to avoid cosmetic surgeons as they consider surgical options more intimidating and expensive so they approach practitioners who claim to treat them nonsurgically.

The esthetic plastic surgeon is at the helm to provide body-contouring services, and if surgery remains the only focus, the opportunities to get other prospective patients who are lower down the "ladder" are missed out. Hence, doing body-contouring practice with the entire setup can set you apart from the competitors. This will also help people to approach you asking for treatment options expecting that you would offer all possible options without bias toward surgery.

To setup a successful body-contouring practice, one must focus on the following aspects.

Essential Tools

- *The setup:* First impressions are quite often the last impression. Indeed, one's expertise and results will not even matter if one is not able to "attract prospective patients". Patients desiring body contouring—and any other esthetic procedure for that matter—tend to have a preconceived notion about the plastic surgeon and their "surgical" office. Body-contouring clinic should have some distinct features for it to attract patients/

clients looking for slimming procedures. The office should preferably be located in a prime location, free from noise and other distractions. The decor should be clean, organized and well lit. The first contact person, usually the receptionist, should not only be polite and friendly, but also be able to answer initial queries or, at the very least be able to direct the patient to such a person. Having a television screen in the waiting room displaying "before and after" pictures of commonly performed body- contouring procedures and patient testimonials help in "priming" the patient and generating confidence. The doctor is expected to be well-dressed, calm, confident and a good listener.

Once the client/patient attends your office, the underlying motive for body contouring is important to be identified, as is the commitment of the patient toward treatment and post-treatment compliance. Warning signs, e.g., unrealistic goals and expectation of a guarantee are indicators of underlying psychological disorders such as body dysmorphic disorder or simply lack of knowledge and understanding.

Once the goals are identified, you should then explain the options with their pros and cons and help the patient make an informed decision. If it is a nonsurgical option that the client/patient chooses, then ensure a qualified and trained practitioner applies the treatment modalities with strict protocols that will help achieve some results. If it is a surgical option only qualified doctors in a daycare center or in a hospital setup should give body-contouring services. The patient needs to be explained that many of these procedures can be done under local anesthesia and can be discharged on the same day. Major surgeries such as mega liposuctions, major excision surgeries or bariatric surgeries should preferably be operated in a hospital with adequate backup.

It cannot be emphasized enough that safety and privacy of the patient are paramount, while also ensuring that the entire experience is a pleasant one.

Marketing is an important part of an esthetic setup and is always beneficial as long as it is done in good taste. Overarching claims and "100% guarantees" have to be avoided. Offering the entire spectrum of procedures and services under one roof is essential to retain the patient. Frequent vacations and absence should be avoided, at least in the initial days of practice.

- *Diagnosis:* All clients approaching for weight loss, slimming or body-contouring procedures should be treated with strict medical protocols. A thorough medical history will help identify the cause of the problem. A standard physical examination and general workup of every patient remains the essential. With respect to body contouring, analyzing the percentage of body fat and other components is useful not only to plan a procedure but also to monitor effect of treatment. If the patient is made conscious about the extent of the problem, their compliance to treatment will increase.

  Once a diagnosis is established, you can help prepare a treatment plan for the patient be it nonsurgical or surgical.

- *Nonsurgical treatments:*
  - *Medical line:* It is important to have a thorough knowledge of what is available in the market with their pros and cons. This will help you explain the patient well and will help you gain their confidence on you and your

practice. Lets have a look at what is available.
- Newer drugs such as sibutramine and orlistat have been approved in parts of the world, but their role in body contouring is yet to be ascertained. Metformin has also been used for weight loss. Appetite suppressant drugs, *isabgol,* herbal and Ayurvedic drugs are available and marketed for their role in weight loss, but their effect is controversial and is not without complications.
- Fillers and volumizers like Macrolane can be used to augment limited areas following surgery and are even useful for a "touch-up" or fine-tuning.
- Newer generation FDA approved drugs, e.g., Kybella (deoxycholic acid) can be used for localized lipolysis for correction of minor deformities.

- *Device-based (noninvasive):* The fear for surgery is real and is often the last resort for many patients. Consequently, and coupled with recent advances in science, the market is flooded with a myriad of devices and techniques. The application of these devices as a primary modality is limited, but they can provide good results in the motivated patient in combination with diet and exercise. They can also be used as adjuncts to a more definitive surgical procedure. It is always good to have at least a couple of such devices in the clinic.
  - U-lipo uses ultrasound energy, which is said to break down fat. It requires multiple sessions and is particularly useful to enhance recovery after surgery.
  - I-Lipo (Energist Ltd., UK) employs low-level laser energy and requires multiple sessions to have a demonstrable effect.
  - VelaShape III (Candela Corporation, USA) makes use of radiofrequency energy along with massage.
  - Cryolipo or CoolSculpting involves precise freezing of subcutaneous fat over multiple sessions.
  - High-intensity focused ultrasound (HIFU) is purported to break fat in very small areas and achieves minimal skin tightening.
  - Physiotherapy devices increase muscle mass and basal metabolic rate (BMR) for weight maintenance and for toning up the abdominal muscle postpregnancy or weight loss.

  There are occasions when patient insists on nonsurgical procedures due to apprehension to surgery, financial issues, etc. In such cases, offer no guarantee on the nonsurgical outcomes and offer them a discount if the patient subsequently wishes to go for surgery. In this way, the patient is satisfied of having tried the nonsurgical option and you do not lose the patient. In future, this same patient will turn up for surgery and will increase your footfall and reduces dependence on referrals. Once nonsurgical treatment options are also offered, your opinion as an expert will be valued more as compared to "beauty clinics" run by non-doctors who offer tall claims and less substance.
- *Surgical procedures:* This is where a plastic surgeon should be well-trained and skilled. You need to understand the

procedures thoroughly to be able to offer them these options.

- *Liposuction:* Liposuction is perhaps the most common surgical procedure performed for body contouring and can be used in almost every region of the body. The technique *per se* has a moderately low-learning curve and its results are fairly reproducible. The introduction of tumescence has further decreased the complications and allowed for "mega liposuctions" to be done.

  Liposuction is most useful when there is extra fat, but the overlying skin and underlying muscle are grossly normal. Smaller volumes can be suctioned under local anesthesia, but higher volumes (>500 mL) generally require general or regional anesthesia. "Mega liposuction" requires higher expertise and is safe if done cautiously in a hospital setup. In conjunction with a dietitian, physiotherapist and psychiatrist, this can be a moral booster for the young, healthy patient and can avoid excisional surgeries in the future.

  Following are some notable modifications developed overtime:
    - *Tumescent liposuction:* It is now considered as the gold standard and renders the procedure less traumatic.
    - *Mechanical liposuction:* This involves use of an oscillating or rotating cannula, which in return reduces surgeon fatigue and is more controlled.
    - *Laser liposuction:* Lasers of various wavelength have been used. This technique is useful for smaller areas, for example, double chin deformity. It also gives a better skin tightening effect.
    - *Ultrasound liposuction:* Ultrasound energy is said to selectively break fat with minimum damage to the surrounding structural tissue. The downside of this technique is the steeper learning curve and the higher risk of causing burns.
    - *Waterjet liposuction:* This technique entails injection of fluid injected with controlled pressure, which helps separate fat cells with relatively fewer traumas. Hence, it is believed to be useful for large volume fat harvest for buttock and breast augmentation.
    - *Radiofrequency liposuction:* It has the benefit of achieving better skin tightening.

  All the newer liposuction methods entail a higher cost and are useful for marketing. However, it is worth noting that similar or occasionally better results are achievable with the traditional liposuction which is much more cost-effective in the initial years of practice. The man behind the machine remains ultimately the most crucial factor.

- *Lipofilling:* Fat obtained from liposuction can be transferred to augment or sculpt other areas of the body such as the breast and buttocks. This additional advantage can go a long way in exceeding expectations set by a cosmetically inclined patient.

- *Excisional surgeries:* When the skin envelope is in excess or of a poor quality, excisional procedures may be a better option for body contouring. These can be combined with liposuction in adjacent areas and it also helps in homeostasis and faster recovery. Muscle tightening can also be done during surgery.

The abdomen is the most common region to be subjected to excisional treatment. Apart from standard abdominoplasty, the procedure can be tailored to fit the needs of the patient, viz., mini abdominoplasty for milder cases and extended lipoabdominoplasty for the more severe cases. Belt lipectomy or body lift can be considered depending on the amount of excess skin.

Other areas that are amenable to surgical correction are thighs (thighplasty or thigh lift), arms (brachyplasty), chest (upper body lift) and breast (breast lift).

- *Bariatric surgery:* Morbid obesity with associated metabolic syndromes and comorbidities call for evaluation for bariatric surgery for weight loss. Excess skin tissue after massive weight loss can then be tackled by various excisional surgeries. This group of surgeries completes the armamentarium to offer the best treatment to every patient. However, you need to refer the patient to a specialized bariatric surgeon who can perform it safely.

Other surgical procedures depend on the region of the body to be contoured. These techniques can be performed in isolation or combined with other surgical or nonsurgical techniques.

Exemplary Team

Body-contouring practice entails involvement of a multidisciplinary team apart from the cosmetic surgeon, depending on the needs and requirements of the patient.

Availability of multiple medical and paramedical specialists under one roof increases patient confidence and comfort. A good teamwork will improve results and credibility of the center and gives an edge compared to others. Science is ever-evolving and newer drugs, machines and procedures enter the market almost every other day. It is important to stay abreast with the latest developments to maintain the lead. A dedicated team goes a long way.

- *Bariatric surgeon*: In the treatment of obese and morbidly obese patients who require a more permanent solution.
- *Endocrinologist*: For evaluation of underlying hormonal disturbances such as hypothyroidism, polycystic ovary syndrome (PCOS), etc., which may have led to obesity or abnormal fat deposition.
- *Dietitian*: Indispensable, especially, in the management of obesity-related procedures. Dietary management is important in both the pre- and postoperative periods. In the preoperative period, the focus is on a balanced, reduced-calorie diet with an objective to produce a net calorie deficit to induce gradual weight loss. Dietary restriction continues in the postoperative period and is monitored regularly for long-term management.
- *Physiotherapist*: Postoperative physiotherapy is critical for a good outcome, early return to work and to prevent weight gain. Muscle building exercise and increasing the BMR will better help maintain weight than diet alone. A qualified therapist best handles nonsurgical lipolysis machines.
- *Psychiatrist and behavioral therapist:* This is an integral part of the treatment and ensures wholesome recovery of the patient after surgery. Behaviors that are contributing to the gain in fat should be

identified and, with the help of regular counseling, the patient needs to be made self-conscious about such behavior. Modification of such behavior is then attempted in a strategic manner.

Quintessential Patient

Body contouring largely remains an elective and subjective surgery, as there are no clearly defined indications or contraindications. However, for practical purposes, patients can be broadly categorized into four categories and the treatment varies accordingly.

Group 1—patients with normal or near-normal weight with good skin quality and muscle tone: These patients are generally motivated and are looking for removal of stubborn fat. They can benefit from liposuction or one of several nonsurgical methods described above.

Group 2—obese patients with good skin tone: Surgical procedures can drastically improve contour and motivate them toward a healthy lifestyle and to reduce weight further.

Group 3—postpregnancy or postmassive weight loss patients: This group of patients requires excision of extra skin and frequently muscle tightening as well.

Group 4—morbidly obese patient: It is not uncommon to find associated comorbidities in such patients. These patients require a truly multidisciplinary approach in the form of bariatric surgery, diet modification, exercise and behavioral therapy. One should approach such patients with caution and ensure that their demands are realistic.

A word of caution: Some patients have unrealistic expectations, which could be due to personal reasons, lack of education/awareness, underlying medical or anatomical condition, tall/false claims of others, if you feel the result is not achievable, it is better to stay away because it is better to be safe than sorry.

It is not uncommon to get a patient who "asks" for liposuction, but would actually benefit from an excisional surgery (abdominoplasty, belt lipectomy, etc.). In such cases, the patients have to be counseled about the benefits of the latter and factors such as muscle tone and skin excess, which would affect the final outcome. Counseling can be supported by "before and after" photos to alleviate the patient's apprehension. However, if the patient is still adamant, polite refusal is the best way forward to avoid long-term regret.

The true test of a physician's character is in the wake of complications and an unhappy patient. Avoid verbal retaliation, instead make yourself available, give them a patient hearing, stand by them and offer them your complete support. The patient will definitely feel comforted and develops a bond with you. Good intention and a positive attitude is what will set you apart from the competition.

SUMMARY

Fuelled by an increase in consciousness among people and professional expertise in body contouring surgery, new devices and machines are being developed and procedures being described everyday. However, irrespective of all the advances, a point to note is that it is not the machine itself, but the brain behind the one who operates it, that gives the best outcome. The future holds tremendous promise in this field with increased research in genetic modification and newer specific drugs. Patient selection, proper counseling and meticulous planning and execution are the key to obtain a desired outcome.

13.6 Building a Breast Surgery Practice: "Reconstructing" the Doctor-Patient Relationship

Neeta Patel

INTRODUCTION

Breasts embody the essence of womanhood and development of these secondary sexual organs at the onset of puberty initiates the awareness of femininity, transitioning into an innate sense of sexuality as she matures into a woman. Like the rest of the animal species, they are meant to provide primary nourishment to the infant and create the first bond between mother and child, but in humans, they also complete their identity as *a woman* throughout their life. The breasts signify femininity, beauty and significantly influence her body image and perception of self-worth. This is evident throughout history and modernity, in the fine arts, sculptures, cinema and the written works, eulogizing their grace and beauty.

Surgery of the breast, therefore, can be a very emotional experience for a woman. The emotions vary from feelings of insecurity, poor self-image and fear of rejection when removal is contemplated for disease, to hope and anticipation when done to enhance esthetic appeal. The physician, therefore, needs to be sensitive, caring and nonjudgmental during counseling, allaying her fears while simultaneously keeping her expectations within the realm of reality. The surgeon, though unbiased, must wear the mantle of friend, philosopher, guide and it cannot be emphasized enough that a humane approach to the patient can greatly assist in building trust in the long-term relationship between patient and doctor.[1]

UNDERSTANDING THE NEED OF YOUR PATIENT

Traditionally, it has always been assumed that the doctor plays the role of the consultant and treatment provider and the patient is always the eternal recipient. However, the doctor-patient relationship can be considered to span three types:
1. The *active-passive* model
2. The *guidance-cooperation* model
3. The *mutual participation* model[2]

The first model is suitable for emergencies and situations wherein the patient cannot be relied upon to give an informed consent due to the urgency to save life. The second model places the doctor in a higher position than that of the patient due to possession of medical knowledge, thus making him/her eligible to work in the patient's best interests.

However, it is the third model that is most suited toward building breast surgery practice. This model entails equal participation of doctor and patient because the patient is an "intelligent" entity having her own expectations and perceptions about the procedural outcome, while the doctor will integrate patient ideology in tailoring an outcome maximally suited to the expectations of the patient. In the end, though the satisfaction of both is ideally desired for best results that, of the patient must always take the priority.

In this regard, breast surgery can also straddle the fine line between the second and third models of the doctor-patient

relationship, as it comprises two aspects albeit with converging outcomes:
1. One, as part of cancer treatment/treatment of some underlying pathology with or without reconstruction
2. Two, breast surgery purely for esthetic reasons.

In the former, while considering surgery, the doctor, has superior knowledge of the possibility of postoperative disfigurement/asymmetry/recurrence. He must make the patient aware of the same in as gentle a manner, as is possible. It is imperative to understand that the patient cannot be "talked-down to" but is informed of these consequences well before hand and it is here that the four basic pillars of any surgical practice need to be enshrined, namely: trust, knowledge, regard and loyalty.[3]

These are often interdependent as trust is developed over time and requires sustained effort on the part of the surgeon, through effective communication of the knowledge he/she possesses in a way that will engender mutual regard between patient and surgeon. Here, the patient should be given every opportunity to air her concerns in a safe, nonjudgmental environment. Lastly, loyalty reflects in the surgeon "walking hand-in-hand" with the patient through the entire course of the treatment and not abandoning her at any stage. This significantly contributes to the patient perception of the surgeon as positive, dependable and honest, leading to reciprocal patient loyalty. In today's world of crumbling doctor-patient relationships, the onus lies with the physician to reinstate faith in the patient, through effective use of his/her emotional intelligence, as much healing is dependent on human contact. In this context, therefore, we deal with both aspects of plastic surgery herewith, describing their nuances in the following sections.

NEW TRENDS

Surgery on the breast purely for esthetic purpose is gaining footfall among women worldwide. This is due to factors that have to do with body-image, perceived appearance in society, enhanced self-worth, sexual satisfaction and other social factors such as level of education and even quality of relationship with parents, in the case of young (18–35 years old) girls.[4] On the other hand, cost, fear of a negative outcome and sociocultural factors preclude many women from actually undergoing breast enhancement surgery even though they may genuinely benefit from it.[5] Evidently, therefore, this is a deeply personal matter and needs careful delicate probing by the surgeon.

In any scenario, when a patient approaches the surgeon, building trust with a nonjudgmental attitude by the surgeon toward the motives for surgery is important. In all cases, one would be well advised to trust the patient's insight as to her concerns and expectations regarding the appearance of her breasts, without dismissing them as frivolous. This is an important but often overlooked aspect of the doctor-patient relationship in practice.

PATIENT EDUCATION VERSUS MARKETING

An appraisal study conducted in UK, France and Germany[5] to understand the reasons why women consider breast augmentation surgery (BAS) but delayed the choice of a surgeon, revealed the finding that almost half the women surveyed simply could not find a surgeon they could trust at the outset.

Among women who had already undergone surgery, the primary cause of dissatisfaction with their initial options among surgeons, was the fact that they perceived the surgeon to be nonattentive toward them and/or disrespectful—again delineating the importance of empathy in the relationship.

Another factor was the distrust that the patient would not get good postoperative care. Ultimately therefore, though almost 75–88% of the women interested in BAS sought information, the numbers finally undergoing surgery were dismally few and not surprisingly, the bottleneck was the consultation with the surgeon.[5]

This study also highlighted the importance of accurate dissemination of information regarding the pros and cons of esthetic plastic surgery to clear the air over myths commonly promulgated by media, advertising and other information sources, as this was a significant deterrent to actually undergoing surgery. Overall, Hedén et al. (2009)[5] proposed laying down a consistent set of guidelines for consultation that will comprehensively (as much as possible) cover mutual patient-doctor queries as to the patient expectations, compatibility of patient-procedure and risks involved.

Esthetic breast surgery is fundamentally different from other forms of surgical intervention in that it is desired by the patient to improve her appearance and consequently her self-confidence. Hence providing adequate biomedical information, including them in the planning of surgery and allowing them to express their concerns/doubts, together with honesty and transparency regarding the surgical outcome, would go a long way in the cementing of the doctor-patient relationship.[6] Lastly, abiding by the ethics of esthetic surgery is of paramount importance. The surgeon must remember that a good sustained practice can only be achieved if honest and efforts are made to "educate" and not "sell" procedures to prospective patients, as in the long run, this field is meant to help people achieve their personal goals and not promote the business of vanity.[7] Breast reconstruction following cancer treatment is an entirely different scenario altogether, as it involves either breast-conserving surgery (BCS), in the early stages of cancer, or types of mastectomy depending on the severity/staging of breast cancer. The course of cancer treatment may range from only mild disfigurement to removal of the entire breast. Needless to say, this involves a great deal of psychological and physiological trauma for the woman, which invariably manifests in anxiety about her future appearance and apprehension regarding further complications of secondary reconstructive surgery. Here too therefore, while the four basic principles of healthy doctor-patient relationship are applicable together with the considerations as described earlier, the main need of the hour is the allaying of fear regarding disfigurement.

ROLE OF COUNSELING

In a survey conducted among women undergoing BCS after early stage cancer removal at the University of Michigan Medical Center,[8] patients expressed the most retrospective procedural dissatisfaction and surgeon distrust, with increasing risk of breast asymmetry after BCS. Factors such as postoperative complications and recurring need for surgery were additional contributors to patient distrust of surgeons.

In this context, the study revealed that proper presurgical counseling by the surgeon to sensitively inform her the risk of asymmetry could help alleviate distrust, regret and dissatisfaction. This was seen for certain mastectomy cases wherein the women were surprisingly accommodating of the loss of the breast because of prior counseling.

A good plastic surgeon should therefore try to achieve a balance in his goals to satisfy both the categories of patients coming to him (reconstructive/esthetic) and enables them to realistically match their expectations with the outcome. Whatever may be the primary reason of our involvement here, patient satisfaction should be the sought after goal.

Emotional needs of a patient increase after surgery and should be borne in mind by the surgeon even after the treatment is over. Though not emphasized upon, in our opinion, the study's investigators also indirectly raised the importance of ethnicity and socioeconomic cultural factors in assessing patient perspectives toward BCS, as they noted that not all ethnic groups responded equally. This may also reflect communication gaps between doctor and patient due to such constraints that inhibit effective bonding.[3] In another study of breast cancer outpatients,[9] patients were assessed for their perception of mutual participation in the brief meetings held with the physician, based on three variables: (1) patient participation (discussing her concerns), (2) physician collaboration (physician encouraging patient to participate in the consultation) and (3) communication success (whether she felt understood/not). Their responses were also compared with audio recordings of physician-patient meetings to obtain perception behavior correlates.

ESSENTIALS OF PATIENT CONSULTATION

The length of consultation, educational background of the patient, her intention to speak and counseling by the physician determined her perception of participation. Her perception of physician collaboration was correlated with the extent to which she was allowed to voice her opinions, fears and other psychosocial talk as well as inclusivity demonstrated by the physician. Lastly, her perception of communication success was correlated with her level of preconsultation anxiety and examination results. Overall therefore, this study too highlights the need for the physician to take multiple factors into account when assessing the patient, including her level of information about her disease, her perception of the ways it has changed her life and shaped her body image and gauge her emotional state prior to consultation. While long outpatient consultation duration per patient may not be feasible, managing the time one spends with the patient in an effective manner could help offset the time crunch. Maintaining eye contact and a welcoming, not intimidating attitude are ways to engender regard for the physician in the patient. The patient should be made an active participant in the discussion of treatment and procedures, so that she feels more empowered to face the consequences and willingly allows transference of responsibility to the physician.

Though the average patient is trusting, changes in marketing trends, social networking sites propagating detrimental rumors about doctors in general may increase the strain on the surgeon. Another point to be noted here is that it is often wise to have a female attendant or nurse during a consultation especially when the doctor happens to be a male.

Besides this many of us do not directly work for the patient but are employed by a healthcare system or firm whose dictates we may have to follow. Unhappy patients, insensitive insurance companies and overall pressure of external economic forces, together with fear of litigation may have also contributed to many surgeons seeking early retirement.

A patient coordinator could get all the pertinent data (past history, details of previous surgery, etc.) from the patient beforehand and must pass all the information to the surgeon prior to the first consultation. The costs and payment for the procedure should be clear to the patient before she leaves. Separate fees for individual services rendered may help consolidate a patient's faith by giving her the freedom to refuse treatments as opposed to combination of procedures offered as a package, which may increase patient paranoia of costly treatments not included at all. Here minimizing unavoidable conflicts in insured patients and acting more as advocates for the patient may help strengthen the weakening patient-doctor bonds.

Research updates coming from patient opinions regarding treatment outcomes is an extremely valuable guide in providing necessary feed back and thus improving our clinical practice. Being a part of a good team that includes specialists of all the concerned fields can prove to be an additional bonus in giving the best possible results.

Educational materials that in the past played a significant role in patient perception of procedural success, along with the interpersonal communication skills of the surgeon have now been largely taken over by the Internet. Solutions now being available on every search engine, choosing an option is easier if one is well informed. Ethical marketing in the form of informative websites with patient testimonials and generous FAQs, have often helped many patients who are anxious or hesitant to undergo a procedure take the bold step forward. Information about the surgeon including his qualifications, affiliations and experience here often helps a patient separate the grain from the chaff. Last but not the least, a successful surgeon cannot have a clinic without the support of the office staff. These people are diplomats for the surgeon and have a big influence over her first impression. The person who answers the phone is the person who sets the table...and a messy table is not the way to start an excellent dinner. They should be dressed appropriately and the facility should be modest but elegant.

By embracing and encompassing the guidelines offered, we can play a significant role in improving overall quality of life for the patient rather than merely providing a skilled service.

REFERENCES

1. Boyd C. Breast cancer: the value and meaning of breasts. In: Cancer Forum 2001. Sydney: The Cancer Council Australia; 2001. p. 160.
2. Szasz TS, Hollender MH. A contribution to the philosophy of medicine: the basic models of the doctor-patient relationship. AMA Arch Intern Med. 1956;97(5):585-92
3. Chipidza FE, Wallwork RS, Stern TA. Impact of the doctor-patient relationship. Prim Care Companion CNS Disord. 2015;17(5):10.
4. Javo IM, Sørlie T. Psychosocial characteristics of young Norwegian women interested in liposuction, breast augmentation, rhinoplasty, and abdominoplasty: a population-based study. Plast Reconstr Surg. 2010;125(5):1536-43.
5. Hedén P, Adams WP, Maxwell P, Nava M, Scheflan M, Stan C. Aesthetic Breast Surgery: Consulting for the Future—Proposals for Improving Doctor–Patient Interactions. Aesthetic Plas Surg. 2009;33(3):388-94.
6. Khoo C. Risk reduction in cosmetic surgery. Clin Risk. 2009;15(6):237-40.
7. Atiyeh BS, Rubeiz MT, Hayek SN. Aesthetic/cosmetic surgery and ethical challenges. Aesthetic Plas Surg. 2008;32(6):829.
8. Waljee JF, Hu ES, Ubel PA, Smith DM, Newman LA, Alderman AK. Effect of esthetic outcome after breast-conserving surgery on psychosocial functioning and quality of life. J Clin Oncol. 2008;26(20):3331-7.
9. Takayama T, Yamazaki Y. How breast cancer outpatients perceive mutual participation in patient–physician interactions. Patient Educ Coun. 2004;52(3):279-89.

SECTION 14
Essentials

14.1 Financial Management

Viral Desai

INTRODUCTION

The need for the doctors to be familiar with financial management cannot be overemphasized. India has a large underserved demand for healthcare services. As doctors, it is our mandate to make healthcare available across the nation. While we are prepared to fulfill this mandate, many of us are often restricted by the financial resources at our disposal. Prudent financial management can help us overcome this challenge to a large extent.

This chapter has three key learning objectives: first, to familiarize you with the legal structure of a medical practice; second, to introduce you to the prudential system of cash flow management in a clinical practice setup; and third, to acquaint you with the management practices that could help you to take the right decisions concerning the growth of your practice.

BASICS OF CLINICAL PRACTICE

Legal Structures and Taxation

A clinical practice can be setup as a proprietorship, partnership, limited liability partnership (LLP), or a private limited company (PLC).

- No special procedure is required to start a *proprietorship* business. The entire income and expense of the clinic are considered to be those of the proprietor, and the resulting profit is taxed as per the tax bracket in which the proprietor falls. The major drawback of this form is that the clinic and the doctor are one and the same legal entity and so in the case of a liability of the practice which cannot be met by the assets of the clinic, personal assets of the doctor can be attached to fulfill such liabilities.
- In the case of a *partnership*, two or more doctors pool their resources to setup the clinic. Income tax is charged on the profits of the partnership at a flat rate (present effective rate is 30.9%), without the benefit of slabs. Interestingly, salary paid to partners, interest paid to partners, and the share of the partners in the total income of the firm is not taxable in the hands of the partners. It is important to note that a partner is legally liable for the actions of the other partner(s). Also, in case the partnership firm is unable to pay its tax dues, each of the partners can be held personally liable for recovery of the tax dues.
- As the name suggests, *LLP* is a special type of partnership in which the liability of the partners is limited to amount agreed by each of them. This form of partnership

requires filing of certain forms and periodic returns with the Registrar of Companies. LLP with an annual turnover of over ₹ 40 lacs or capital contribution of over ₹ 25 lacs is required to be audited by a Chartered Accountant.

- A *PLC* is generally not an advisable form for a clinical practice as it is a highly regulated and is required to fulfill several legal compliances. That said, financial investors in clinical practices would generally require that the practice be structured as a PLC, for ease of control. It is possible to convert an existing practice to a PLC at such a time. The present effective tax rate for PLC is 25.17%.

A Bit about GST

As mentioned earlier, Income Tax is applicable at different rates of each of the above structures. In addition, in certain cases a clinic may also be liable to charge and deposit Goods and Services Tax (GST). Let us have a quick look at the GST system. The GST law requires that any business with turnover of more than ₹ 20 lacs in a year must register itself with the Central Board of Indirect Taxes and Customs (CBIC). Turnover in this case means the total income of the clinic (and in the case of proprietorship, of the proprietor) earned during the financial year. However, if the turnover comprises solely of income from delivery of "healthcare services" by a "clinical establishment" or "authorized medical practitioner" or "paramedics", such income is exempt from GST. The **Figure 14.1.1** explains the important terms related to GST.

Clinics which are engaged only in exempt healthcare services are said to be providing only exempt services and thus, they are not required to register under GST. However, clinics providing both healthcare and nonhealthcare services (say, medical training for doctors) are required to consider their total turnover from healthcare and nonhealthcare services. If this total turnover exceeds ₹ 20 lacs, the clinic has to register under GST.

Once a doctor or a clinic is registered under GST, it is mandatory to file a GST return (called GSTR 3B) every month as well as a consolidated return every 3 months (called GSTR-1). The principle of paying or claiming GST is explained in **Figure 14.1.2**.

Notification No. 9/2017 exempts healthcare services by a clinical establishment or authorized medical practitioner or paramedics from GST

Healthcare services means diagnosis, treatment or care for illness, injury, deformity, abnormality or pregnancy
- Includes two-way transportation of the patient
- Excludes hair transplant or cosmetic or plastic surgery, except to reconstruct bodily functions affected due to congenital defects, injury, trauma, or developmental abnormalities

Clinical establishment means a hospital, nursing home, clinic, etc. that offers services requiring diagnosis or treatment or care for illness, injury, deformity, abnormality or pregnancy or diagnostic or investigative services of diseases

Authorized medical practitioner means a medical practitioner registered with any of the medical councils in India

Paramedic is a trained professional such as a nursing staff, physiotherapist, technician, or lab assistant

Fig. 14.1.1: Important terms related to GST.

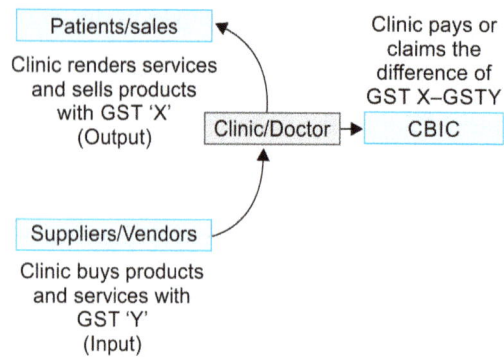

Fig. 14.1.2: Principle of paying or claiming GST.

It must be noted that the penalty for failure to take GST registration is the higher of (a) ₹ 10,000, (b) the amount of tax evaded, and (c) short tax liability.

MANAGING THE CASH FLOW

Cash is popularly called the lifeblood of an enterprise, and very aptly so. Just as prudent blood pressure management is vital for the physiological wellbeing of a human being, a sensible management of cash flow is necessary to maintain the health of a business system. Let us have a quick review of the basics of cash flow management.

Sources and Uses of Finance

There are three sources for a clinic to generate money for its operations and growth, explained here:
1. *Capital:* Capital is the corpus that is required to setup the clinic and is the first source of finance for a business or profession. Capital may be procured by way of equity (owners' funds) or as debt (borrowed funds).
2. *Revenues from operating activities:* Operating revenue is the continuing source of finance for a business. For doctors, operating revenues are generally the fees that are charged to patients and professional fees that are received from hospitals for services provided. Operational revenues depend on the amount of time invested into the practice and so they should ideally be complemented with other sources of finance.
3. *Revenues from financing activities:* These are the earnings from investments made and are generally in the form of interest, dividends, or growth in value of financial assets [such as the net asset value (NAV) of a mutual fund]. Revenues from financing activities are a passive source of income.

Just as it is important for us to focus on the sources of funds, we must also understand the three categories of use of funds by a clinic:
1. *Capital expenditure (or CAPEX):* This is the money spent on purchasing and maintaining assets with an expected useful life of over 1 year. These assets include the clinic premises, furniture, computers, and medical equipment.
2. *Operating expenditure (or OPEX):* This is the expense that is required for the clinic to run its operations. Examples of OPEX are payment of salaries paid, purchase of consumables, rent paid for leased assets, insurance premia, and marketing costs.
3. *Investments:* Like any prudent business, a clinic should invest its retained earnings in a way that risk and returns are favorably balanced. The important things to be aware of in "treasury management" are the various avenues of investments available, the inflation-adjusted rate of return that each investment vehicle provides, the risk profile of the investment vehicle, and time frame for which one can invest the funds **(Fig. 14.1.3)**.

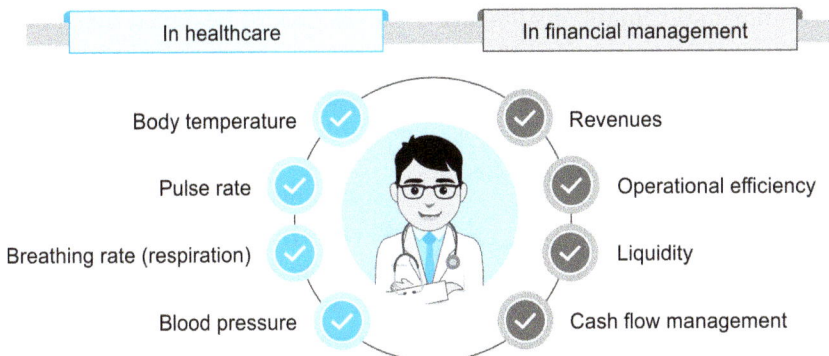

Fig. 14.1.3: Basic vital parameters.

Striking a Balance between Sources and Uses of Funds

A smart practitioner ensures that the revenues of the clinic are greater than its expenses. This surplus can be achieved by tweaking our working methods.

- Reduce inventory of assets (consumables). Apart from locking up funds, carrying an inventory increases the risk of obsolescence. If possible, negotiate with your suppliers for purchase of consumables on consignment basis.
- Get a business credit card issued in the name of your clinic and use it for incurring all official expenses. The usage statement will enable you to track the "invisible" expenses of your practice.
- Track the productivity of your staff to ensure against overstaffing. Communicating KPIs (key performance indicators) for each of your employees. Each KPI reflects your expectation from the concerned employee and should be specific and measurable. An example of KPI for an employee in charge of administration is "*Average admission time of a patient should not exceed 30 minutes from the time of reporting*".
- As much as possible, instead of hiring employees, engage consultants, especially in noncore areas such as website management and digital marketing. Consultants can be held to strict SLAs (service level agreements) which is often not possible with employees. In case of continuing nonperformance, terminating a service contract is easier than firing an employee.
- Consider offering services on a retainer basis. An example is an annual engagement comprising predefined investigations and a calendar of consultations for a recurring fee. This model, known as "the concierge model" in the West, ensures convenience for your patients (they might be protected against a spike in medical costs arising from to a sudden condition) and ensures recurring revenues to the clinic.

MANAGING GROWTH

Frameworks of Financial Management

There are several models that are used by financial experts to evaluate critical business decisions. For the purpose of this chapter, we consider the following four strategic questions that are relevant for a growth-oriented clinic.

- How can you plan finances for long-term growth of your practice?

- How is the monetary value of your practice estimated?
- How do you choose between two projects which seem equally profitable?

How can you finance long-term growth of your practice?

Growth implies an expansion in capacity or in the suite of service offerings. The most common source of financing growth is accumulated profits (also called "retained earnings"). These are the clinic's own funds that can be used for expansion. However, financing long-term growth may require looking beyond internal resources. Debt, private equity, and strategic investment are the two most common forms of growth funding.

Debt financing may involve borrowing money by taking a bank loan or by issuing a debt instrument. The principal amount of the debt has to be repaid as per the payment schedule. This is unlike private equity and strategic investment, which invests funds as nonreturnable equity capital. However, the terms of private equity and strategic investment are often more stringent than that of debt. The choice between the alternatives has to be made keeping in mind factors such as how much are you willing to dilute your ownership and control, are your future cash flows stable, do you have assets that you can leverage, and the impact of taxation (**Table 14.1.1**).

Some of the nonfinancial means of achieving growth of your practice are *franchising* (if your practice is process-intensive), *licensing* (if your practice involves proprietary intellectual property, such as a brand name), and *forming joint ventures* with synergistic businesses.

Table 14.1.1: Common forms of growth funding.

Parameter	Own funds	Retained earnings	Bank loan	Private equity	Strategic investor
Availability	Immediate	Immediate	1–2 months	3–6 months	6–9 months
Quantum	Low	Low	Depends on assets	High	Medium
Cost of Funds	Low	Low	Medium	High	High
Repayment period	No repayment required	No repayment required	1–5 years	3–8 years	5–15 years
Constraints	• Not always available • May not be enough to fund growth	May not be enough to fund growth	Requires assets on the balance sheet	Invests mostly in rapidly-growing medical practices	Can be difficult to find a suitable investor
Advantages	No dilution of ownership	No dilution of ownership	Temporary relationship	Brings in support ecosystem	A good investor can accelerate growth
Risks	Lack of discipline may result in haphazard fund management	Impacts liquidity (availability of funds) in the business	• Pledge of assets • Strict interest payments	• Expects high growth and return • Loss of control in some situations	• Loss of control • May interfere in strategic decisions

How is the monetary value of your practice estimated?

The determination of value of an enterprise is made by one of the three widely-used methods:

1. *The Discounted Cash Flow (DCF) method* estimates the value of an enterprise based on the present value of its future cash inflows and outflows. These future cash flows are "discounted" to a present value using a discounting factor. The resulting sum of the present value is the value of the enterprise. The Table below shows a simplified DCF model for valuation of a clinical practice **(Table 14.1.2)**.

2. *The Asset Valuation Method* is used when the business primarily contains assets such as medical devices, real estate, furniture, etc. The basic principle of this method is to subtract the total external liabilities of the business from its assets **(Table 14.1.3)**. As the outcome of this method is based on the basket of assets owned by the enterprise, this method is

Table 14.1.2: DCF model for valuation.

Assumed growth rate of revenues	12%
Assumed growth rate of operating expenses	10%
Discounting factor	7%
(Discounting factor should represent the risk involved in the business and must be more than inflation rate)	

Table 14.1.3: Asset valuation method.

(All amounts in ₹)

Financial years	Legend	2019–20	2020–21	2021–22	2022–23	2023–24	2024–25	2025–26
Year no.		1	2	3	4	5	6	7
Revenues								
Estimated revenue from operating activities	A	9,60,000	10,75,200	12,04,224	13,48,731	15,10,579	16,91,848	18,94,870
Total revenues	B = A	9,60,000	10,75,200	12,04,224	13,48,731	15,10,579	16,91,848	18,94,870
Expenses								
Capital expenses	C	3,00,000	-	-	12,00,000	-	-	15,00,000
Operating expenses	D	3,50,000	3,85,000	4,23,500	4,65,850	5,12,435	5,63,679	6,20,046
Total expenses	E = C + D	6,50,000	3,85,000	4,23,500	16,65,850	5,12,435	5,63,679	21,20,046
Profit before tax	F = A-E	3,10,000	6,90,200	7,80,724	–3,17,119	9,98,144	11,28,170	–2,25,177
Tax (@35%)	G = F × 0.35%	1,08,500	2,41,570	2,73,253	-	3,49,350	3,94,859	-
Profit after tax	H = F-G	2,01,500	4,48,630	5,07,471	–3,17,119	6,48,793	7,33,310	–2,25,177
Discounted cash flows (DCF)	I = H/[(1.07%)^(Year No.)]	1,88,318	3,91,851	4,14,247	–2,41,929	4,62,581	4,88,636	–1,40,229
Enterprise value (Sum of DCF)	J = ΣI$_{(1, 2,...,7)}$	15,63,475						

used mostly in cases where the business is being liquidated and where the practice is being sold without including its goodwill and future business.

3. *The Market Multiple Method* is a "quick and dirty" valuation method which adopts the premise that the value of similar enterprises is similar, when adjusted for scale **(Table 14.1.4)**. A multiple factor (generally, revenue) is computed on the basis of observed recent transactions. This multiple factor is then applied to other enterprises within the same industry. The table alongside considers a case involving the (Enterprise Value/Revenue) multiple. In this table, the value of Enterprise A is seen as ₹ 1.15 crore on an annual revenue of ₹ 9.60 lacs. This works out to an EV/Revenue, multiple of (1,15,20,000/9,60,000) = 12x. We can use this multiple to compute the value of Enterprise B by using the known revenue of Enterprise B and the industry multiple, to arrive at a valuation of ₹ 86,40,000. While this method is simple, it suffers from two main drawbacks: (1) this method does not evaluate the effects of various factors affecting the valuation and (2) it does computes value on the basis of a single instance of a company's parameters rather than a period of time and disregards the enterprise's growth rate.

How do you choose between two mutually exclusive projects which seem equally profitable?

Sometimes, we are faced with choosing among two or more capital-intensive projects. For example, the purchase of a new medical device versus setting-up of a new clinic. In such a case, a financial framework called the "NPV (net present value) Rule" is useful to select the more profitable project. This method helps us compare the total present value of the anticipated future cash flows of the various projects. The project with the higher total present value is the preferred project. To calculate the present value, the cash flows of each project are discounted using the cost of capital of that project. Here is a simplified example.

In this example, the purchase of a medical device requires an upfront payment of ₹ 75,00,000 and involves maintenance costs of ₹ 50,000 a year. The expansion of the existing clinic requires an upfront investment of ₹ 40,00,000 and annual expenses of ₹ 9,25,000. The finance for the purchase of the medical device is available at an interest rate of 12% per annum, whereas a loan for the expansion is available at 18% per annum interest. In a 5-year span, the expenditure and the income from both the options are same. Yet, despite a higher cost of its finance, the NPV of the option for expansion is higher; it is, therefore, the more profitable of the two alternatives **(Table 14.1.5)**.

Of course, the above is a simplified model for the purpose of education that disregards several important factors such as taxation, depreciation, residual value, etc.

Table 14.1.4: Market multiple method of valuation.

Enterprise A		
Company A	Legend	Amount
Revenue	A	9,60,000
Observed valuation	B	1,15,20,000
Computed multiple	C = B/A	12

Enterprise B		
Parameter	Legend	Amount
Revenue	D	7,20,000
Observed multiple	E = C	12
Computed valuation	F = D×E	86,40,000

Table 14.1.5: Planning of expenditure for a clinic setup.

Option 1: Purchase a medical device

Capital required	75,00,000				
Equipment loan rate	12%				
Year >	1	2	3	4	5
Expenses	75,00,000	50,000	50,000	50,000	50,000
Revenues	23,72,500	25,55,000	25,55,000	25,55,000	25,55,000
Net cash flow	–51,27,500	25,05,000	25,05,000	25,05,000	25,05,000
Discounted cash flow	–45,78,125	19,95,971	17,83,010	15,91,973	14,21,404
Total DCF/NPV	22,15,232				

Option 2: Expand clinic's premises

Capital required	40,00,000				
Personal loan rate	18%				
Year >	1	2	3	4	5
Expenses	40,00,000	9,25,000	9,25,000	9,25,000	9,25,000
Revenues	23,72,500	25,55,000	25,55,000	25,55,000	25,55,000
Net cash flow	–16,27,500	16,30,000	16,30,000	16,30,000	16,30,000
Discounted cash flow	–13,79,237	11,70,641	9,92,058	8,40,736	7,12,488
Total DCF/NPV	23,36,696				

THREE SINS OF FINANCE WHICH DOCTORS SHOULD AVOID

Not paying attention to money

Money is considered by many of us to be the "elephant in the room". Unlike other professionals, we doctors do not focus as much on matters of money as on serving mankind at large. For many of us, our punishing work schedules barely leave us with any time to go beyond the demands of our craft. This approach needs to change

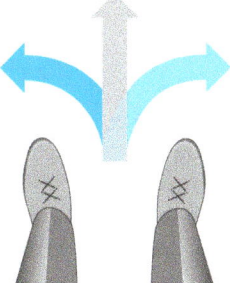

Not planning for growth

After setting up a clinical setup, many doctors depend solely on word-of-mouth for growth. This is because in the past, the path traversed by successful doctors was to build a reputation after years of successful practice. In today's fast-paced times, however, not having a plan for growth may make matters quite difficult

Not seeking professional help

We understand the value that specialists add to a medical case, yet we ourselves do not seek expert help when it comes to finance. It is important that you get references of suitable professionals from your existing network (such as your CA) and take some time to discuss and identify the right professional

SOME DO'S AND DON'TS FOR DOCTORS

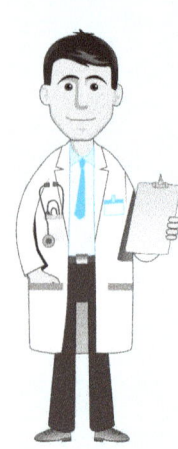

For young doctors who are starting out
- Have a rough plan forecasting your expenses and income
- Resist the temptation to make huge purchases at the start of your career
- Actively network with peers and seniors at conferences and over Linkedin, etc.
- Make sure you are covered under an effective insurance policy for a suitable amount

For doctors who are expanding their practice
- Standardize and document as many of your operating processes as possible
- Consult an intellectual property rights (IPR) lawyer and ensure that your IP is secure
- Actively use IT as an enabler; it will help you be present everywhere at the same time
- Create a second level of managers from within your team to help you oversee matters

For doctors who are opening a chain of clinics
- Ensure that you do not overextend yourself and your resources
- Be familiar with investment contracts, especially clauses relating to loss of control
- Implement an Enterprise Resource Planning (ERP) software for overall management
- Have a plan for upholding the standard of service quality across the newly-added clinics

- *Do not mix business and personal expenses:* Very early in my practice, I used to charge my clinic's expenses to my personal credit card out of the belief that it did not matter—after all, those payments had to be made one way or the other. I immediately corrected this practice once I noted that it would inflate my clinic's net income, leading to a higher business tax outflow!
- *Pay all vendors in full and on time:* This has helped my clinic avoid having to pay interest on delayed payments. It has also enhanced my reputation as a prompt client, which has in turn attracted high-quality vendors and advantageous commercial terms.
- *Book early:* My staff follows a Standard Operating Process (SOP) to immediately reserve my flights and hotels every time I accept an invitation to attend a medical conference or schedule a business trip. This ensures that we get the early-bird rates which are often substantially lower than last-minute fares.
- *Do not trust your memory with expenses:* I would advise you to build the habit of submitting your expenses to your accountant at the earliest opportunity. I have been tardy in the past on this count, especially after long international trips, and have often missed out on later fully recollecting the official spends that should have been recorded as expenses.
- *Plan your unavoidable spends:* If you plan your routine business purchases beforehand, you may be able to get concessional rates. I have found Amazon Business Account to be a great resource that offers good discounts on bulk orders for clinic stationery.
- *Revisit your expenses:* Walk through your banking account statement once a calendar quarter. If you are anything like me, you will discover several "invisible costs" (these are mostly lifestyle expenses) that seem pretty inconsequential by themselves but add up to a large number pretty quickly.

CONCLUSION

Financial management is a vast subject in itself. If this chapter has been able to familiarize you with some of the techniques in managing your practice, it would have served its purpose. I would end by recommending further reading books available for enthusiastic learners: Cash flow for Dummies discusses the basics of cash flow management, valuation by Aswath Damodaran is a great resource for finance novices and experts alike, and financial decision making by Narayanan and Nanda would be helpful if you wish to delve deeper into the intricacies of finance.

14.2 Legal Issues in Clinical Practice

Satish Bhat

INTRODUCTION

Laws relevant to a doctor in medical practice include both to regulate the work/duty as part of the professional services, and those to protect or safeguard the interests/rights of the doctor. Law is an obligation expected by society of individual/groups of individuals and enforced by a competent authority. Healthcare being included in the concurrent list of the Constitution of India, empowers both the state and the central government to enact laws for the same.

Rules to regulate the professional services of a medical practitioner, have been made by the Medical Council of India (MCI) under provisions of the Indian Medical Council (IMC) Act 1956. Though the National Medical Commission (NMC) Act has been notified on 9.8.2019, till the rules are framed and notified, rules under the IMC will stay in force. What makes such professional services of a doctor unique is that even the ethical norms are enforceable by law as prescribed in the Code of Medical Ethics Regulations 2002. Other professional services such as law, architecture, chartered accountants, company secretaries, etc., do not have such clear-cut ethical guidelines that are legally enforceable.[1] Such is the high level of accountability society expects of doctors.

Despite this, the IMC Act 1956 does not have the word "welfare" in objectives of MCI, unlike the Lawyers Act or Journalist Act. Hence, laws to protect the rights of a doctor are only the same as that of an ordinary citizen. Only special law for medical practitioners, is the prevention of violence in Hospital Act passed by various state legislatures. Despite a long standing demand by IMA to have a central law passed by parliament for prevention of hospital violence, this is yet to materialize.[2]

OVERVIEW OF LAWS RELEVANT TO MEDICAL PRACTICE[3]

These have been grouped into laws to regulate duties and protect rights.

Duties

Regulation of services provided: There are a wide spectrum of various aspects in medical practice and healthcare services, with laws that govern them, and are mentioned ahead. Though these laws have been grouped into those relevant to individual doctor and those applicable to hospitals, such segregation is fluid.

Laws relevant as an individual medical practitioner:
- Registration of medical practice
- Emergency healthcare laws
- Law regarding conduct of medical professional
- Criminal liability in medical profession
- Laws regarding management of patients
- Common medicolegal laws

For the hospital:
- Laws regarding commissioning of hospital
- Certifications, licenses and ongoing reports regarding hospital work
- Laws regarding storage, safe medication and sale of drugs and devices
- Laws regarding environmental safety
- Laws regarding employment and manpower
- Laws related to safety of doctors, patients and common citizens in hospital premises
- Laws governing professional training and research
- Laws governing hospital business

Rights/Needs

Few common scenarios where doctors/healthcare providers' rights and welfare are of concern, include:
- Abuse and defamation of doctors/hospital in media
- Recovery of hospital bill
- Protection against abuse and violence
- *Healthcare needs of the medical practitioner*: Doctor as a patient
- Medical indemnity (medicolegal protection) and social security

HEALTHCARE AT CROSSROADS

It is beyond the scope of this chapter to discuss the entire spectrum of laws relevant in medical practice. Since details of laws/regulations for doctors are available easily, the focus ahead is on the rights/needs of doctors while in medical practice. Before we go into the details of each of these, an overview is due to few aspects common to all.

Woefully inadequate public healthcare services, rising population and poor funding of public healthcare is a long-standing issue. In this background, increasing cost for providing healthcare in private sector, ineffective regulation and judicial remedy along with rising expectations of citizens have all led to skyrocketing of dissatisfaction with healthcare services in the last two decades. This is reflected simultaneously as:

- *Defamation, abuse and incidents of violence for healthcare service, doctors and hospitals*: IMA survey has shown 75% of doctor having faced abuse at least once in their lifetime.
- This is compounded by the attitude of media to jump to conclusions and sensationalize allegations of negligence regarding doctors and hospitals.
- 110% annual rise in incidence of medical negligence cases, which further form 12% of all cases in consumer forum.
- Increasing number of criminal complaints against doctors.

All these have together resulted in increased stress for practicing doctors. One study by Kerala IMA reveals that average life span of practicing doctors is 10 years less than the average citizen in society.[4,5] For most doctors, illness that keeps them away from work inevitably means a significant loss of regular earning. This applies even for those in a full time job in private multispecialty hospitals, unless they happen to be government employees. However, number of doctors who have availed a social security scheme, that provides for financial support in case of temporary or permanent loss of earning capacity, is likely to be very low. In the absence of a personal mediclaim policy, doctors (or family members) will need to pay from their pocket to take care of medical expenses, which adds to the burden following loss of earning when the doctor him/herself is a victim of illness.

While healthcare service provided by doctors even in private practice is considered as a public and essential service in various judgments, denial of which is punishable by law, the complementary right of those who provide this service has not been considered at all. The same essential service when provided in the government system, the service providers (doctors, nurses and other staff employed in the healthcare system) are provided various benefits as welfare needs, with statutory laws to regulate the same. In the absence of any such laws for doctors in the private sector, but with similar responsibility as those in public setup, the medical associations need to take the initiative to manage welfare programs and schemes for their member doctors.

PATIENT'S DISSATISFACTION, ALLEGATIONS OF INCOMPETENCE AND MEDICAL NEGLIGENCE

A common narrative that connects all scenarios where rights of doctors comes under threat, the moment there is any unfavorable outcome, is when doctors are assumed guilty in a casual manner, aspersions cast, and the consequences thereof. Hence, it is worth understanding the key nuances of judging competence, and in turn negligence.

Since the 1995 judgment of IMA versus VP Shantha, medical profession has been brought under the ambit of Consumer Protection Act 1986.[6] This has opened the avenue for nonmedical people to form an opinion on the healthcare services. While the compensations awarded by consumer forums are steadily rising, as is the tendency to file a complaint in consumer forum, the pendency of cases and lack of clarity regarding "competence in a given case" is only adding to the chaos. Lack of faith in judicial system, and inevitable delay, makes many aggrieved ones to abuse doctors verbally and physically, even by taking law into their own hands. An overview of the prevailing laws and rules, and understanding the forces that prevail in society, will help the doctor stay clear of such issues, and comply with the Law.

Three basic requirements of medical negligence:
1. Duty of Care
2. Lapse (due to breach/deficiency in skill, care or knowledge)
3. Resulting injury

Despite these guidelines, there is ambiguity in applying them, on account of:
- Wide spectrum of scenarios resulting from lapse
- Scenarios that mimic negligence
- Uncertain benchmark/yardstick to decide competency in a given case
- Poor knowledge of the strict inclusion criteria for criminal negligence.

Despite an initial mention in 2002 Ethical Guidelines of MCI, guidelines in deciding on negligence or competence in a given scenario are not available. This leads to an ambiguity in the reference/yardstick/standard applied, to decide whether there is a lapse in skill, knowledge or care in the given scenario.[7]

This is followed as per Bolam principle:
- The standard to be applied would be that usually held by an ordinary *competent* person exercising ordinary *skill* in that profession.

- It is not possible for every professional to possess the highest level of expertise or skills in that branch/field which he practices.
- A highly skilled professional may be possessed of better qualities, but that cannot be made the standard for judging the performance of the professional proceeded against on indictment of negligence.

Despite these clear guidelines, confusion commonly arises when a doctor is called to give an expert opinion, due to ambiguity in either:

- *Standard applied (Bolam test)*: Medical training primes us to deliver *the best*, legal guidelines expect only what can be done by doctor with *average* skill, not the best. Unless this difference is consciously understood, those in the decision making seat may erroneously call a competent person with average skill as negligent.
- *Civil versus criminal negligence*: Police mainly want to know whether negligence amounts to offence under criminal law. *Without appreciating the difference in civil versus criminal negligence*, medical experts report is as just "negligence", implying civil negligence. Police take it as criminal negligence.

COMMON MISCONCEPTIONS IN SOCIETY AND FACTS (TABLE 14.2.1)

Table 14.2.1: Common Misconceptions in Society and Facts.

	Misconceptions	Facts
1.	Every adverse outcome is a negligence for which doctor is responsible	People seem to have forgotten that death can happen after an AMI in the ICCU of even a top corporate hospital, AIIMS or even mayo clinic. Even adverse outcome of death may simply be a natural outcome of disease rather than negligence
2.	With any doubt of negligence, police complaint will lead to criminal action	Unless the actions resulting in the lapse amount to gross recklessness, the incident do not come within the ambit of gross negligence defined by Criminal Law. Police complaint in such cases will be dismissed
3.	Any doctor or hospital staff can identify when adverse outcome is due to negligence by a doctor	Loose comments by peers, lead to label of "negligence" by patient's family, when it may actually be a medical accident or error where no single person can be held responsible
4.	If patients are unhappy with the treatment they will complain to the authorities	Lack of faith in "justice" by legal process, often leads to them taking law into own hands, verbal abuse and violence in hospital or defamation through media, "to get even" with the doctors
5.	Once complaint is lodged with authorities, anger and hostility will settle down	Often, complaint lodged with police simply to pressurize doctor to give immediate compensation/hospital bill waiver or use as a negotiating tool in case doctor files a complaint against the patient's attenders/family for hospital violence

The Ultimate Myth

Healthcare is a noble profession and doctors should serve society without expecting monetary benefits, regardless of the hardships they may face. If patients are unhappy with the service, the doctor can be pulled up for same.

Fact

Healthcare is a service provided for a fee bound by a contract. Though doctors can enforce the contract and recover their fees in case patient do not pay, this is cumbersome given the judicial inertia. Doctors have their rights, just like any other citizen, and can ensure they are protected. Allegations regarding the professional service can be evaluated only with reference to the set professional standards, and not by some casual opinion.

Eventual Situation

Since sympathies lie with the patients and citizens, doctor's situation:
- Duties are expected as a noble profession
- Lapse in duty is punishable as a service provider
- When there is a question of doctors' rights/welfare, there are no takers.

LEGAL REMEDY TO PROTECT DOCTOR'S RIGHTS

Abuse and Defamation in Media

Let us see the common ways in which this happens, the remedy available, and some case examples

- *Type A*: Social Media Defamation—SM
- *Type B*: Defamation due to poor/inaccurate mention of facts or misinterpretation by Media (MSM)
- *Type C*: Defamation by someone else— reported as it is in Print/Online Media website (MSM)

A primigravida underwent an obstetric hysterectomy following uncontrolled PPH. When her condition did not stabilize, with consumptive coagulopathy added, she was referred to the medical college hospital 5 km away, where she passed away despite all possible care. All done with due consent at every stage, and counseling and

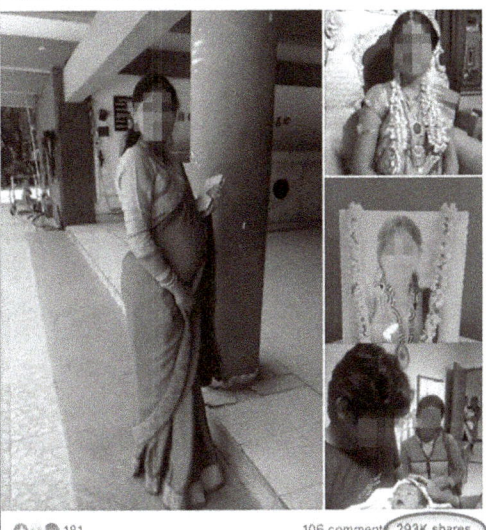

communication on record. Despite all this, a criminal complaint was made with police against the gynecologist, besides the defamation seen above on social media. Note the 2.93 lacs shares, and views by each person on the time line of each of these 2.93 lacs people.

Suggested response: Since the abuse was premediated and done consciously, it amounts to a criminal defamation punishable under IPC 499, 500. However, for FIR to be registered by the police, complaint and approval by the local magistrate is a prerequisite. Complaint needs to be done by the victim (the Gynecologist), failing which complaint only by IMA or anyone else does not hold ground.

Fake cardiologist blamed for leader's death

UDUPI: The family members of Janata Dal(S) Udupi district former president Mahim Kumar Hegde alleged that the leader had died due to the recklessness of the doctor who claimed himself to be a cardiologist and treated him.

Speaking to the media persons here on Friday, the counsel for the family Latha C S Holla claimed that the Dakshina Kannada Consumer Forum Court had upheld the allegation and slapped a fine of Rs 15 lakh against the doctor who had treated the politician since 2004. She said that Hegde died on June 10, 2010.

The leader shared friendly relationship with the doctor. He believed him and his way of treatment.

Although the deceased suffered heart-related complications, the physician Dr Ashok Kumar Y G working in Okude Diagnostic in Kunjeebettu in Udupi did not reveal the fact that the former had blocks in two arteries.

She added that to practice as the nephrologist or cardiologist, one must have qualification from the recognized University and the above said physician just claimed himself nephrologist or cardiologist, which is utterly fake.

Latha said that the doctor always prescribed medicine for acidity and failed to recognise the heart problems suffered by the leader.

She said the Consumer Court gave the verdict on April 29, 2015, following which the fact of his lack of proficiency in the field was clear.

When Hegde suffered severe complications, he was referred to the Gandhi hospital and later the experts in Gandhi hospital referred the patient to Yenepoya hospital in Mangaluru and not to KMC, which was nearby.

The court has ordered for Rs 15 lakh compensation from the accused to the wife of the victim and slapped a fine of Rs 10,000 on Gandhi Hospital for its failure to refer the patient to the nearest hospital and the ambulance that was provided lacked the medical facilities, she alleged.

DH News Service

Physician can't be called fake cardiologist: AMC

MANGALURU: The Association of Medical Consultants (AMC) has clarified that a physician cannot be called fake cardiologist as there are no prevailing guidelines in India, as to what is the precise domain of one speciality versus another similar speciality.

This segregation becomes all the more difficult when it is a matter of a broad speciality and a sub (super) speciality. Even though the Indian Medical Council Act of 1956 empowers the Medical Council of India (MCI) to frame guidelines in these matters, there are none laid down so far, according to a release issued by AMC President Dr M C Suvarna and Secretary Dr Ullasa Shetty.

The AMC was reacting to a news report published on August 8, 2015 with headline "Fake cardiologist blamed for leader's death," based on a statement by the family members of JD(S) Udupi district former president Mahim Kumar Hegde. The family had alleged that the leader had died due to recklessness of a "fake cardiologist," who claimed himself to be a cardiologist and treated him.

The reference was made against Physician Dr Ashok Kumar Y G, then working at Okude Diagnostic in Kunjibettu in Udupi.

The AMC said that prior to the advent of super speciality training in India, the services of a super specialist like a cardiologist were provided by the broad speciality doctor - the physician in this case.

Stating that even a qualified medical graduate is expected to provide the primary care in case of emergencies, including cardiology, the AMC stressed the need for a change in attitude of society.

DH News Service

Following death during angioplasty in a cath lab, patient's family got a favorable judgment to their complaint against the referring doctor in the local District Consumer Forum. The aggrieved doctor filed an appeal right away in the State Forum. However, the patient's family held a press meet the next day, and gave subjective comments to media. One of the reports in leading English daily was seen as quite offensive by the media of the region. One local medical association, AMC Mangalore wrote to the Bureau Chief of the newspaper and met him. They understood the situation and promptly published an update with the alternative version of the events.

In case they had failed to respond, complaint of criminal defamation was the next option, with documents to support that the media publication failed to take corrective action despite being requested.

Examples of defamatory comments by those holding public office, published verbatim by media, are also very damaging. Comments by political leaders are very difficult to take up through the judicial system, and drag on for even decades when taken up.

- Jan Adhikar Party (JAP) chief and Lok Sabha legislator from Bihar Rajesh Ranjan alias Pappu Yadav has called for the social boycott of doctors charging arbitrary fee at their private clinics and nursing homes.[8]
- "Resign and stay at home if you are so scared" Smt. Majula Chellur, Chief Justice of Bombay High Court while hearing

a petition against Resident Doctors for striking work following repeated episodes of violence and assault while at work in Government Hospitals.[9]

Such events reinforce the negative image about the healthcare community, and the impression the doctors can be taken to task by anyone and everyone in society. This eventually leads to worsening of the doctor-patient relationship, which manifests as increased hospital violence and cases against doctors.

Recovery of Hospital Bill

- *One*: Common scenario is when patient expires after complicated illness, with mounting Hospital Bill or when patient discharge is due after complicated illness and treatment. In either case it is against the law, to withhold either the discharge or handover of the dead body on account of pending hospital bill.[10]
- *Two*: Free of cost treatment in case of emergency—Section 12(2) of Clinical Establishment Act makes it obligatory for hospitals and doctors to treatment cases that is brought to them, but without any provision regarding payment for the same.[11]

The Supreme Court of India as long back as 1989 observed in Parmanand Katara v. Union of India AIR 1989 SC 2039 that when accidents occur and the victims are taken to hospitals or to a medical practitioner, they are not taken care of for giving emergency medical treatment on the ground that the case is a medicolegal case and the injured person should go to a Government Hospital. The Supreme Court emphasized the need for making it obligatory for hospitals and medical practitioners to provide emergency medical care. This is not the only reason for not attending on injured persons or persons in a medical emergency; for sometimes such persons are turned out on the ground that they are not in a position to make payment immediately or that they have no insurance or that they are not members of any scheme which entitles them to medical reimbursement.[12]

So, what the Clinical Establishments Act expects from the doctors is neither new nor unfair or unjust. Alleviation of pain and suffering and saving human lives is the primary purpose and a patient is the "raison d'etre" of medical profession.

Failure to comply with the regulation may not only invite legal action but may also cause loss of respect and sympathy in the eyes of the public. *Yes, the issue of non-payments (for treatment of many emergency cases) is a matter of serious concern, which has not been addressed by the IMC Regulations, the Government or the Supreme Court Judgment quoted earlier.*

This uncertainty got extended further following the Ministry of Road Transport notification dated May 12th, 2015 regarding Good Samaritans who bring road side accident victims to the hospital. Section 10 of the notification specifically states that all public and private hospitals are not to detain bystander or a Good Samaritan or demand payment for registration or admission costs. It is unfortunate that once when amendments were being made to fill a lacuna which existed so far and resulted in countless deaths it could have been made more comprehensive and not left an important question hanging as to "Who will bear the cost of treatment"?[13]

A suggestion to take care (recover) treatment cost was provided by Dr Neeraj Nagpal (Hope Clinics <hopeclinics@yahoo.com>). This is by providing cashless treatment to all accident cases by the insurance companies, and appears to be quite reasonable and workable. All the vehicles on Indian roads are insured and if the Government passes on the liability of cashless treatment to these Insurance companies, the scheme could be implemented nationally in one stroke. More than 99% of the victims could be saved with this decision and the purpose of insurance served.

Insurance companies routinely take help of loss and claim assessors for the vehicles involved in the accident, and settle the claim immediately to repair the vehicles involved and bring it back on the roads within a week. Why cannot the same insurance companies have their own medical personnel as injury and disability assessors to look at the interests of accident victims and approve their proposed bill at the private hospital? Until this is done, does it not give the feeling that the car involved in the crash is more valuable than the life of victim as far as insurers are concerned?

Until this, a solution to this is provided, these are the common scenarios, when a doctor goes to court for recovery of unpaid bills for emergency services provided:

Possibility 1: Keep going to hearings and waste your time till you get tired.

Possibility 2: The patient may be very poor and the court finds that the patient has no money to pay you. What next?

Possibility 3: The court asks the patient to pay money along with litigation charges (say around ₹ 20,000/-). Now would you get a good lawyer below ₹ 50,000/-? So what have you finally gained? Nothing.

Possibility 4: The patient might file a negligence case against you to avoid the above case. In that event your name will be splashed all over the newspapers and you will have another case on your hands.

- *Three*: One common method used by patients to waive off the unpaid bill is to file a frivolous complaint with the Consumer Forum. Section 26 of the CPA covers dismissal of false complaints, where a complaint instituted before the District Forum, the State Commission or, as the case may be, the National Commission is found to be frivolous or vexatious, it shall, for reasons to be recorded in writing, dismiss the complaint and make an order that the complainant shall pay to the opposite party such cost, not exceeding 10,000, as may be specified in the order. An accusation may be frivolous or vexatious without being wholly false. A "vexatious" charge may be partly true, but the object of the person making the accusation should be primarily to harass the persons accused.

Protection against Abuse and Violence

Whether or not grievance regarding treatment provided is valid or not, abusing the healthcare provider (Doctor, Hospital staff or Medical Establishment) is unacceptable, and in violation of the Law. Given that healthcare services are an essential part of society, special laws have been made to safeguard this service from violence and abuse. Let us see what are the options available to the doctor in such a scenario:

- *One*: Preventive measures: Few of them include
  - Have CCTV coverage in your premises
  - Have a counseling/discussion room close to critical areas like casualty, OT, ICU where patient/attenders/family

can be called to sit and discuss, while the same is recorded.
- Display prominently the provisions of Hospital Violence Act, and it is stringent non-bailable and imprisonment provisions
- Make a designated Code White/Purple as an alert for summoning hospital staff to the venue of a potential violence/abuse in the hospital. The moment this is announced on the public address system of the hospital, all staff not in a critical position should reach the venue of the incident immediately.
- Have a SOP prepared in advance, and display for hospital personnel to use when needed.
- Have an emergency medicolegal response team as part of the Local Association (IMA), with few members who can reach the venue at short notice, in case of a crisis.
- Have an indemnity policy, both for individual doctor and for the medical establishment, with adequate cover.

■ *Two*: Remedial measures
- Dial 100 to inform the police. Call station/personal number of officers only after dialing the 100 which has an automated system to inform Police vans that are on the streets
- Document the incident by audio-visual means
- Do everything possible to diffuse the confrontation
- In case of physical abuse, remember each doctor has a right to protect themselves from bodily harm, by all means including offensive defense. IPC sections 96-106 have provisions where causing injury to someone for protecting self *is not an injury*. Do remember that even a person walking on the street has a right to protect themselves in case they are assaulted, and same is applicable to a doctor in the hospital.
- Register a formal complaint with the police, including all supportive evidence and collect an acknowledgment. Always make the local association as a party to the complaint, to help better manage any pressure to withdraw that may come later.
- Offer all hospital documents to the patient attenders and police personnel, after taking time to ensure it is suitably complete. Any damage to records must be mentioned in the police complaint.
- In case there is a counter complaint filed with the police against the doctors/hospital, alleging negligence leading to grievous injury, do not be worried even if an FIR is filed. Politely remind the police officials, that to proceed against the doctor, they need to have an opinion by a designated Medical Board. Violation of the same will amount to violation of Supreme Court Guidelines and contempt of Court.
- Do not offer/agree to make any suggestion of making a monetary payment to the family for settling the case. Despite the payment as agreed, the patient's family can file a complaint while mentioning the payment done as an admission of guilt.
- Cases registered against culprits should be given wide publicity through media, and the case pursued as per law till the culprits are punished. In case the doctor or hospital contacts any media, call them to meet in person and provide all details and evidence. In case media publishes the incident

without the correct version of facts, with/without contacting the hospital or doctor, make it a point to write them a letter asking to publish a corrected version of events.

Long-term initiatives by IMA/Associations needed to control hospital violence:
- A Central Hospital Violence Act with punishment at least 7 years to ensure the culprits do not get bail under any circumstances. This act to have a provision such that evidence provided by the victims (of violence) need not be as a routine asked to be corroborated evidence provided, unless there is some doubt about its credibility.
- Guidelines by media for reporting on healthcare events, to protect the identity of the accused and victim, avoid sensationalism
- Amend the IMC Act 1956 to include the "welfare of doctors" as one of the objectives of the MCI. Even though the NMC Act 2019 has been notified, this is still missing from the preamble of the act, and will need an amendment in the Parliament to include this.

Healthcare and Insurance Needs of the Medical Practitioner: The Doctor-Patient

Just like anyone else, a doctor too falls sick and may need hospitalization. It is a common practice (professional etiquette) among doctors not to charge any professional fees, for the services provided to the medical treatment of any colleague. This obligation at times is so strong, it may dissuade treating doctor from providing the service to a colleague, knowing the usual monetary benefit will be missing. Whether or not such a reluctance is there, every doctor who provides a professional service is due to receive his professional dues. A simply way to address this situation is to have a medical insurance policy for the doctor and his/her family. This will ensure that hospital costs besides the professional services provided during treatment do not become a burden for the doctor who is hospitalized.

Thus came the idea for a mediclaim policy designed for doctors. Once discharged from hospital, there will be a period of recovery at home before getting back to work. This may take a few months in case of major illness and especially accidents. A good medical indemnity policy may include a monthly compensation for this period when the doctor is unable to get back to his remunerative work. Some policy may even have a compensation for any permanent deformity/disability that interferes with the future revenue generating potential of the policy holder (Doctor in this case). Alternatively, this may be included in the benefits of a social security policy also.

Having seen the issues faced by our patients, when they wish to avail of benefits of their medical insurance policy, a good medical policy by any medical association will convey as many of these issues in a policy for their doctor members. Few of these include:
- Cover for preexisting diseases
- Cover for congenital diseases
- Cover for outpatient procedures
- Cover for common diseases in the initial 1 or 2 years of beginning the policy
- Extending the same benefits for family members of the doctor who avails the policy for association members.

Such a policy for doctor members, will have a team of doctors within the association itself, who initially will approve any claims that may arise from the policy holding members. This committee/team has to ensure that the professional and other charges in the hospital bill are realistic, failing which the premium for all members in the subsequent years can increase significantly. Purpose of any insurance scheme is distribution of risk/burden among all members, and it should stay just at that. Any deviation, and the scheme can become nonviable.

Professional Indemnity and Social Security

Any insurance policy by an association for its members, is a group insurance where the insurance provider typically is one of the four public sector general insurance companies in India. In today's litigation prone era, beginning a medical practice without adequate indemnity is like driving a vehicle on the road without vehicle insurance. In fact, medical indemnity should be mandatory just like having a medical license. Unfortunately, the regulatory body that issues medical license is yet to see the situation thus, and it is left to medical associations to ensure their members have a suitable indemnity cover. Public hospitals, trust hospitals, general practitioners, medical students are all various scenarios where one would not have expected to be sued years ago, but reality is that the medical practitioner working in all these scenarios needs indemnity cover. In case of a compensation that needs to be paid, which courts are increasingly awarding in amount of few crores of late, any payment out of own pocket/savings is likely to make the doctor and family financially bankrupt, as they would need to sell of their assets including immovable ones (property).

Few cautions while availing an indemnity policy include:

- *Adequate cover*: Minimum rupees 1 crore is recommended. This is the compensation that even the District Forum can award as per draft of the Consumer Protection Amendment Act 2019.
- *Covers the appropriate spectrum of work*: Cosmetic procedures, whether by plastic surgeon, dermatologist or dentist, will not be covered by the conventional policy for any members of that specialty. A well-planned policy will provide cover for these additional services, by collecting an additional premium on account of the higher risk of litigation/compensation involved with these cosmetic procedures.
- Retroactive date is maintained. This is the date from which cases treated with be covered in case of any claims that may arise. Avoiding delay in annual renewal and any gap in period of cover is the simplest way to get the earliest retroactive date.
- Cover is needed for a senior doctor even after they retire from practice, to account for any claims arising from incidents in the previous few years. (Run-off cover)
- *Out of court settlement*: Any adverse outcome that simply cannot be justified in any way other than medical negligence, will eventually have compensation awarded by the Consumer Forum. Alternatively, deciding on a mutually agreeable compensation amount, without the stress and delay of court proceedings is in the interests of the petitioner and respondent also. This can be done through a legally established procedure called "Out of Court Settlement."
- *Cover for penalty other than by Consumer Forum*: Compensations may be awarded by Human Rights Commission, Civil Courts, and rarely other authorities. Conventional policy may cover only compensations awarded by Consumer Forums
- *Cover for criminal proceedings*: A good policy will take care of the expenses in defending the doctor against criminal charges regarding treatment provided,

provided the doctor is proved innocent at the end.

A Social Security scheme, by an association is similar to a life insurance policy available for the general population, which provides financial support in the event of an untimely demise of the policyholder member. But unlike a typical life insurance policy available for all, in a social security scheme, even after the scheme member does not pay annual premium after initial few years of payment, there is a lump sum benefit the family receives, in the event of demise.

Details of few schemes from prominent Medical Associations include:
- Indian Medical Association (IMA) Schemes
- IMA Health Scheme (www.imanhs.com)
- IMA PPF (http://www.nimapps.com)
- IMA Social Security Scheme (https://www.imansss.org)
- Medicos Legal Action Group (MLAG) Chandigarh Indemnity Scheme
- MLAG Indemnity (https://www.mlag.in/index.php/mlag-indemnity)
- Association of Medical Consultants (AMC) Mumbai Schemes
- AMC Mumbai Professional indemnity (https://amcmumbai.com/professional-indemnity/)
- AMC Mumbai Health Scheme (https://amcmumbai.com/professional-indemnity/)
- AMC Mumbai Social Security Scheme (https://amcmumbai.com/cbs-consultants-benevolent-scheme/)

THE WAY AHEAD

Legal issues faced by doctors in medical practice can be addressed keeping in mind the healthcare needs of society. There are many issues that can be addressed within the fraternity, especially matters of self-regulation, without waiting for any external inputs. Evaluating an adverse medical outcome, and grading the severity of the lapse if any, along with the prescribed penalty, is a long pending matter. In fact, failure to self-regulate leads to guidelines being made by those outside the medical profession, and then we are left with the job of course correction. With policy decisions on healthcare, while authorities and elected government will always have their own political compulsions, medical professional bodies need to give the facts that are scientific and realistic, without any bias or fear. And given the current trend where doctors are portrayed as the whipping boy, and responsible for most of the ails in healthcare, unless the facts are taken directly across to society and the masses, we will continue to bear the brunt of hostility and anger that prevails with the common citizen, for the woeful condition of healthcare seen today.

REFERENCES

1. INDIAN MEDICAL COUNCIL (Professional Conduct, Etiquette and Ethics) Regulations, 2002. Available from https://www.mciindia.org/documents/rulesAndRegulations/Ethics%20Regulations-2002.pdf
2. IMA threatens to launch countrywide ceasework. Available from https://www.deccanherald.com/national/national-politics/ima-threatens-to-launch-countrywide-ceasework-759003.html
3. Laws Applicable to Medical Practice and Hospitals in India: MM Singh et al International Journal of Research Foundation of Hospital and healthcare Foundation, 2013;1(1):19-23. Available from http://www.imalko.in/downloads/laws.pdf
4. Kerala Doctors die earlier than General Public: Study. Available from https://timesofindia.indiatimes.com/city/kochi/docs-die-early-than-gen-public-study/articleshow/61716443.cms
5. Pandey SK, Sharma V. Doctor, heal thyself: addressing the shorter life expectancy of doctors in India. Indian J Ophthalmol. 2019;67:1248-50

Section 14: Essentials

6. Indian Medical Association vs VP Shantha and Ors on 13 November, 1995. Available from https://indiankanoon.org/doc/723973/
7. A Guide for Expert Opinion: Is every Adverse Outcome a Medical Negligence? Satish Bhat, Chapter 22, Textbook on Medicolegal Issues in Dermatology and Plastic Surgery, Jaypee Publishers New Delhi, 2019.
8. Socially boycott doctors, they are worse than hangmen: Pappu Yadav. Available from https://www.hindustantimes.com/india-news/socially-boycott-doctors-they-are-worse-than-hangmen-pappu-yadav/story-AEzr08ApvU3m6bddcnIRAL.html
9. Resign and stay at home if you are so scared: High court to doctors. Available from https://timesofindia.indiatimes.com/city/mumbai/resign-and-stay-at-home-if-you-are-so-scared-hc-to-docs/articleshow/57761819.cms
10. Hospitals can't hold patients hostage for unpaid bills: Delhi High Court. Available from https://economictimes.indiatimes.com/news/politics-and-nation/hospitals-cant-hold-patients-hostage-for-unpaid-bills-delhi-high-court/articleshow/58381822.cms?from=mdr
11. Clinical Establishement Registration and Regulation Act and treatment of Emergency Cases. Available from https://www.mciindia.org/documents/rulesAndRegulations/Ethics%20Regulations-2002.pdf
12. Pt. Parmanand Katara vs Union Of India and Ors on 28 August, 1989. Available from https://indiankanoon.org/doc/498126/
13. Guidelines for Protection of Good Samaritans, Union Ministry of Health and Family welfare, GOI August 24, 2015. Available from https://www.mca.gov.in/Ministry/pdf/Guidelines_07sep2015.pdf

14.3 Practice Management in Skin and Plastic Surgery: Challenges and Roadblocks Commonly Faced—How to Overcome them?

Rakesh Kalra

INTRODUCTION

A fresh medical graduate beginning his esthetic practice faces peculiar problems, vastly different from those faced by freshers in any other branch of medicine. It needs to be understood what makes setting-up a cosmetic practice so different and so difficult. Let us begin by understanding the four main ingredients required before a cosmetic practice can be setup.
1. Professional development
2. Facility development
3. Clientele development
4. Relationship and trust development

(*For the purpose of ease in defining the cosmetic surgical practice for plastic surgeons, as well as setting-up a cosmetic dermatological practice for dermatologists, the rest of the text in this chapter is going to refer to it commonly as setting-up a "Cosmetic Practice"*)

PROFESSIONAL DEVELOPMENT

- There is no formal cosmetic practice training in either surgical or medical stream. In no department across the country, is there a special department of cosmetic surgery or cosmetic dermatology.

  There is no course, no predefined syllabus. Most faculty of medical colleges with a postgraduate department of plastic surgery or dermatology, belong to a period when they themselves were not fully trained in this stream.

All this means that it is very difficult for a postgraduate trainee to train himself sufficiently for cosmetic practice at his first academic training where he gets his basic training. At the end of his curriculum, at best he has only a degree in General Plastic Surgery or Traditional Dermatology.

- To setup a practice, lack of basic training in cosmetic practice means the trainee has to depend upon Fellowships, and training under individual mentors, or in private centers. This has its own challenges. Finding the right mentor is one problem. Usually, the mentors are experts in one area or one field of cosmetic only. Hence, finding a mentor or a center that provides a wholesome training is difficult.
- Thirdly, this sort of a training is expensive. The trainee has to possibly pay for his training. And also look for boarding and lodging at his own expense, much more expensive than the hostels that are inexpensive at medical colleges. Lastly, it means spending a fair amount of time at each separate center where he trains himself in a variety of procedures. Even in the modern era, there is thus a requirement of the traditional, age-old style of "Guru-Shishya" kind training for one of the most advanced and modern sorts of treatments.
- Moving ahead from here and considering that the trainee has finally armed himself with enough observation of the mentors and that too at good centers, comes the next question of sufficient hands-on experience. Some centers give hands-on experience, while others do not. At the time of setting-up the cosmetic practice, the doctor often considers himself a novice, and is not confident enough to carry out the cosmetic procedures. The clients are demanding, and expect perfect results. The training, therefore, has to be very good, and the results excellent. It is like the first day at the box office. The initial few patients either make or break the whole future of practice. The doctor has to feign sufficient experience, even if the next case is the very first one he does. Then, the doctor has to deliver the very best at the first go itself. In cosmetic practice, the results are on the skin surface and nothing is hidden. This is what gives anxious moments to anyone doing a cosmetic procedure for the first time.

FACILITY DEVELOPMENT

- The next question is: When and where to start a practice. Usually, a very swanky clinic is required to match competition. But a swanky clinic, self-owned, is usually very expensive, especially difficult for a new comer to afford. Adding to this are the high rates of EMIS on loans taken.
- Present day practice is much more complicated as well. One needs several licenses, accreditations, government regulations, etc.
- Human resource selection for a fresh practice is also a challenge. Gathering together the correctly qualified staff, with adequate experience in the required field, is an uphill task. Competition is so much that holding back the desired manpower means paying them adequate to better salaries, to prevent attrition and keep the turnover low.
- Dealing with the vendors and suppliers of various expensive equipment in the correct manner, getting the best deals out of them, learning the intricacies of machine functionalities, understanding and properly conducting the legal

formalities of purchase and subsequent maintenance and even affording the high costs of equipment are all a daunting task that a fresher has to look into, with no such prior experience.

CLIENTELE DEVELOPMENT

Add on to all these are the requirements for a social media presence as well, which is the new demand of cosmetic practice in these modern times. And even the social media presence is not restricted to one forum, but must be on several forums, together with digital marketing and a good website.

RELATIONSHIP AND TRUST DEVELOPMENT

- Keeping yourself going and growing, developing relationships, maintaining contact details of patients and reminding them through sweet letters for their next sittings, sending out good wishes on birthdays and anniversaries—all are important aspects of developing personal relationships in a cosmetic practice.
- A personal touch with each and every patient goes a long way. The idea is to develop more friends than just patients. However, this friendship should not compromise the professional relationship. A center where the staff looks after even the petty needs of any person at all, not necessarily a patient, is always a successful center. A kind word from the doctor, expressing a genuine concern regarding the patients' family or self, make all the difference.
- The ultimate challenge is to develop trust, which is a long-term investment of the doctor. This alone shall go a long way in making a doctor and his cosmetic center successful over a long innings.
- Finally comes that unhappy patient, who are greater in number at the beginning of a practice. Developing the maturity to deal with them patiently is an art that needs to be picked-up almost simultaneously. One has to learn to tackle such patients in such a manner that they do not harm the reputation to any degree.

CONCLUSION

So, what are the answers to the above problems?
- A doctor proposing to take-up cosmetic practice as a career, should, even during his postgraduation, focus on cosmetic surgery and cosmetic dermatology with greater interest in learning from his regular faculty.
- He must attend as many cosmetic conferences as possible during the tenure of PG training. These are almost always subsidized for PG students.
- The trainee should speak to seniors, make friends with cosmetic practitioners, etc., to learn as much as possible from them.
- He should seek out long periods of observation and fellowships under well-known practitioners. While doing so, financial reimbursements should not be the criteria, but value learning, ease of getting questions answered, hands-on exposure, etc., should be the main criteria.
- The location where practice is begun needs to be well chosen. You may choose a location where no competition is nearby. On the other hand, seeking out a location among several similar clinics as in metros has its own advantages too, as a kind of market place of similar therapy develops in the neighborhood, and one can position oneself in the midst of readily available clientele.

- Your clinic should be affordable. It is not good to stretch yourself too much financially. However, it is a good idea to consult a financial consultant as well as your Chartered Accountants, who can advise you on the advisability of loans, and balance the expected returns over your investments.
- Within limits of financial prudence, fully equipping your clinic is a better idea than going slow and one by one. But once again you have to balance it shrewdly.
- Branding yourself, branding your clinic are important aspects too. This needs to be artistically done. Take the help of a professional.
- IT professionals can also help with websites and pumping up your net-presence by logging in your center to various social media platforms. This also needs care though.
- Your availability at your center, sincere, ethical practice, keeping the patients' pocket uppermost in mind, rather than yours own; and ultimate patient satisfaction even if it requires that extra mile, are all very important mantras to ensure success and longevity of your cosmetic practice.
- If, unfortunately there is an unhappy patient, then never hesitate in spending extra time with him, even reoperating at a heavily subsidized cost. Returning the fee taken is not a good idea, instead do offer a revision and absorb most of the costs.

14.4 Incorporating Research into your Practice

Anil Kumar Garg, Seema Garg

HOW TO DO RESEARCH?

To perform research only two things are needed:
1. A keen observant nature and questioning why, what, how
2. A consistent effort to prove yourself

Introduction

Research is imperative for advancement. Usually if there is a dissertation or thesis during residency, the quality of dissertations is very important. It is the mentor's responsibility that work done by the resident shall be new, innovative and shall add to research rather than be generic. Research papers should be published during residency.

Residents should be encouraged to stimulate new ideas, innovation and lateral thinking.

Residents can certainly innovate cheaper and user-friendly alternatives suitable to their respective circumstances. There is a need to overcome the thought block of "limitation of time and facility in India". When Newton gave the concept of gravitation, he just saw an apple falling to earth. Similarly, A Einstein gave many concepts which during his time were not proved experimentally. So, to innovate a concept or method all that is needed is to think. Especially due to digital technology which has made the whole world as one.

The author has innovated many such instruments and methods.[1]

One has to be motivated to do research. The thought should be "We are using instruments and procedures which were created by someone, so it is our responsibility to add to this." The sense of responsibility and innovation will certainly activate our research mind. All concepts and ideas are born in our own minds, and for that, nothing external is needed. I live in a second-tier city and am a private practitioner but just by this approach I have innovated many instruments and did research.[1-5] I modified a liposuction machine. I replaced 0.25 horsepower motor of routine suction machine to one horsepower to increase the suction pressure. This cost me only a few thousand, and I am using it for the last 15 years.

When I started hair transplant, I realized there was a vacuum for instruments and training facilities. The instruments were very expensive which made them out of reach. I used to think about those who have just finished residency, do not have money to buy and want to learn. This thought stimulated me and I started innovating many things. The simple FUE machine which was sold cost 3–5 lacs, I was using a dental motor for maxillofacial surgery. Immediately I used this at low RPM and thought to modify the torque which was a very simple thing to do. Similarly, I saw there were no trained assistant for hair transplant and no training modules. I thought there was a need for it and innovated the training module by just leaf, paper, pencil, and foam and trained my all staff using this module.[1] There was a common problem of graft desiccation during dissection, I noticed this and innovated a dynamic hydration follicle dissection board just by keeping a saline wet foam below wooden spatula.[2]

When I used to draw the hairline, I noticed that the mark on a flexible scale every day is at the same distance whatever irrespective of the head size. I took more than 6 months to explain this and designed a hairline concept.[5]

HOW TO DO A STUDY?

Only thing is that we need to be vigilant every time and identify the problem and then ask ourselves: How do we solve it?

This I will explain by showing how I did my study on use of plasma as graft holding solution.

Be Vigilant and/or Observant

Example: I was using platelet-rich plasma (PRP) for my patients during hair transplant for recipient area. After PRP, I use to discard the platelet poor plasma. One day I thought why not keep my grafts in this plasma, after all it is a part of blood having negligible cellular content but other contents of blood are present, and certainly it should be better than saline. Hence, there was a strong evidence in my thinking process based on already existing data about plasma. The idea evolved with my observant thinking. I started using plasma as a graft holding solution. After few cases, I observed that the incidence of posthair transplant anagen effluvium decreased and there was early and better hair growth. This was subjective evidence. To have an objective evidence we need to plan a study.

Study Model Planning

I had to prove my observation objectively or based on scientific data. What were the factors I was examining?
- Incidence of decreased anagen effluvium
- Early hair growth
- Good quality of hair, hair thickness
- Density of hair
- Is there any effect of plasma on hair follicle survival, does it prevent ischemic injury?

The Challenges and Answers

- For anagen effluvium and early hair growth, simple good quality photographs. For hair thickness and hair density tricoscan, or digital dermoscopy

  Above were easily available and I had to just make a plan at what interval these data should be recoded.

- The next thing was—does plasma affect graft survival? Does hair follicle can survive longer?

  For that, the routine studies done before were to implant grafts after different ischemia times. If I were to do the same, then my study result would come quite late. I was wondering if there was anything which could tell me immediately if follicle cells were surviving or not. Again the answer was there by immunoassay or other complicated methods, I still wanted a simpler solution in my midcap city. In today's era we are blessed by Google. I searched on the internet and I found MTT stain which stains live cells only. I discussed with a histopathologist who agreed to do it. Finally, we achieved success in staining live cells. To my utter surprize the hair follicle cells were viable even up to 72 hours of ischemia time. That is how we could present the histological evidence that hair follicle can survive longer in plasma than in saline.

  So, I had all parameters to be measured at different intervals. Then what I needed were the patients.

  I have a good volume of patients. I read some other studies, and finally decided to plan for split scalp study instead of two groups of patients.

- Finally the question of consent arose. This was really difficult, but fortunately being a mid-cap city and my seniority with the long standing personnel relationship I could take consent without much problem. This was easy to convince that one side grafts will be stored in plasma which is not going to harm at all and same number of grafts we will do extra.

  The consent for esthetic surgery patients is bit tricky.

  Select patients who are easy to deal with. It is better if they are known to you and or in some relation. Explain that the study is not going to harm them in any way, third is extra care in terms of finance, free medicines and free procedures, etc.

- Then another very important factor was taking ethical committee permission. This I think is the most difficult part to manage, especially if you are practicing in private. I advise you, if you inclined to do such research work it is better you join any private medical college where an ethical committee is present. Another option is there are some agencies who do this job for you. But it is mandatory to take permission. I believed that for my study it was not necessary as I was using autologous plasma. But I was wrong, ideally it should have been taken. This was the main reason I could not publish this study in reputed international journal, but finally, the paper has been accepted for index peer-reviewed journal. Another option was that you can publish it under heading of innovations or short cases studies where ethical permission is not needed.

- Follow-up visits. This was also not difficult for me as most of the patients were in close contact. My advice is select such patients who are easy to deal with and easily contactable and include at least 25% extra numbers of patients.

- Statistical analysis of data and "p" value. Initially, it was bit difficult but finally we got a teaching faculty in the department of preventive and social medicine in local

medical college, but you can find any qualified professional.
- Citations and other related articles to support your study is another important aspect. Again, in today's era of internet it is easy to find the references related to your work. Read all important articles and correlate with your findings.
- Extend your study. Once you have done the basic study and do not stop it here. Increase the sample size, add more variations and other parameters.
- Try to make your study multicenter, so final outcome in terms of random control multicenter trials to prove evidence basis so it is recommended. In my study, these last two things are still left which I am planning to do so.

So the problems were many, but at the same time every problem was solved but it took time and it was more than 3 years to complete the study to bring up to level of publication.

I presented the same in the international conference of International Society of Hair Restoration. The study was very well appreciated by even the most senior surgeon Dr Rassman. It was then sent to Association of Plastic Surgeons of India for the research paper award. I was given the Sam C Bose research award of the year. Now it is finally accepted to be published in the indexed peer-reviewed journal of Indian Journal of Plastic Surgeon.

I am very well-known just for one study and The International Society of Hair Restoration Surgery (ISHRS) invited me to their international conference to present in a workshop and it was kept for 2 days. This is the first study across the world and for future it will be cited in all articles related to this.

Looking back at the effort we put in, we also realized how much we gained. This is highly encouraging and what led to this study? Only because of a keen observant nature and basic questioning of why, what, how and finally, a consistent effort to prove yourself.

Both these ideas were applied in Newton's gravitation theory. Newton saw that the apple was falling, he asked why it is falling. Then he proved his own question and came with an answer that gave birth to gravitational force. That person is still alive among us through his work.

CONCLUSION

What we are is the result of research and innovations done before and you can usher in tomorrow only by today's research. By Anyone and anywhere "research and innovation" can be done. Only two things are needed for this, one is keen observant nature and questioning yourself why, what, how and another is consistent effort to prove yourself.

REFERENCES

1. Garg AK. Garg S. A learning module in hair restoration surgery: A simple and economic method to learn all steps of strip method of hair follicles harvesting and implantation. Indian J Plast Surg. 2017;50:230-5.
2. Garg AK, Seema G. A histological and clinical evaluation of plasma as a graft holding solution and its efficacy in terms of hair growth and graft survival. Hair Transplant Forum International. 2018;28:94-6.
3. Garg AK, Seema G. Dynamic hydration follicle dissection board: An innovative device. Hair Transplant Forum International. 2014;24:214.
4. Garg AK, Seema G. The use of body hair with scalp hair for "combination grafting" to enhance visual density of hair transplantation and increase coverage in advanced alopecia. Hair Transplant Forum International. 2018;28: 217-23.
5. Garg AK, Seema G. Decoding facial esthetics to recreate an aesthetic hairline: A method which includes forehead curvature. J Cutn Asthet Surg. 2017;10:195-9.

Index

Page numbers followed by *b* refer to box, *f* refer to figure, *fc* refer to flowchart, and *t* refer to table.

A

Ablative fractional lasers 74, 75
Abuse and violence, protection against 408, 414
Academic work 87
Academy and Association of Cutaneous Surgeons 19
Acanthosis nigricans 84
Accident reporting 52
Accreditations 43, 44, 126
   benefits of 46
   challenges for 47
   fulfillment 123
   qualifying criteria for 46
   timeline 46, 47*t*
Acne 84, 136
   flare-up with isotretinoin 242
   scar
      reduction 136
      surgical treatments 379
   surgery 136
Acquired immunodeficiency syndrome 17, 49, 163, 217
Adding procedures 40
Additional medical qualification, registration certificate for 314*f*
Adrenaline 31
Advanced life support skills 270
Advertisement 349
   misguiding 178
   misleading 178
Advertising expenses 118
Advisory Council 210
Air (Prevention and Control of Pollution) Act, 1981 45
Air conditioning 262
Albert Einstein stated 282
Allergic rhinitis 258
Allergy clinic, managing 258
Allopathy 164, 165
Allowable Expenses under Income Tax Act 118*b*
Alopecia
   areata 74
   diffuse 84
Amazon medical quackery 171
Ambience 250, 329
   in clinic 355
American Academy of Dermatology 9, 190, 358
   practice 55
American Board of Cosmetic Surgery 33
American College of Mohs Surgeons 11
American College of Surgeons 44
American Fellowships and Training Programs in Dermatopathology 14*t*
American Marketing Association 21
American Medical Association 188
American Society of Dermatologic Surgery 11
Anesthesia machine 340
Anesthetic purpose, suction machine for 340
Anesthetist 341
Anger management 213
Angioedema 259
   severe 84
Animal waste 53, 54
Annual maintenance contract 265, 314
Annual report 51
Anxiety 213
Appointment system 64, 328
Arms Act 45
Artificial intelligence 42
Artificial tears 31
Asian Dermatology Congress 9
Asian Society for Pigment Cell Research 9
Asset valuation method 403, 403*t*
Association of Cutaneous Surgeons 9, 200
Association of Hair Restoration Surgeons 358
Association of Medical Consultants 113
Association of Plastic Surgeons 358
Asthma 258

Atomic energy regulatory body approvals 45
Atopic dermatitis 258
Atopic eczema 258
Atopic patch test 259
Atropine 31
Attitude 310
Audit fees 118
Authorized medical practitioner 399
Autoclave and ethylene oxide sterilization machine 340
Autologous serum skin test 259, 260
Autonomy, respect for 189
Ayurveda, Yoga and Naturopathy Unani, Siddha Homeopathy (AYUSH) 164

B

Baldness 379
Bank charge 118
Bar-code system 51
　establish 50
Bargainers 370
Bariatric surgeon 391
Bariatric surgery 391
Basal metabolic rate 389
Basic dermatology clinic, service provided in 29
Basic skin clinic, architecture of 28
Basic vital parameters 401f
Basophil activation test 259
Beauty clinics 165
Behavior 230, 310
Benzyl benzoate 273
Betamethasone 31
Billboards for distributing educational content, use of 131f
Billing 40
Biomedical waste 48, 51
　generators 52
Biomedical waste management 48, 49, 50fc, 51
　handling rules 45, 49
　rules 51
　　salient features of 50, 52
　　steps of 52
　system, evolution of 49
Biopsies 253
Blepharoplasty 136
Blogging 349
Blood
　dyscrasias 84
　pressure apparatus 31
　tests 254

Body contouring
　practice 386
　scenario 387
Body dysmorphic disorder 221
Boilers Act 45
Bolam test 410
Boosts love and bonding 214
Botox 136
Botulinum toxin 136
Braces 136
Brand 347
　building 80
Breach of duty owed 174
Breast
　augmentation 136
　surgery 394
　conserving surgery 395
　implant
　　insertion, funnel for 340
　　search volumes of 364f
　surgery of 393
　tourniquet 340
Brochure 131, 357
　listing 136b
　sample highlighting technology 249f
Broken glass 54
Brow lifts 379
Budget 136, 367
Building breast surgery practice 393
Building bridges 83
Building plan and infrastructure 345
Building rhinoplasty practice 383
Business
　models, comparison of 82t
　plan 343
　types of 82
Buying equipment 265

C

Cable Television Networks Act 45
Calamine lotion 273
Cancer 238
Capital expenditure 400
Carbon peel 136
Case law 205
Cash book 118
Castellani's paint 273
Catheters 54
Central Board of Indirect Taxes and Customs 399
Central Consumer Protection Authority 210

Central Consumer Protection Council 210
Central Council of Indian Medicine 165
Central Hospital Violence Act 416
Central Information Commission 149
Central Pollution Control Board 52, 54
Central Sales Tax Act 45
Centrifugation machine 340
Certificates issued 320
Challenges 271
Changing room 340
Chartered Institute of Marketing 21
Cheek augmentation 136, 379
Chemical
   liquid waste 54
   peels 107, 136
   waste 53, 54
Chest diseases 200
Chief executive officer 376
Chief operating officer job purpose 98
Child dentistry 136
Chin
   augmentation 379
   enhancement 136
Chloroquine 280
Chronic diseases 100
Civil Court 205
Civil law and negligence 173
Civil procedure code 148
Civil versus criminal negligence 410
Clientele development 419, 421
Clinic building documents 77
Clinic expenses 118
Clinic locator 140
Clinic management software 38
Clinic plan 34
   client record management 36
   closure room 35
   flooring 36
   furniture 36
   hair
      transplant room 35
      wash space 35
   lighting 36
   office 34
   pharmacy 35
   photography space 35
   reception 34
   restrooms 35
   staff and pantry room 35
   storage 34
   technology and treatments 37
   treatment rooms 35
   waiting room 34
Clinic space 29, 248
Clinic staff 133
Clinic, equipment, and staffing 355
Clinical dermatology 19, 55
Clinical Establishments Act 29, 43, 148, 148*t*
Clinical examination 253
Clinical laboratory waste 54
Clinical photographs 318
Clinical practice
   basics of 398
   empathy and ethos of 238
   legal issues in 407
Clinical skills 291
Clofazimine 280
Code of Criminal Procedure 211
Code of ethics 200, 211
Code of Hammurabi 188
Code of medical ethics 147, 188, 191, 198
   for dermatologists 190
   legal implications of 200
   regulations 127
   technical principles of 188
Collateral materials 357
Collective responsibility 70
Comfortable consulting room 248*f*
Commercial space utilization 27
Common biomedical waste treatment facility 49, 50
Communication 15, 234
   skills 291, 305, 311
      strong 96
   ways of effective 239
Community participation and integration 44, 45
Compelling information 139
Competition analysis 28
Computer during medical interview 243
Computer repair and maintenance 118
Connective tissue diseases 84
Consent
   forms 250, 322
   validity of 143
Consistency 351
Constitution of India 147
Consultants 89
   fee 118
Consultation 65, 251
   and follow-up visit notes 316
   fee and expenses 283
   room 29

Consumer Commissions 210
Consumer forum 148
Consumer Protection Act 43, 45, 148, 201, 208, 209, 354
Consumer Protection Bill 116
Content management system 139
Continuing medical education 88, 335
   and conferences, pharma support for 89
Continuing medical exams workshops 24
Continuous quality improvement 45, 46, 279
Contract Act 45
Contravention of Provisions of Drugs and Cosmetics Act 196
Conveyance expenses 118
Copies of bills 118
Copyright Act 45
Corporate practice 7
Cosmetic 171, 255f
   dentistry 379
   dermatology 3, 116
     practice 5
   practice, parameters of quality of 328
   surgeon 199
   surgery 136, 200, 332
     assessing suitability for 335
     safety in 334
Cosmetology Society 200
Cost negotiation 77
Cost of service 333
Counseling 99
   role of 395
Counselor 102
   and technician
     advantages of 103
     qualities required for 104
     role of 99
     chamber 338
Credentials and achievements, display of 357
Criminal Court 205
Criminal law and negligence 175
Criminal Procedure Code 148, 166
Criminal proceedings, cover for 417
Current Indian healthcare, problems of 239
Customer relationship management 376
Customs Act 46
CUTIS Academy of Cutaneous Sciences 286
Cytotoxic
   drugs 53, 54
   wastes 54

D

Dapsone 85, 280
Data safety 41
Dawn 286
Day care esthetic surgery clinic 337
Dealing with unreasonable clients, dilemma of 327
Deep vein thrombosis pumps 340
Defamation, abuse and incidents of violence 408
Defibrillator 340
Deformity and execution of surgery, evaluation of 335
Dental services 136
Dentist regulations 46
Depo-Medrol 176
Deriphyllin 31
Dermabrasion 379
Dermascope 31
Dermatologic laser surgery 11
Dermatological lasers 74
Dermatological practice 86
Dermatological research 17
Dermatological Surgery and Laser Unit Programme 11
Dermatology 3, 16, 85, 100, 184, 199, 225, 229, 273, 280, 281
   and quackery 164
   center, categories of 95t
   diagnostic 17
   medicolegal cases in 173, 175
   roots of 3
   significance in 100
   technicians in 102
Dermatology and Aesthetic Surgery International League 9
Dermatology practice 3, 238, 283, 288
   evolution of 3
   levels of 56t
   models of 4, 55t
   trends in 55
Dermatology Society 239
Dermatopathology 3, 17-19, 280, 281
   fellowships and training in 13
Dermatopreneurs 229
Dermatoscopy 19
Dermatosurgery 3, 6, 17, 19, 200
Dermoscopy 6, 17, 254
Designated partner identification number 81
Designing esthetic clinic 33
Desperation 163

Device quackery 162
Dexamethasone 31
Diet and trichology 255
Dietary supplements 171
Dietitian 391
Digital marketing 137*t*, 138, 361, 362
    tools 365*f*
Digital single lens reflex 340
Dimple creation 337, 379
Diploma in Clinical Dermatology 169
Diploma in Practical Dermatology 169
Direct health hazard 163
Director identification number 81
Discarded glass 54
Discarded medicines 53, 54
Discharge card/notes 322
Disclaimer 160
Discoid lupus erythematosus 216
Discounted cash flow 403
Diseases, epidemiological data of 23
Dissection room 271
District commission 211
Doctor and clinic, accreditations of 357
Doctor and staff, grooming of 309
Doctor attire and conduct 357
Doctor consultation chamber 338
Doctor empathy 235
Doctor references 322
Doctor relations 187
Doctor-patient
    interface 213
    relationship 234
Doctors, registration of 198
Documentations 312
Double chin reduction 379
Drawbacks and limitations 85
Dressings 253
Drug
    hypersensitivity syndrome 84
    rashes 84
Drugs and Cosmetics Act 46, 149, 165

E

Ear setback 379
Economic hazards 164
Eczema 100, 136, 259
Education and licensing of surgeon 335
Educational commission 14
Educational items 92
Effective communication 72

Electricity Act 46
Electricity rules 46
Electrodes 340
Electronic medical records 66, 254, 286,
    316
Electroporation 382
Emergency drug kit 31
Emergency kit 260
Emergency medicine 84
Empathy 96
Employees Provident Fund Act 46
Employees' State Insurance Act 46
Employment Exchange Act 46
Encounter special situation 242
Endocrinologist 391
Endocrinology 84
Endoscopic surgeries, monitors for 340
Endotracheal tubes 341
Energy-based devices 340
ENT surgeon 85
Enterprise resource planning 363
Enterprise value/revenue 404
Entrepreneurship cycle 59*fc*
Environment Protection Act 46
Enzyme-linked immunospot 259
Eosinophilia 84
Epidemiological research 313
Epidermal cell suspension 107
Equal identity, establishing 72
Equal Remuneration Act 46
Equipment 355, 382
    and disposables 331
    depreciation on 118
E-resources, utilization of 108
Erythema
    multiforme 84
    nodosum 84
Established practices 24
Establishing clinic 119
Esthetic 183
    dermatologist 109
    medical procedures, classification of 183
    practice 379
Esthetic dermatology 17, 19, 136, 247
    significance in 101
Esthetic medicine 33
    evidence-based 293
Esthetic procedure 182
    room 248*f*
European Academy of Dermatology and
    Venereology 9

Evidence-based medicine 25
Excimer laser 74
Excisional surgeries 390
Exemplary team 391
Expansion dilemma 79
Explosives Act 46
Ex-servicemen Contributory Health Scheme 43
External marketing 354, 354*t*, 358, 359
Eye drops 31
Eyelid tucks 379

F

Face craft program 136
Facelifts 379
Facial esthetic 379
   clinic 382
   plastic surgery 378
   surgery 378
     practice, structure of 381
Facility development 419, 420
Facility management and safety 44, 45
Factories awarding unauthorized and illegal diplomas 169
Family dermatology practice 68
Family practice
   advantages of 68
   disadvantages of 70
Family vacation, lack of 71
Fast decision making 279
Fat grafting 307, 379
Fatal Accidents Act 46
Fee and subscription 118
Feedback forms 251
Fellowships 9
Fever 84
Fight fear 214
Final disposal, transportation for 54
Finance 14, 263
   and planning 109
   getting 344
   sources and uses of 400
Financial and facility resources 48
Financial aspects 57
Financial management 73, 398, 407
   frameworks of 401
Financial planning 121
   strong 73
Financial resources 79
Finding staff 283
Flap surgeries 253

Follicular unit
   extraction 105
   transplant 281
Food
   allergy 258
   and drug administration 168, 331
Foreign materials 336
Foreign medical graduates 14
Foundation 33, 288
Franchisee-type peripheral clinic 62
Fundamental rights 147
Funds, sources and uses of 401
Fungal infections 136

G

Gastroenterology 85
General dentistry 136
General dermatology practice 253
General practitioner 123
Generic names of drugs, use of 192
Genodermatoses 84
Geriatric dermatology 17
Gianotti-Crosti syndrome 266
Golden rule of success 308
Goods and Services Tax 40, 399
   registered for 314
Google drive 363, 364*f*
Google search analytics 24
Great stress reliever 214
Griseofulvin 280
Group practice 56
   management 56
   seven Ps of 57*b*, 58*f*
   types of 61
Growth 372
   funding, common forms of 402*t*
   organ 281
   phase 60
Gynecological history 317

H

Hair
   accessories 255
   card test 254
   care 136, 252
   cosmetics 252
   counts, daily 254
   dermoscopy 254
   fall 136
   grooming 252

Index

growth, unwanted 252
loss 252, 257, 269
microscopic examination of 254
mount test 254
pull test 254
restoration surgery practice, establishing 269
shaft abnormalities 252
Hair disorders 29
consultation for 29
Hair practice
difficulties in 256
evolving 256
Hair removal 106
laser 74, 264
Hair transplant 136
and liposuction 110
back table with lights and microscope for 340
room 35
search volumes of 363f
setup 284
technician 341
Hair transplantation 19, 170, 172, 253, 270, 280, 281
fellowships and training in 12
practice, requirements for 269
Hair wash
space 35
test 254
Handheld torch 31
Handling online reviews 226
Hay fever 258
Hazard warnings, labels of 54f
Hazardous waste 49
basel convention on 49
Health care 209, 343
waste management 49
Health hucksters 162
Health Insurance Portability and Accountability Act 332
Health quackery hazards 163
Healthcare
and insurance of medical practitioner 416
at crossroads 408
facility 45, 49
marketing 130
practice 213
Professionals and Consumer Protection Act 208

service 208, 399
waste 48
Healthy lifestyle 297
Hematology 84
Hepatitis 49
B virus 49
C virus 49
management of 85
High power system 75
High-intensity focused ultrasound 264, 389
Hindu Undivided Family 119
Hippocratic oath 188
Hiring and managing staff 94
Hirsutism 84
Hormonal evaluation 254
Hospital administration manager responsibilities 98
Hospital bill, recovery of 408, 413
Hospital Violence Act 415
Hospital/healthcare facility 51
Housekeeping staff 341
Human anatomical waste 53, 54
Human disease 208
Human immunodeficiency virus 17, 171, 217
medicine 17, 19
Human resource 341, 376
management functions 97
manager job description 97
planning 94
Human Rights 195
Commission 205
Hydralift treatment 136
Hydrocortisone 31

I

Ideal practice management software 38
Immunobullous conditions 84
Immunofluorescence 17, 19
Implant
dentistry 136
use of 336
In-clinic queries 24
Income tax
returns 77
slabs and rates 118
Incompetence and medical negligence, allegations of 409
Indemnity subclauses 114
Indian Association of Aesthetic Plastic Surgeons 358

Indian Association of Dermatologists,
    Venereologists and Leprologists 8, 14, 19,
    200, 358
Indian Council of Medical Research 197
Indian Journal of Plastic Surgeon 425
Indian Medical Association 149, 167, 205
    schemes 418
Indian Medical Council 143, 191, 407
    Act 166, 191
    Register 200
Indian Scholarships and Fellowships 8
Indirect health hazards 163
Infant mortality rate 162
Infection control 44
Infiltration 270
Inflammatory hair disorder 252
Infliximab 84
Information 251
Informed consent 143, 144, 176, 236
    lack of documentation of 143
Infrastructure 256, 258, 267, 271
In-house facility plans and equipment 344
Inpatient documentation and medical records 321
Instrument 256, 271
    and equipment 385
    trolley 340
Insurance Companies Regulation 43
Insurance Regulatory and Development Authority 47, 113
Integrated health care delivery system 4
Intense pulsed light 74, 75
Internal marketing 132, 354, 354t
Internal medicine 84
International Congress of Dermatology 9
International Master Course on Aging Sciences Academy 12
International Observership Program in Dermatology 10
International Organization for Standardization 357
International Society of Aesthetic Plastic Surgery 358
International Society of Dermatology 12
International Society of Hair Restoration Surgery 12, 358, 425
International Training Opportunities 10
International Traveling Mentorship Program 11
Intralesional injections 106
Intramuscular injections 176
Intravenous tubes and sets 54

Invasive procedures 184
Itch 85, 258
Itemizing and billing services 125, 126

J

Joint Commission on Accreditation of Hospitals 44
Journal of Cutaneous and Aesthetic Surgery 76
Judgment, error of 160
Junior member, advantages to 61

K

Karnataka Private Medical Establishments Act 124, 148
Karnataka Prohibition of Violence Against Medicare Service Personnel and Damage to Property in Medicare Service Institutions Act 151, 152, 154
Karnataka Violence Act 151
Knowledge, sharing of 69

L

Lab expenses 118
Laboratory medicine 85
Laboratory tests 254
Landing page 363, 364, 365f
Laser
    and esthetic dermatology 19
    clinic, managing 260
    company background 78
    liposuction 390
    medicine 17, 18
    peel 136
    procedure room for 248f
    room lights 262
    safety protocols during 249f
    setup 284
    specifications 75
    technician 341
    toning 136
Laser hair
    reduction 136
    removal 75, 249f, 253
        patient, clinical record of 330t
    systems 75
Laundry 340
Law enforcement 167
Law in negligence, process of 203
Laws relevant to medical practice 407

Leaflets 131
Ledger 118
Legal aspects 256
Legal awareness 147
Legal education 147
Legal liability 143
Legal references 166
Legal restrictions, evasion of 192
Legal status 169, 172
Legal structures and taxation 398
Legally bound service 334
Leprology 199
Leprosy 184
Lesions, clearing of 239
License/Regulations under Biomedical
	Management and Handling Rules 45
Licenses and insurance 346
Light microscopy 254
Limited liability partnership 80, 81, 119, 398
Lip enhancement 136
Lipofilling 390
Liposuction 136, 390
Liquid waste 53
Live media important 365
Local area network 41
Logo and concept 34
Low level laser light therapy 253
Lymph nodes 84

M

Making eye contact 235
Male breast surgery 136
Management information system reports 98
Market multiple method 404, 404*t*
Market research 356
Marketing 15, 21, 127, 271, 347, 354
	and evaluating practice 346
	goals 373
	plan 356
	spend, return on investment for 360
Master technical aspects 354
Mastering art of plastic surgery 304
Mastering personality development 308
Masters in clinical dermatology 169
Maternal mortality ratio 162
Mechanical liposuction 390
Media, abuse and defamation in 411
Medical and surgical history 317
Medical audits and statistics 313
Medical business professional 327

Medical cosmetology 17
Medical Council of India 32, 127, 134, 147, 148,
	167, 184, 191, 209, 354, 407
Medical Council Registration 77
Medical Counselor Job Responsibilities 97
Medical dermatology 116
Medical education 313
Medical indemnity
	and social security 408
	insurance 315
Medical negligence 158
	concept of 148
	essential ingredients of 159
Medical practice 303, 326, 379
Medical practitioner
	healthcare of 408
	investments for 109
Medical profession 127
Medical professionals 181
	and clinical establishments 149
Medical quackery 162
Medical records, maintenance of 191
Medical representatives 88
	management of 72
Medical students 152
Medical Termination of Pregnancy Act 196
Medicare service institutions 152
Medicine 231
	clinics practicing modern system of 44
	expired 54
	practicing, modern system of 44
Medicolegal aspects 15
	in practice 143
Medicolegal cases 43
Medicolegal cell 205
Medicolegal rounds 15
Medicolegal situation, warning signs of 203
Medicos legal action group 418
Mega liposuction 388, 390
Melanoma, malignant 85
Mentoring, importance of 215
Mesotherapy 136, 253
Metallic body implants 54
Methotrexate 85
Microaire and ultrasound-assisted liposuction
	342
Microbiology and biotechnology waste 53
Microdermabrasion 107, 136
Microneedling 136
Minamata convention on mercury 49
Minimally invasive procedures 184

Minimum alternate tax 81
Misconduct 195
Mobile expenses 118
Mobile responsive sites 140

N

Nail
   diseases 136
   disorders 29
     consultation for 29
Narcotics and Psychotropic Substances Act and License 45
Narrow-band ultraviolet B phototherapy treatment 25
National Accreditation Board for Hospitals and Healthcare Providers 44, 208, 321, 357
National Accreditation Board for Testing and Calibration Laboratories 124
National AIDS Control Organization 50
National Commission 211
National Consumer Disputes Redressal Commission 212
National Medical Commission 407
   Act 211
National Medical Council 184
National Skin Centre 13
Neck lift 379
Neodymium-doped yttrium aluminum garnet 177
   laser 75, 264, 284
Nerve blocks 270
Net asset value 400
Networking 268
New techniques in practice, adopting 291
Nicolau syndrome 179
No objection certificate 45, 346
   under Pollution Control Act 45
Nonablative fractional lasers 74
Noneducational and practice-related items, prohibition of 91
Noninflammatory hair disorder 252
Noninvasive procedures 183
Non-steroidal anti-inflammatory drugs 258
Nuremberg code 188
Nurses
   and technicians operating lasers 177
   registered 152
Nursing mothers, baby-feeding area for 267f
Nursing staff 341
Nursing students 152

Nutritional quackery 162
Nutritionist 85

O

Offence, cognizance of 153
Offline software 41
Omission and error policy 114
Oncology 85
Online and social media marketing 361
Online booking 139
Online software 41
Onychology 6
Operation
   notes 322
   room 345
Operation theater 250, 271, 340, 345
   inpatient clinic with 343
   set up 26
   technician 341
Operative plan 386
Oral surgeon 85
Oral surgery 136
Organization 352
   challenges 48
   types of 94
Out of box thinking 370
Out-of-court settlement 202, 417
Outpatient department 64
   procedure consent forms 319
Outpatient documentation and medical records 316
Ownership models 125, 126
Oxygen and nitrous oxide cylinders 340
Oxyhemoglobin 76

P

Palpation 254
Paramedical workers 152
Partnership firm 79, 80
Patch testing 107
Patient coordinator 338, 341
Patient counseling 255
Patient counselor 341
Patient demanding immediate results 220
Patient disappointment 242
Patient education 371
Patient education
   and knowledge 243
   versus marketing 394
Patient information 317

Patient questionnaire 316, 317f
Patient rights and education 44
Patient's dissatisfaction, allegations of incompetence and medical negligence 409
Patient-centered communication 241
Patterned baldness 84
Payment issues 222
Pediatric dermatology 3, 17-19, 266
   clinic, managing 266
   practice 267, 269
   training in 267
Peer-to-peer group practice 62
Penalty 153
Permanent account number 117
Permissions, registrations and insurance 314
Persistent organic pollutants 49
Personal documents 77
Personal hygiene 310
Personal protective equipment 54
Personality
   development 308
   disorders 221
Pharma industry, interaction of 88
Pharmacist and chemist-based quackery 165
Pharmacy 35, 45, 255, 339
   and hair cosmetics 255
   and laboratory 279
Pheniramine maleate 31
Photodermatology 19
Photographic trichogram 254
Photography room 338
Phototherapy 107
Physicians
   duties of 192
   in consultation, duties of 193
   to colleagues, duties of 190
   to patients, duties of 190
   to public and to paramedical profession, duties of 194
Physicians-motivation-adaptation 292
Physiotherapist 391
Picosecond lasers 74
Pigmentary lasers 74
Pigmentation 136
Plastic ampoules 54
Plastic surgeons, digital marketing for 362
Plastic surgery 85
   addicts 370
   practice 303
Plateau phase 60

Platelet rich plasma 106, 135, 136, 253, 340
Platysmaplasty 379
Policy retroactive 114
Polyclinics 55
Polycystic ovarian syndrome 84
Postage and courier expenses 118
Postdiagnostic support 213
Postgraduate Diploma in Clinical Cosmetology 168, 169
Postgraduate Diploma in Medical Trichology 168
Post-inflammatory hyperpigmentation 76, 236
Post-inflammatory pigmentation 112
Potassium
   hydroxide 107
   mount 254
Power-assisted liposuction 340, 342
Practice, types of 383
Practitioners of Indian medicine 164
Practitioners views 227
Pre-accreditation entry level certification 47, 48
Precocious cutaneous metastasis 85
Preconsultation promotional activities 357
Prediagnostic support 213
Premises, calculate cost of 344
Preoperative instruction sheet 318
Presumptive taxation 119
   advantages of 119
Presurgery instructions 319f
Prevention of legal implications of code of medical ethics 201
Print media 130, 358
Private limited company and proprietorship firm, differences between 120t
Procedure consent form 323f
Procedure room 30, 248, 248f, 339
Product selection 294
Professional development 419
Professional indemnity 336
   and social security 417
   for dermatologist 112
   individual policy 113
Professional interactions 329
Professional misconduct 143
Professional services, payment of 192
Professional skills 250
Prohibition of violence 153
Promotion 278, 295
Proof lies with patient, burden of 180
Proper informed consent, components of 144
Psoriasis 74, 84, 100, 136
   vulgaris 112

Psoriatic arthritis 84
Psychiatric comorbidities 221
Psychiatrist and behavioral therapist 391
Psychological medicine 85
Pulse dye lasers 74, 76
Punch biopsy probes 31
Punishment and disciplinary action 197
Purchase contract 77
Purchasing laser system 78*b*

Q

Q switched lasers 23, 74
Quack 164, 166
   listen 163
   medicines 161
   training of 165
   types of 161
Quackery 149, 161, 164, 170, 256
   fighting against 167
   prevention of 167, 172
Qualitative factors 25
Quality Council of India 208
Quality family time, lack of 71
Quotation from company 77

R

Radiation protection certificate 45
Radiofrequency 106
   liposuction 390
   technology 110
Randomized controlled trials 244
Ranitidine 31
Rash 84
Rebates and commission 195
Reception 65, 262*f*
   area layout 30*f*
   cum waiting area 29
   desk 338
   room 34
Records, maintenance of 51
Recovery room 250, 340
Reflective listening 240
Registrar of firms 80
Registration certificate 315*f*
Registration numbers, display of 192
Regulatory fulfillment 123
Relationship and trust development 419, 421
Relieves pain 214
Research 422
Restroom 35, 339

Retail drug license 45
Retinoid dermatitis 242
Revenue streams 124, 126
Revision of limits 115
Rheumatology 84
Rhinoplasty 307, 379
   practice 385
   skills 383
   surgeon 384
   training 383
Right to Information Act 149
Rituximab 84
Root canal therapy 136
Runoff cover 115

S

Safe documentation practices 185, 186
Safe heart 214
Safe hygiene practices 185, 186
Safe medical practice 185
Safe patient relations 185, 186
Safe prescription practices 185, 186
Safe staff practices 186
Safe surgery operation theater practices 185, 186
Safeguards against litigation 160
Safety 369
   code building permit, rules of 45
Sales tax registration certificate 45
Sample collection 253
Scabies 273
Scalp
   dermatoscopic examination of 254*f*
   tumors, excision of 253
Scars and rejuvenation 74
Scholarships and educational funds 91
Sclerotherapy 106
Scrubbing area 340
Search engine 350
   marketing 350
   optimization 141, 228, 350
      fundamental of 351
Security and comfort, sense of 215
Segregated waste, collection of 53
Service providers 112
Setting up allergy clinic 260
Setting up clinic 21, 283
Setting up goals 372
Severity index 259
Sexual medicine 17
Sexually transmitted disease 135, 187, 273

Index

Shops and Establishment Act 314
Signboards and advertisements 198
Simple partnership 80
Site marking 322, 324f
Skill 270
   based group practice 62
Skin
   and plastic surgery, practice management in 419
   biopsy 136
   disorder 29, 136, 258
      consultation for 29
   dryness of 84
   prick test 259
   tag removal 136
   tightening 136
Small healthcare organizations 208
Smell 309
Smile designing and makeover 136
Smile line reduction 136
Social communication and interaction 213
Social media 363, 365f
   channels 365
   feedback 24
   links 140
   marketing 141
Social security scheme 418
Soft skill training 15
Software, disadvantages of 42
Sole proprietorship firm 80
Sonoporation devices 382
Sound 309
South Asian Regional Conference of Dermatology 9
Space requirement 261
Speaker programs 90
Speaker training meetings 90
Spectrum of services 378
Squamous cell carcinoma 85
Staff 233, 250
   recruitment and team building 385
   uniform expenses 118
   welfare expenses 118
Stand-alone and platform systems
   advantages of 77t
   disadvantages of 77t
Standard dermatology clinic 29
Standard operating
   procedures 87, 105, 149, 154
   process 406
Standees and posters 132

State Commission 211
State Consumer Protection Council 210
State Government's Authorities 166
State Medical Acts 165
State Medical Council 143, 209
State Medical Register 198
State Pollution Control Boards 52
State Pollution Control Committees 52
Sterilization room 340
Steroids, excess dosage of 176
Stethoscope 31
Stevens-Johnson syndrome 84, 177
Stockholm convention 49
Stress 213
Stretch mark reduction 136
Study model planning 423
Surgeon's assistant 341
Surgical area 339
Surgical goals 374
Surgical light source 340
Surgical procedures 389
Suture removal 253
Switches position 263f
Systemic lupus erythematosus 84, 216

T

Target clientele 349
Taste 309
Tattoo
   reduction 136
   removal 106
Tax
   auditing 119
   planning 117
Technical knowledge 96
Teledermatology 3, 108
Telemarketing 132, 132f
Telephone 118
Television 132, 359
Television commercials 131
Tetracycline 280
Therapeutic lasers 74
Thermometer 31
Third-party educational professional membership 89
Thyroid
   diseases 84
   profile 254
Touch 309
Toxic epidermal necrolysis 176

Traditional marketing 130, 137t, 353, 354
   advantages of 133
   aims of 133
   billboards 131
   broadcast 131
   direct mail 131
   disadvantages of 134
   internal marketing 132
   print media 130
   telephone 132
   word of mouth 130
Training 87, 270
   options 19
   under senior dermatologist 7, 8
Trichloroacetic acid 232
Trichogram 254
Trichology 6, 17-19
   photography in 255
   practice 252, 253
     components of 252
   unit 252
     infrastructure of 253f
Trichometry 254
Trichoscan, dermatoscopic examination of 254f
Trichoscopic examination 254
Trichoscopy 254
Trichotherapists 272
Trichotillometry 254
Trust, levels of 134
Tuberculosis 200
Tumescent liposuction 390
Tummy tuck 136

U

Ultrasound liposuction 390
Unethical Acts 194
Unethical conduct, exposure of 192
Unique selling proposition 306, 333
Urine bags 54
Urticaria 19, 136, 258
   chronic 258, 259

V

Vampire facelift 136
Vascular lasers 74
Vascular surgeon 85
Vasculitis 84

Vehicle running and maintenance 118
Venereology 184, 199
Video-dermoscopy 254
Violence 149, 152
   against medical professionals and medical care establishments, nature of 155
Viral exanthems, atypical 266
Vision 136
Visitors lounge 338
Vitiligo 74, 136, 217
Vitiligo surgery 7, 136

W

Waiting room 34, 271
   well-planned 34f
Wart and corn removal 136
Waste
   bags, weighing of 54
   contaminated 54
   management 250
   pretreatment of 52
   segregation of 52
   sharps 53, 54
   soiled 54
   solid 53
   transportation of collected 53
Waste after categorization
   color coding of 54t
   disposal of 54t
Waste disposal 340
   protocols, safe 185, 186
Waterjet liposuction 390
Website 138, 350, 363, 364, 365f
   types of 139
Weighing scale 340
Well-lit consulting chamber 249f
Wellness 382
Wireless operation certificate 45
Wood's lamp 31
   examination 29
Workload, division of 71
World Congress of Dermatology 9
World Congress of Hair Research 9
World Health Organization 49, 99
World Medical Association 188

Y

Yellow pages 359

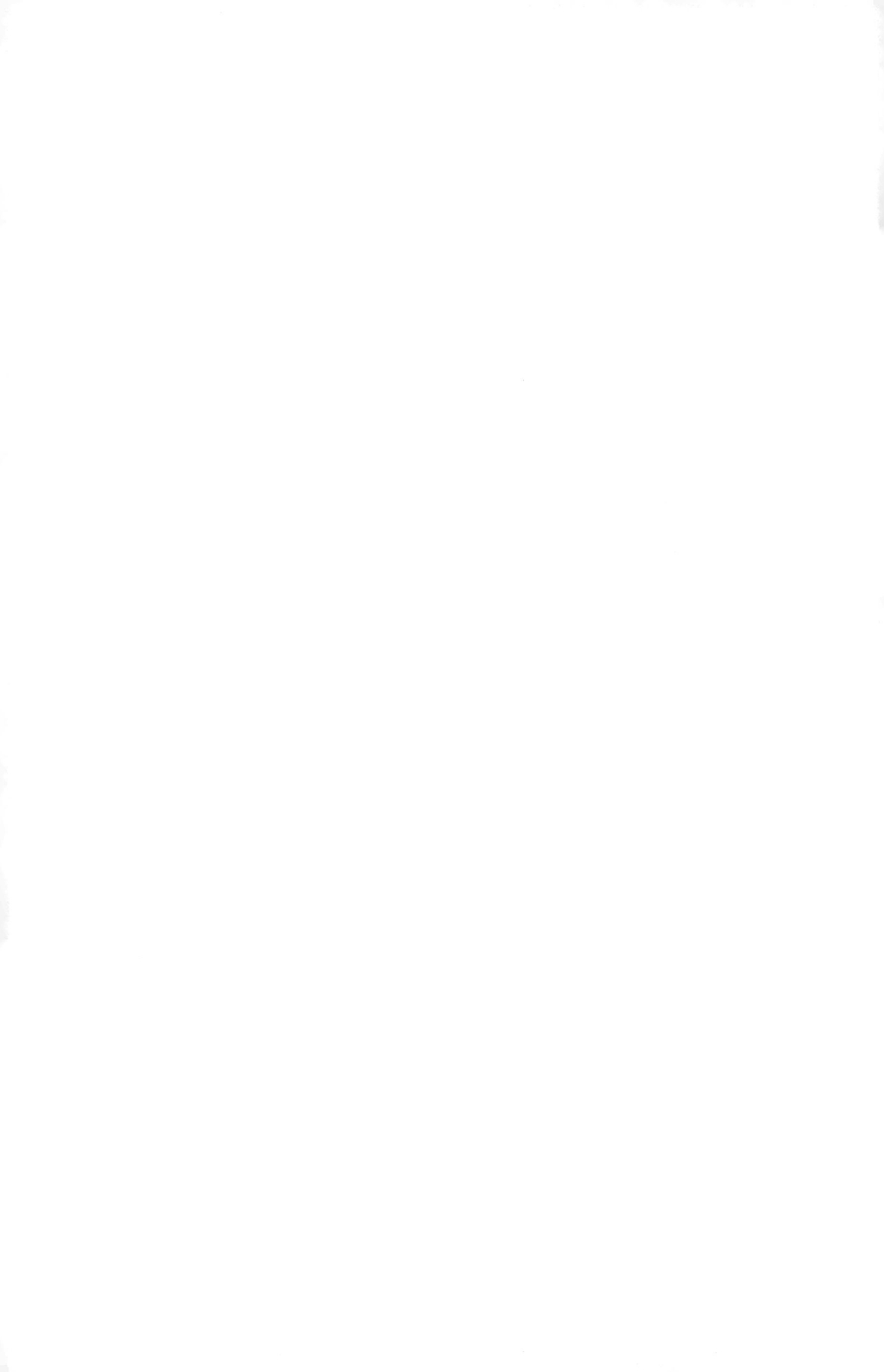

EU GSPR Authorised Reprsentative
Logos Europe, 9 rue Nicolas Poussin
1700, La Rochelle, France
Phone: +33 (0) 6 67 93 73 78
E-mail: contact@logoseurope.eu

www.ingramcontent.com/pod-product-compliance
Ingram Content Group UK Ltd.
Pitfield, Milton Keynes, MK11 3LW, UK
UKHW050429150426

5217IPUK00019B/1315